Imaging Anatomy of the Head and Spine

A Photographic Color Atlas of
MRI, CT, Gross, and Microscopic Anatomy
in Axial, Coronal, and Sagittal Planes

Imaging Anatomy of the Head and Spine

A Photographic Color Atlas of MRI, CT, Gross, and Microscopic Anatomy in Axial, Coronal, and Sagittal Planes

H. N. Schnitzlein, Ph.D.
Professor of Anatomy

F. Reed Murtagh, M.D.
Associate Professor of Radiology

University of South Florida
College of Medicine
Tampa, Florida

With contributions by

Carlos R. Martinez, M.D.
Clinical Associate
Professor of Radiology

John A. Arrington, M.D.
Clinical Associate in Radiology

Laurence P. Clarke, Ph.D.
Associate Professor of Radiology

University of South Florida
College of Medicine
Tampa, Florida

C. P. Shah, M.D.
Assistant Professor of Radiology

Timothy Reid, M.D.
Clinical Associate in Neurology

Fred J. Hodges, III, M.D.
Professor of Radiology

Mallinckrodt Institute of Radiology
Washington University School of Medicine
St. Louis, Missouri

Urban & Schwarzenberg · Baltimore–Munich 1985

Urban & Schwarzenberg, Inc.
7 E. Redwood Street
Baltimore, Maryland 21202
USA

Urban & Schwarzenberg
Pettenkoferstraße 18
D-8000 München 2
West Germany

Printed in Germany by Kösel, Kempten

NOTICE

The Editors (or Author(s)) and the Publisher of this work have made every effort to ensure that the drug dosage schedules herein are accurate and in accord with the standards accepted at the time of publication. The reader is strongly advised, however, to check the product information sheet included in the package of each drug he or she plans to administer to be certain that changes have not been made in the recommended dose or in the contraindications for administration.

Library of Congress Cataloging in Publication Data

Schnitzlein, H.N.
Imaging anatomy of the head and spine.
Includes index.
1. Head–Anatomy–Atlases. 2. Spine–Anatomy–Atlases. 3. Head–Radiography–Atlases. 4. Spine–Radiography–Atlases. 5. Nuclear magnetic resonance–Diagnostic use–Atlases. 6. Tomography–Atlases. I. Murtagh, F. Reed. II.Title. [DNLM: 1. Head–radiography–atlases. 2. Head–radionuclide imaging–atlases. 3. Nuclear Magnetic Resonance–atlases. 4. Spine–radiography–atlases. 5. Spine–radionuclide imaging–atlases. 6. Tomography, Emission Computed–atlases. 7. Tomography, X-Ray Computed–atlases. WE 17 S361i]
QM 535.S36 1985 611'.91 84-10365
ISBN 0-8067-1881-1

ISBN 0-8067-1881-1 Baltimore
ISBN 3-541-71881-1 Munich

To Our Wives
Harriett and Dede

Preface

Sectional anatomy has become increasingly important for the interpretation of computed images including the noninvasive computed axial tomography (CT), magnetic resonance imaging (MRI), and positron emission tomography (PET). Magnetic resonance imaging (MRI), which may be displayed in any plane with differing modalities, has become more available and of growing clinical usefulness.

The display of the transverse (axial) computed image has become standardized with the patient supine (face up). The visualized section is usually shown as if viewed from the inferior surface, i. e., with left and right reversed. The most common CT axial image of the head is in a plane approximately 15° above the infraorbitomeatal (IOM) line but the current MR axial image is more nearly parallel to the IOM line. MR images may be displayed in additional coronal planes (viewed from the front) and sagittal planes (usually viewed from the left). Variations from these standard planes may be diagnostically advantageous or may result from technical necessity. Although there are many excellent anatomic and radiologic atlases available to demonstrate the human central nervous system, the adoption of the supine, coronal, and sagittal orientations and especially the innumerable permutations of MRI, requires the presentation of normal structure in comparable perspectives. It has been our purpose in preparing this atlas to photograph the anatomy of the head and spine in formats commonly used and to select comparable CT and MRI scans for optimal visualization of the brainstem and spinal cord. The correlation of MRI with CT and cadaver anatomy is presented to facilitate interpretation, since MRI provides entirely new modes for the illustration of anatomy and pathology.

The authors have found the experience of preparing this atlas very rewarding and the contributors have all been most cooperative and helpful. The continuous support of Dr. Martin Silbiger, Chairman of the Department of Radiology, University of South Florida College of Medicine, has been a necessary encouragement. The CT images of the cadavers were made by Mr. Keith Ladd, who had to fit his work into those irregular times when the scanner was not being used for patients. We are grateful to him and the James A. Haley Veterans Administration Hospital for providing this invaluable contribution. The patient CT scans were selected from the files of the James A. Haley Veterans Administration Hospital and from Tampa General Hospital. Most of the patient MRI scans of the head were kindly provided by Dr. Fred J. Hodges, III, of the Edward Mallinckrodt Institute of Radiology in St. Louis. The MRI scans of the lumbar spine are from Dr. Roger G. Schnell and the Broward NMR facility, Ft. Lauderdale, Florida. The microscopic sections were prepared by Mrs. Ruth Reese and the initial graphics were completed by Mr. L. Dale Britt. The CT and MRI scans were photographed by Mr. Paul Glass who also provided expert assistance in preparing the prints. Typing of the manuscript was done by Rhonda Tuttle, Lucy Penn, and Charlene Krissman. Without such capable and willing assistance, this atlas could not have been completed.

A special word of thanks is due Drs. John Arrington, Brian Cornell, James F. Benenati, Michael T. Donohue, Derryl L. McLeod, Michael H. Owens, Timothy Reid, and Daniel Jones, now in residencies in radiology, pathology, otolaryngology, and neurology. Their meticulous proofreading of the original figures not only corrected errors but greatly enhanced the selection of useful labels.

We are particularly grateful to the entire staff of Urban & Schwarzenberg for their encouragement and for their special efforts toward producing an atlas of quality.

H. N. Schnitzlein, Ph. D.
F. Reed Murtagh, M. D.

Contents

Introduction

The anatomy of the head and spine is presented photographically in those planes and orientations of increasing clinical usefulness. The gross anatomy of the brain and the microscopic anatomy have been taken from our earlier atlas *(Computed Tomography of the Head and Spine,* © 1983 Urban & Schwarzenberg). Seven additional cadavers were sectioned and photographed for this volume. CT scans of patients and examples of patient MRI scans were selected and are arranged together for easily accessible comparison study. The designation "nuclear magnetic resonance" (NMR) has not been used in this work. Instead, "magnetic resonance imaging" (MRI) is used throughout. "MRI" appears to be the term of choice in the literature as well in the American College of Radiology, and the authors find a number of practical disadvantages with the use of "NMR."

Following CT imaging in the desired plane, the cadaver heads were embedded in gelatin, frozen, and sectioned at 7 to 10 mm on a fine-toothed band saw. Some distortion and pathology are inevitable in nearly all cadaver specimens and an attempt was made to select only those with minimal distortion. Photographs were made with an adjacent centimeter scale and under fluid to avoid highlights. Initial labeling of color prints was facilitated by the efforts of senior medical students and residents in neurology and neuroradiology.

Innumerable CT scans (GE 8800 or Siemens Somatom) and MRI scans (Siemens Magnetom or Technicare Teslacon) of patients were studied in an effort to select those most nearly comparable to the gross anatomical specimen or those which best displayed the structures to be illustrated. The CT scans in the axial plane correlate with the gross section but the available MRI scans are more nearly horizontal. The MRI scans in the coronal plane correspond to the gross specimen but the CT angle on patients is rarely a true coronal. Coronal CT scans of the cadaver illustrated are included for comparison with the MRI since the interpretation of CT is currently better established. Similarly, sagittal CT scans of the cadaver are illustrated since the sagittal CT reconstructions of patients usually lack the anatomical detail for contrast with the MRI scans. All identifying numbers and names have been removed from the CT and MRI scans.

Traditional scans in axial planes are viewed as if looking up from the feet; in coronal planes as if viewed from the front looking at the face, and sagittal planes are more commonly displayed with the nose to the observer's left. Orientation of the temporal bone may be in several modifications as well as the usual planes. The spine is usually best studied in planes parallel to the disc spaces. Variations in the angle of the cut will obviously result in some differences in the anatomical structures revealed. This can be used to great advantage or may mask some features and result in misinterpretations. It must always be borne in mind that the CT or MRI scan is a computer average of all structures within the thickness of the slice.

Since the cisterns and ventricles are well visualized on CT and MRI scans and because they have some constant anatomical relationships and contents, a section illustrating these CSF spaces has been incorporated. Although some structures cannot be definitely discerned on CT or MRI, their identification can be implied if certain related anatomical structures can be seen. The blood vessels of the brain are frequently well visualized on MRI scans. An additional illustration of the veins has been made to accompany the basic arterial channels which were presented in the previous volume. The orbit, the temporal bone, and the larynx may be examined with thin-section CT scans. The detailed anatomy of these regions as displayed by CT is also presented in separate sections to enhance their review.

Concise descriptions accompany the photographs of CT and MRI displays with the intent of emphasizing pertinent anatomical features or clinically relevant signs and symptoms. Tables summarizing the tracts and ventricles and cisterns have also been added to expedite their review.

The authors have had as their goal the compilation of illustrative material in an atlas that would be helpful and easy to use for the clinician and the radiologist in training or practice. As such, we hope to present, between one set of covers, the anatomical information needed to interpret most neurologically oriented studies performed with the major imaging modalities of CT or MRI.

The Gross Brain

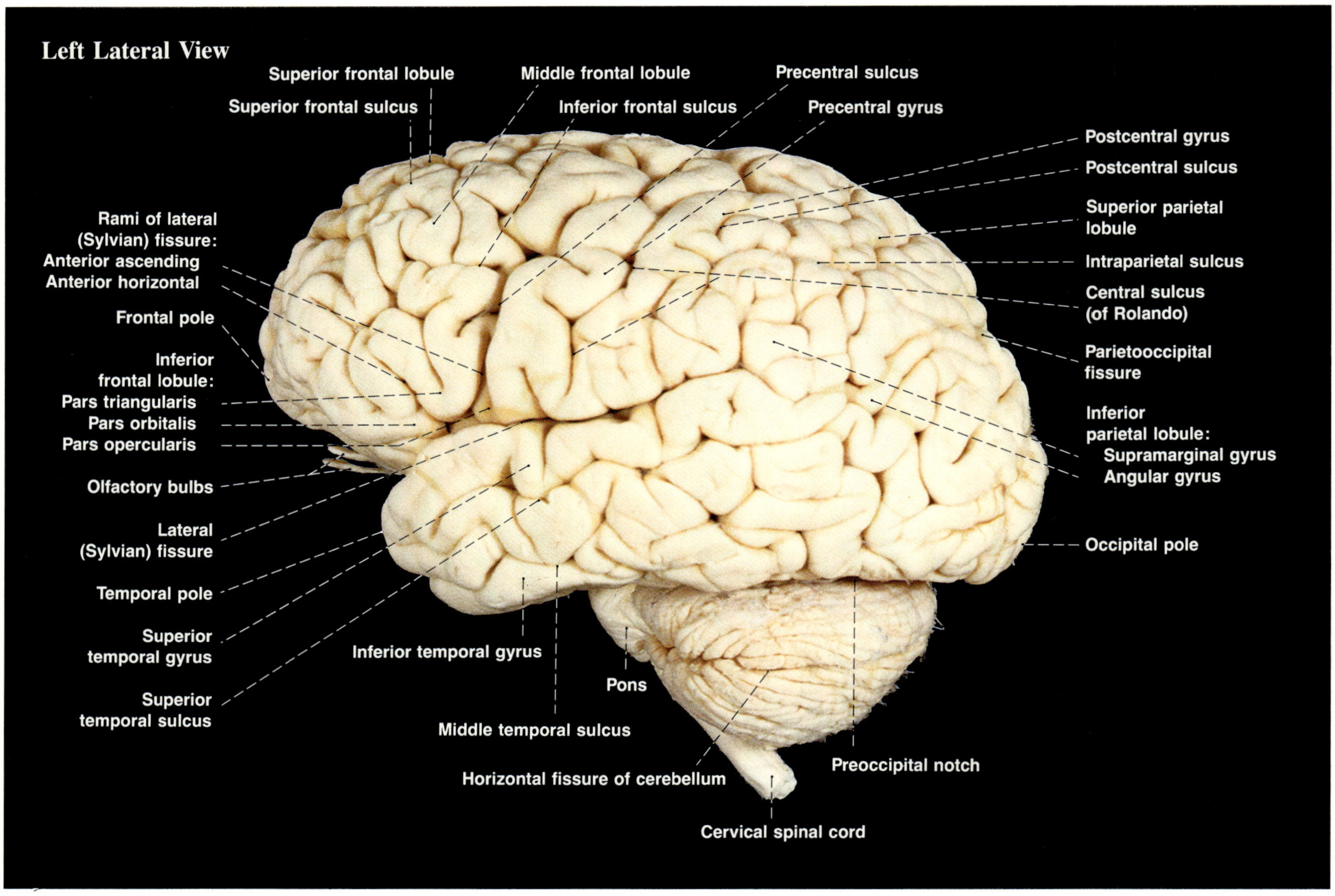

Left side of the brain. The orientation approximates its anatomic position.

2 cm

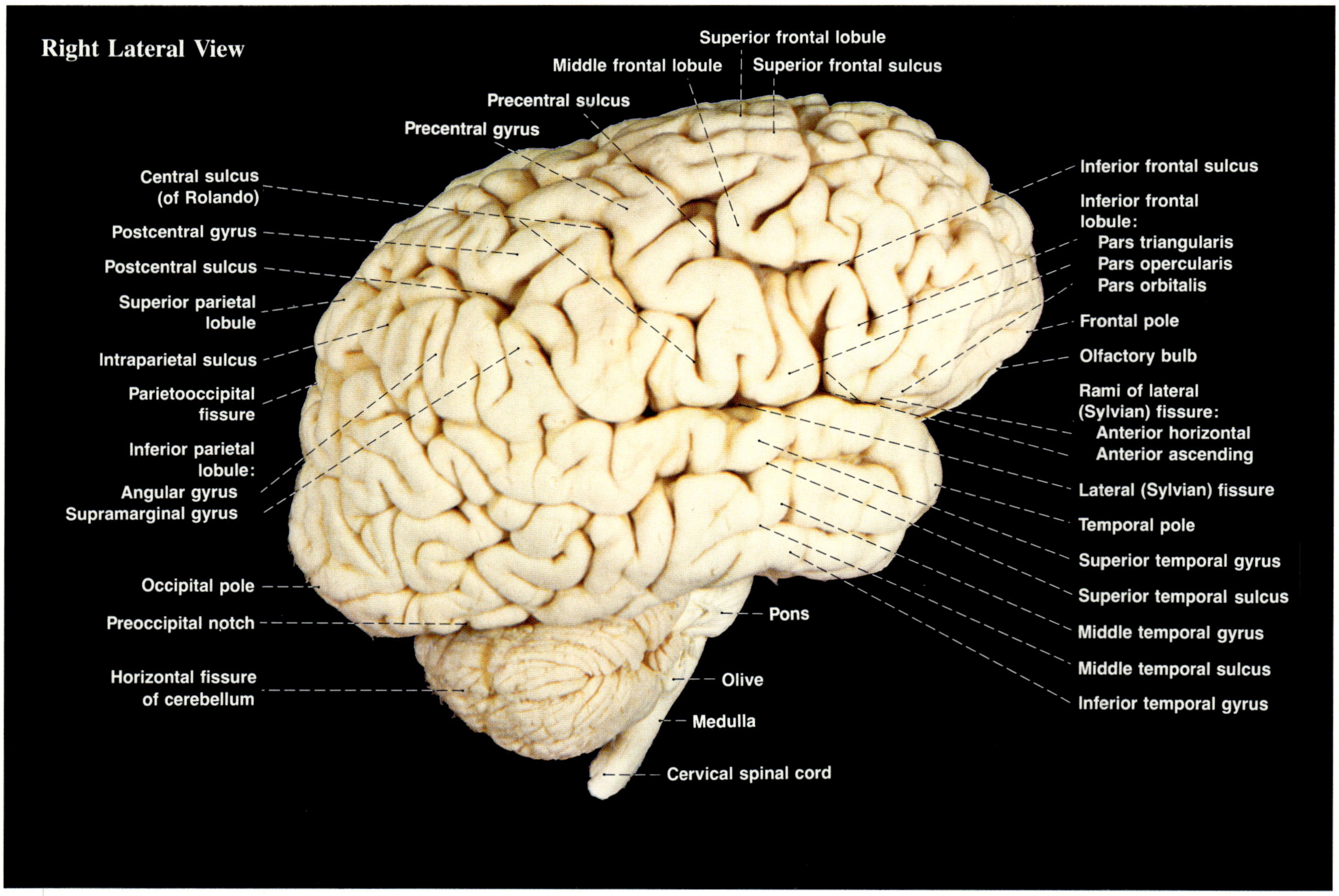

Right side of the brain. This figure may be compared with the left surface of the same brain.

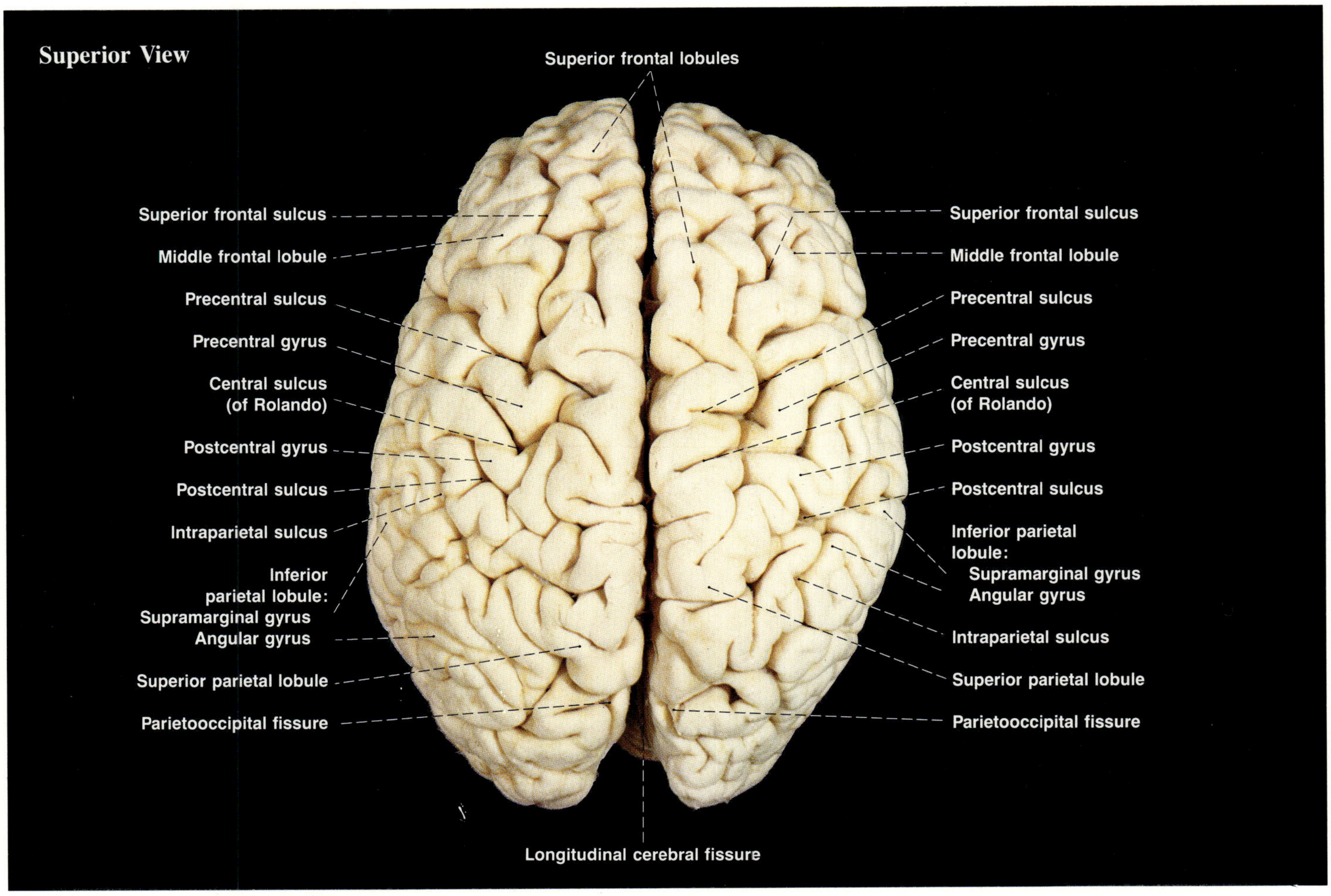

The brain viewed from above. The difference in the pattern of gyri and sulci between the right and left cerebral hemispheres is apparent.

2 cm

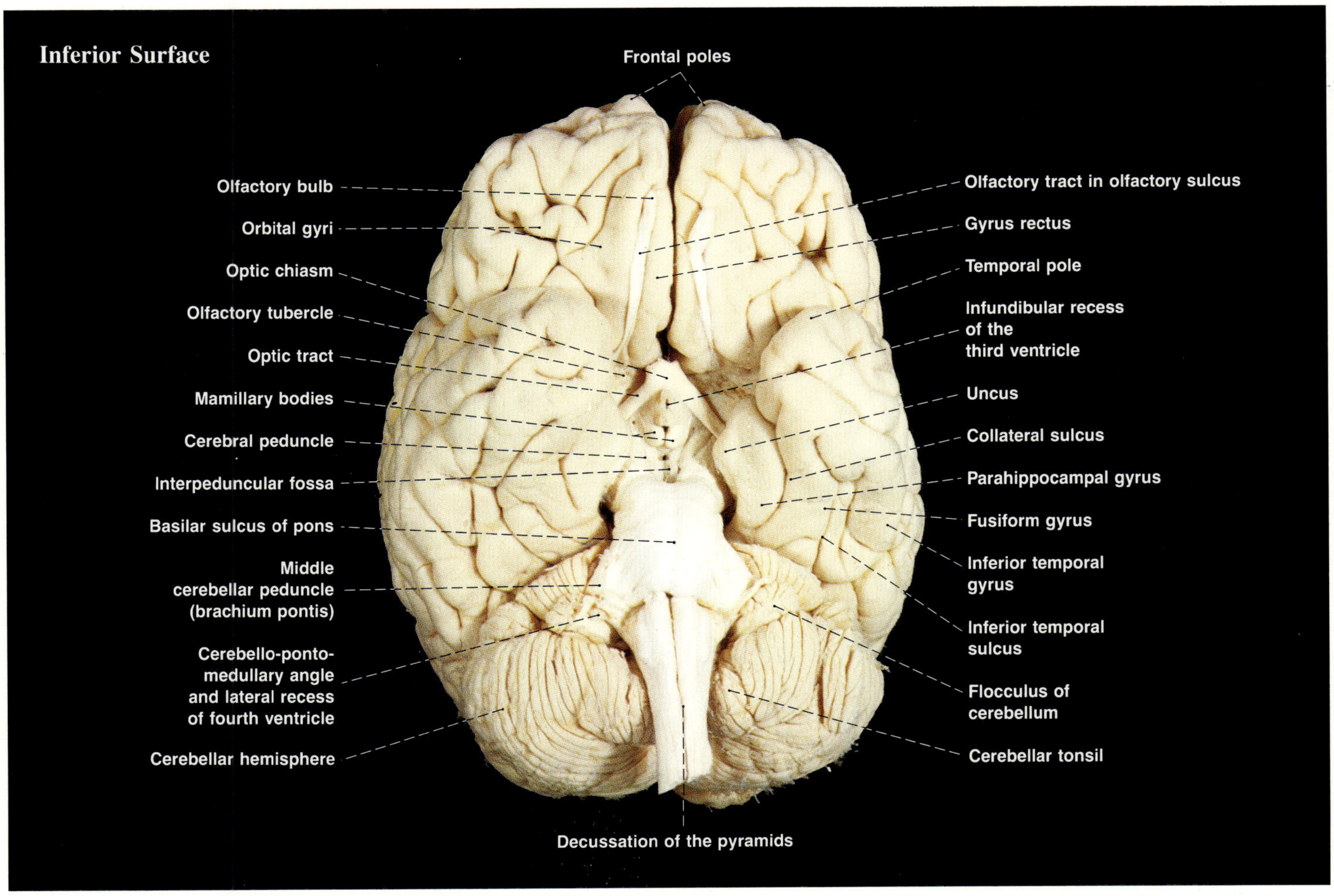

The brain viewed from below. The pia and arachnoid have been removed to better demonstrate the gross anatomic features.

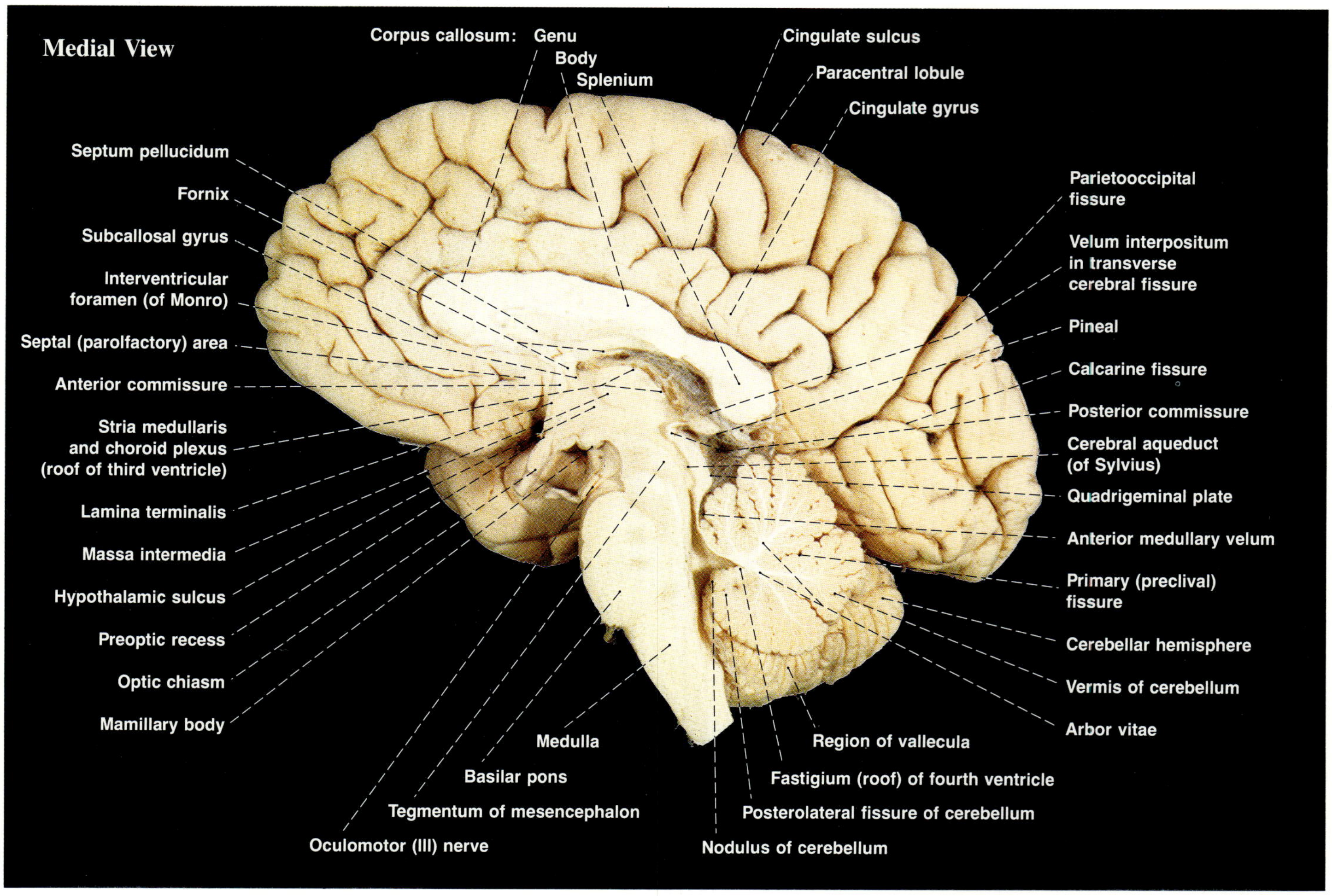

The medial aspect of the right side of the brain. The sagittal cut is just to the left of the midline anteriorly, leaving the septum pellucidum between the corpus callosum and the fornix intact.

2 cm

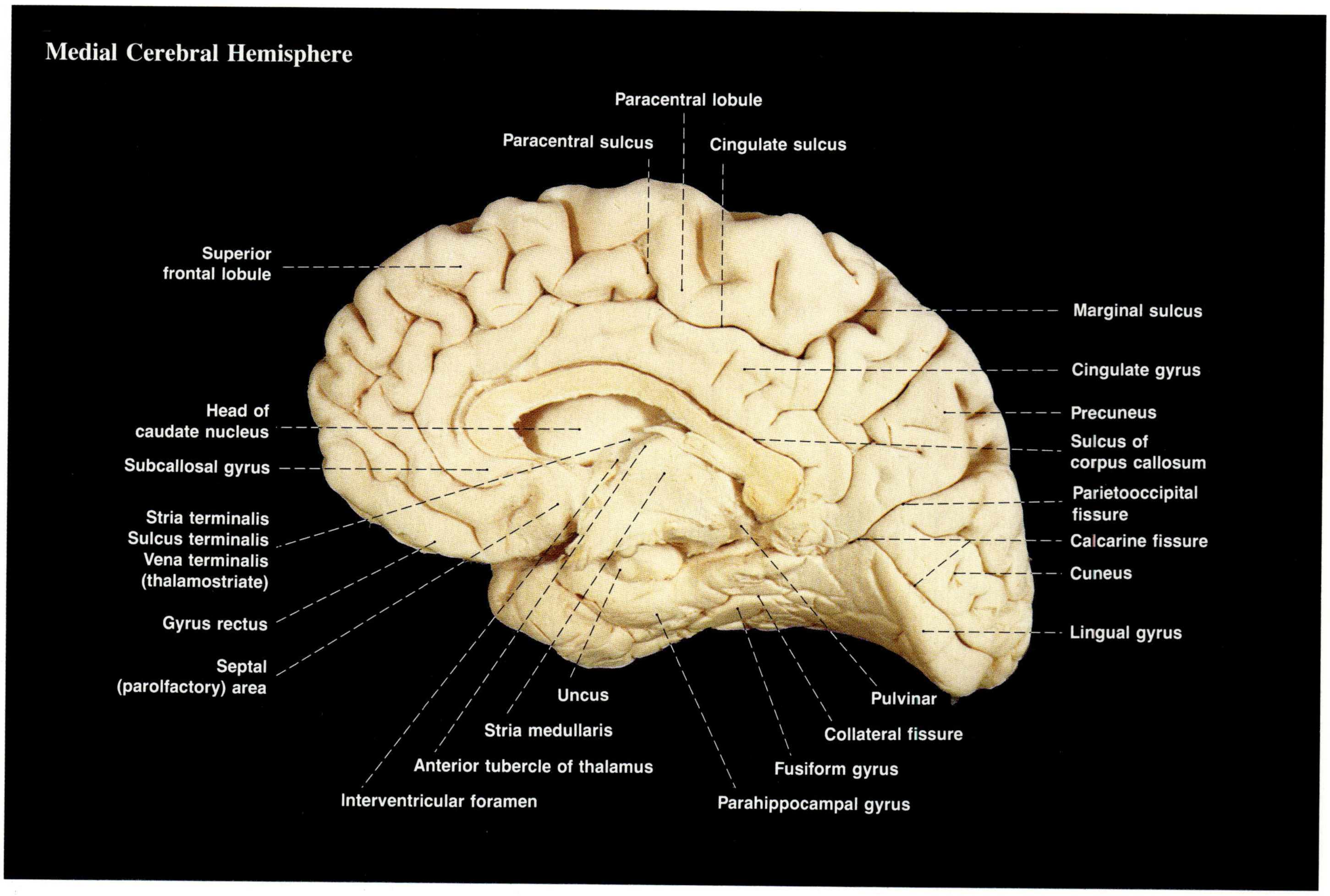

The medial aspect of the right cerebral hemisphere. The plane of the section is just to the right of the midsagittal plane and septum pellucidum anteriorly, exposing the right lateral ventricle. Note differences in cortical pattern from brain above.

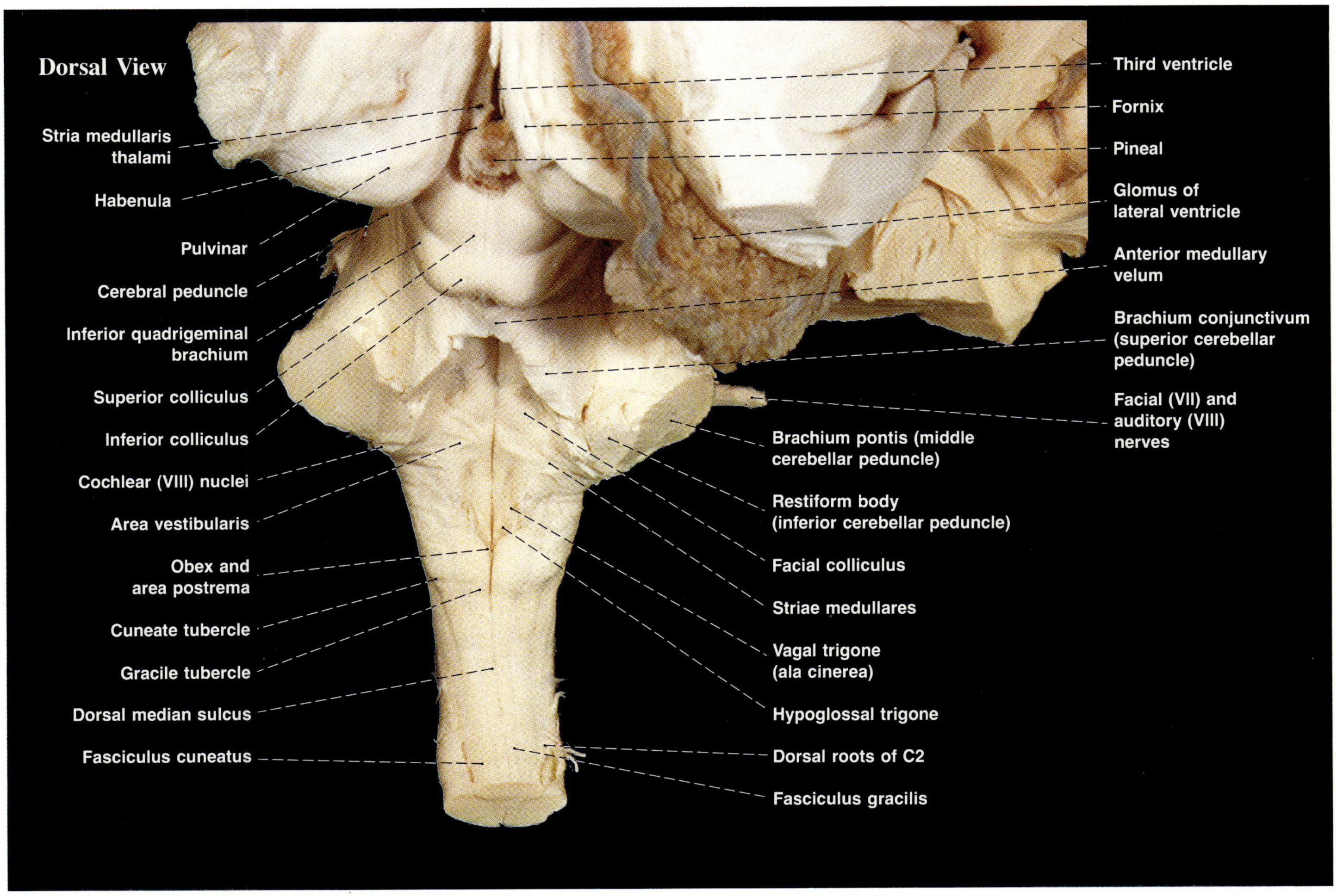

The dorsal aspect of the brainstem and floor of the fourth ventricle, following removal of occipital lobes of the cerebrum and section of the cerebellar peduncles and removal of the cerebellum.

2 cm

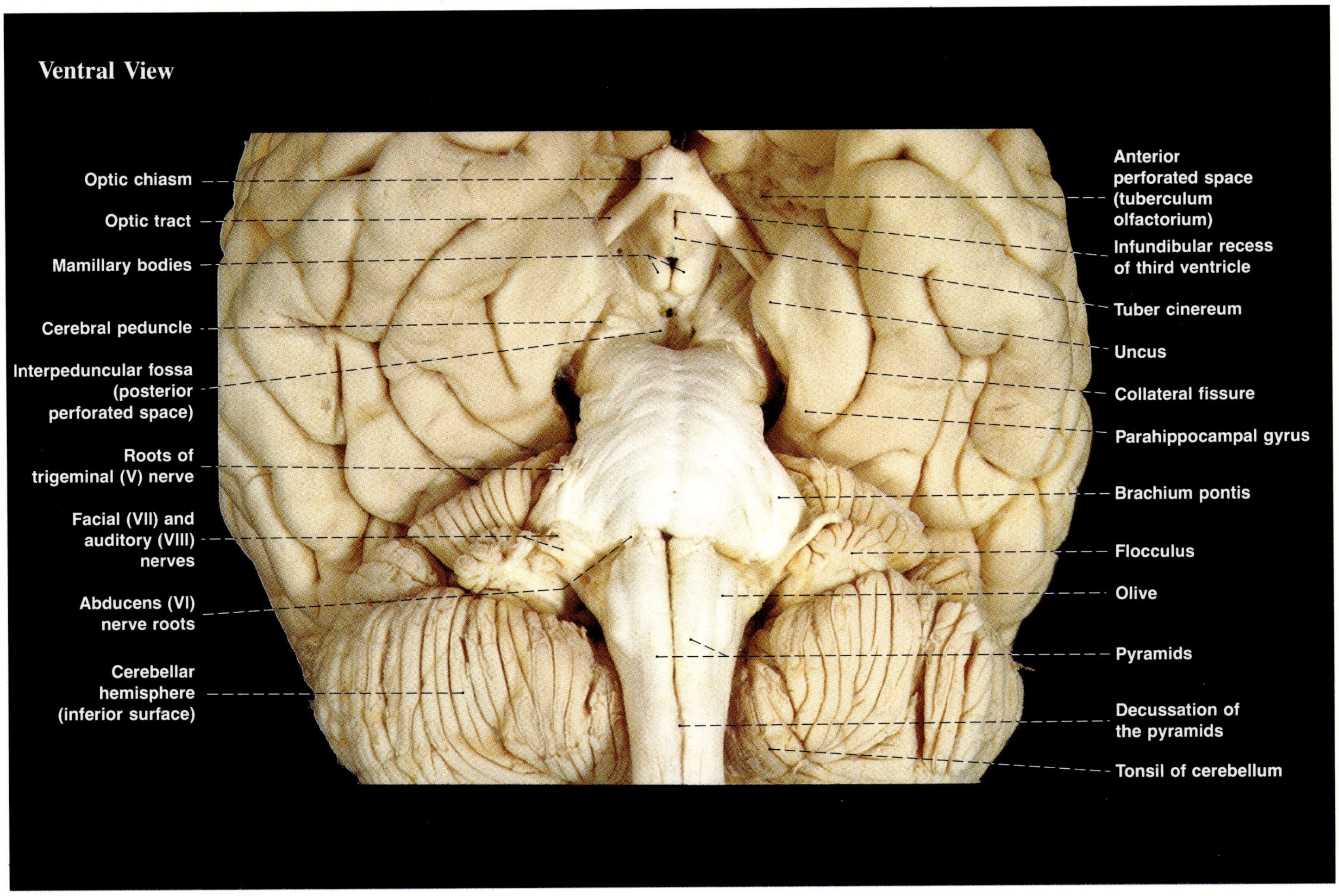

2 cm

The ventral surface of the brainstem. The pia, arachnoid, and blood vessels have been removed.

Selected Bibliography

Ariëns Kappers, C. U., G. C. Huber, and E. C. Crosby. *The Comparative Anatomy of the Nervous System of Vertebrates, including Man*. The Macmillan Co., New York, 1936.

Brodal, A. *Neurological Anatomy in Relation to Clinical Medicine*. Oxford University Press, New York, 1981.

Carpenter, M. B., and J. Sutin. *Human Neuroanatomy, 8th ed*. Williams & Wilkins, Baltimore, 1983.

Clemente, C. D. *Anatomy, A Regional Atlas of the Human Body, 2nd ed*. Urban & Schwarzenberg, Baltimore and Munich, 1981.

Crosby, E. C., T. Humphrey, and E. W. Lauer. *Correlative Anatomy of the Nervous System*. The Macmillan Co., New York, 1962.

Dandy, W. E. *The Brain* (Reprint). Hoeber Division of Harper & Row, New York, 1969.

DeArmond, S. J., M. M. Fusco, and M. M. Dewey. *Structure of the Human Brain: A Photographic Atlas*. Oxford University Press, New York, 1976.

Ferner, H. *Eduard Pernkopf Atlas of Topographical and Applied Human Anatomy, 2nd Revised ed. Vol. I, Head and Neck*. Urban & Schwarzenberg, Baltimore and Munich, 1980.

Ferner, H., and J. Staubesand. *Sobotta Atlas of Human Anatomy, 10th English ed.,* Translated by W. Hild. Urban & Schwarzenberg, Baltimore and Munich, 1983.

Gluhbegovic, N., and T. H. Williams. *The Human Brain: A Photographic Guide*. Harper & Row, Hagerstown, 1980.

Haines, D. E. *Neuroanatomy, An Atlas of Structures, Sections, and Systems*. Urban & Schwarzenberg, Baltimore and Munich, 1983.

Lang, J. *Clinical Anatomy of the Head, Neurocranium, Orbit, Craniocervical Regions*. Trans. by R. R. Wilson and D. P. Winstanley. Springer-Verlag, Berlin, Heidelberg, New York, 1983.

Penfield, W. and T. Rasmussen. *The Cerebral Cortex of Man*. The Macmillan Co., New York, 1950.

Smith, C. G. *Serial Dissections of the Human Brain*. Urban & Schwarzenberg, Baltimore and Munich, 1981.

Stephan, H., R. Bauchot, and O. J. Andy. *The Primate Brain*. Appleton-Century-Crofts, New York, 1970.

Taveras, J. M., and E. H. Wood. *Diagnostic Neuroradiology, 2nd ed. Vols I* and *II*. Williams & Wilkins, Baltimore, 1976.

Warwick, R., and P. L. Williams. *Gray's Anatomy, 36th British ed*. W. B. Saunders Co., Philadelphia, 1980.

Willis, W. D., and R. G. Grossmann. *Medical Neurobiology, Neuroanatomical and Neurophysiological Principles Basic to Clinical Neuroscience, 3rd ed*. C. V. Mosby Co., St. Louis, 1981.

Axial Planes

Fundamental differences in the mechanics of image generation between CT and MRI have resulted in obvious differences in the exact planes of the images in this section. On axial CT, the convention has been, and probably will continue to be, the orientation of an axial plane at a 15-20° tilt to the orbitomeatal (infraorbitomeatal, IOM) base line. Almost all CT images of the head are generated and displayed in this manner as it insures maximum information (i.e., anterior fossa and posterior fossa structures on one cut) per slice. MRI scans, on the other hand, are being generated and displayed in a configuration usually parallel to the orbitomeatal line or some angle other than that employed for axial CT. The reason lies in a combination of technical factors peculiar to MRI, including the fact that the patient lies in the resonator coil and the bore of the magnet in a position comfortable for the patient and images are then gathered (either single slice or volume collection methods) in a true axial plane. To obtain an image oriented 15° to the orbitomeatal line, the patient must keep his chin flexed for many minutes and this has proven physically difficult for many patients to perform. Images are therefore obtained in a true axial plane to whatever position the patient can maintain his head for the relatively long periods of time necessary to generate the image.

Patient CT Scan

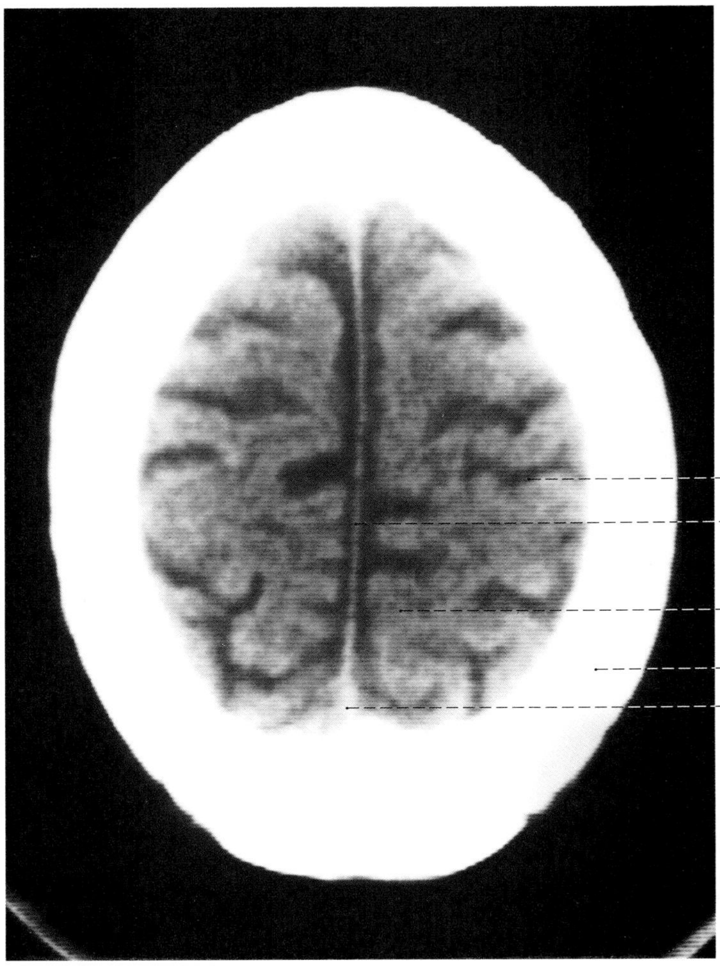

Patient MRI Scan

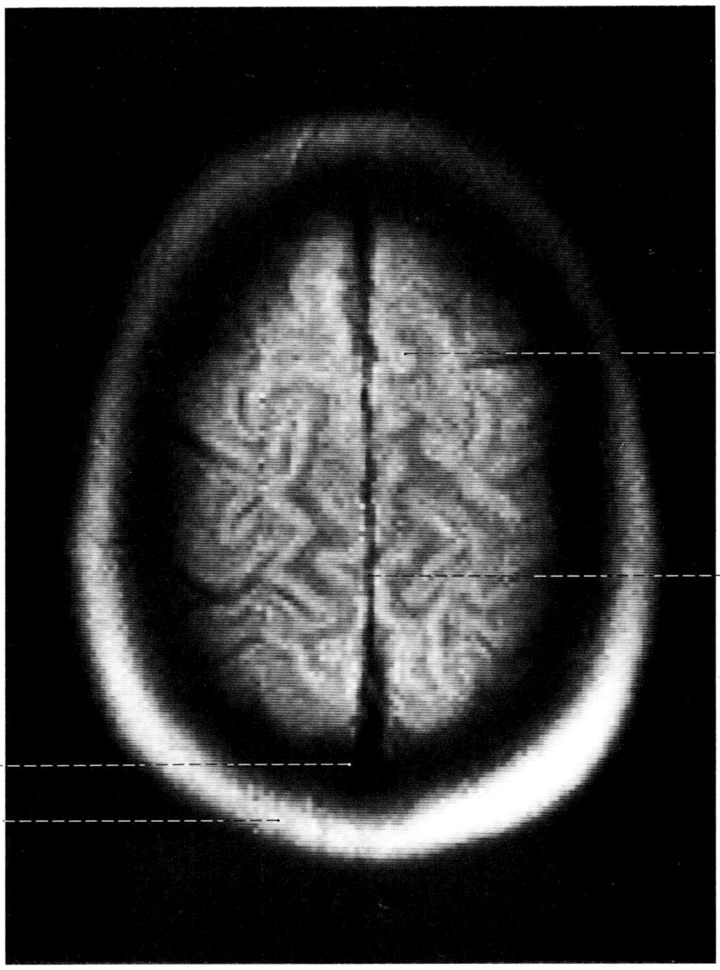

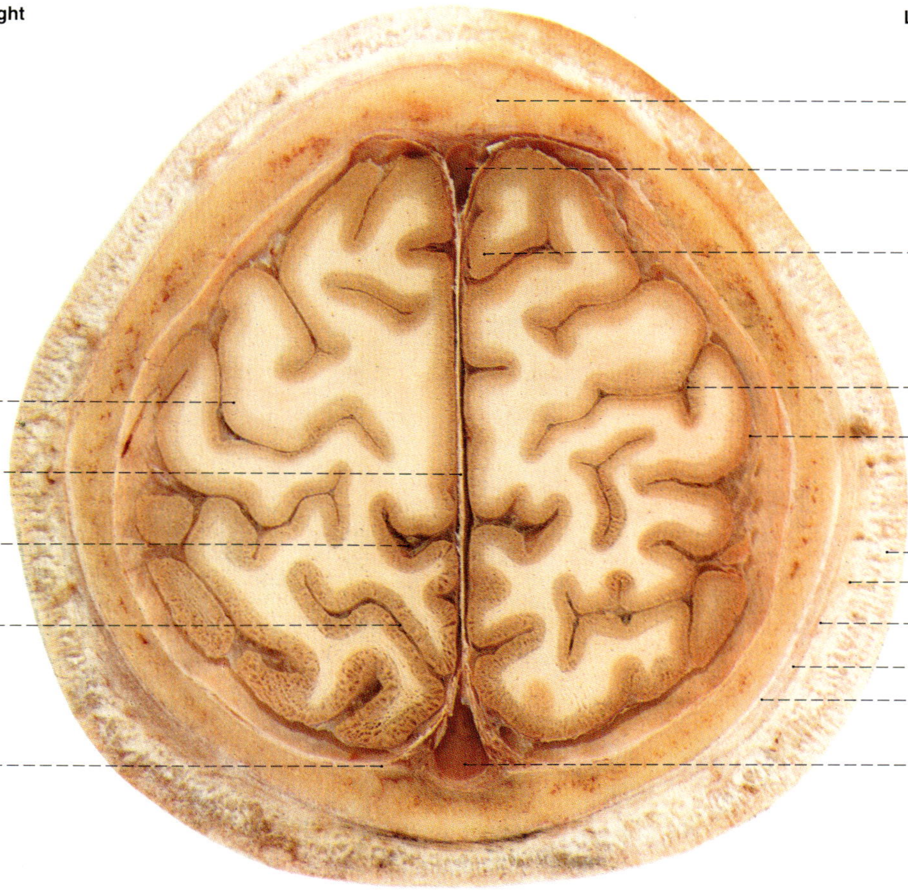

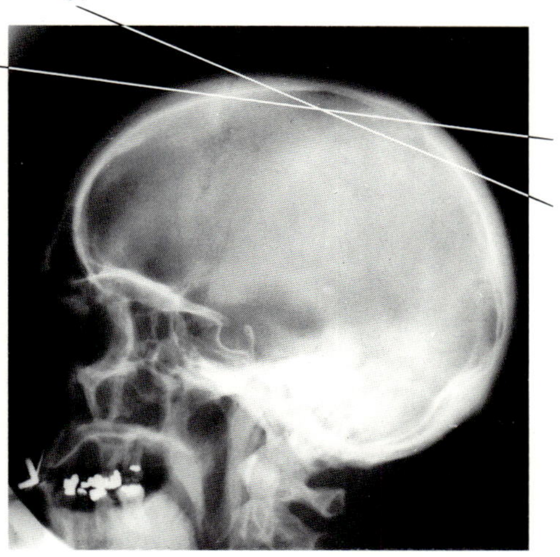

Planes of Sections

Any axial section through the superior 5 cm of the adult head will usually pass above the corpus callosum and the lateral ventricles. Such planes will, however, demonstrate the gyri and sulci of the superior frontal and parietal lobes, the longitudinal cerebral fissure containing the falx cerebri, and the superior sagittal sinus. The plane of the MRI approximates the infraorbito-meatal line (IOM) but the CT is in the more common 15° angle from the IOM line.

The cortical sensory and motor areas adjacent to the falx cerebri are those representing the lower extremities and perineum. The subcortical fiber bundles include projection paths from the precentral motor areas (corticospinal), thalamocortical fibers to the postcentral gyrus (sensory radiations), and frontoparietooccipital association tracts. The anterior cerebral artery supplies the areas adjacent to the falx and the middle cerebral artery perfuses the lateral cortex.

Lack of visualization of sulci containing cerebrospinal fluid may indicate cerebral edema in older age groups, although representing a normal finding in earlier years. Narrowing of the gyri and enlargement of the sulci must be interpreted with caution, and diagnoses of cortical (and subcortical) atrophy or senile dementia should not be made solely on the basis of this observation, since a wide normal range has been recorded radiographically.

Patient CT Scan

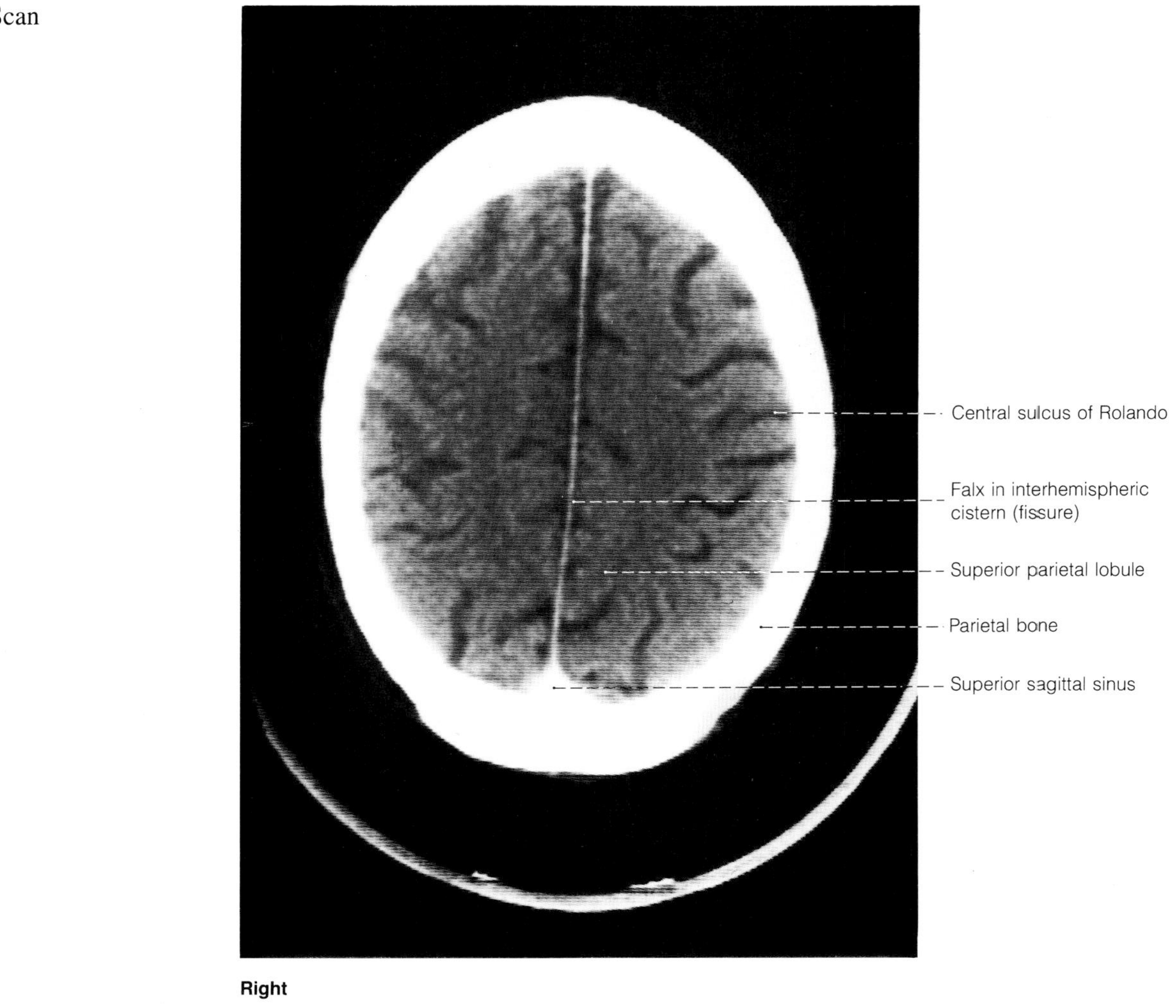

Patient MRI Scan

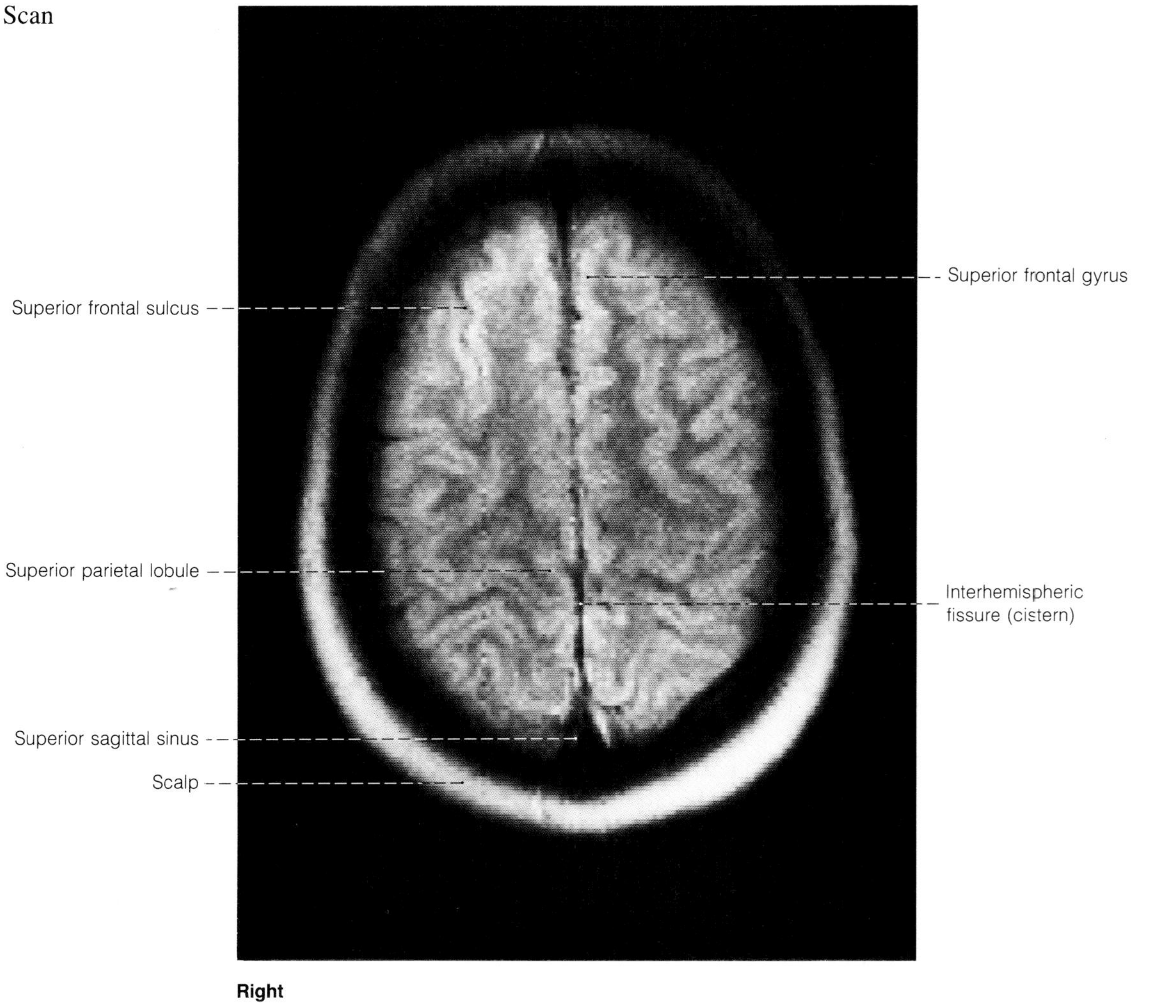

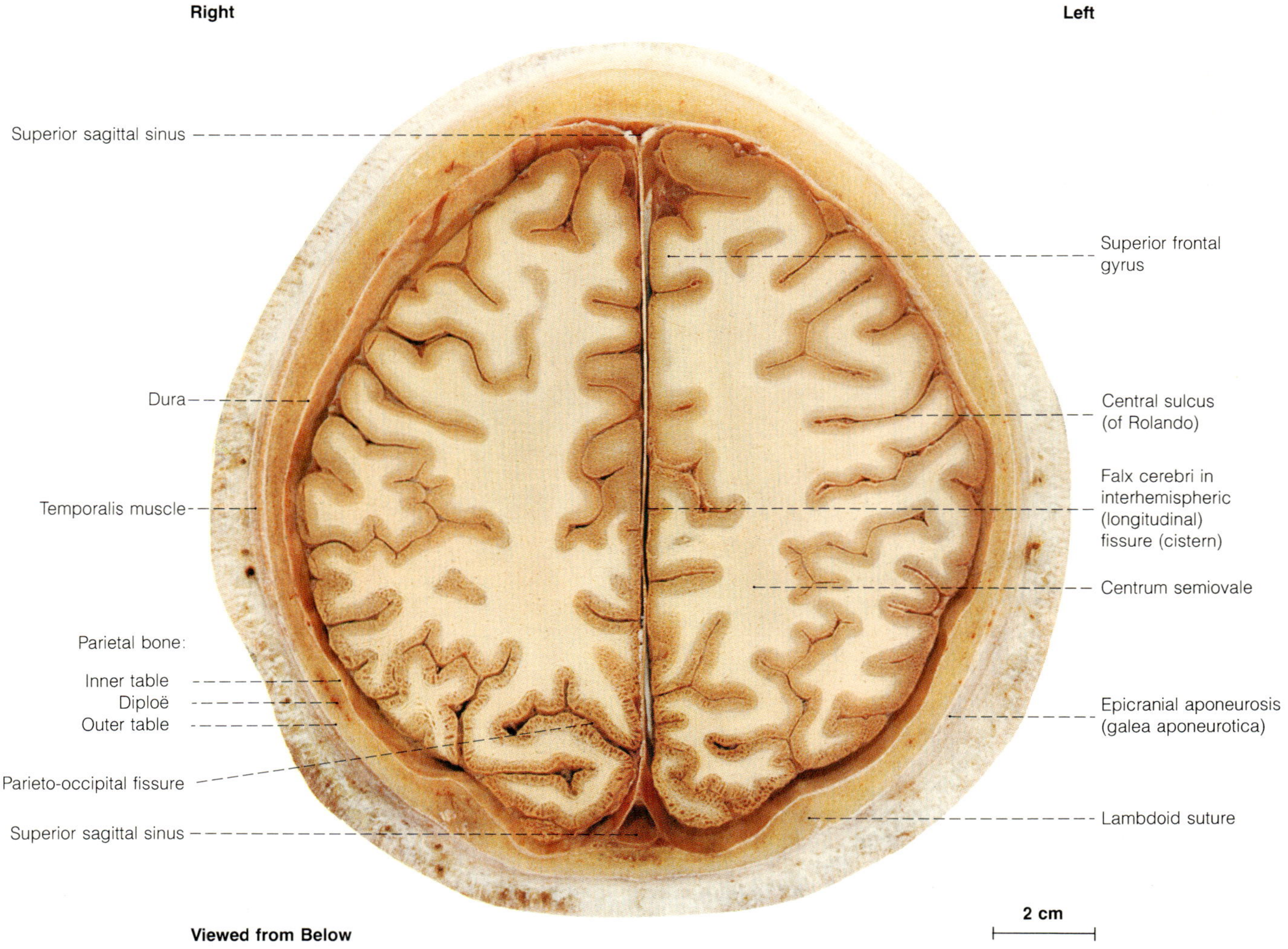

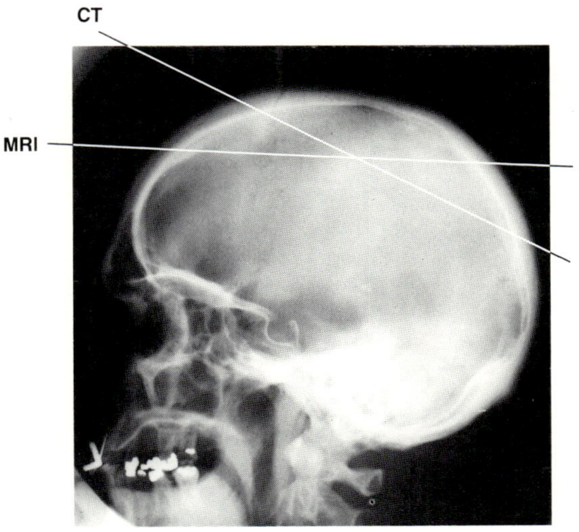

Planes of Sections

One of the distinct advantages of MRI imaging is the ability to differentiate distinctly cortical and subcortical gray (e.g., striatum and thalamus) from the white matter of the hemisphere. Such differentiation can be obtained with spin echo images and delayed pulsing giving T2 weighted information. In planes above the corpus callosum, the subcortical white matter (centrum semiovale) contains not only the projection tracts but also (and largely) both short and long subcortical association paths. Involvement of these tracts alone by limited pathological processes may or may not produce overt symptoms. It is now frequently possible to demonstrate such lesions with MRI.

The peripheral ring of white around the head on the CT image represents the dense bone at this window setting; however, on MRI this is the soft tissue of the scalp. Since there is a large amount of fat in subcutaneous layers of the scalp and since fat has long T1 and T2 values, this is perceived as white on our MRI viewing scale. The dark area beneath the fat of the scalp is a combination of CSF (including the CSF of the sulci) and bone. Neither gives off a detectable MRI signal at this pulse sequence and both therefore appear black. The dense dura of the falx also gives off very little signal and is also denoted in black. A sharp delineation between bone, CSF, and brain is not obtained in this section because their interfaces overlay each other and are therefore averaged together in a 1 cm cut.

Patient CT Scan

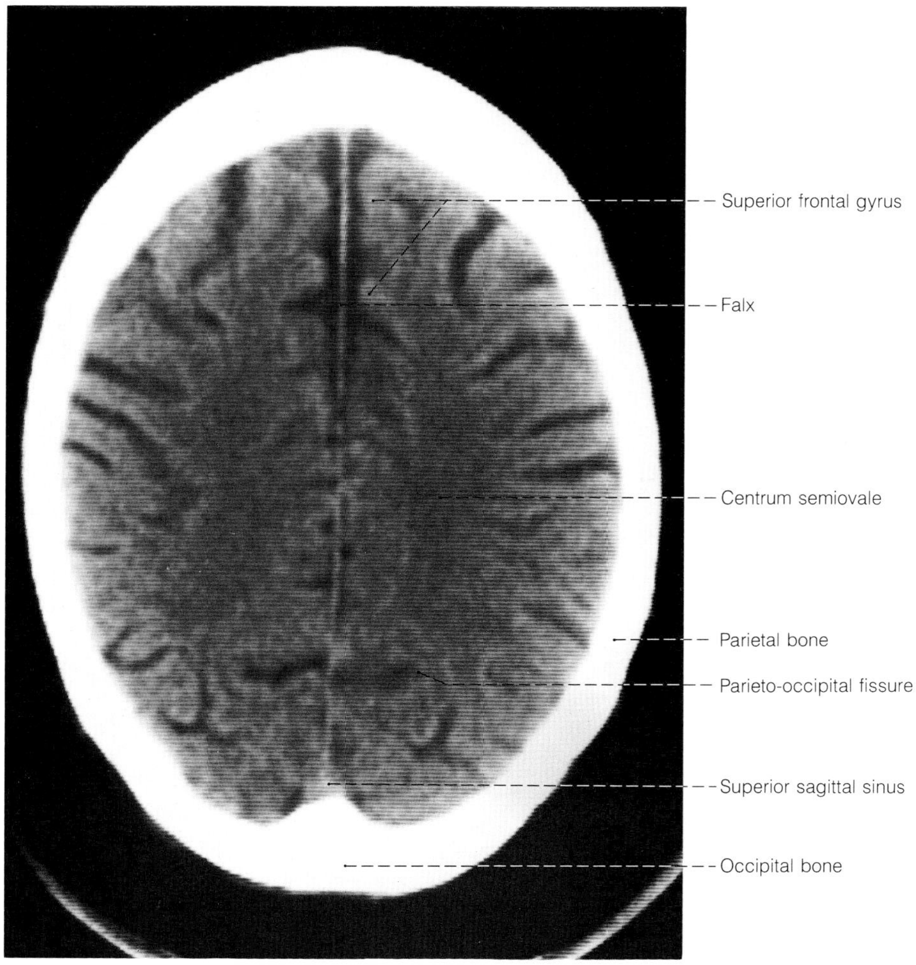

Right

Patient MRI Scan

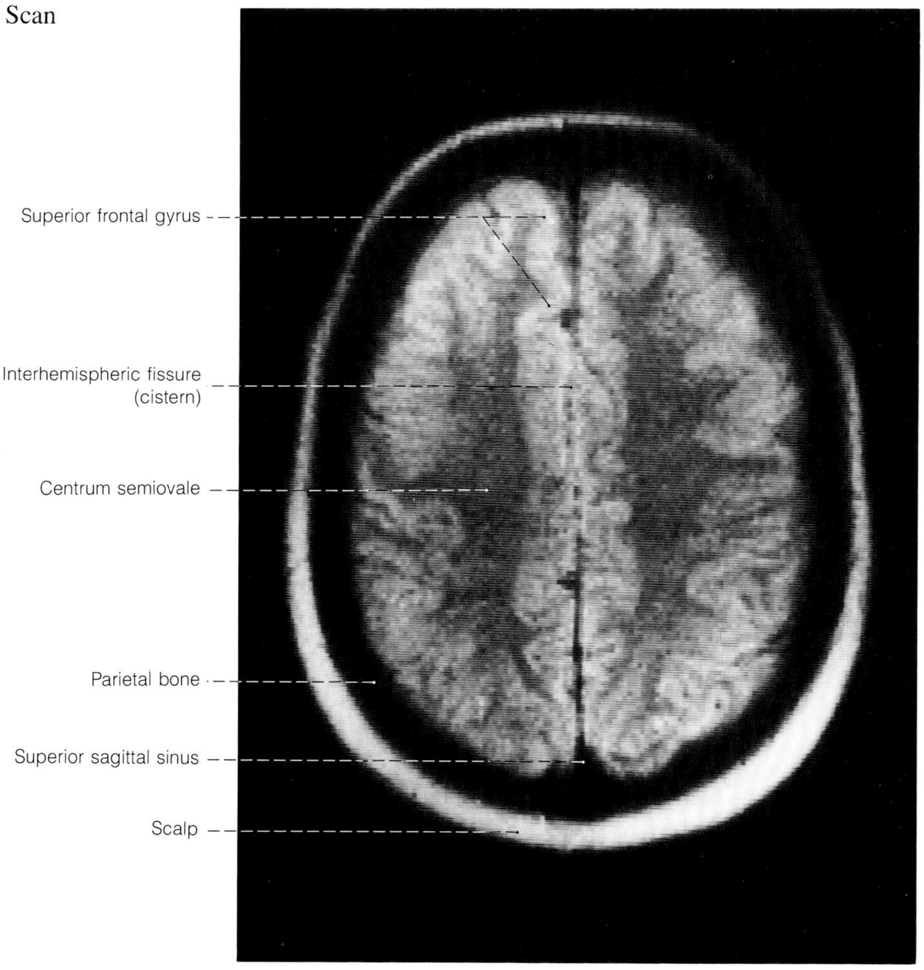

Right

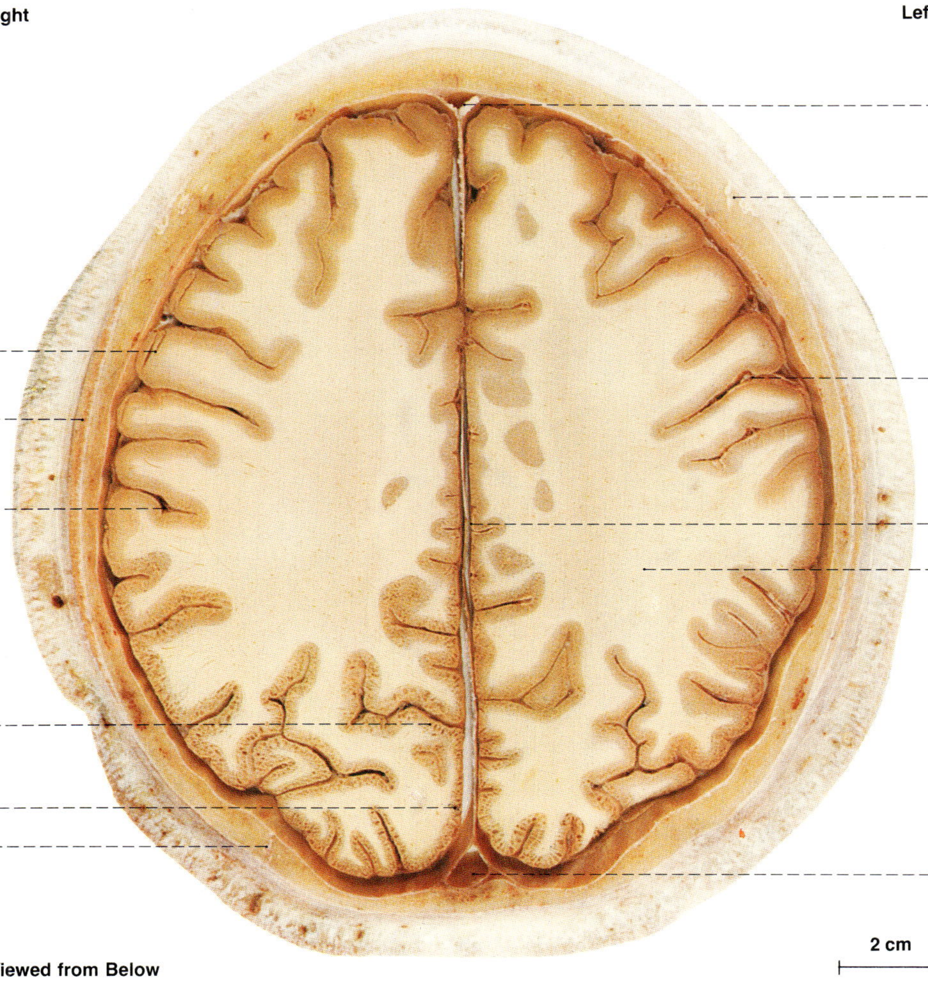

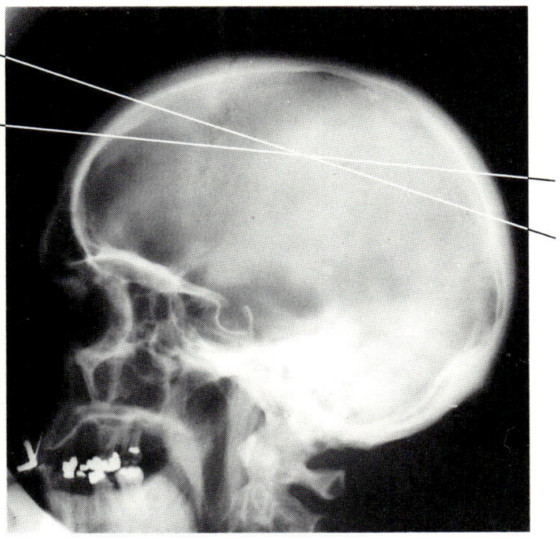

Planes of Sections

The head illustrated in the gross photograph and those selected for the CT and MRI displays demonstrate normal variations in the shape of the skull. The gross specimen is quite brachycephalic (cephalic index, > 80) and the patient shown in the CT image is definitely dolichocephalic (cephalic index < 75). Since the surface of the hemispheres of the brain approximates the inner surface of the skull and variation is not uncommon, absolute measurements for locating specific sulci or gyri are of limited value. In comparing right and left hemispheres in a single patient, there are also some normal differences in sulci and gyri in the two sides, some of which may be attributable to handedness.

Posteriorly, the cuneus labeled in the gross specimen is the cortical area above the calcarine fissure. It contains areas #18 and #19 as well as the visual radiations from the opposite inferior visual field in the subcortical white matter. The more horizontal plane of the MRI differs from the CT and passes through the frontal and parietal lobes but is largely above the occipital lobe.

Patient CT Scan

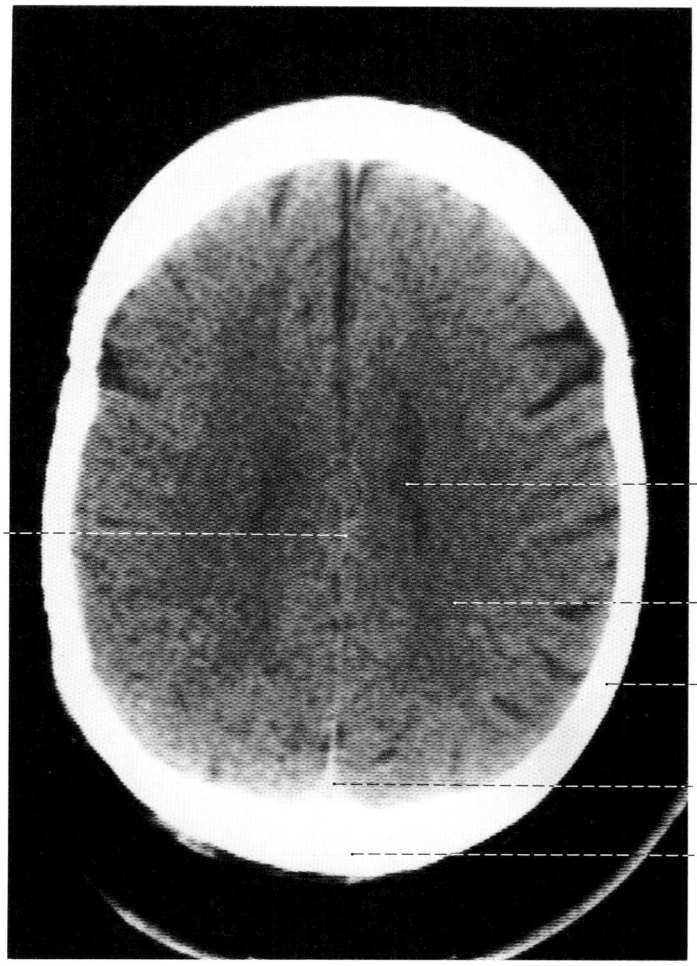

Patient MRI Scan

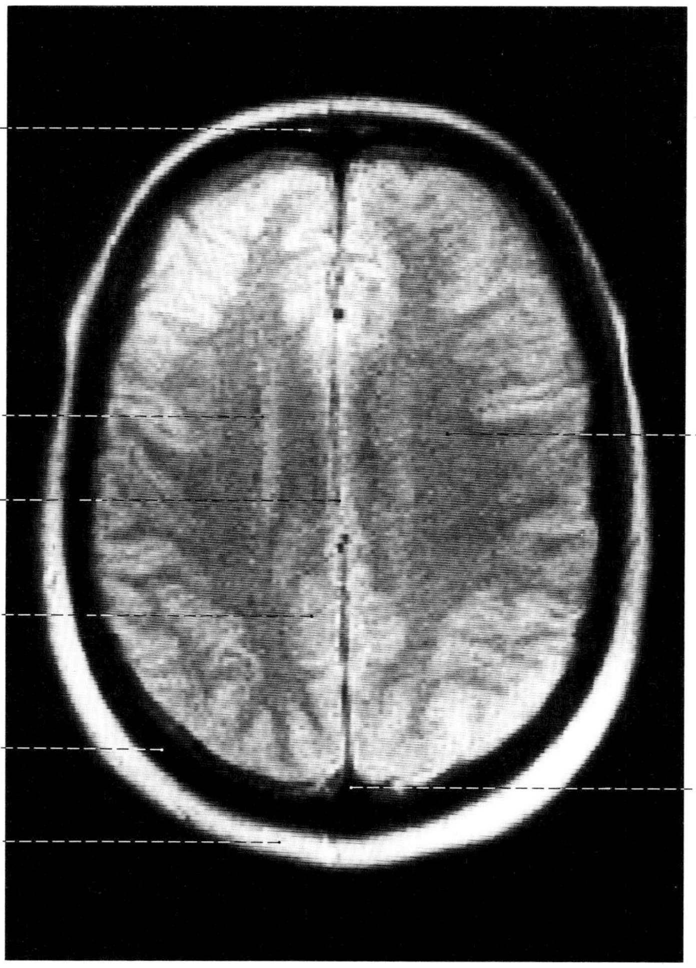

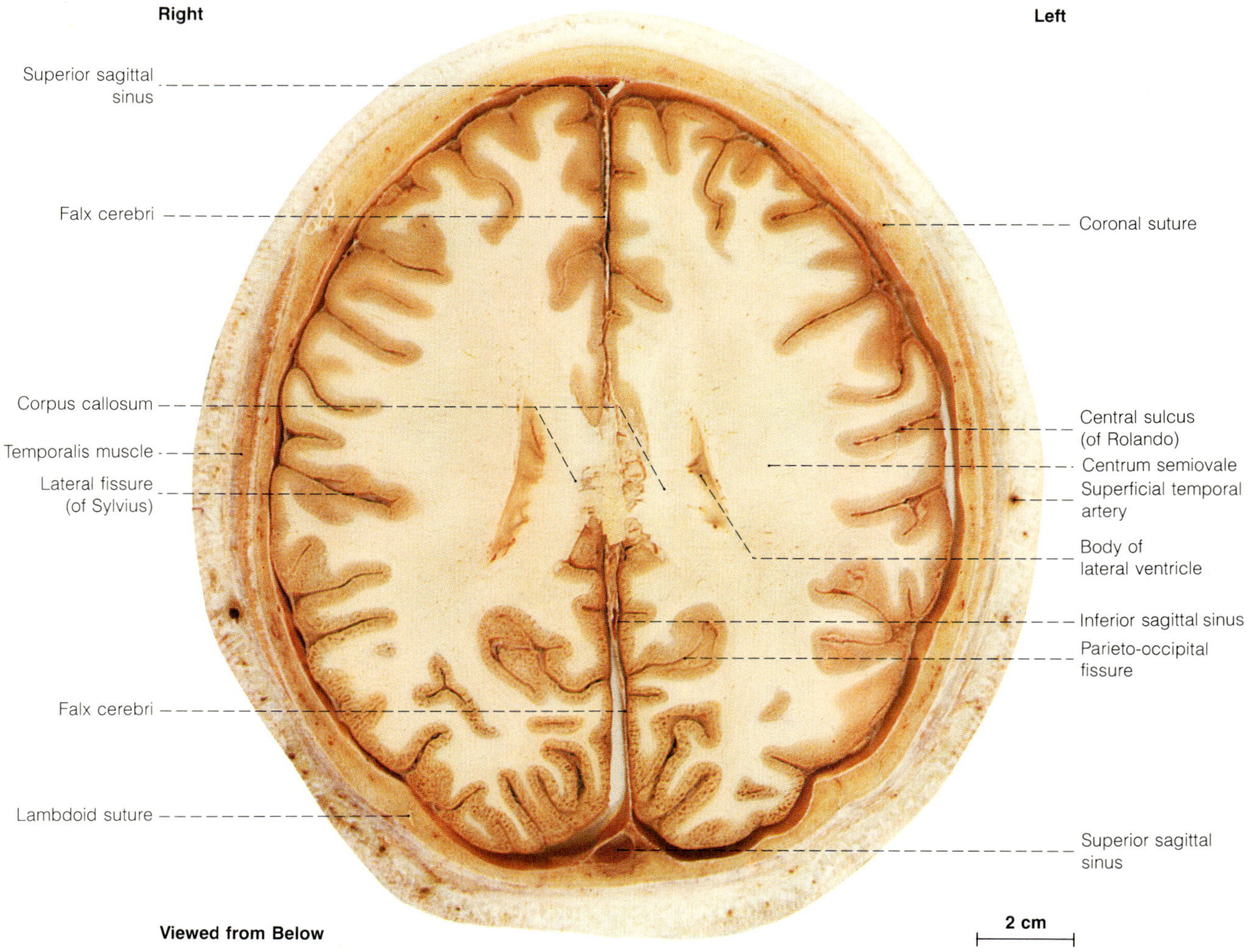

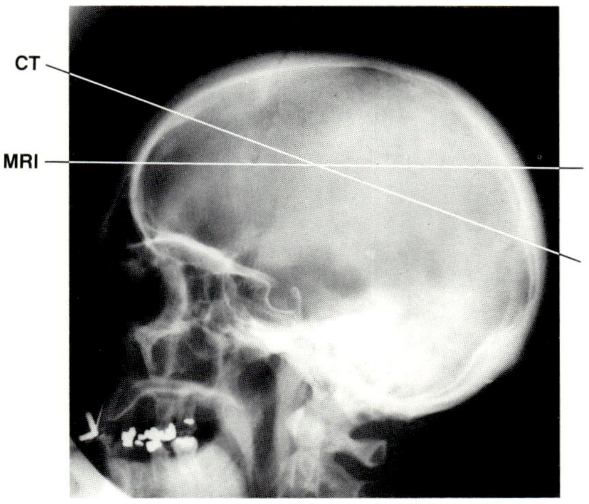

Planes of Sections

A plane 15° above the IOM (infraorbito-meatal) line, 6 to 7 cm from the top of the head and above the tentorium cerebelli will pass through the upper surface of the bodies of the lateral ventricles and the corpus callosum. Cortical areas include the face and/or hand region and part of Wernicke's area (supramarginal and angular gyri). The MRI plane, more nearly paralleling the IOM plane, passes more superiorly through the parietal lobe and more inferiorly through the frontal lobe.

The internal carotid artery supplies the lateral hemisphere by branches of the middle cerebral artery. The medial hemisphere at this level is perfused by branches of the anterior cerebral artery. Only a small part of the medial occipital lobe in this plane may be supplied by the parietooccipital branches of the posterior cerebral artery.

Displacement of the falx cerebri to the right or left from its midline position is an indication of a superior intracranial space-occupying mass. A shift of the cingulate gyrus and pericallosal artery under the free margin of the falx may also occur. Accumulation of blood on either side of the midline may indicate hemorrhage from the superficial (cortical) veins draining into the superior sagittal sinus.

In addition to the superior visual radiations (carrying visual impulses from the contralateral lower visual fields), the subcortical white matter contains the large superior longitudinal frontooccipital and occipitofrontal association tracts. Lateral to the body of the lateral ventricle is the superior extension of the internal capsule with its motor and sensory projection tracts. Infarcts localized to this area may appear as nonenhancing lucencies lateral to the body of the ventricle and are referred to as "lacunar" infarcts if they do not involve subjacent cortical gray matter. This is a radiographic term only and should not be confused with microscopic "lacunar" infarcts seen in the same area on histologic examination.

On the MRI scan, marrow (diploë) in the frontal bones is beginning to be evident and is represented by the band of signal (white) anteriorly, and less distinctly in occipital locations.

Superior Thalamus

Patient CT Scan

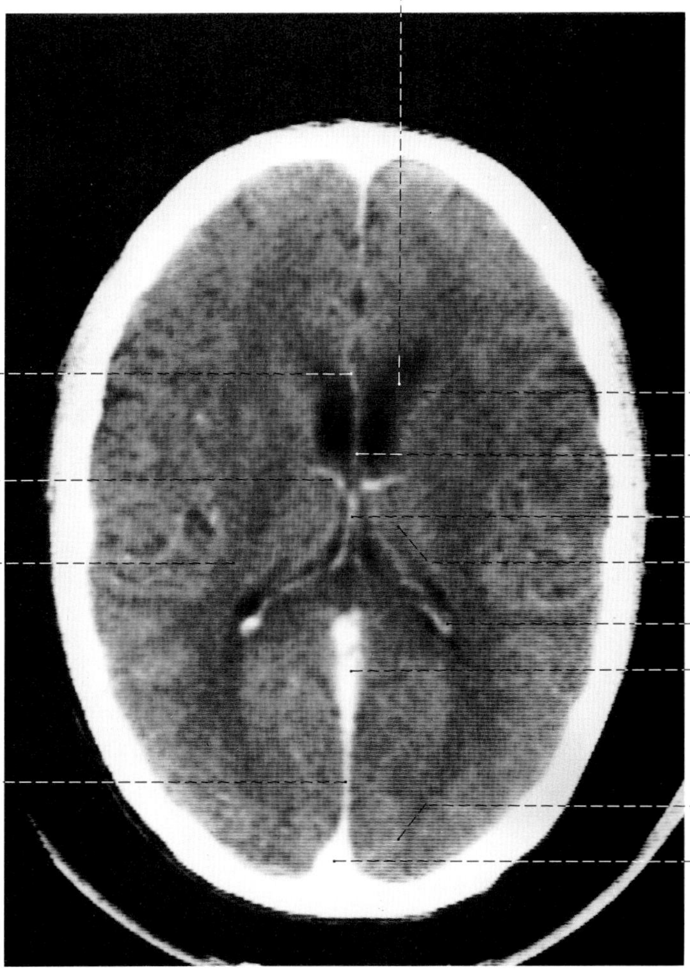

Patient MRI Scan

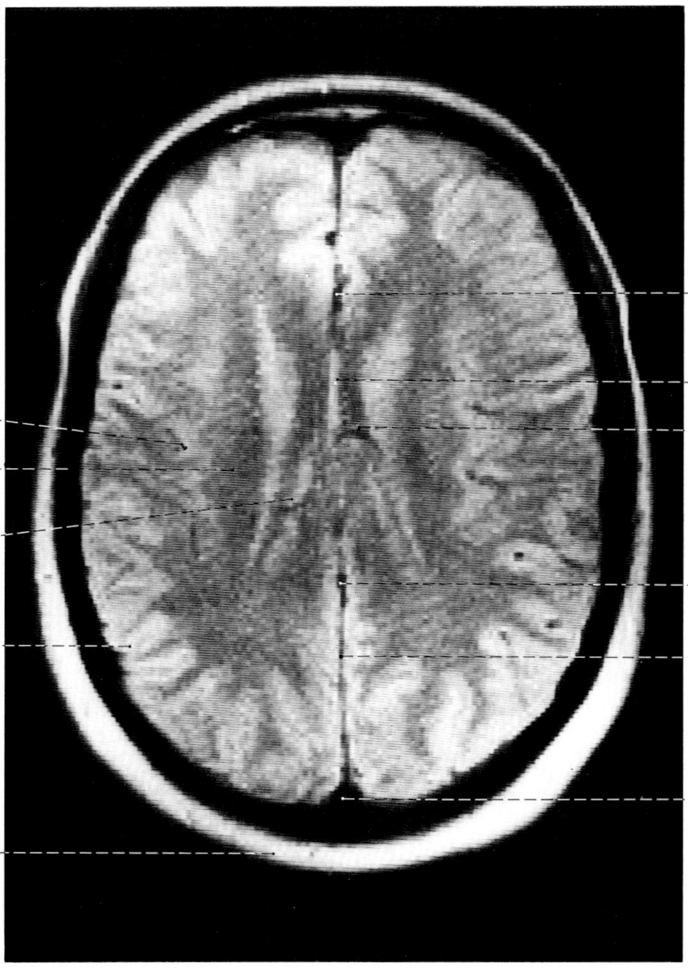

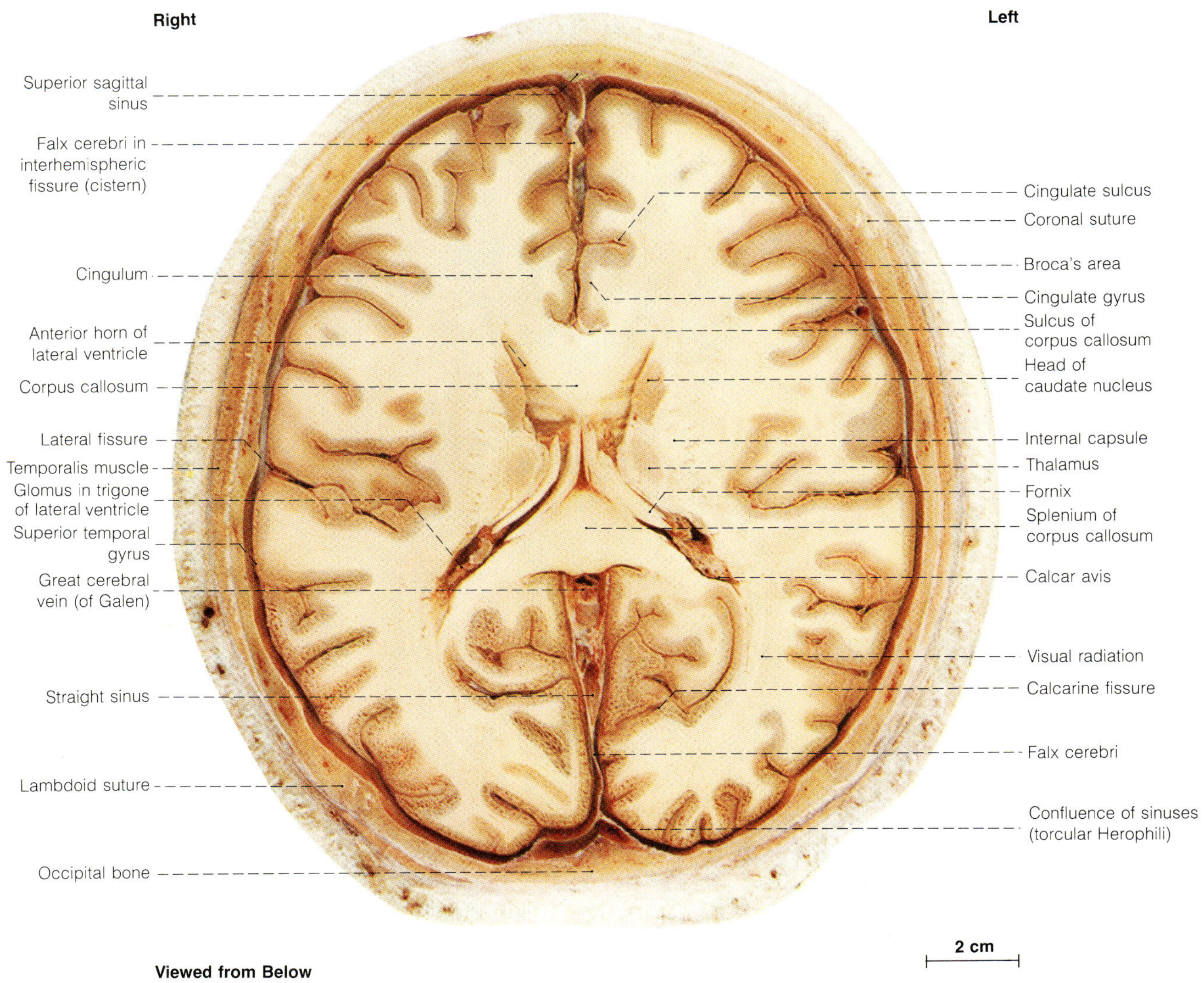

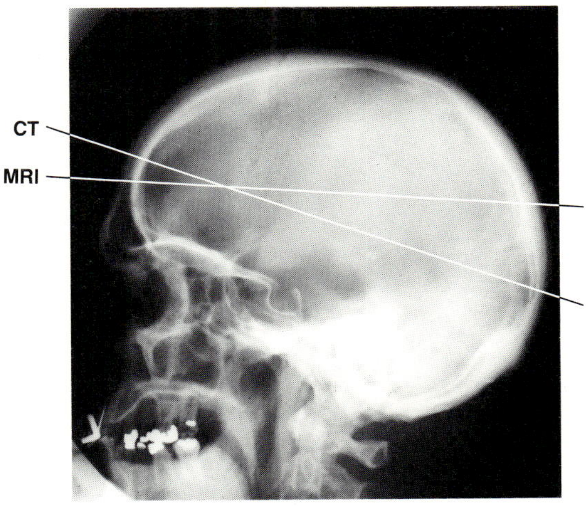

Planes of Sections

The CT and gross anatomical planes are approximately 7 to 8 cm from the top of the head passing just above the tentorium cerebelli and paralleling the long axis of the lateral ventricles. The cortical areas include Broca's area, the face regions of the pre- and postcentral gyri.

The head of the caudate nucleus forms a characteristic convexity in the lateral wall of the anterior horn of the lateral ventricle. Lateral to the head of the caudate is the anterior limb of the internal capsule with its thalamofrontal projections (to and from the "prefrontal" cortex) and frontopontine tracts. The posterior limb with its corticospinal tracts, corticobulbar tracts, and sensory radiations is lateral to the thalamus.

The anterior cerebral artery supplies the medial cortical areas anteriorly, and the posterior cerebral artery perfuses the medial cortical areas posteriorly. The entire lateral cortical region is supplied by branches of the middle cerebral artery. Perforating arteries from the circle of Willis and the adjacent cerebral arteries project into the deep nuclear regions.

The falx cerebri is usually shallow rostrally, having its greatest depth posteriorly where it joins the apex of the tentorium cerebelli. The straight sinus and great cerebral vein (of Galen) are located in this junction in the CT and gross sections but the MRI plane is above these posterior structures while transecting the inferior frontal lobe.

Note the superior detail on the MRI scan as a result of differences in technique of generating images and lack of artifact from bone, as in CT. CSF has a relatively low signal with this pulse sequence and CSF in ventricles and sulci provide major contrast within the brain, as with CT. However, differences in pulse response of white and grey matter also allow for excellent differentiation of anatomic structures.

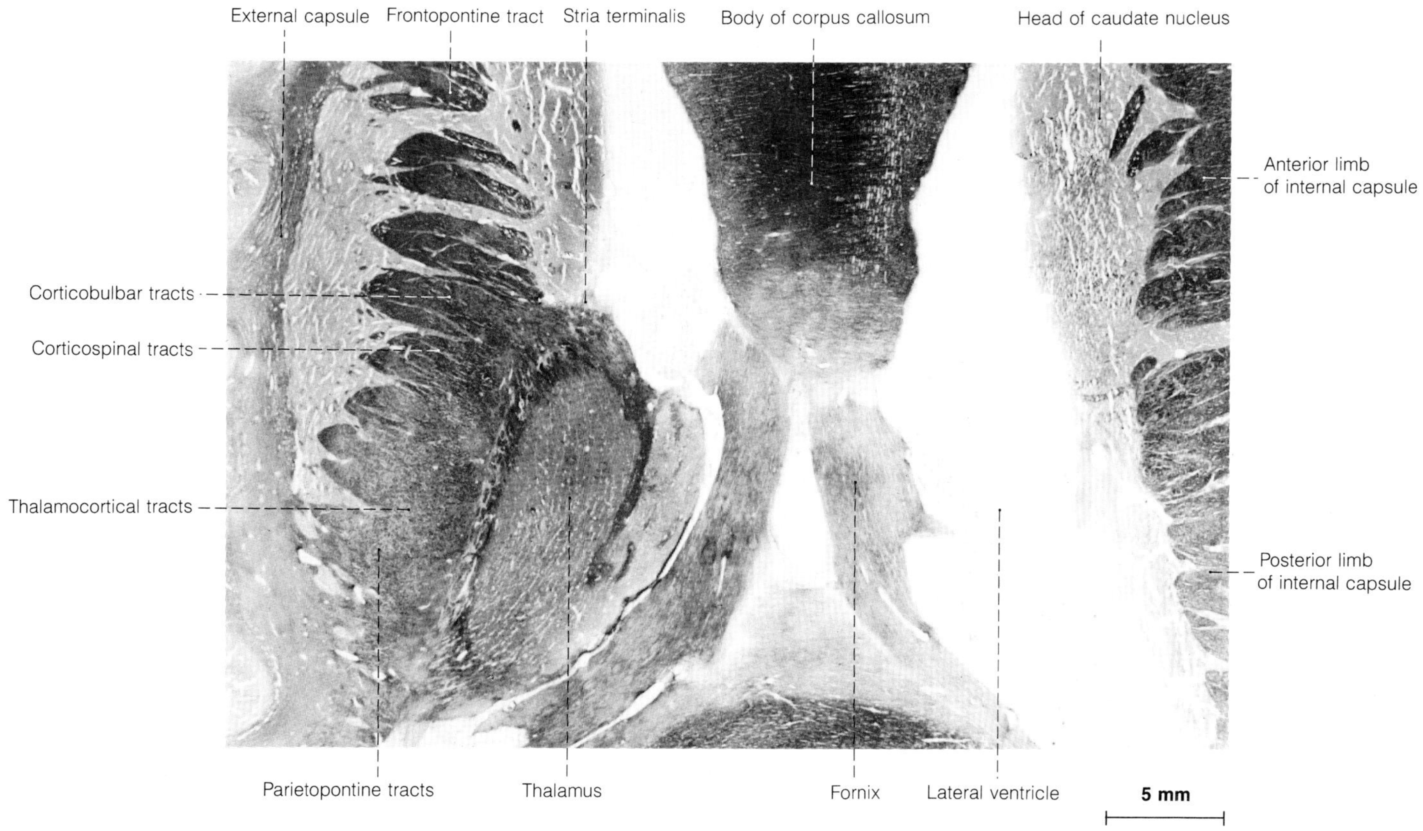
External capsule
Frontopontine tract
Stria terminalis
Body of corpus callosum
Head of caudate nucleus
Anterior limb of internal capsule
Corticobulbar tracts
Corticospinal tracts
Thalamocortical tracts
Posterior limb of internal capsule
Parietopontine tracts
Thalamus
Fornix
Lateral ventricle
5 mm

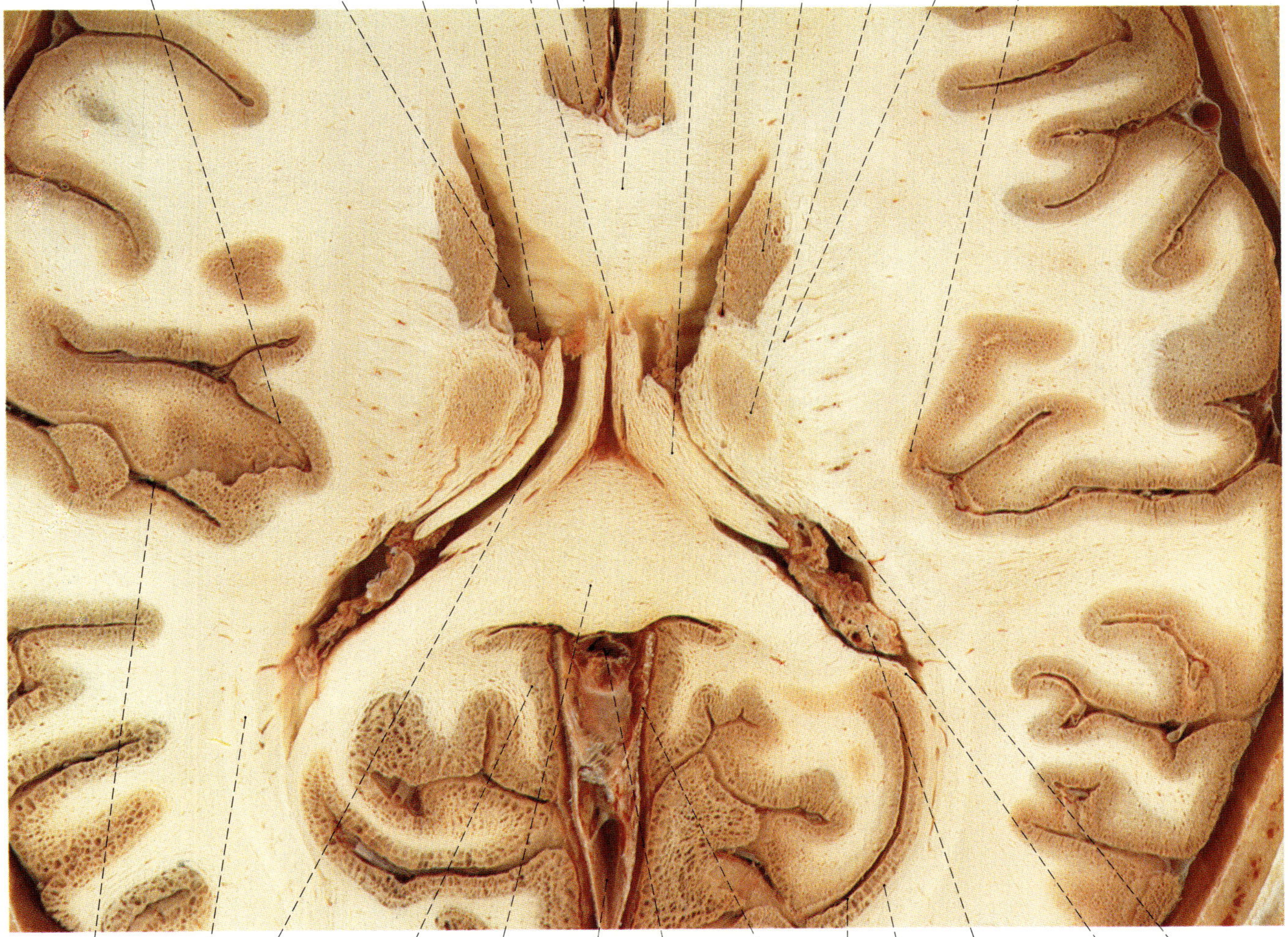

Viewed from Below

The corpus callosum, a large commissural fiber bundle, forms the superior boundary of the lateral ventricles and interconnects the neocortical areas of the two hemispheres. The internal capsule is the major concentration of fibers between the cerebral cortex and more inferior regions of the brain and spinal cord. The nuclear bridges between the caudate nucleus and putamen intersected by the bundles forming the anterior limb of the internal capsule are the basis of the term "striatum". The fornices interrelate the temporal lobe hippocampi with the septal (parolfactory) areas and the hypothalamus.

The ascending tracts of the internal capsule are intermingled with and intersected by other sensory pathways and by motor fiber systems. The descending corticobulbar and corticospinal systems are likewise intimately associated with sensory systems and with other cortico-striatal and cortico-thalamic paths.

Mid Thalamus

Patient CT Scan

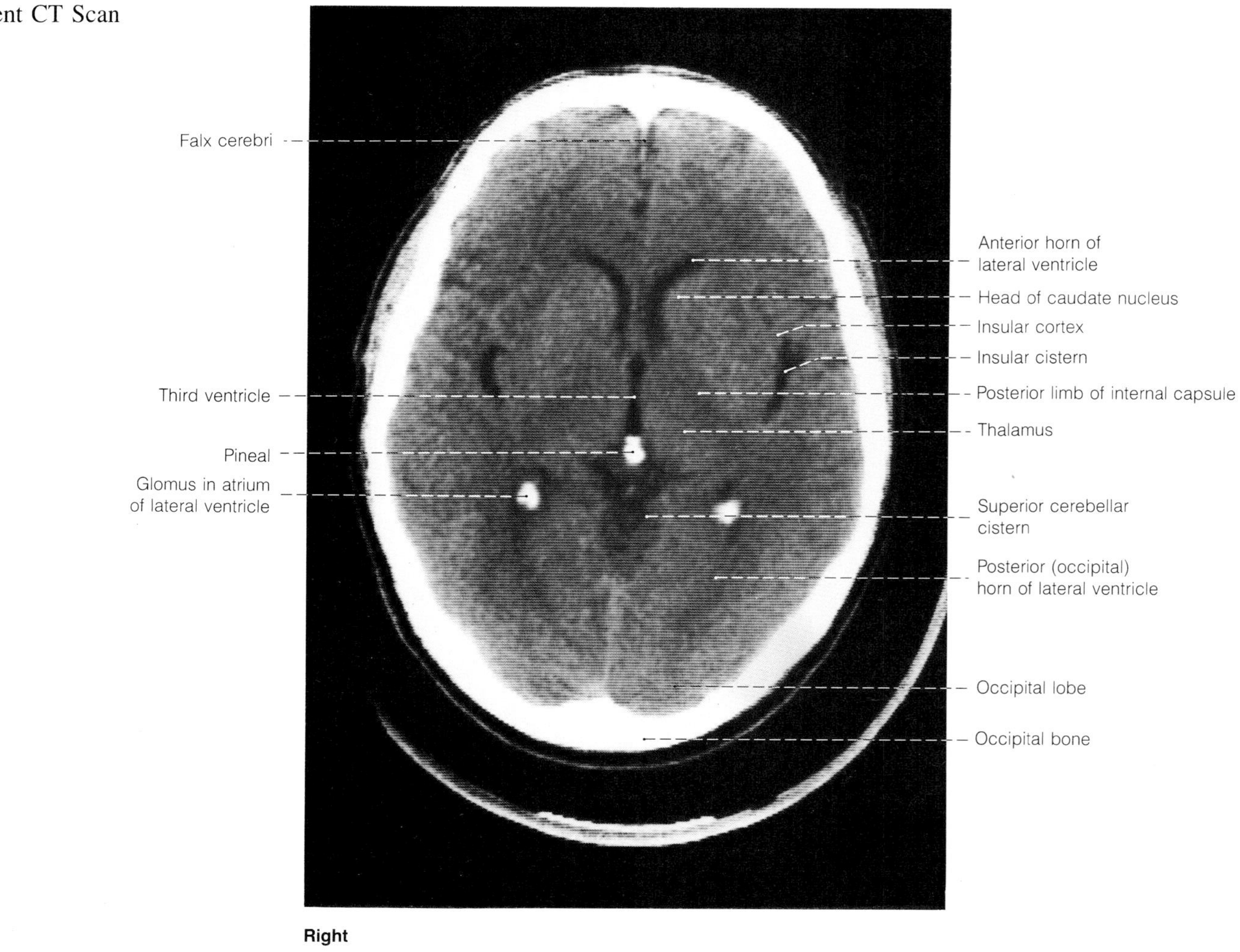

Patient MRI Scan

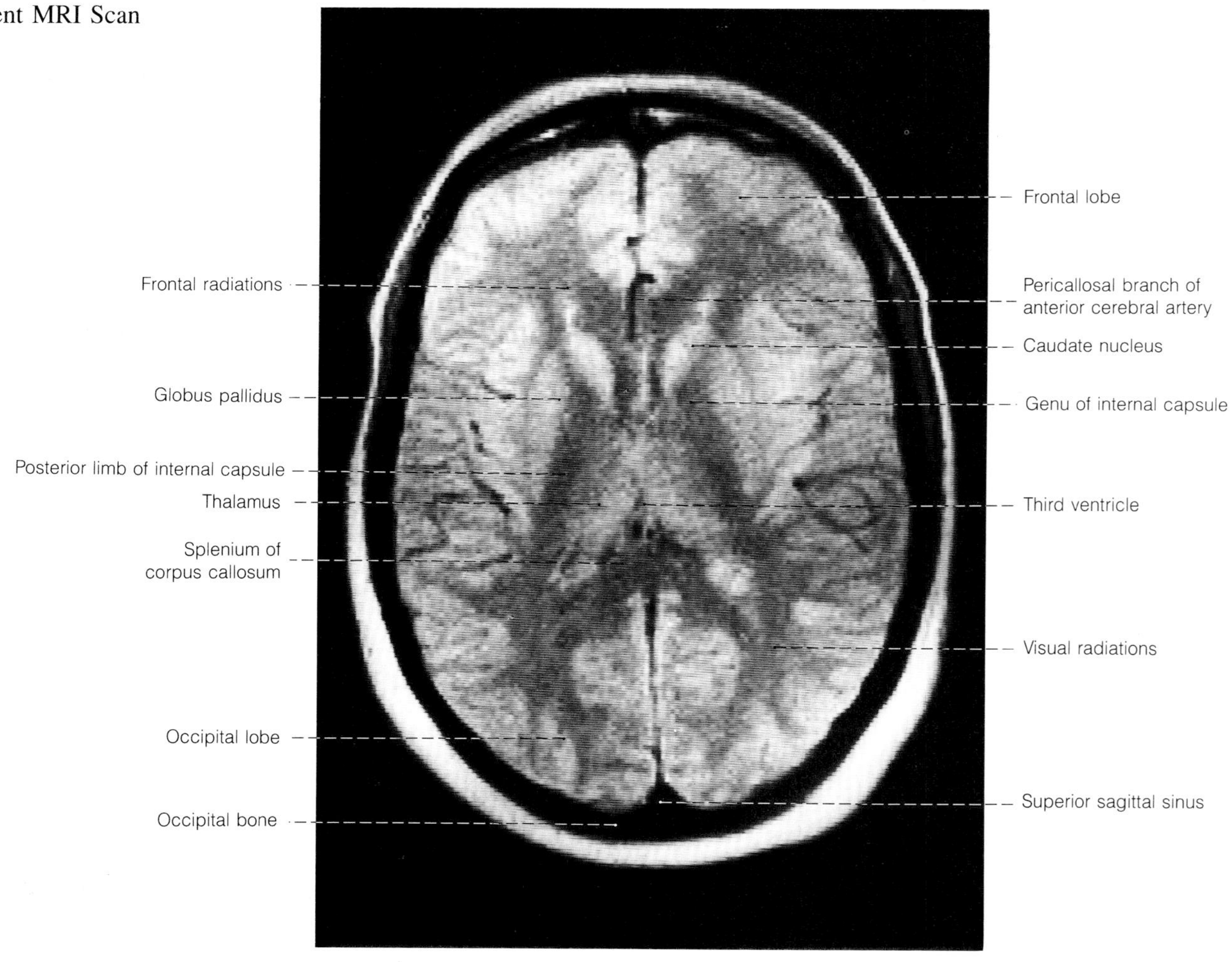

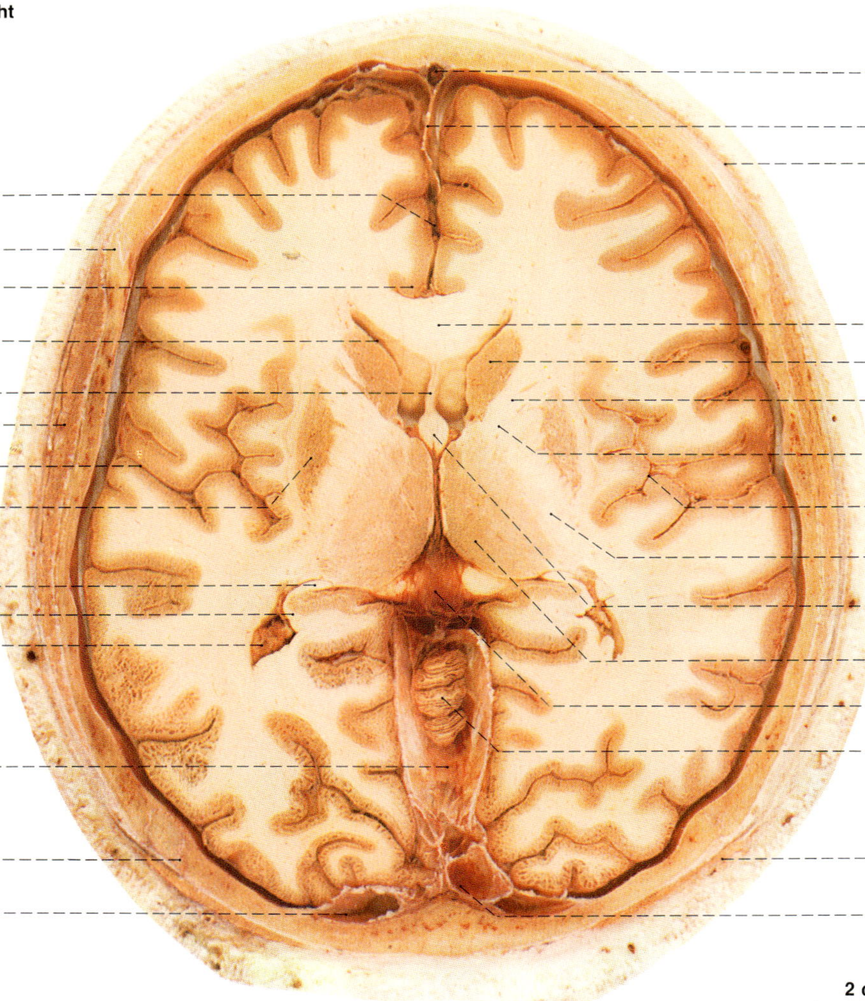

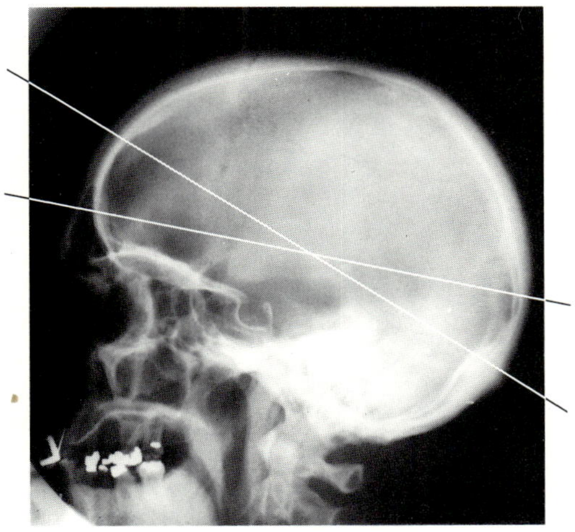

Planes of Sections

The CT, MRI and gross anatomical cuts pass directly through the main body of the thalamic nuclei, showing how the third ventricle exists as a cleft between the two. This is usually quite narrow as illustrated in the MRI scan and in the gross specimen, but may be enlarged as in the CT image in older individuals with some brain atrophy. The more horizontal plane of the MRI passes through the splenium of the corpus callosum and the inferior frontal lobe.

Internal capsule fibers (posterior limb) are aggregated lateral to the thalamus. The anterior limb and genu are bordered on their lateral aspect by the most superior portion of the putamen, external capsule and claustrum. Extremely well demonstrated on the gross specimen are the cut surfaces of the anterior columns of the fornix, and more of the anterior body of the corpus callosum. Branches of the anterior cerebral arteries, the pericallosals, may be noted on the gross specimen and MRI anterior to the corpus callosum running superiorly in close approximation to each other.

With the excellent MRI differentiation of the cellular thalamus and lenticular nucleus from the axons forming the internal capsule, it is possible to locate the interventricular foramen of Monro, anterior commissure, anterior columns of the fornix, genu of the internal capsule, and globus pallidus which are all anatomically contiguous.

The posterior limb of the internal capsule, made up of the thick myelinated corticospinal tract nerve fibers has a decidedly different intensity than surrounding grey matter nuclei, a difference which is felt to be due to relative water content and not to fat content in the myelin. (Note the myelinated fibers are less intense with this pulse sequence.)

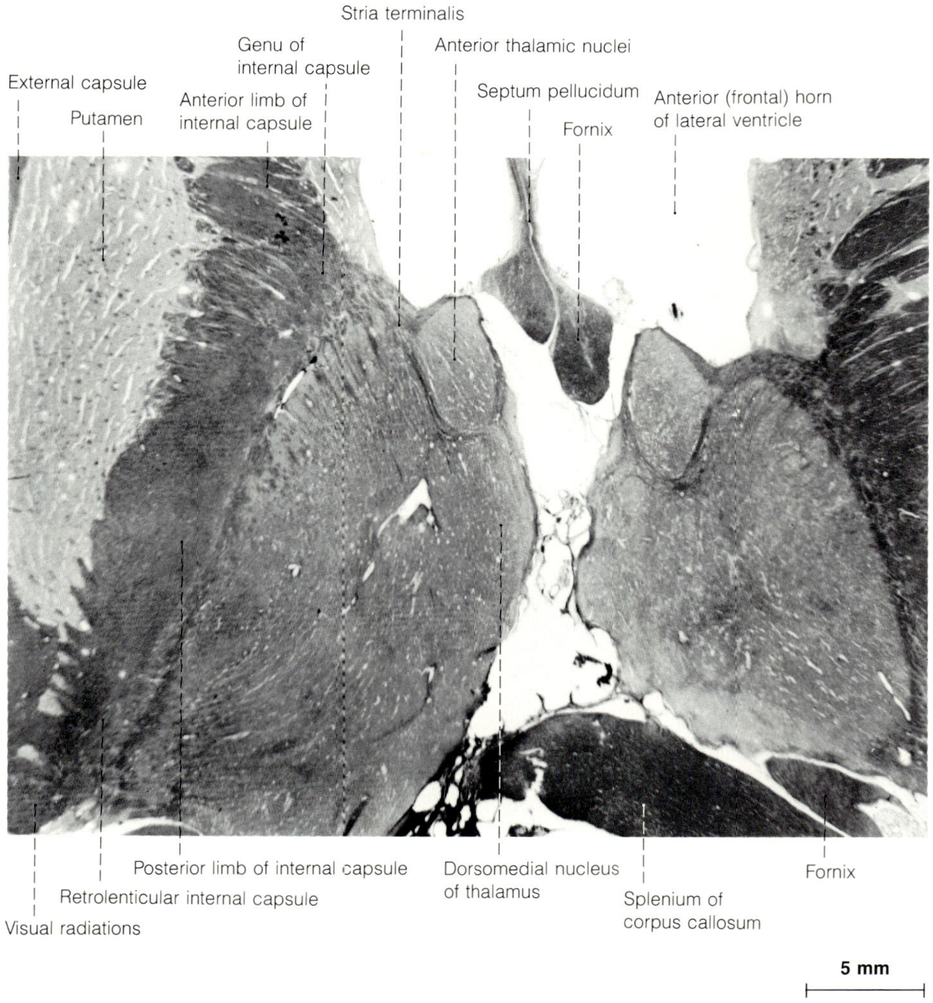
Stria terminalis
Genu of internal capsule
Anterior thalamic nuclei
External capsule
Septum pellucidum
Anterior (frontal) horn of lateral ventricle
Putamen
Anterior limb of internal capsule
Fornix
Posterior limb of internal capsule
Dorsomedial nucleus of thalamus
Fornix
Retrolenticular internal capsule
Splenium of corpus callosum
Visual radiations
5 mm

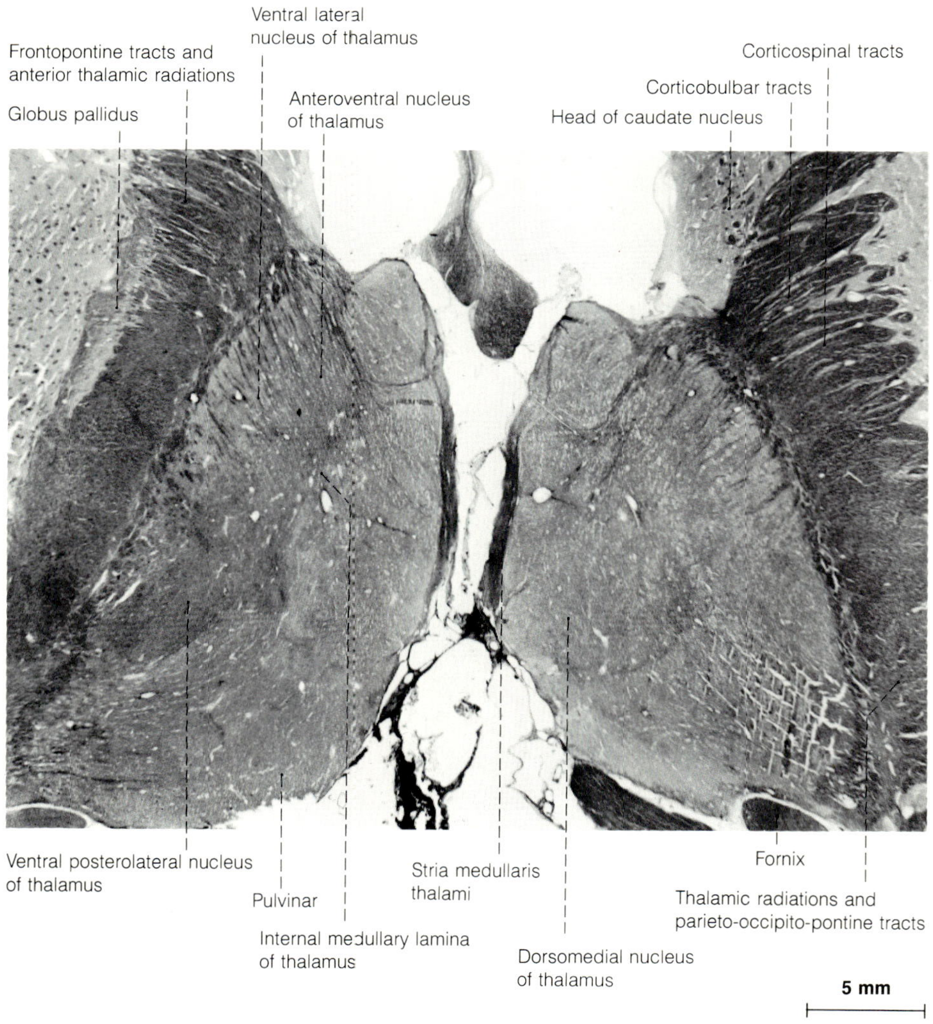
Ventral lateral nucleus of thalamus
Frontopontine tracts and anterior thalamic radiations
Corticospinal tracts
Anteroventral nucleus of thalamus
Corticobulbar tracts
Globus pallidus
Head of caudate nucleus
Ventral posterolateral nucleus of thalamus
Stria medullaris thalami
Fornix
Pulvinar
Thalamic radiations and parieto-occipito-pontine tracts
Internal medullary lamina of thalamus
Dorsomedial nucleus of thalamus
5 mm

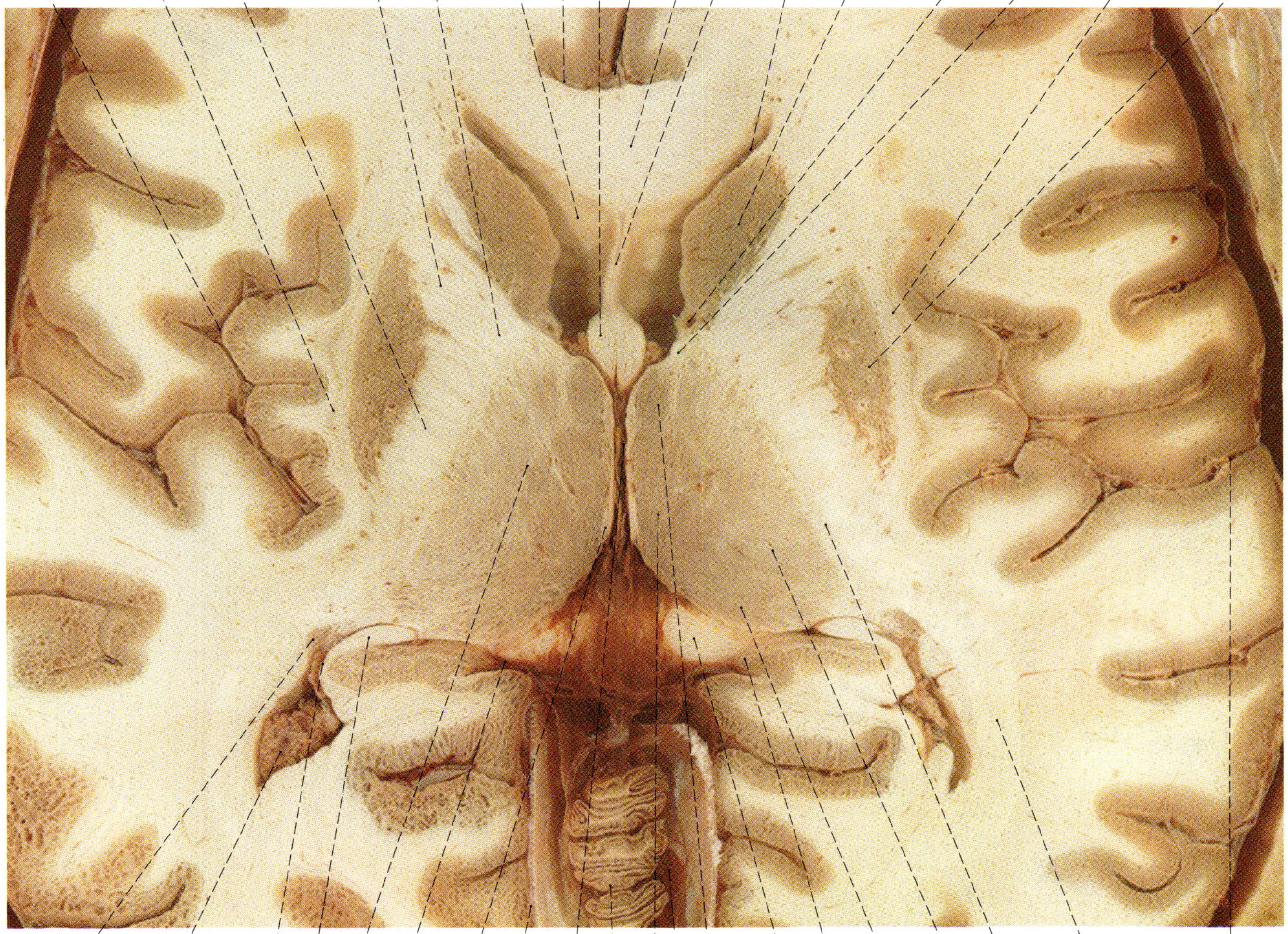

The nuclei of the dorsal thalamus, medial to the posterior limb of the internal capsule, are primarily involved in relaying ascending information to the cerebral cortex. These nuclei also receive fibers from designated cortical areas and develop in conjunction with the cortex.

The anterior nuclei are interconnected with the cingulate and adjacent cortex; the dorsomedial nucleus projects to and receives from the frontal (prefrontal) areas; the lateral nuclei are especially involved in the sensory paths to the postcentral and adjacent cortex; and the pulvinar is intimately interrelated with posterior parietal and occipital areas.

The stria medullaris is a phylogenetically old tract. It projects from numerous rhinencephalic areas to the habenular nuclei but its function in man is obscure.

Patient CT Scan

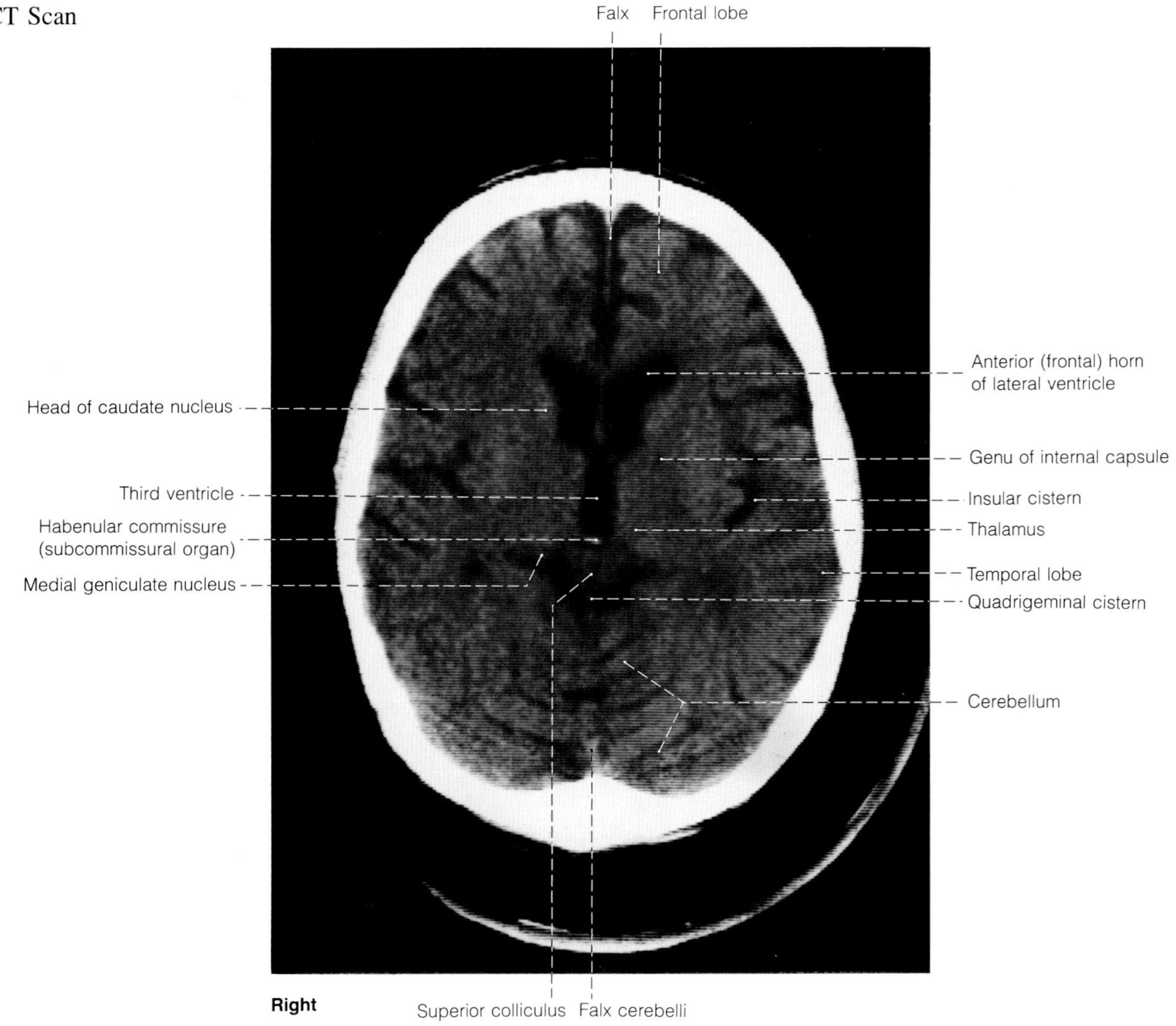

Patient MRI Scan

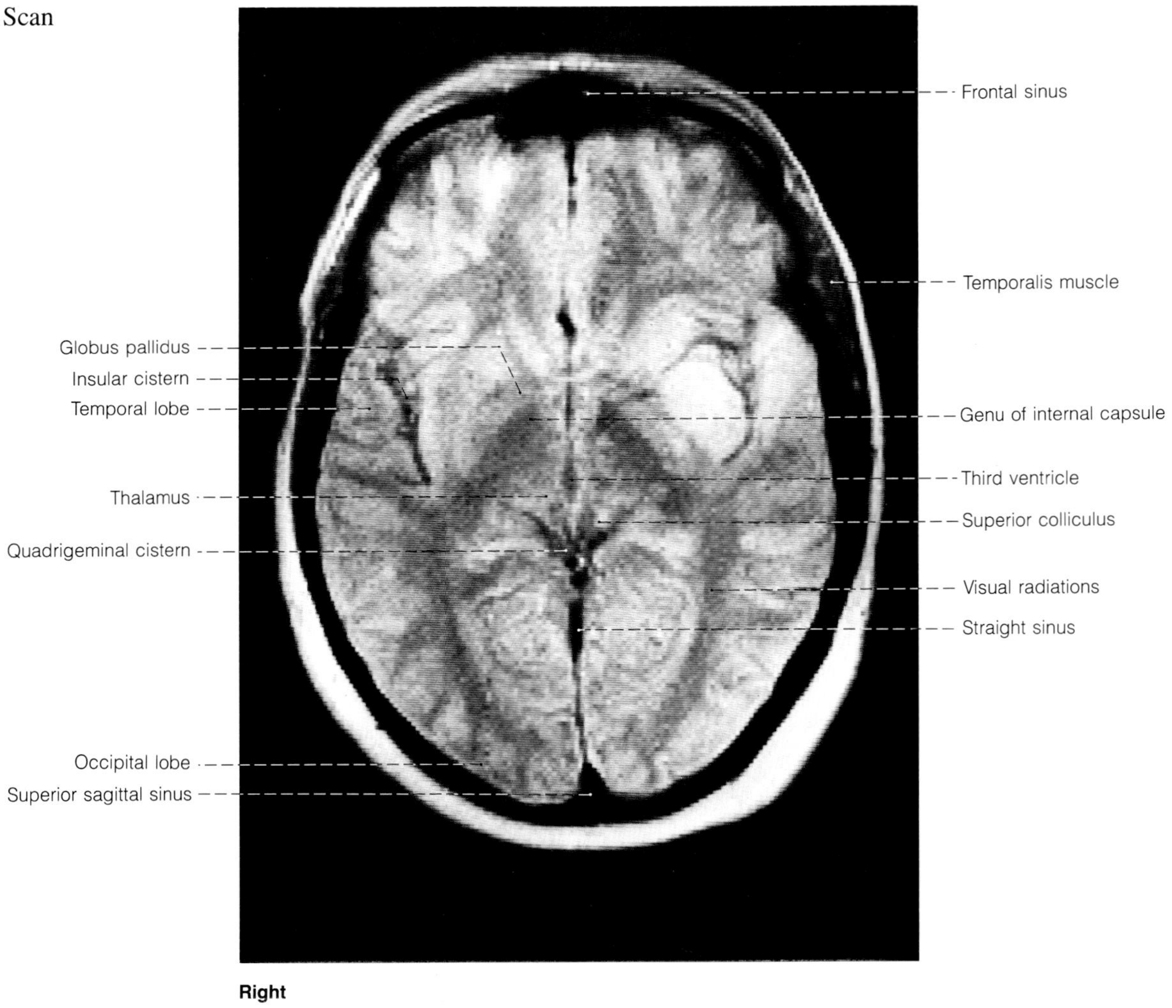

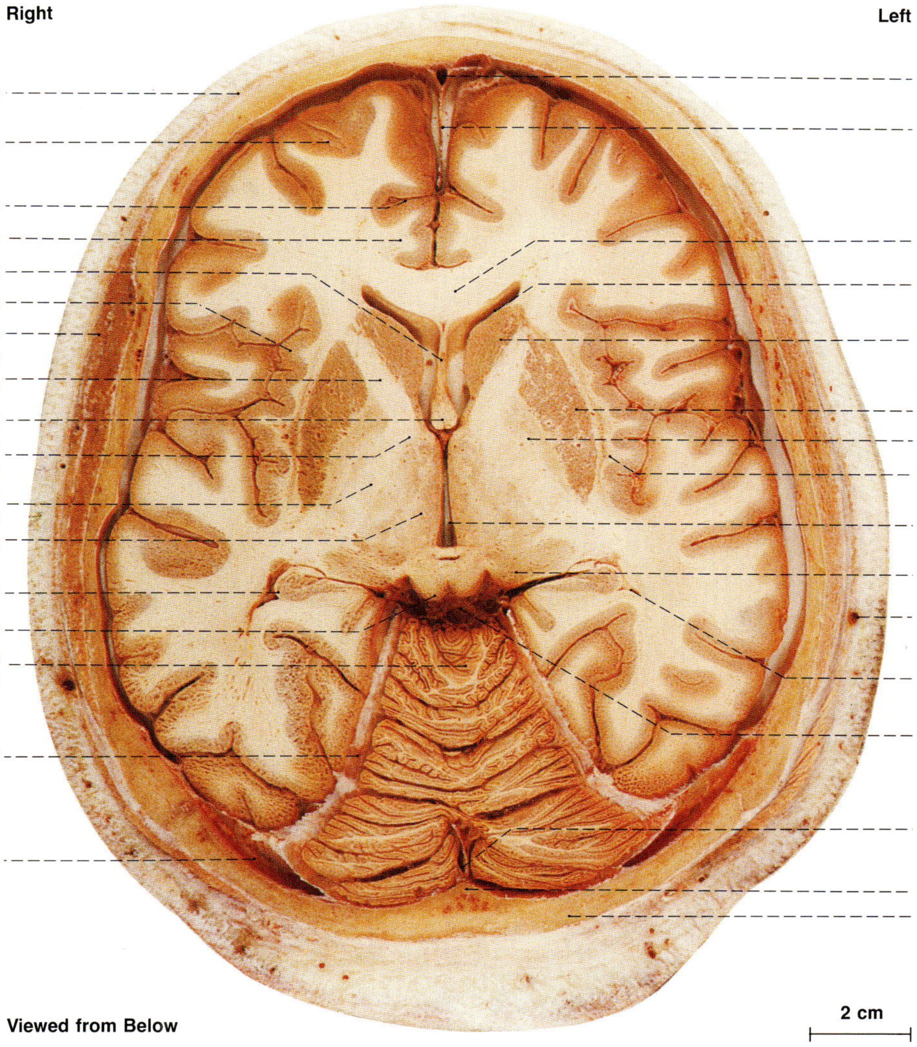

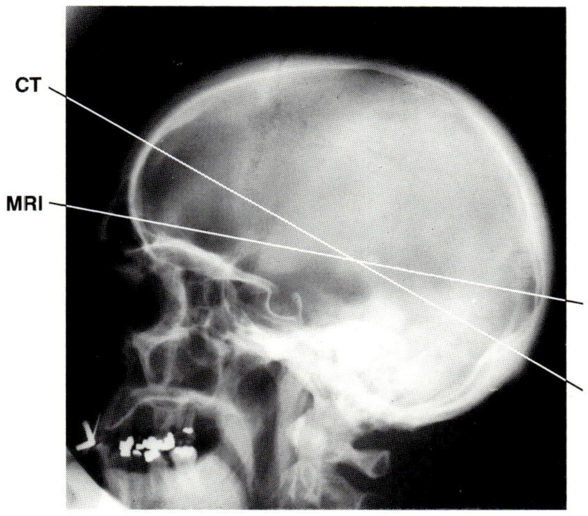

Planes of Sections

The gross anatomical and CT slice show more of the cerebellar structures, but the plane of the MRI section passes through the apex of the tentorium. The two well-defined bulges of the superior colliculi can be seen and their relationship to the medial geniculate nuclei appreciated on CT and gross studies. The dorsal thalamic nuclei are becoming less prominent but the CT plane now includes more of the globus pallidus medial to the putamen. These structures are well demonstrated due to differences in coloration in the gross specimen, but are better demonstrated on histologic stained sections (page 28). The lateral (Sylvian) fissure and insular cortex medial to it are useful landmarks for the middle cerebral artery and the lenticular nucleus.

An interesting feature posteriorly is the transverse cerebral fissure which leads from the quadrigeminal plate cistern toward the lateral horn of the ventricular system and through which may run the vessels supplying choroid of the lateral ventricles, e.g., the postero-lateral choroidal arteries from the basilar circulation. The fimbria and hippocampus are present at the posterio-lateral aspect of the transverse cerebral fissure.

Also well demonstrated at this level in the CT plane is the interventricular foramen of Monro, the sole communication of the lateral ventricles with the third ventricle through which large amounts of CSF must flow at all times.

The ventricular system on the gross and CT studies is more generous than that in the more nearly normal MRI scan. Grey and white matter differences continue to be better seen on the MRI.

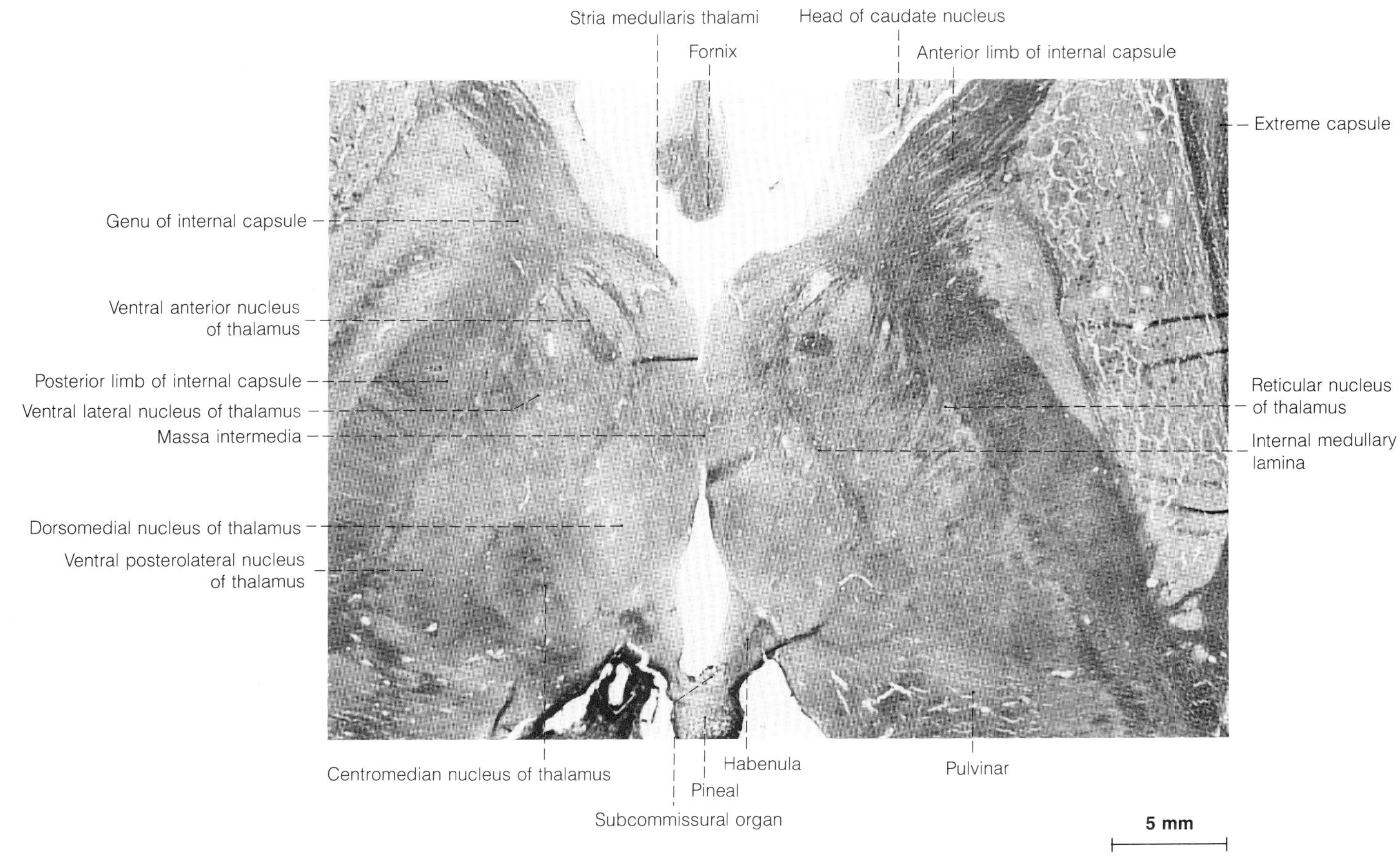
Stria medullaris thalami
Head of caudate nucleus
Fornix
Anterior limb of internal capsule
Extreme capsule
Genu of internal capsule
Ventral anterior nucleus of thalamus
Posterior limb of internal capsule
Ventral lateral nucleus of thalamus
Massa intermedia
Reticular nucleus of thalamus
Internal medullary lamina
Dorsomedial nucleus of thalamus
Ventral posterolateral nucleus of thalamus
Centromedian nucleus of thalamus
Habenula
Pineal
Subcommissural organ
Pulvinar
5 mm

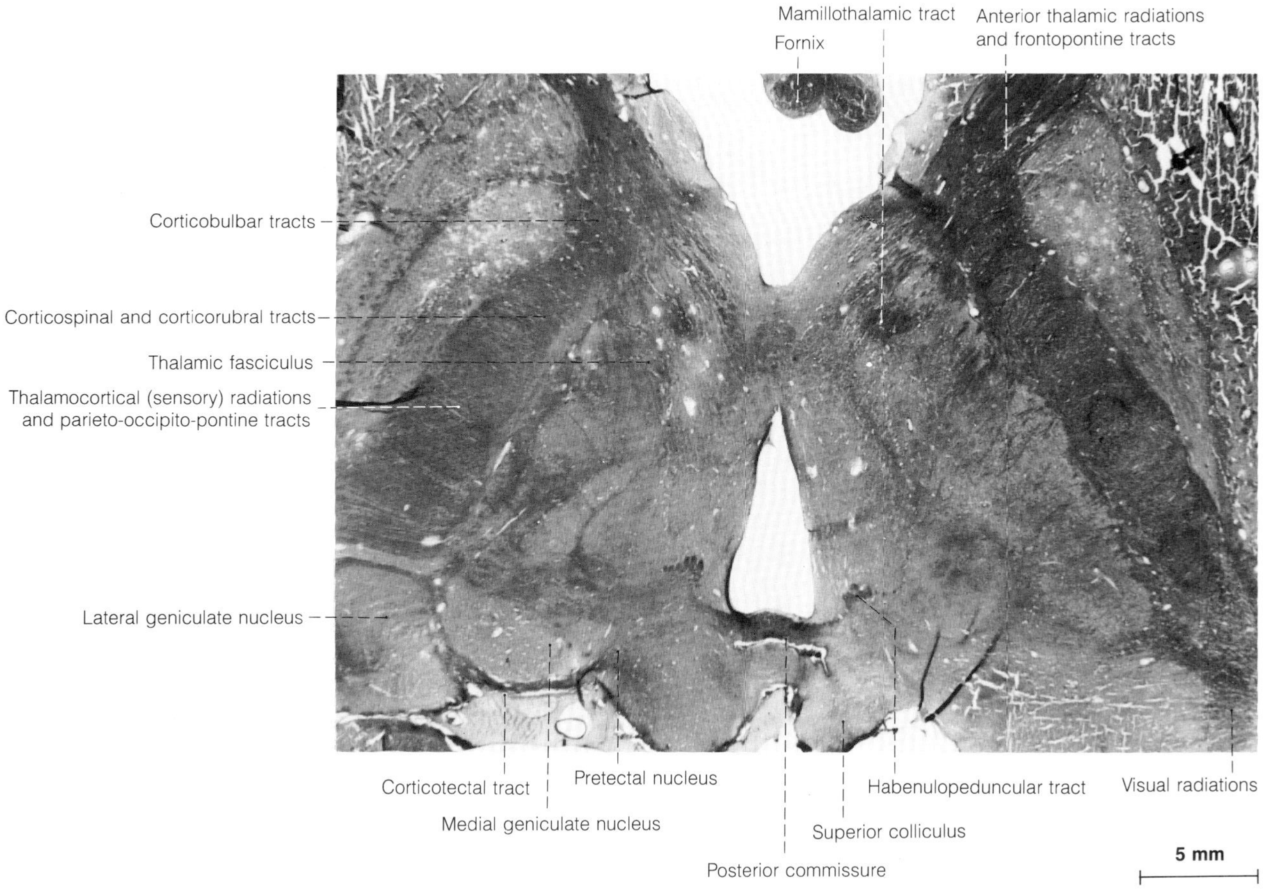
Mamillothalamic tract
Fornix
Anterior thalamic radiations and frontopontine tracts
Corticobulbar tracts
Corticospinal and corticorubral tracts
Thalamic fasciculus
Thalamocortical (sensory) radiations and parieto-occipito-pontine tracts
Lateral geniculate nucleus
Corticotectal tract
Pretectal nucleus
Medial geniculate nucleus
Habenulopeduncular tract
Visual radiations
Superior colliculus
Posterior commissure
5 mm

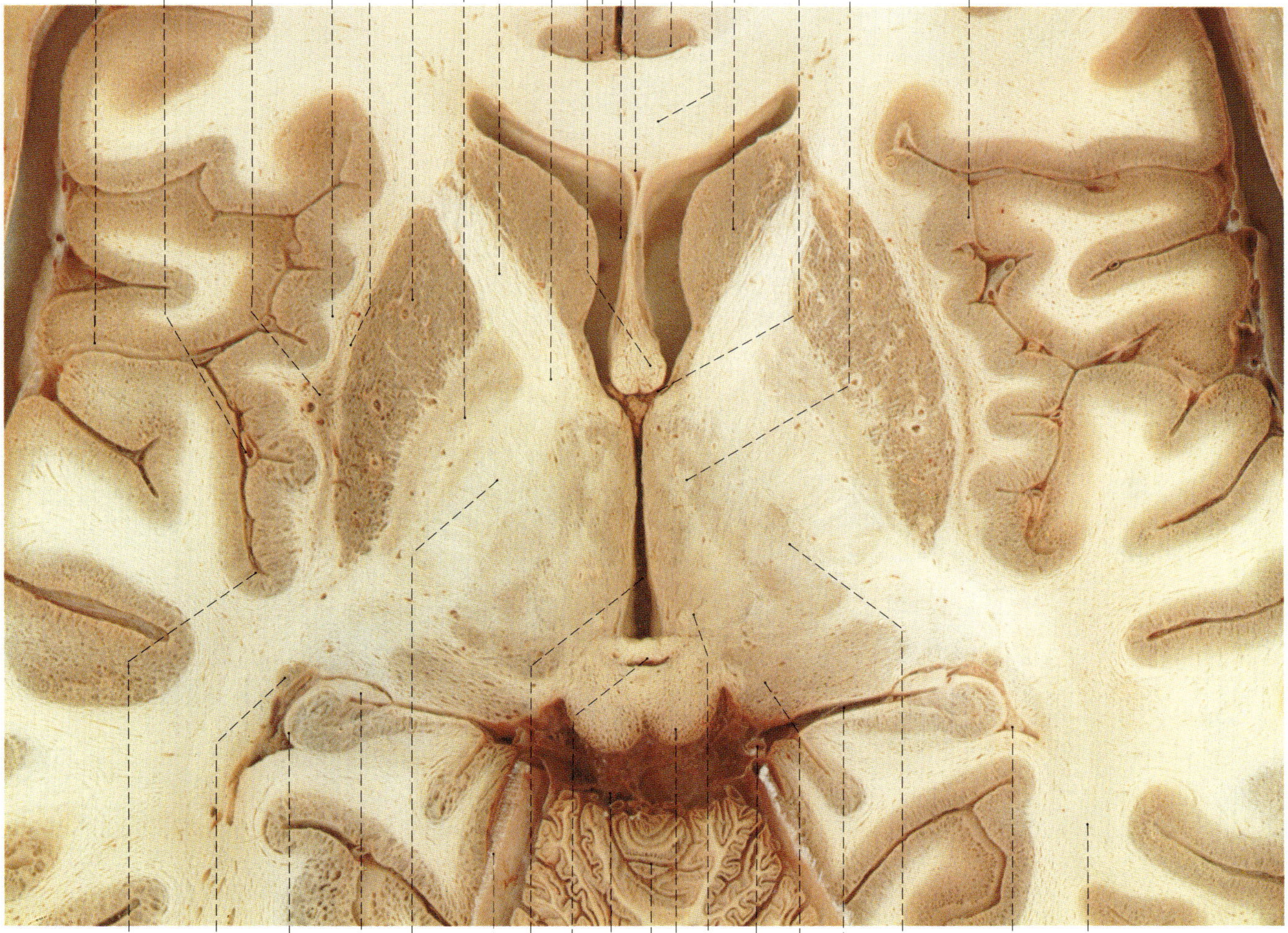

The posterior commissure and habenulopeduncular tracts serve as anatomical boundaries between the diencephalon and mesencephalon. A single CT or MRI section through this region will include both the diencephalon and the mesencephalon. The microscopic section also demonstrates the overlapping and the contiguity of these subdivisions of the brain.

The ependyma below the habenular commissure is modified into the subcommissural organ. It may become calcified in older individuals and appear in unenhanced radiographs or CT displays.

The microscopic connections demonstrate the proximity of corticobulbar and corticospinal fibers to those thalamo-cortical interconnections in the genu and anterior limb of the internal capsule. Lesions in this area may cause not only profound motor symptoms but may also induce personality and behavioral disorders.

Patient CT Scan

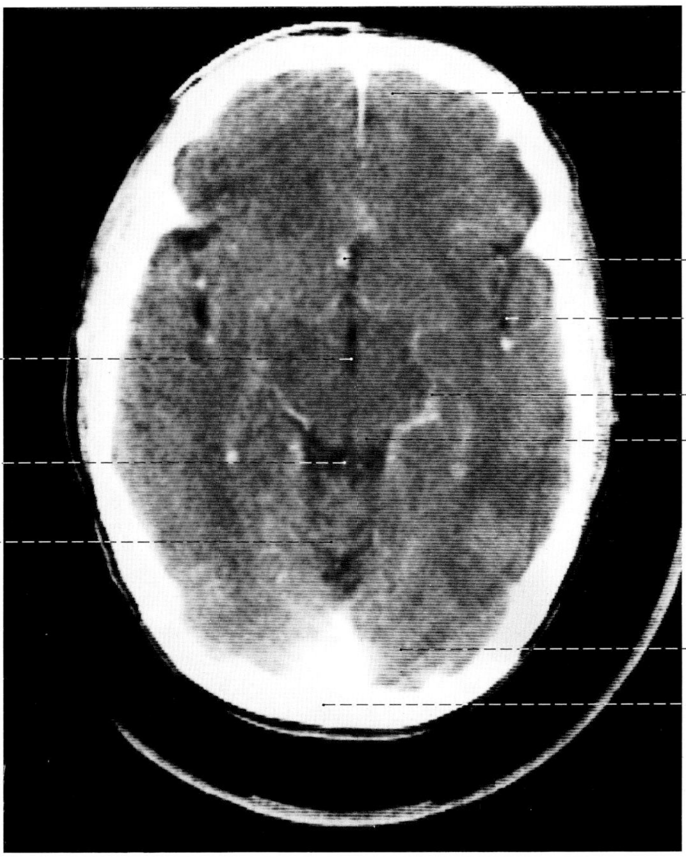

Right

Patient MRI Scan

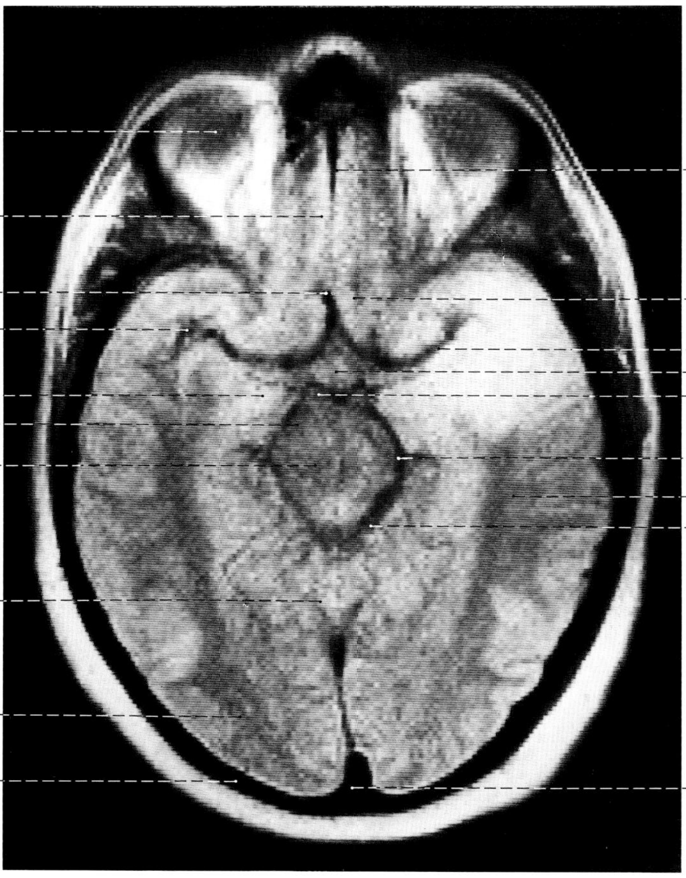

Right

In the CT scan and gross anatomical section there is excellent demonstration of the inferior aspect of the third ventricle. It lies just above the infundibular recess and is in the same plane as the cerebral aqueduct of Sylvius which is located more posteriorly. On the right side of the gross specimen there is a fortuitous demonstration of the anterior commissure. This clearly shows the temporal lobe origin of these crossing fibers and the post-commissural fornix, both located just anterior to the interventricular foramen. The more horizontal angle of the MRI display passes through the pentagonal cistern immediately below the hypothalamus. Some hypothalamic tissue may be present in the anterior part of the cistern.

In the brainstem several important nuclei may be present on the MRI, notably the red nucleus and the substantia nigra between the

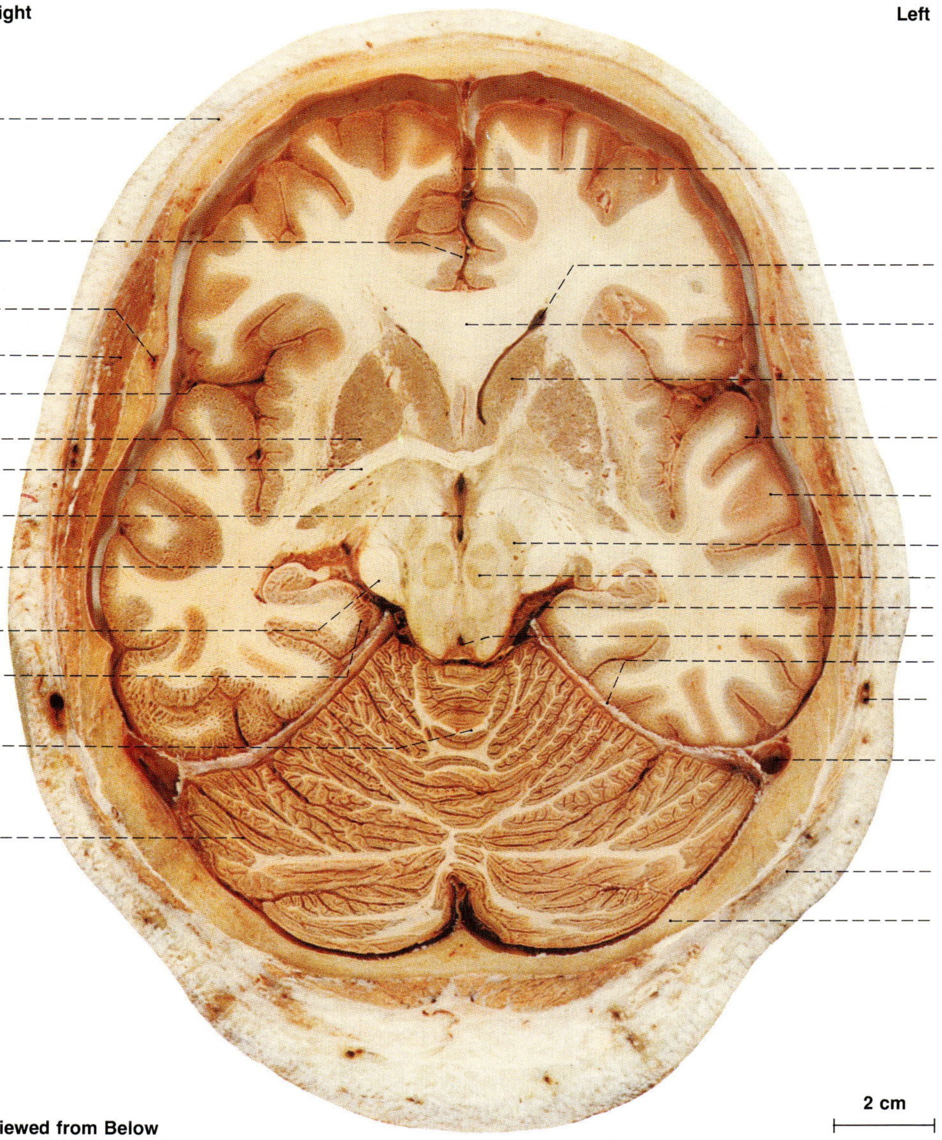

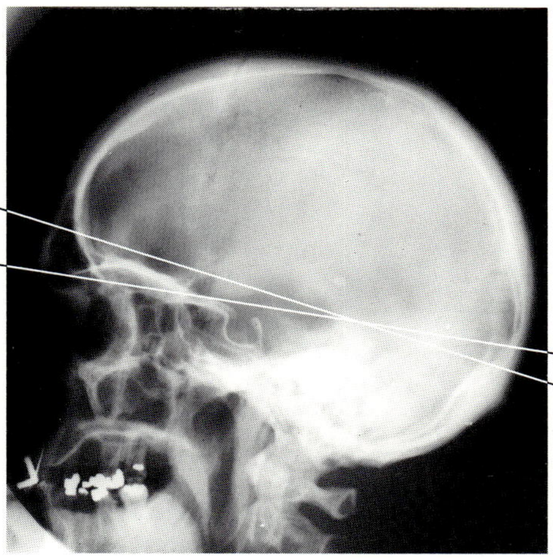

Planes of Sections

cerebral peduncle and brachium conjunctivum. Dorsal to these are the inferior colliculi appearing on both the CT and MRI displays. Fibers of the corticospinal tract in the middle of the cerebral peduncles pass into and out of the plane of the slice.

The MRI scan appears to demonstrate the various nuclei deep within the brainstem to a better advantage than CT, probably because of the close proximity of multiple different structures of grey or white matter. Fiber tracts running perpendicularly through the slice should afford excellent contrast to the scattered small nuclei which will have differing hydrogen content. Thus, nuclear areas such as the colliculi are seen to have a brighter signal than fiber pathways immediately ventral to them. The bright signal in the left temporal lobe is a glioblastoma.

Anteriorly, on the gross specimen the genu or anterior portion of the curved corpus callosum has been reached. The slit in the posterior portion of the callosal fibers surrounded by gray matter is actually outside the brain and is the interhemispheric fissure in the parolfactory area. Another interesting feature laterally in the gross specimen is the demonstration of the middle meningeal artery closely adherent to the inner table of the skull near the squamosal suture. This shows the manner in which the artery runs within the dura and makes a groove in the inner table of the skull. This location is minimally variable, showing the posterior branch of the middle meningeal artery at the level of the lateral fissure of Sylvius.

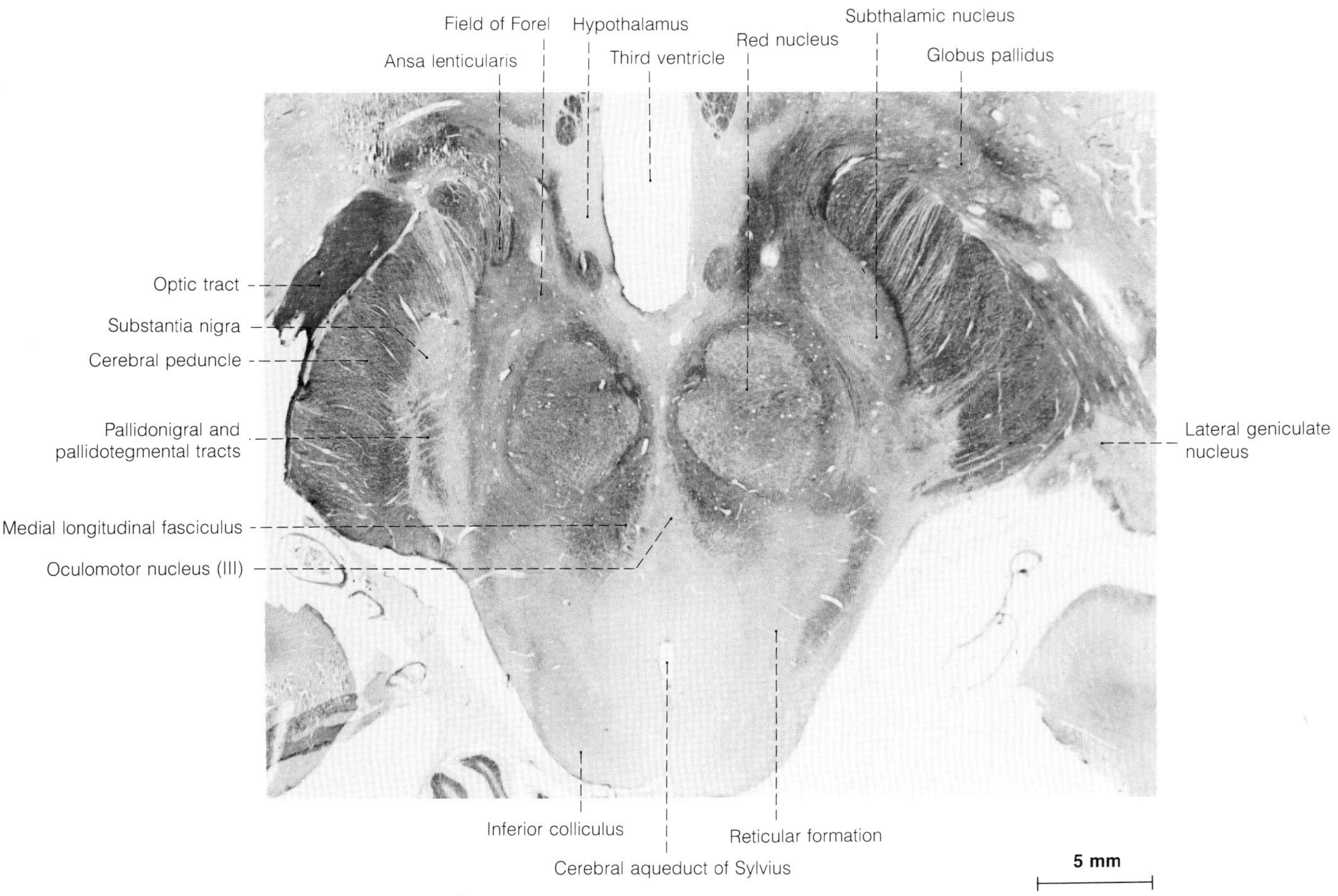
Field of Forel
Hypothalamus
Subthalamic nucleus
Red nucleus
Ansa lenticularis
Third ventricle
Globus pallidus
Optic tract
Substantia nigra
Cerebral peduncle
Pallidonigral and pallidotegmental tracts
Lateral geniculate nucleus
Medial longitudinal fasciculus
Oculomotor nucleus (III)
Inferior colliculus
Reticular formation
Cerebral aqueduct of Sylvius
5 mm

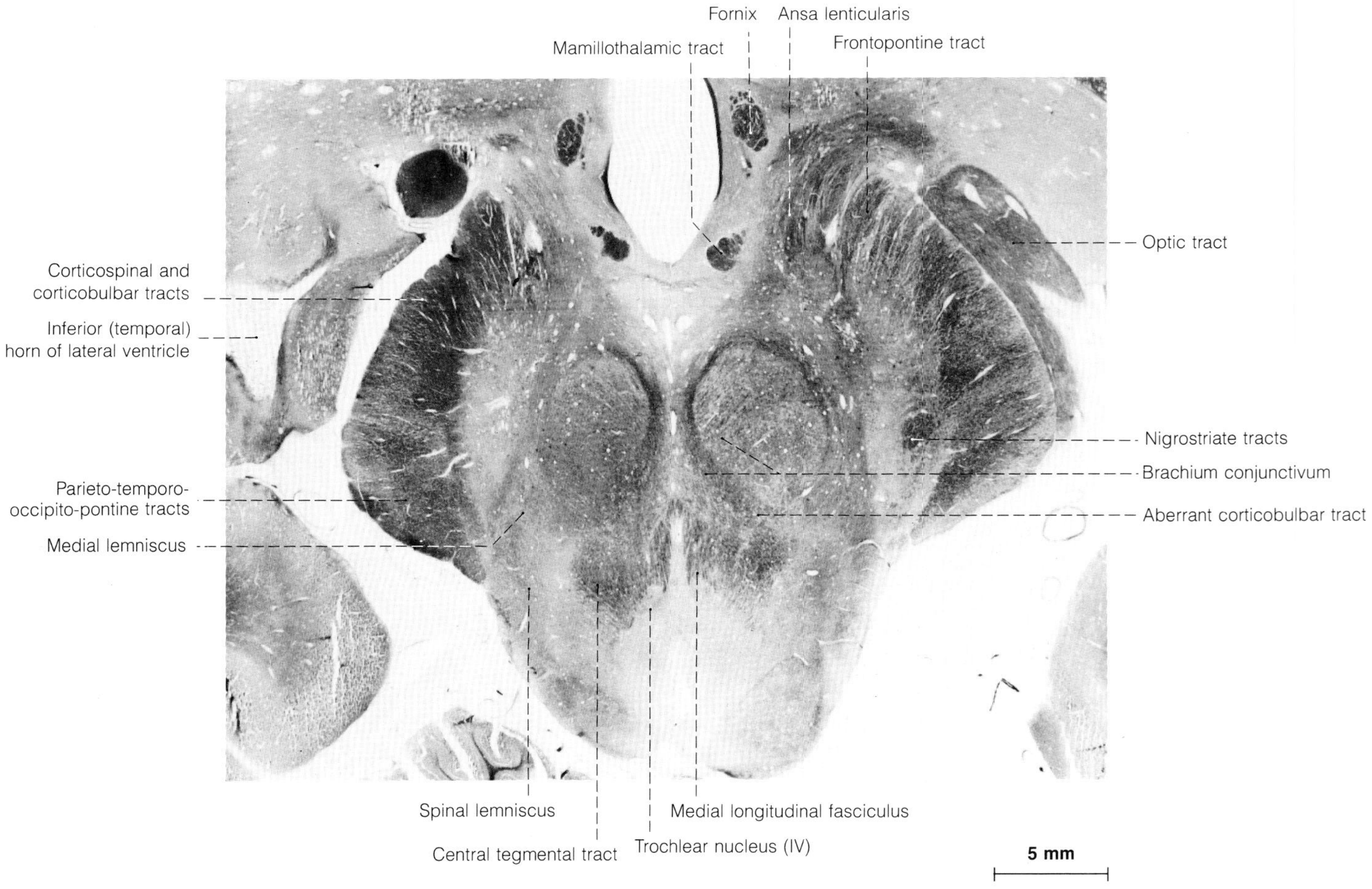
Fornix
Ansa lenticularis
Mamillothalamic tract
Frontopontine tract
Optic tract
Corticospinal and corticobulbar tracts
Inferior (temporal) horn of lateral ventricle
Nigrostriate tracts
Brachium conjunctivum
Parieto-temporo-occipito-pontine tracts
Aberrant corticobulbar tract
Medial lemniscus
Spinal lemniscus
Medial longitudinal fasciculus
Central tegmental tract
Trochlear nucleus (IV)
5 mm

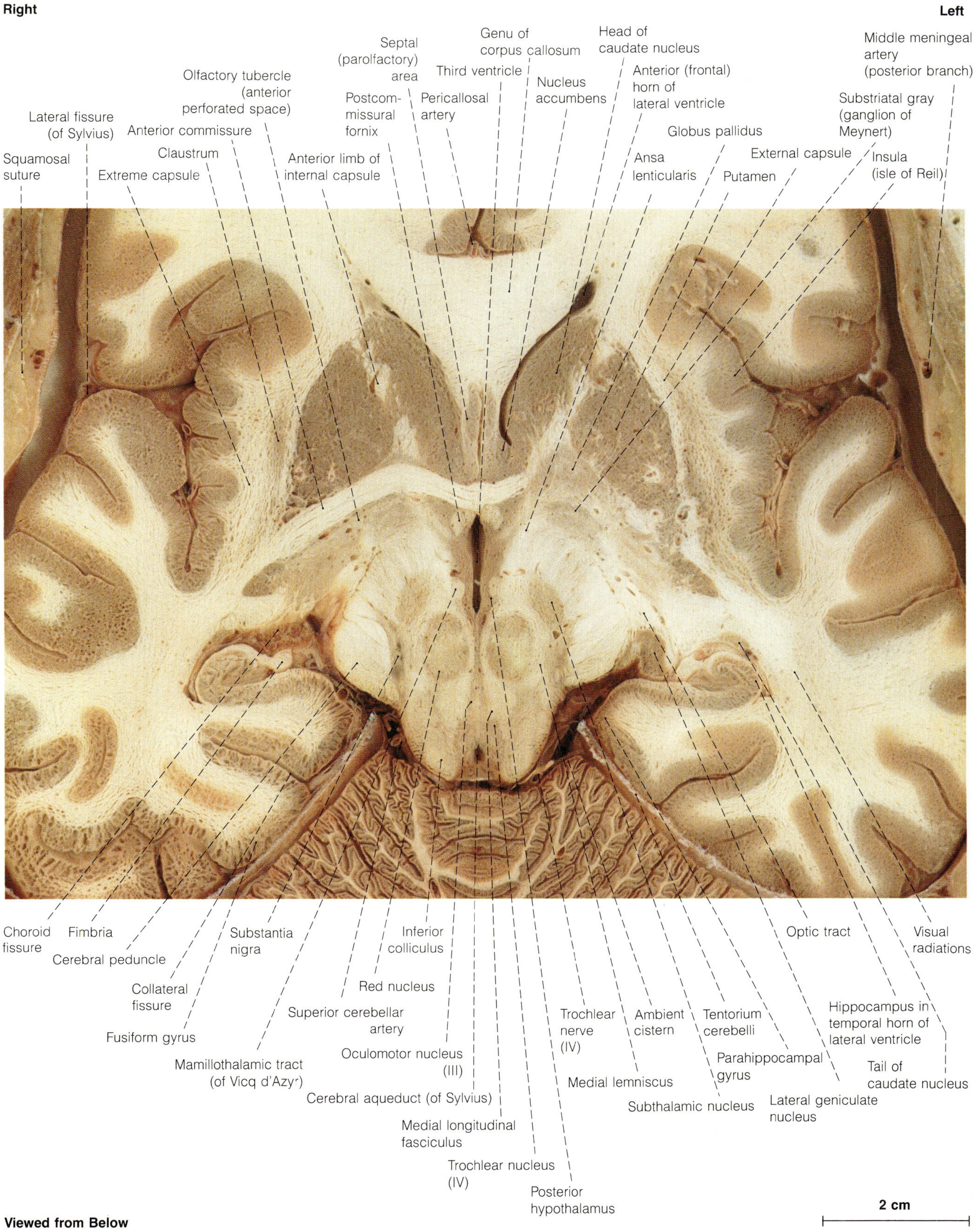

The continuity of the hypothalamus and ventral thalamus (subthalamic nucleus and field of Forel) with the tegmentum of the mesencephalon can be appreciated in these sections. Disturbances in visceral motor activity as well as the typical decerebrate posture and loss of consciousness associated with lesions in this region are easily explained.

The proximity of the optic tracts to the ansa lenticularis as the tracts course lateral to the cerebral peduncles and medial to the hippocampal formation is evident in both the gross and microscopic preparations. Medially, within the tegmentum of the mesencephalon, the brachium conjunctivum surrounds and penetrates the red nucleus. Cerebellar impulses traversing the brachium conjunctivum are interrelated here with descending striatal pathways in the ansa lenticularis.

Interpeduncular Cistern

Patient CT Scan

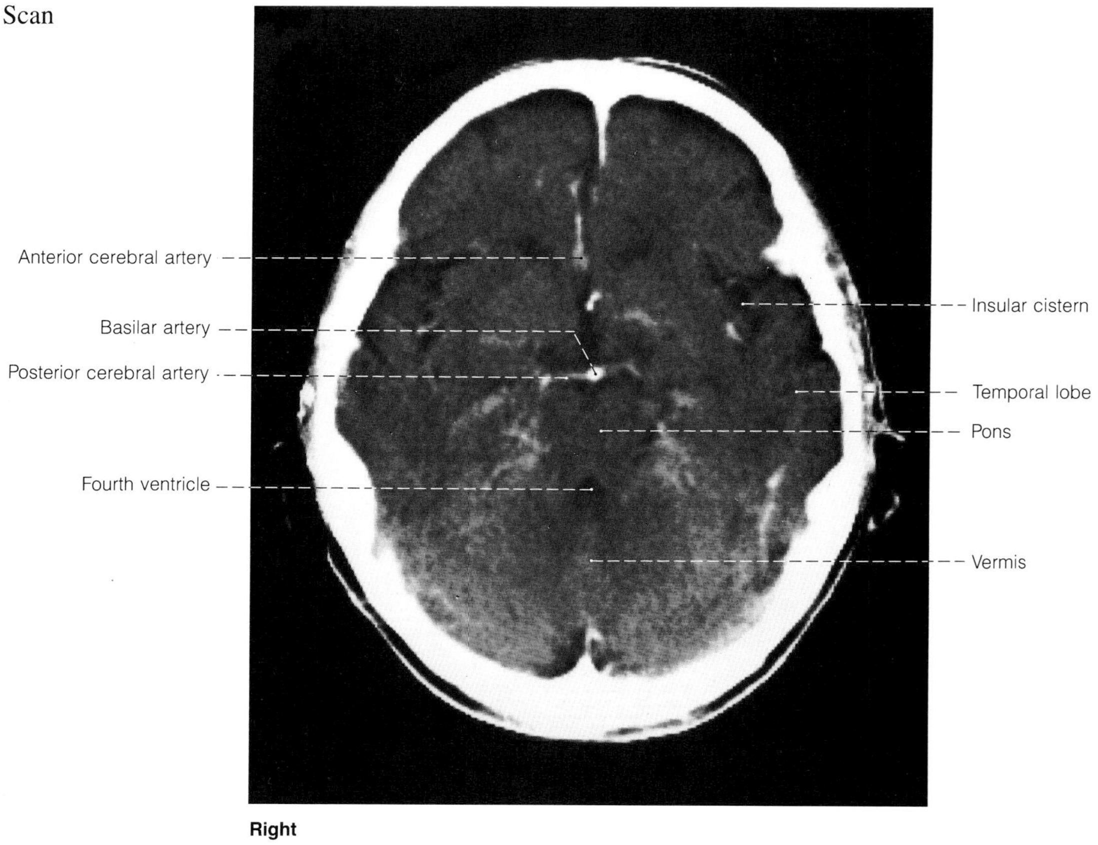

Patient MRI Scan

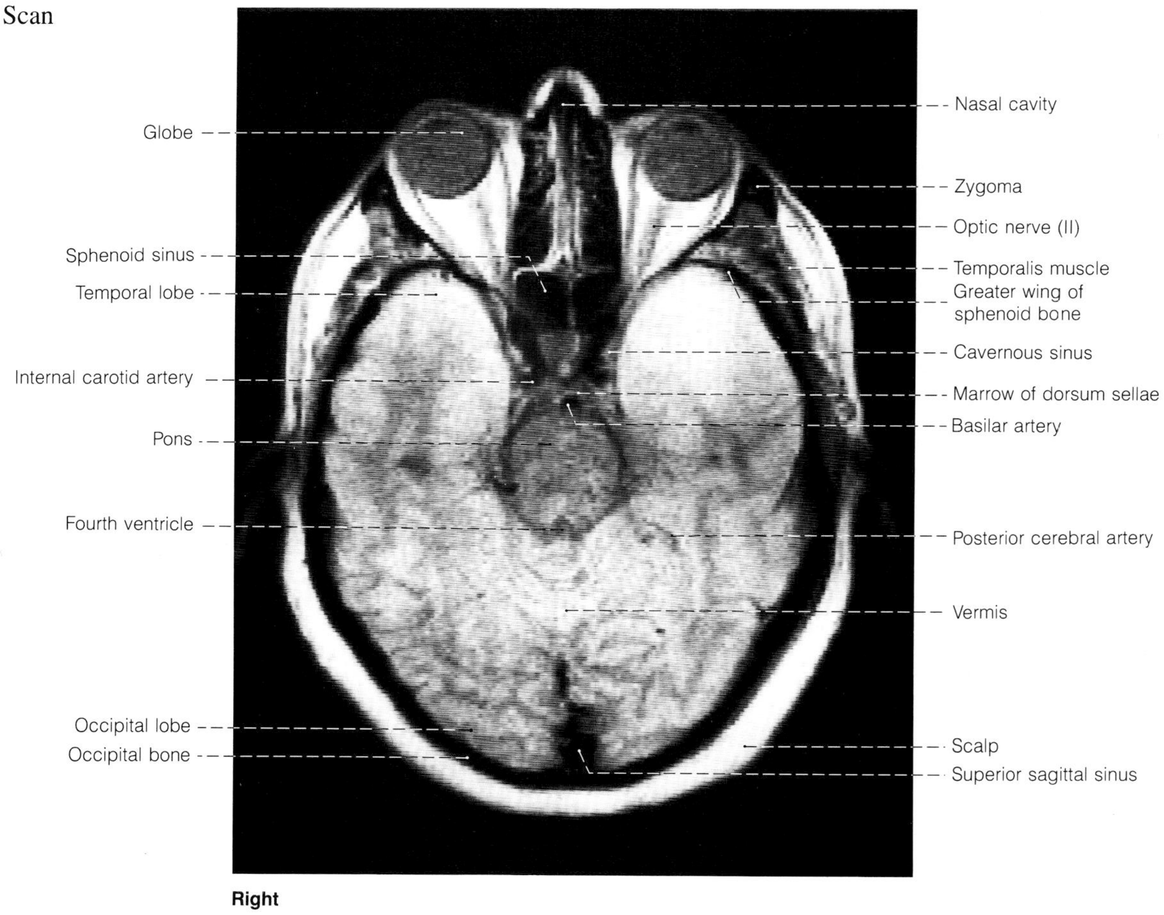

The cerebral peduncles are seen in the gross specimen to have emerged from within the substance of the brain and an interpeduncular cistern now exists between the two peduncles. Just anterior to these lie the mamillary bodies, paired nuclear aggregates, with the infundibular recess of the third ventricle just in front of them. The anterior extent of the caudate nucleus is just antero-lateral to the hypothalamus and the lamina terminalis forms the anterior limit of the third ventricle. Both the CT and MRI images pass through the lower mesencephalon and upper pons, but the difference in the plane illustrates the great differences in the anterior and posterior structures intersected.

The brachia conjunctiva (superior cerebellar peduncles) form prominent supero-lateral pontine extensions at this level, bordering the fourth ventricle bilaterally. Dorsomedial lies the nodulus of the cerebellum. Another interesting feature is the fourth cranial nerve (trochlear) seen traveling around the brainstem beneath the tentorium on the right side of the specimen.

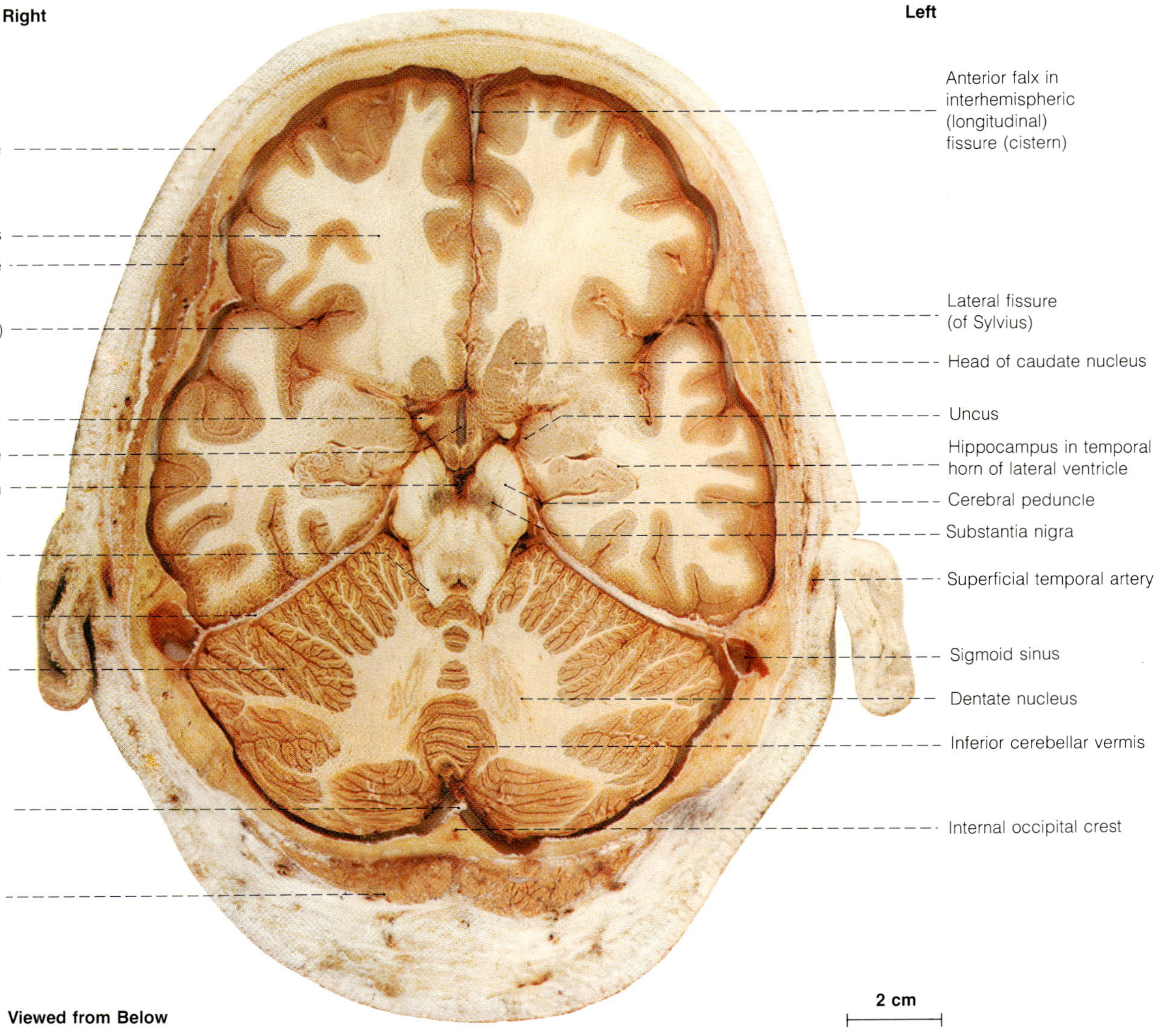

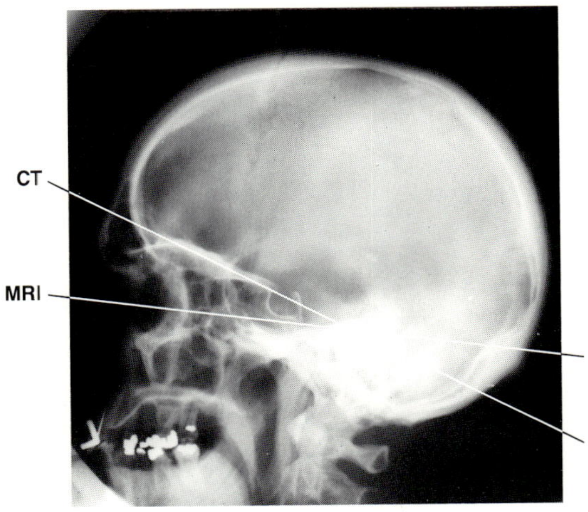

Planes of Sections

Laterally located structures include the sigmoid sinuses, enclosed in their dural envelopes, and generous portions of temporal and frontal lobes anteriorly and anterolaterally.

In the contrast enhanced CT, the basilar artery and posterior cerebral arteries are well demonstrated in white; in the MRI scan, even though taken at a different angle, the "black holes" indicating fastmoving blood (no signal) in the basilar and posterior cerebral arteries can be seen as well as two "black holes" representing the cavernous portions of the carotid arteries.

The brainstem is cut on both CT and MRI at approximately the same level, if not the same angle. Note how clearly the aqueduct appears on the MRI scan. Also of note on the MRI are the black areas representing the sphenoid and maxillary sinuses. Grey-white matter contrast continues to be high with this pulse sequence and is helpful in diagnosing and lateralizing pathological conditions.

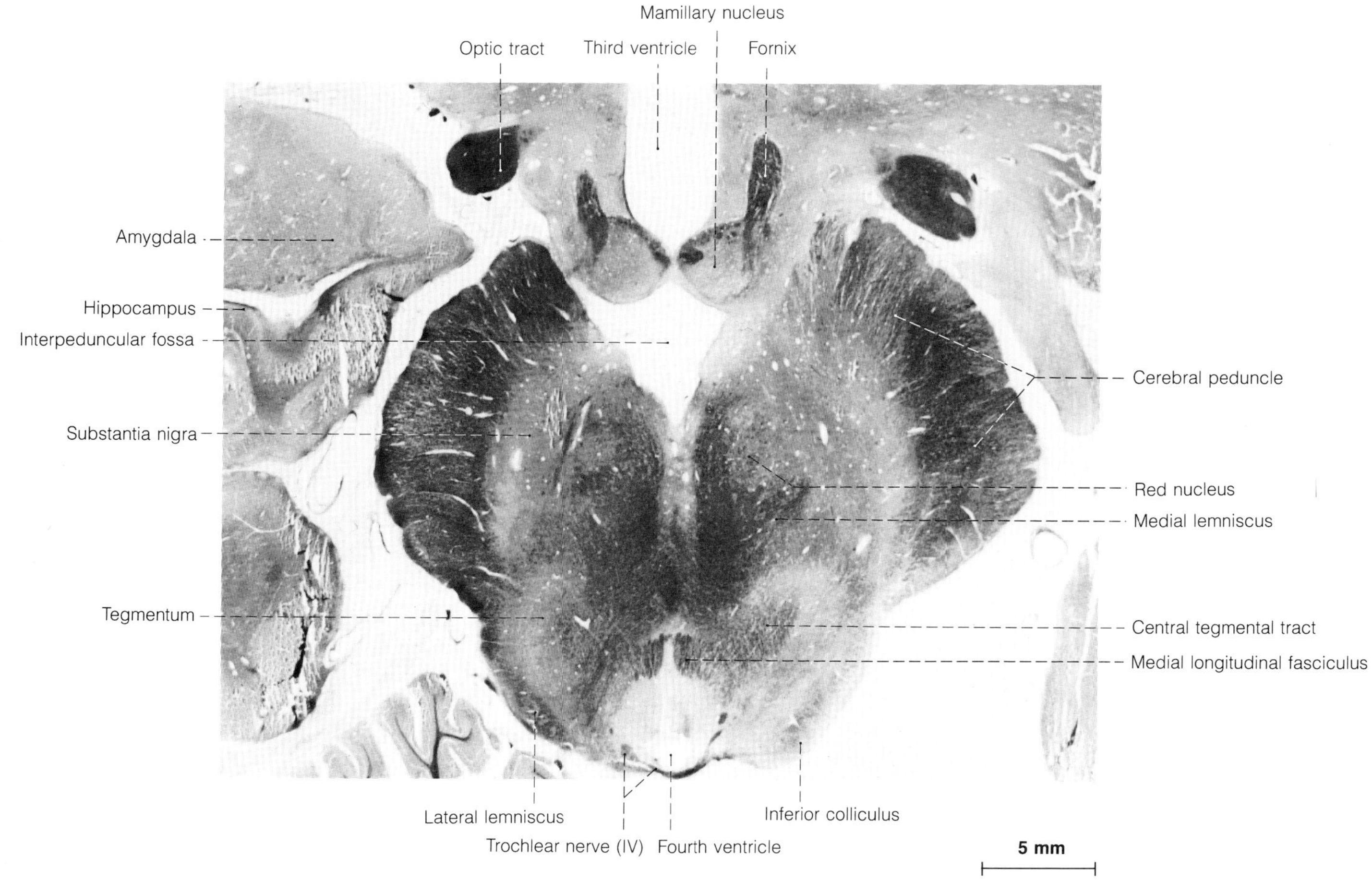
Mamillary nucleus
Optic tract
Third ventricle
Fornix
Amygdala
Hippocampus
Interpeduncular fossa
Substantia nigra
Tegmentum
Cerebral peduncle
Red nucleus
Medial lemniscus
Central tegmental tract
Medial longitudinal fasciculus
Lateral lemniscus
Inferior colliculus
Trochlear nerve (IV)
Fourth ventricle
5 mm

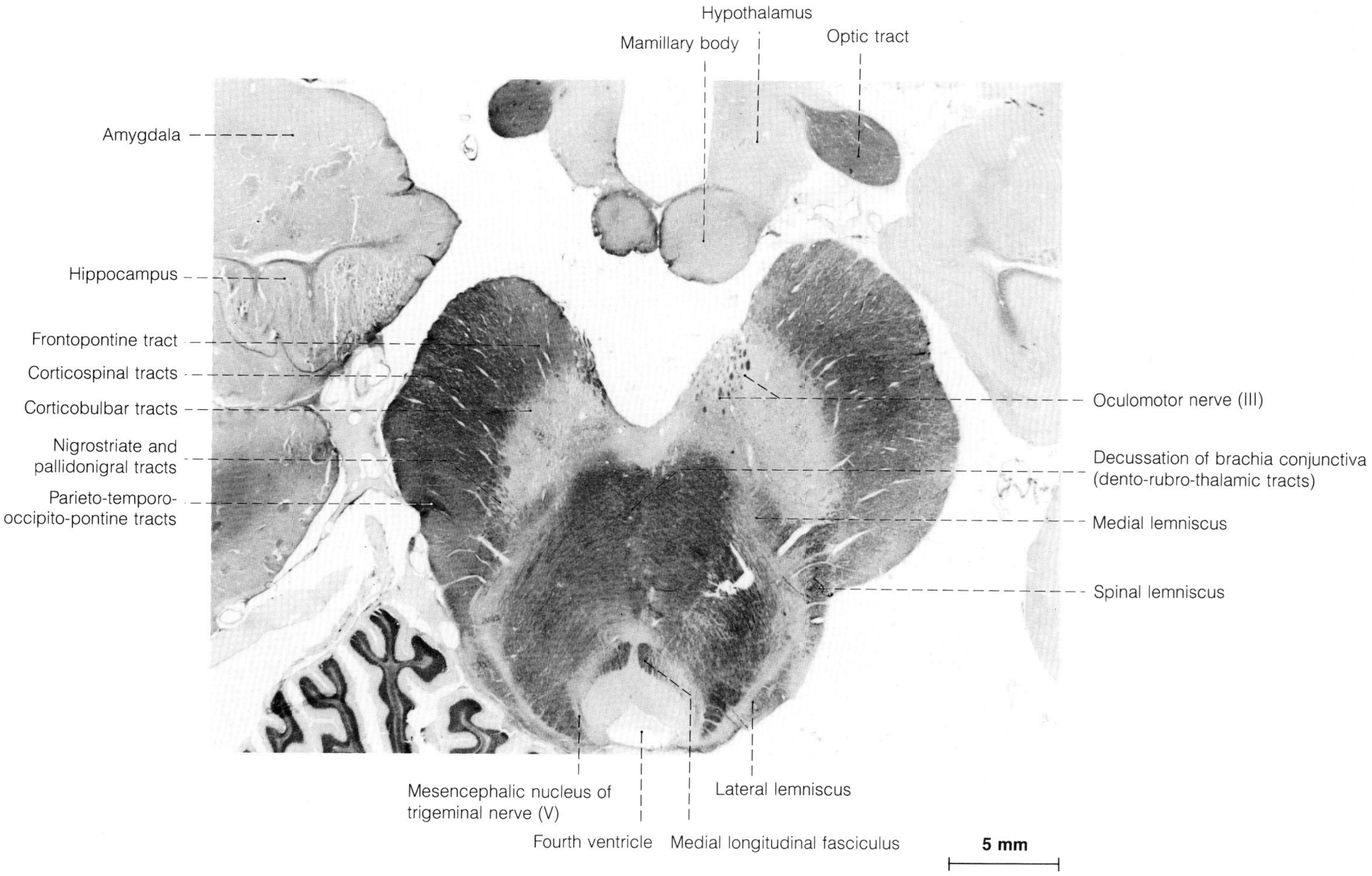
Hypothalamus
Mamillary body
Optic tract
Amygdala
Hippocampus
Frontopontine tract
Corticospinal tracts
Corticobulbar tracts
Nigrostriate and pallidonigral tracts
Parieto-temporo-occipito-pontine tracts
Oculomotor nerve (III)
Decussation of brachia conjunctiva (dento-rubro-thalamic tracts)
Medial lemniscus
Spinal lemniscus
Mesencephalic nucleus of trigeminal nerve (V)
Lateral lemniscus
Fourth ventricle
Medial longitudinal fasciculus
5 mm

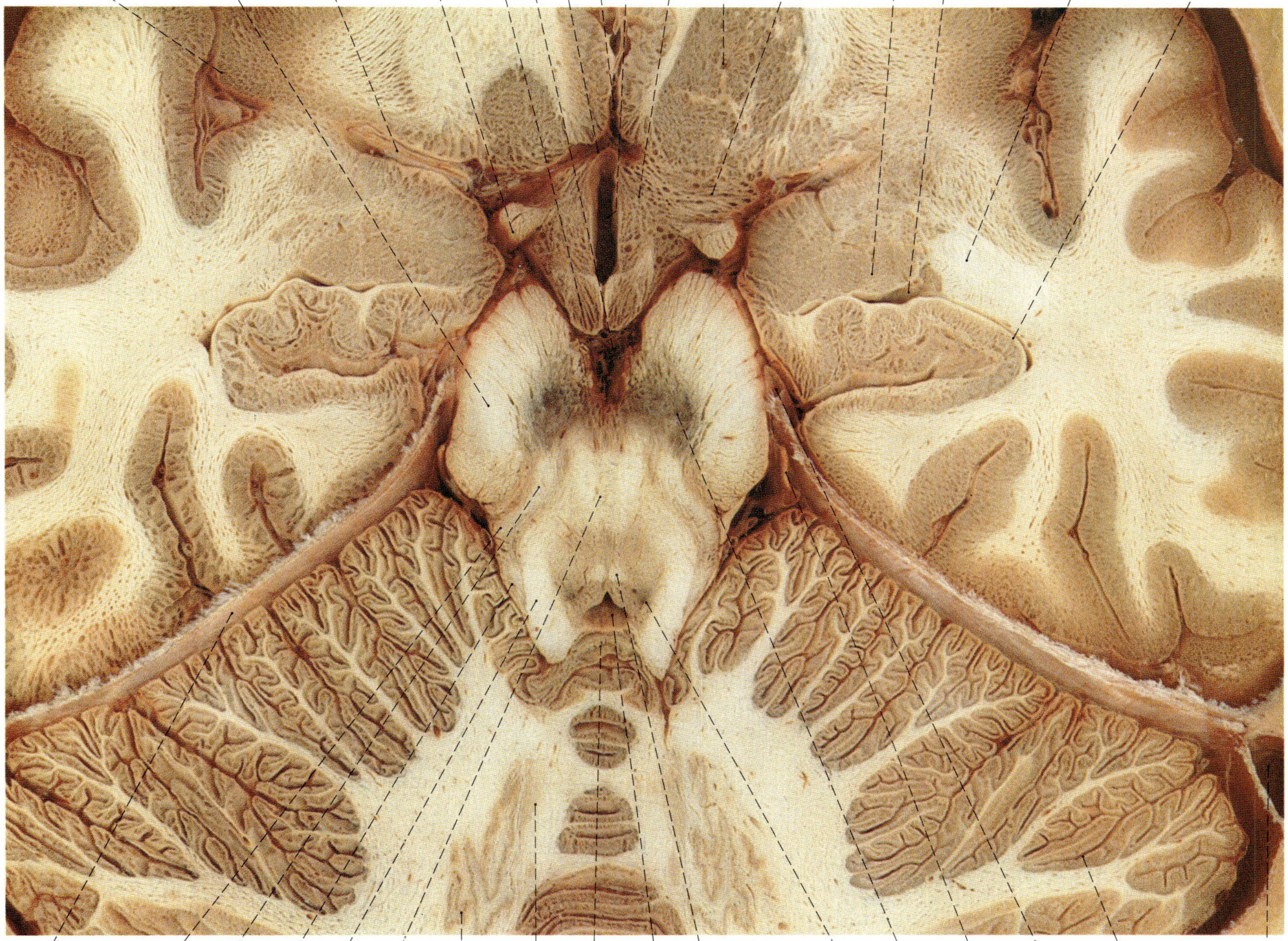

Sections near the inferior colliculus of the mesencephalon contain the decussating fibers of the brachium conjunctivum (superior cerebellar peduncle) as they project from the deep cerebellar nuclei (especially the dentate) to the red nucleus and thalamus of the opposite side. Since descending motor pathways also cross, cerebellar dysfunction is most prominent on the same side as a cerebellar lesion.

The amygdala indents the anterior margin of the inferior (temporal) horn of the lateral ventricle and the hippocampus rolls into the medial wall of the temporal horn. Although the amygdala is usually considered a single structure, it obviously has both cortical and ventricular (striatal) components.

Patient CT Scan

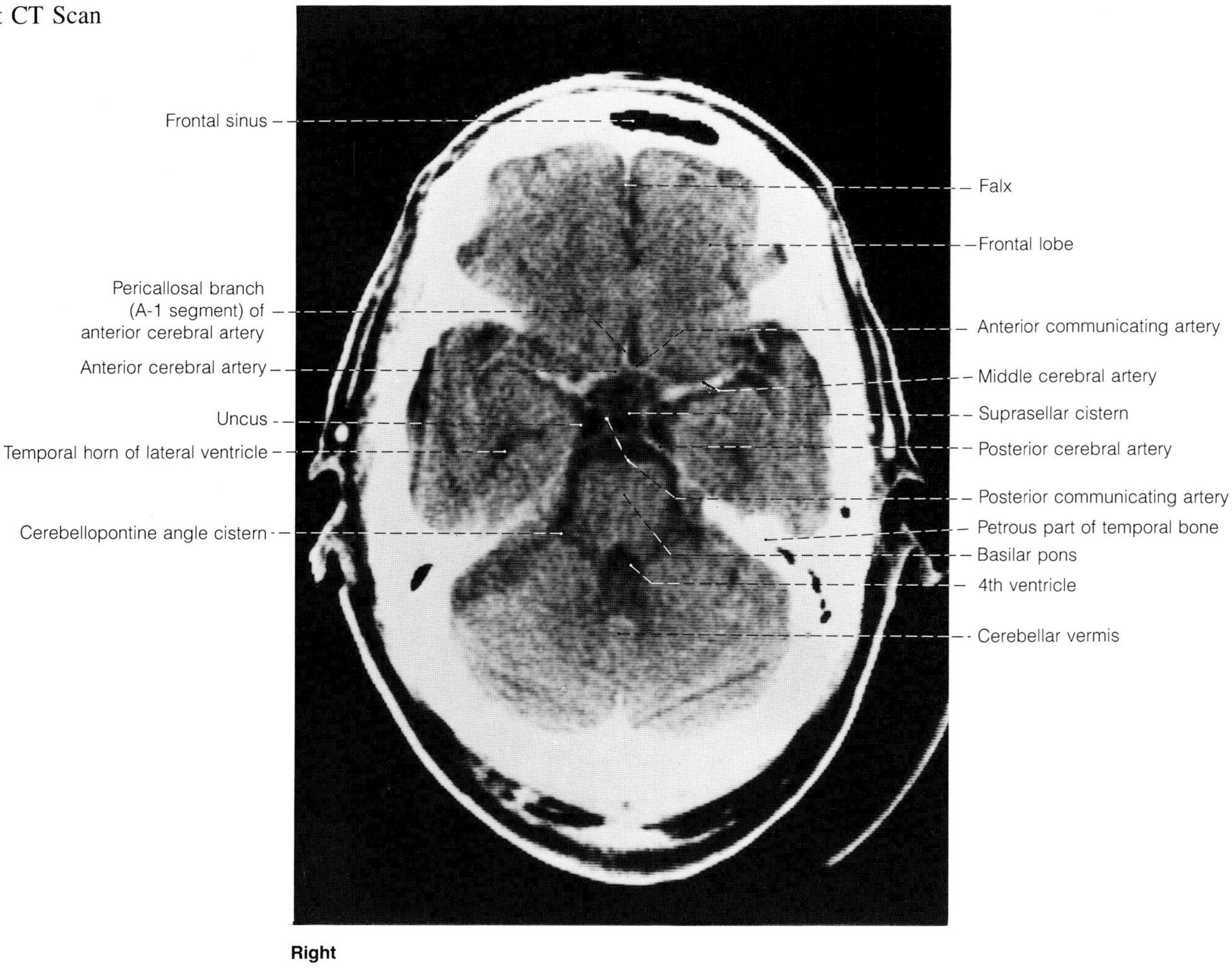

Patient MRI Scan

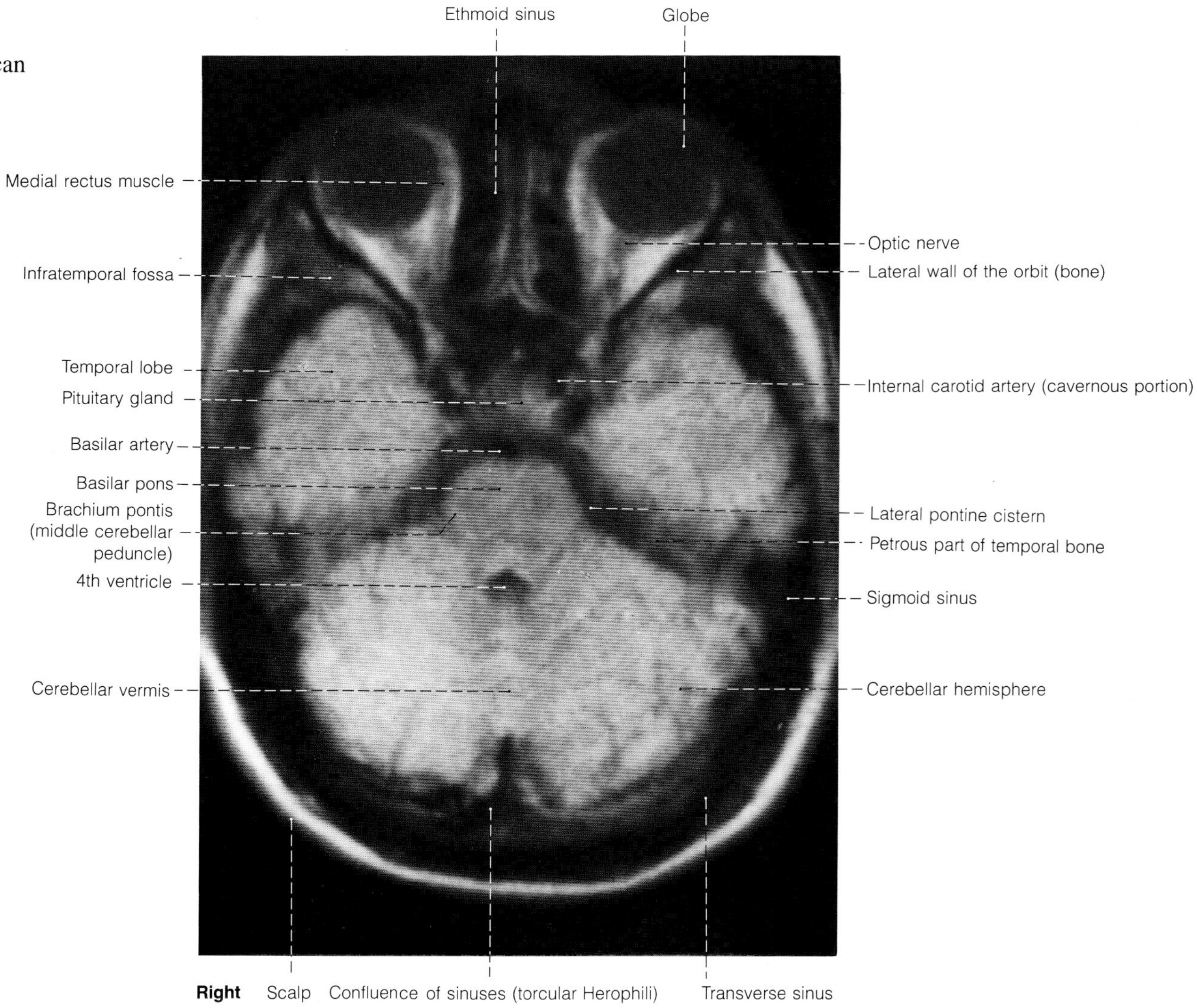

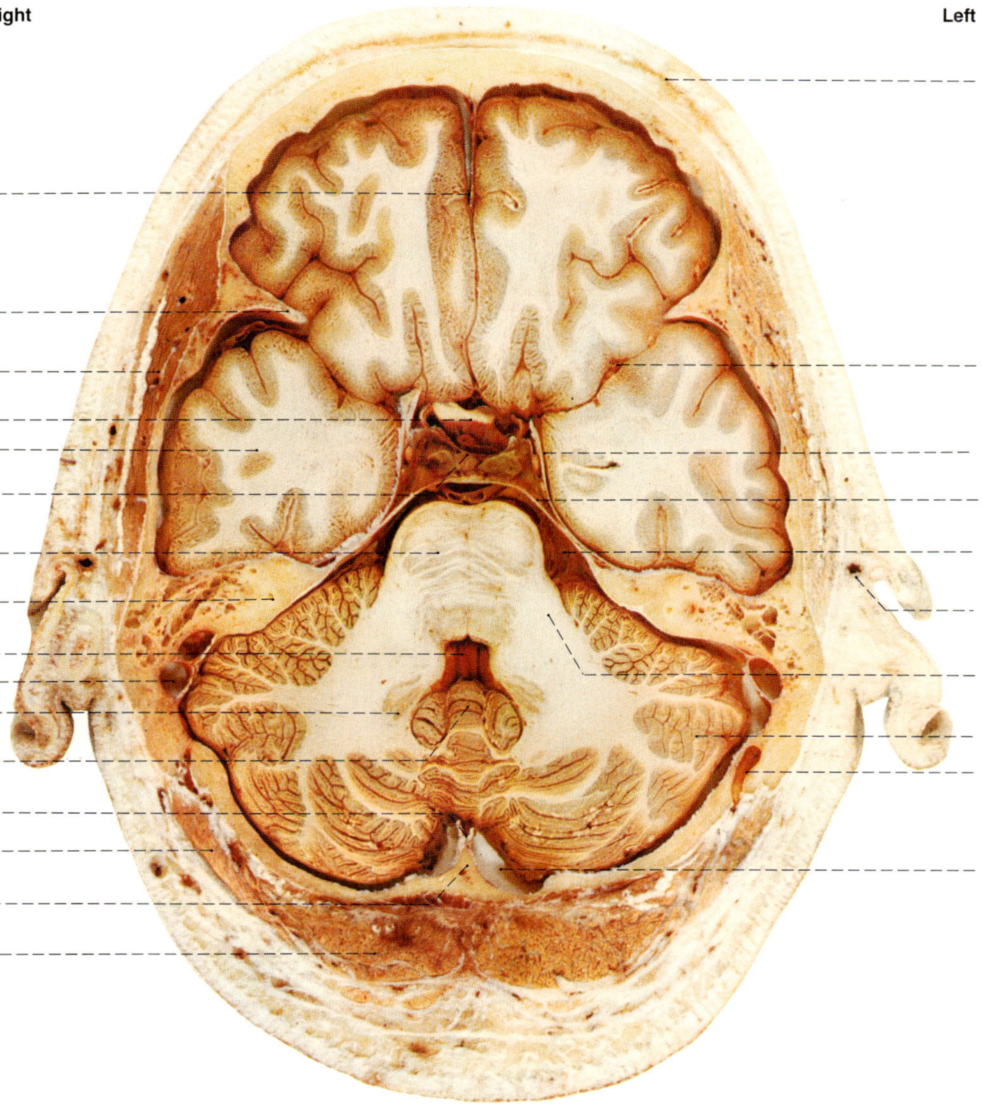

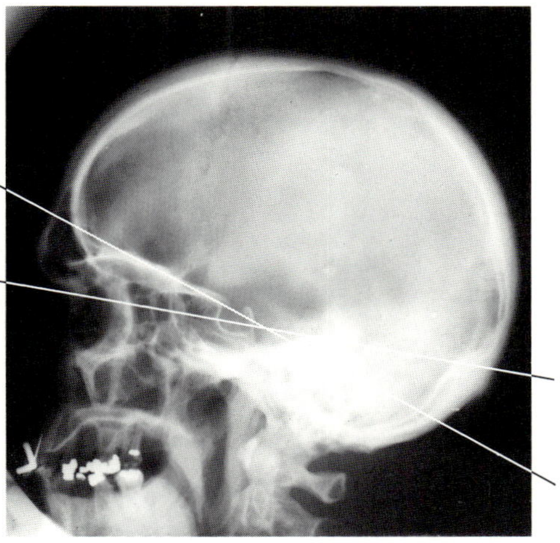

Planes of Sections

The plane of the CT cut is through the pentagonal cistern and the presence of contrast enhances visualization of the circle of Willis. The optic chiasm is in the anterior-superior portion of the pentagonal or suprasellar cistern and the infundibulum of the pituitary is present more posteriorly. The lesser wing of the sphenoid can be seen laterally in the region of the pterion and larger portions of the petrous bone are beginning to be evident. The MRI scan also passes through the upper pons but its more horizontal plane is below the pentagonal cistern and intersects the orbits.

Beneath the tentorium, the base of the pons is a landmark with its lateral wings forming the brachia pontis or middle cerebellar peduncles. The fourth ventricle is recognizable centrally with the nodulus of the cerebellar vermis indenting the posterior roof of the ventricle. Lateral recesses of the 4th ventricle are caudal to this level. Cerebellar hemispheres continue to be the dominant features of the posterior fossa. The MRI has distinct advantages in demonstrating the anatomy within the posterior fossa since the density of the petrous part of the temporal bone frequently causes CT artifacts such as beam hardening.

The tentorium attaches to the anterior and posterior clinoid processes by the anterior and posterior petroclinoid ligaments respectively. These dural folds may infrequently become calcified, but in either case would not be visualized on MRI due to lack of signal.

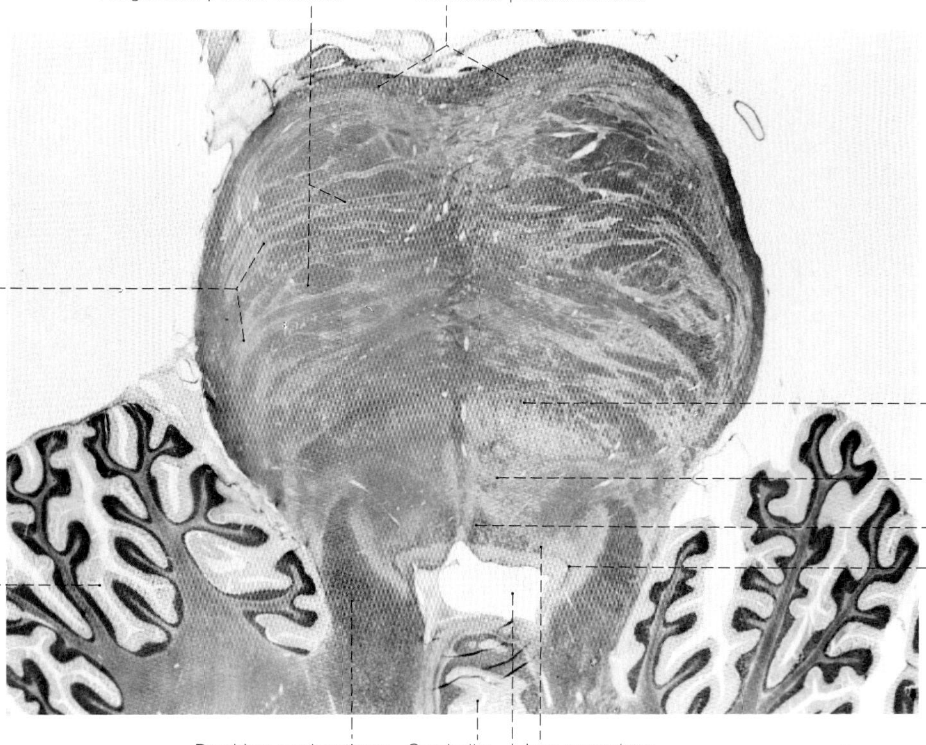
Longitudinal pontine bundles
Transverse pontine bundles
Pontine nuclei
Medial lemniscus
Reticular formation
Medial longitudinal fasciculus
Mesencephalic tract of trigeminal nerve (V)
Cerebellar hemisphere
Brachium conjunctivum (superior cerebellar peduncle)
Cerebellar vermis
Locus ceruleus
Fourth ventricle
5 mm

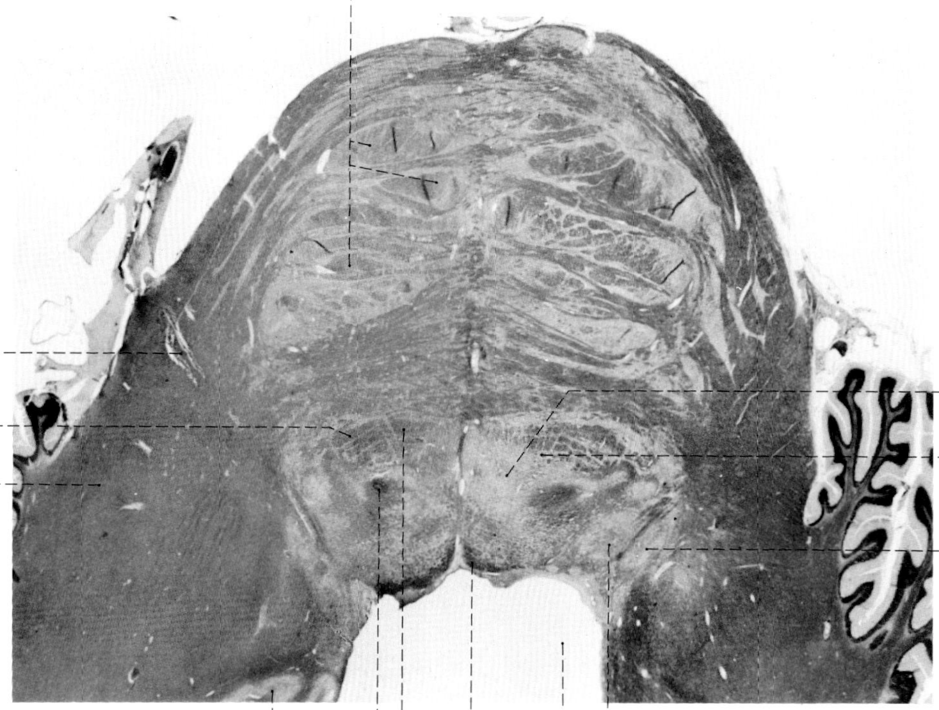
Corticospinal and regular corticobulbar tracts
Trigeminal nerve (V)
Spinal lemniscus (spinothalamic tracts)
Brachium pontis (Ponto-cerebellar fibers)
Reticular formation
Ventral secondary ascending tract of trigeminal nerve (V)
Chief sensory nucleus of trigeminal nerve (V)
Dentate nucleus
Central tegmental tract
Medial lemniscus
Medial longitudinal fasciculus
Fourth ventricle
Motor nucleus of trigeminal nerve (V)
5 mm

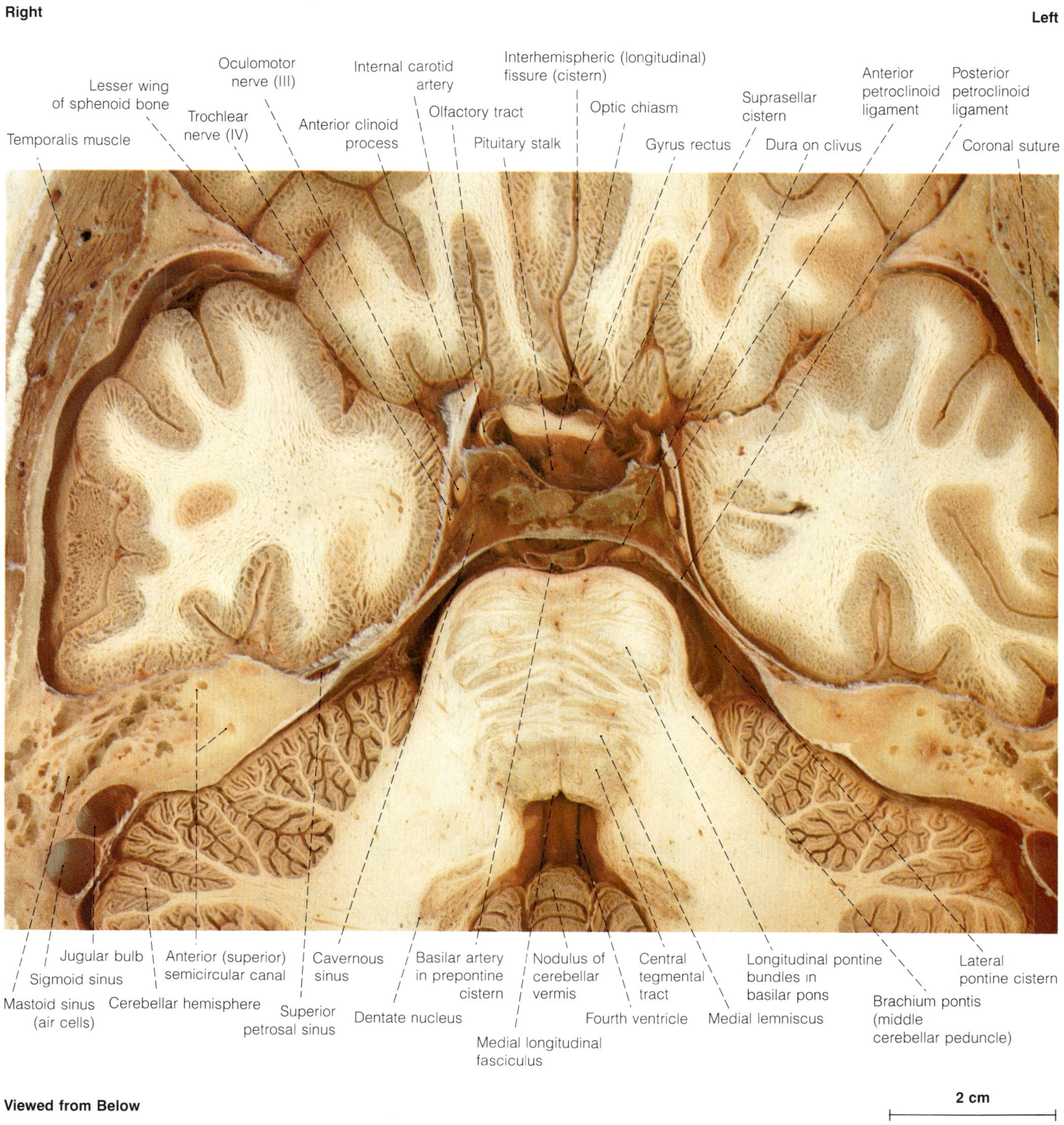

These sections through the upper pons are above and through the trigeminal nerve. The brachia conjunctiva (superior cerebellar peduncles) emerging from the cerebellum are medial to the entering massive middle cerebellar peduncles (brachia pontis). The relatively small size of the tegmental part of the pons may be compared with the greater basilar portion anterior to the medial lemniscus.

Within the tegmentum, the central tegmental tract projecting striatal and tegmental impulses to the inferior olive for relay to the cerebellum is easily identified although it lacks definitive boundaries. The medial longitudinal fasciculi are important bundles at this level in interconnecting the extraocular (III, IV, VI) and vestibular (VIII) nuclei. Destruction of these paths in the floor of the fourth ventricle results in internuclear ophthalmoplegia. Small unilateral lesion of the medial longitudinal fasciculus, although rare, may not be detected by CT or MRI because of the pixel size. It is expected that lesions in this area might be visualized in the future with MRI imaging at high field strengths.

Patient CT Scan

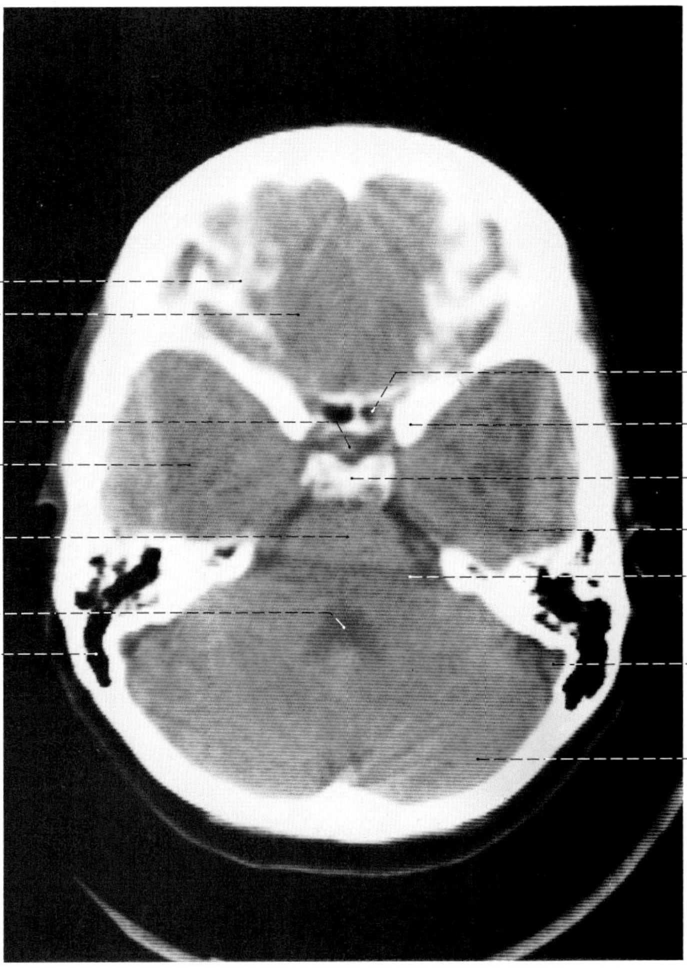

Right

Patient MRI Scan

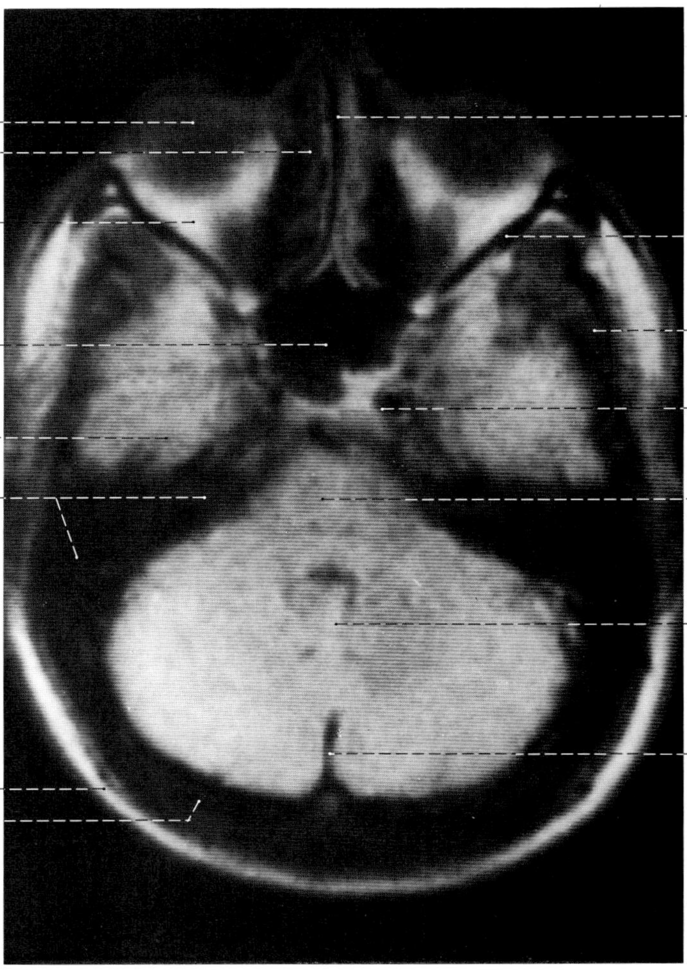

Right

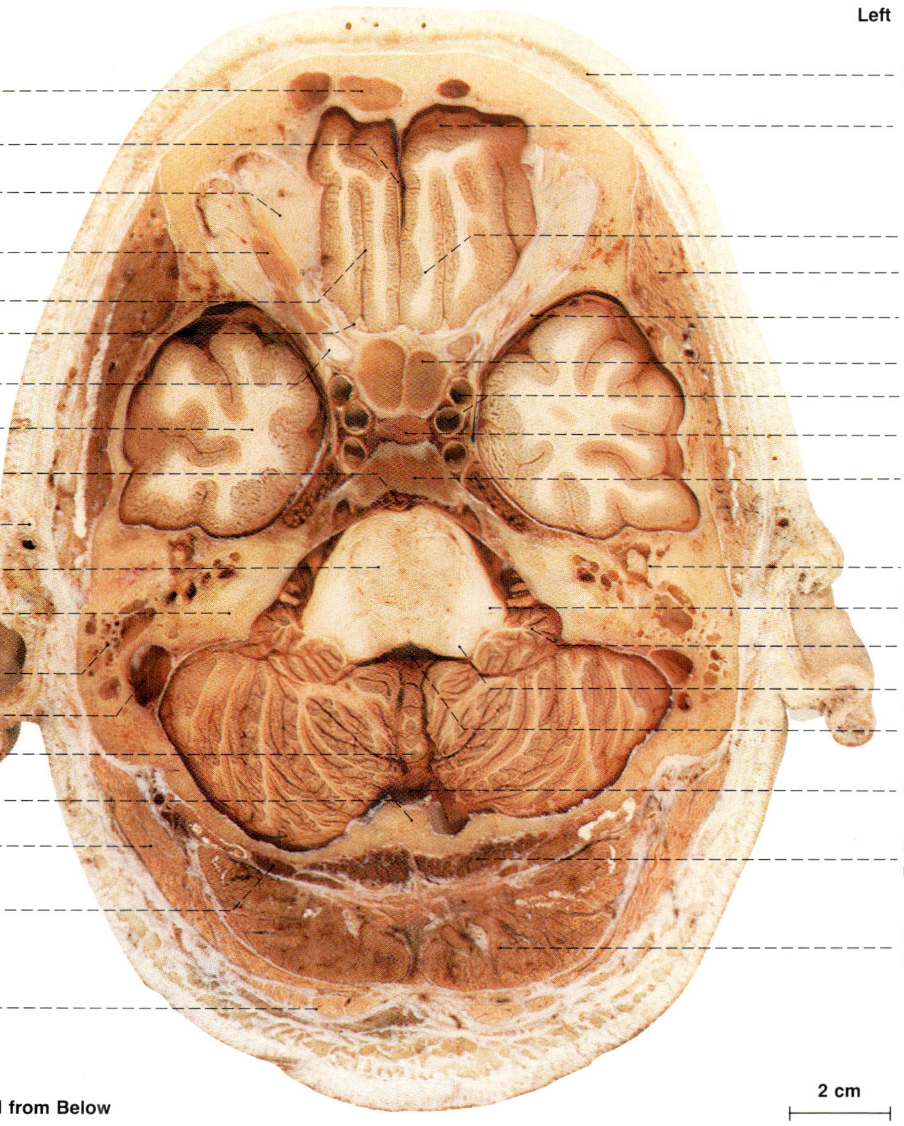

Planes of Sections

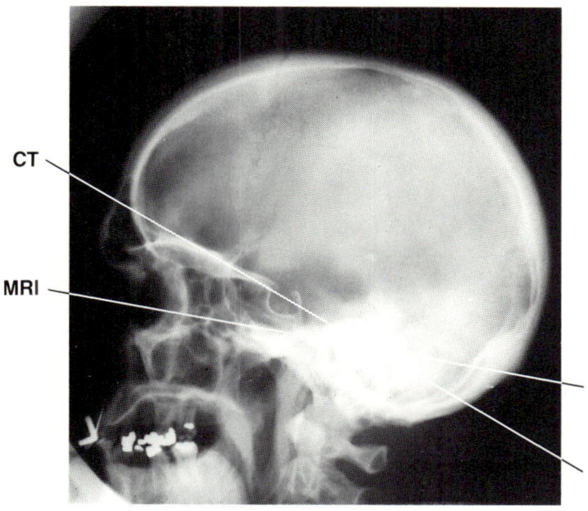

The gross anatomical cut is fortuitously through the cavernous sinus. The sellar contents (pituitary gland) are clearly shown with the lateral walls of the sella recognizable as the medial dural envelope of the cavernous sinuses. The internal carotid artery makes several turns at this level, forming the "siphon" which has been cut in several sections because of this curved course. The sphenoid sinus lies just anterior to the pituitary fossa, separated only by a thin septum of bone. A very nice demonstration of the contents of the optic canal can be seen on the right with the optic nerve (II) flanked by the ophthalmic artery in an infero-lateral location. The other nerves which traverse the walls of the cavernous sinus, notably the oculomotor (III) trochlear (IV), ophthalmic division of the trigeminal (V_1), and the abducens (VI), are posterior behind and lateral to the optic nerve (CN II).

Just dorsally lies the caudal pons featuring the dorsal location of the restiform bodies (inferior cerebellar peduncles) passing into (and from) the cerebellum just medial to the flocculus of the cerebellum. The facial nerve (VII) and auditory nerve (VIII) pass through the cerebellopontine angle cistern at this level to enter the internal auditory canal.

Macro features include the tips of the temporal lobes in the middle cranial fossae and the midline inferior-most extent of the cerebellar vermis in the posterior cranial fossa. These features are separated by the petrous part of the temporal bones.

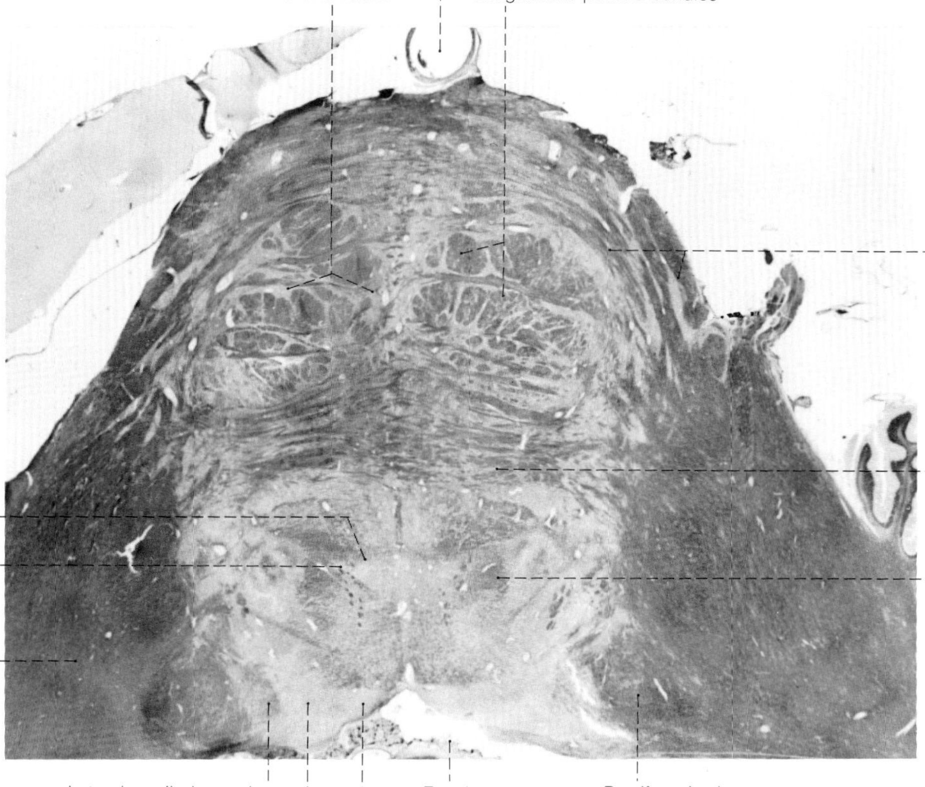
Basilar artery
Pontine nuclei
Longitudinal pontine bundles
Transverse pontine bundles
Trapezoid body
Aberrant corticobulbar tracts
Ventral reticulospinal tract
Central tegmental tract
Brachium pontis
Lateral vestibular nucleus
Medial vestibular nucleus
Abducens nucleus (VI)
Fourth ventricle
Restiform body
5 mm

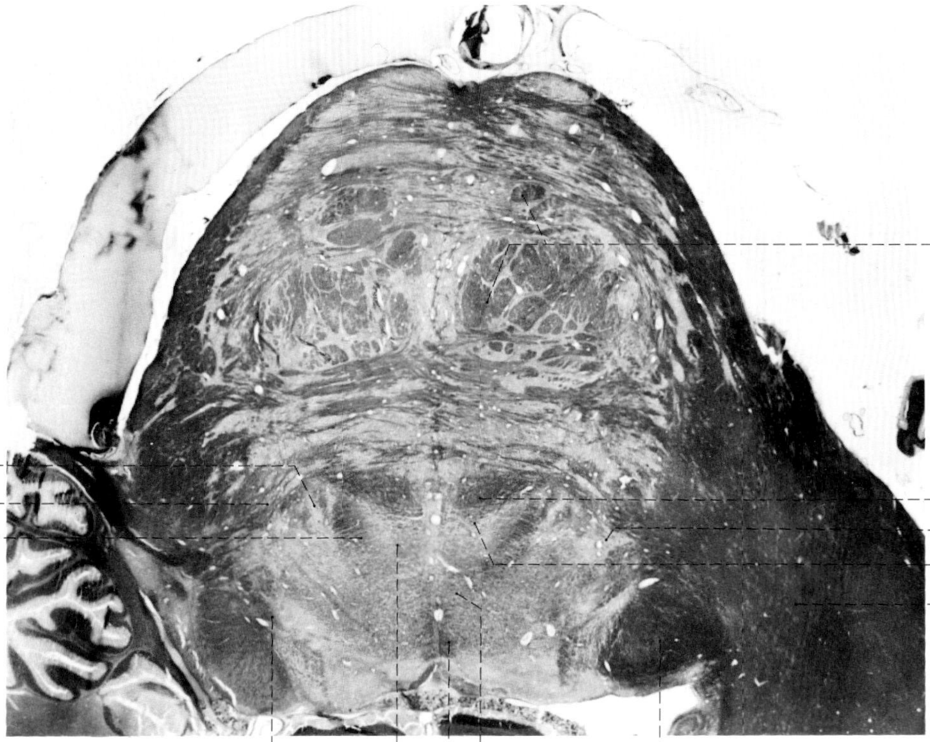
Corticospinal, corticopontine and corticobulbar tracts
Superior olivary nucleus
Spinothalamic tracts
Central tegmental tract
Medial lemniscus
Facial nucleus (VII)
Aberrant corticobulbar tracts
Pontocerebellar fibers
Spinal tract of trigeminal nerve (V)
Reticular formation
Medial tectospinal tract
Medial longitudinal fasciculus
Cerebellovestibular and cerebelloreticular fibers
5 mm

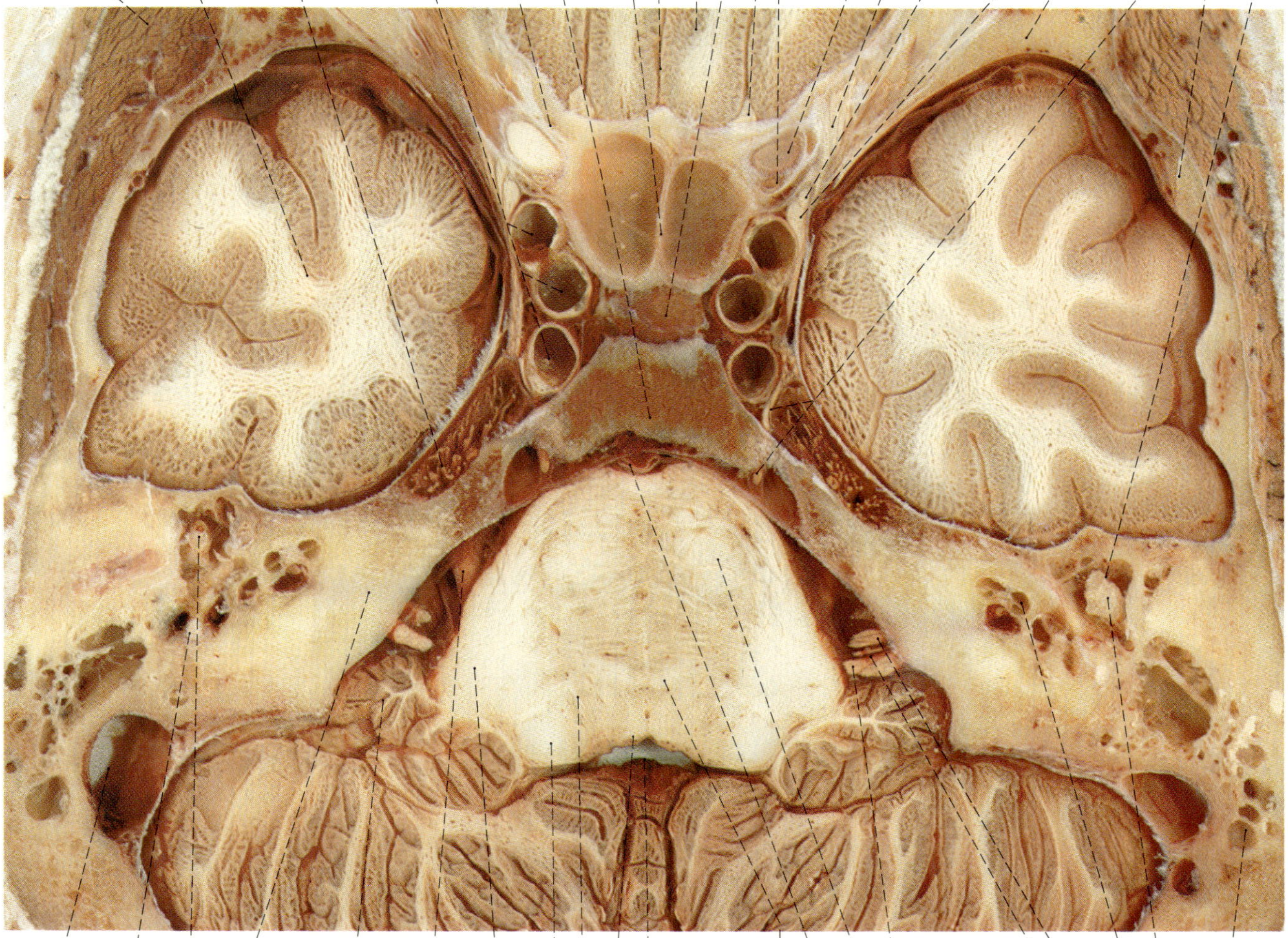

The angle of the usual CT plane at 15° above the IOM line is such that it passes through the upper pons anteriorly and lower pons posteriorly. It illustrates the proximity of the vestibular, abducens and facial nuclei in the tegmental portion of the pons. The ventral pons contains the large descending corticospinal, corticobulbar and corticopontine pathways, as yet largely uncrossed. The major ascending tracts occupy a plane between the basilar pons and tegmentum. The lateral pons at these levels is formed by the middle and inferior cerebellar peduncles. Important respiratory and cardiovascular tracts traverse the pontine tegmentum.

Patient CT Scan

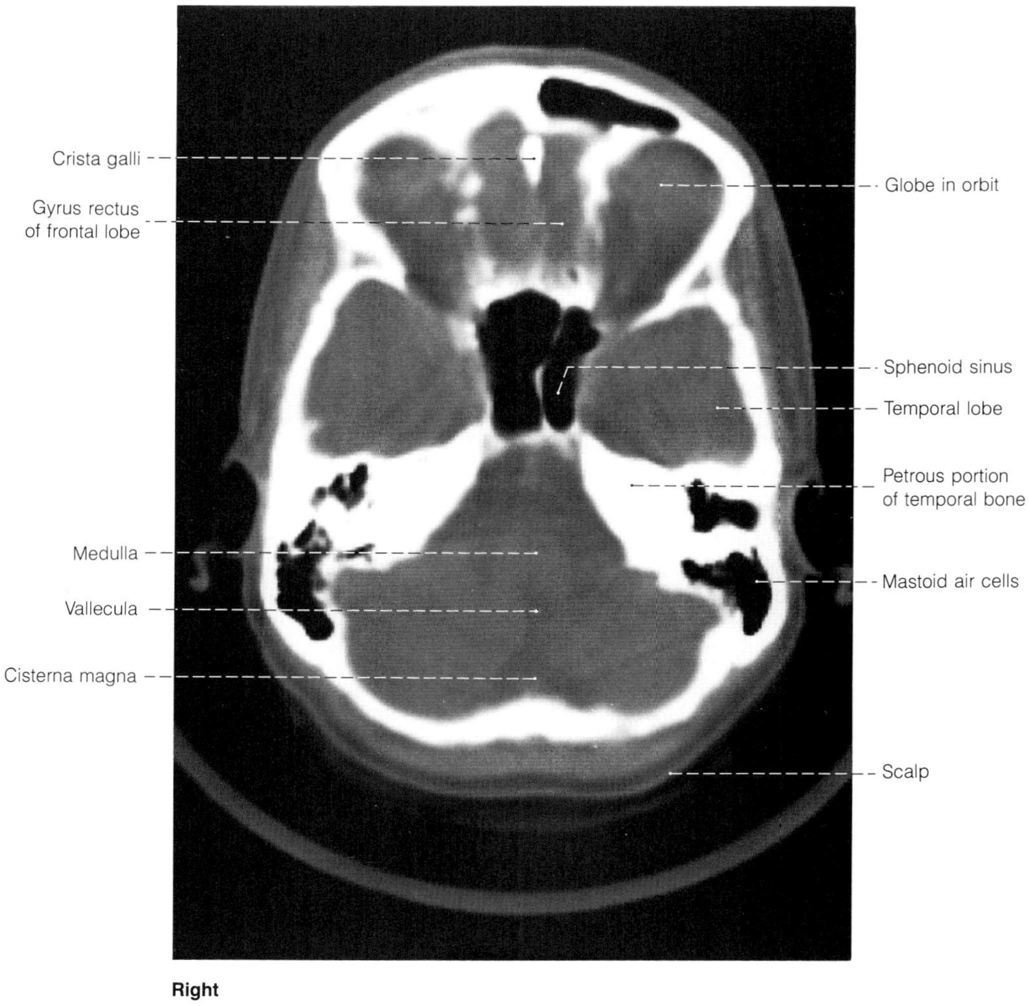

Patient MRI Scan

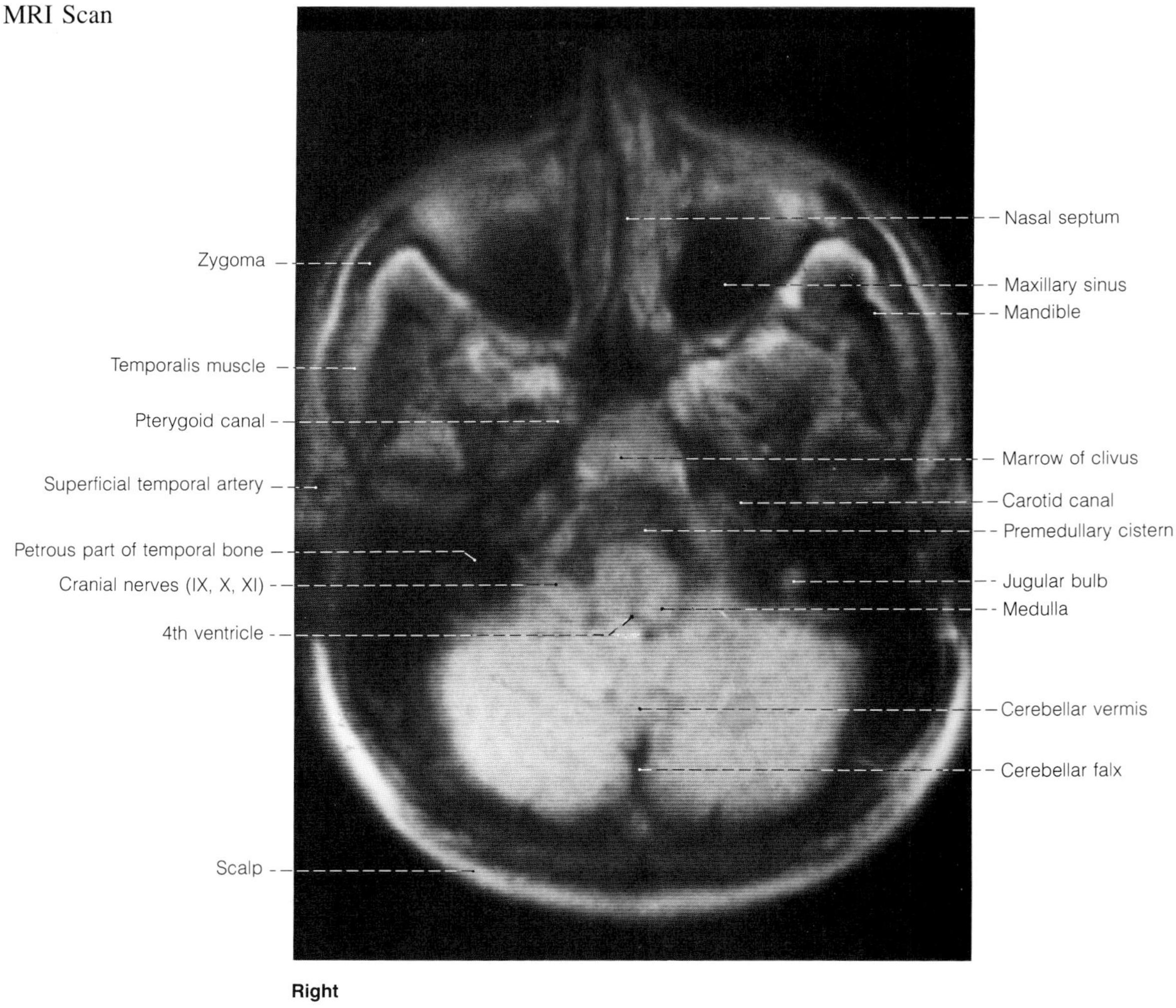

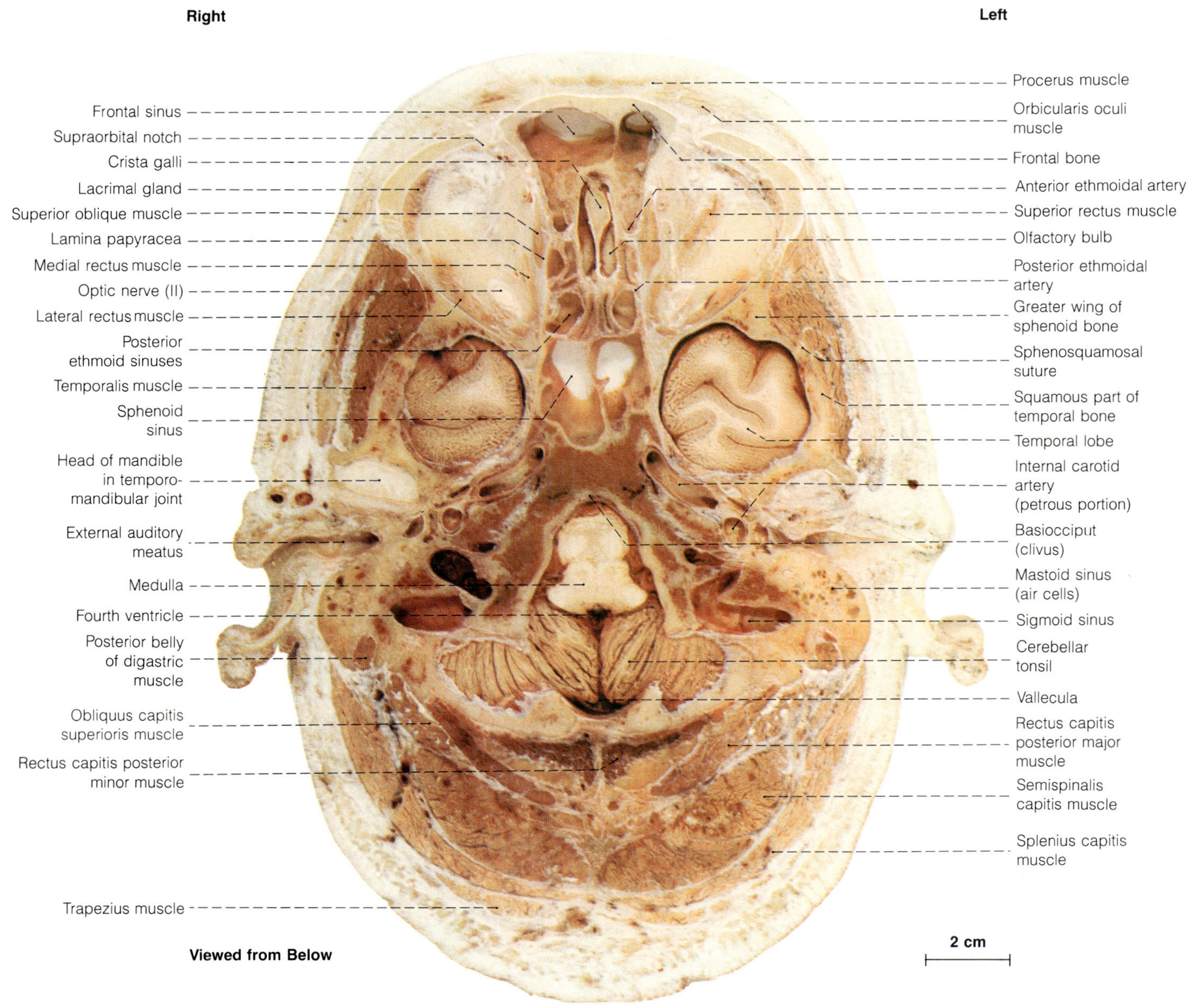

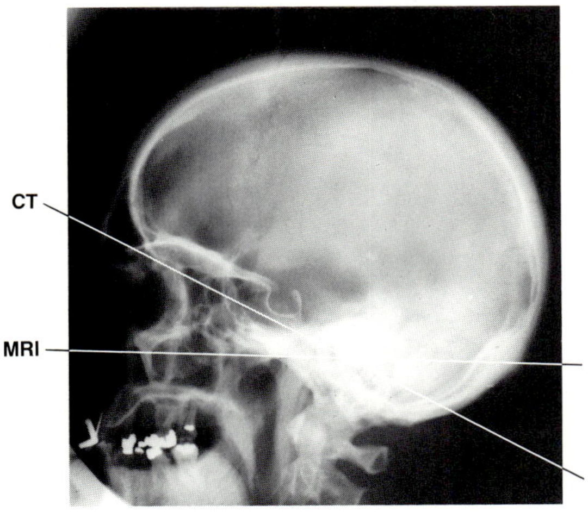

Planes of Sections

This level presents the characteristic quadrangular shape of the upper medulla which can be readily recognized with metrizamide cisternography on CT or without any contrast on MRI. Posterolaterally there are portions of the inferior cerebellar peduncles (restiform bodies). Dorsally, the cerebellar tonsils are in evidence with the vallecula between them. The anatomical slice has fortuitously passed through the horizontal (petrous) portion of the internal carotid artery as it courses anteriorly and medially through the petrous bone with the Eustachian tube just anteriolateral and the tympanic cavity just lateral to it. The jugular bulb is immediately behind the internal carotid artery as it turns forward to become the petrous portion of the internal carotid.

This level also passes through the globe and upper orbital structures illustrating the large amount of orbital fat which is normally present at this level. Orbital fat is demonstrated as a very white area on most MRI sequences due to its very high signal characteristics. Because of its low density on CT, the fat permits excellent differentiation of other orbital structures (muscles, globe, vascular channels) with this imaging medium. The position of the olfactory bulbs on either side of the crista galli and medial to the upper orbit is well illustrated.

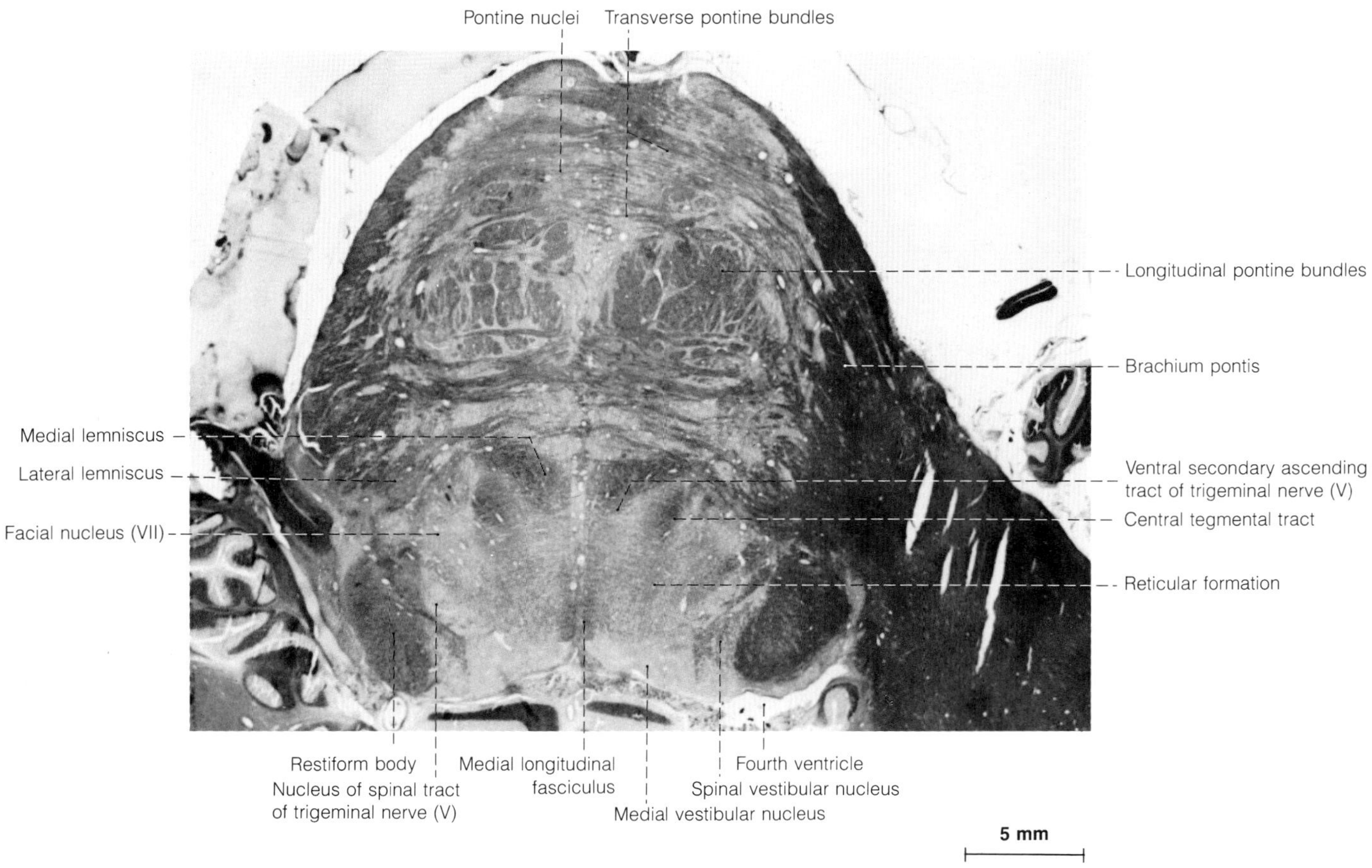
Pontine nuclei
Transverse pontine bundles
Longitudinal pontine bundles
Brachium pontis
Medial lemniscus
Lateral lemniscus
Ventral secondary ascending tract of trigeminal nerve (V)
Central tegmental tract
Facial nucleus (VII)
Reticular formation
Restiform body
Nucleus of spinal tract of trigeminal nerve (V)
Medial longitudinal fasciculus
Fourth ventricle
Spinal vestibular nucleus
Medial vestibular nucleus
5 mm

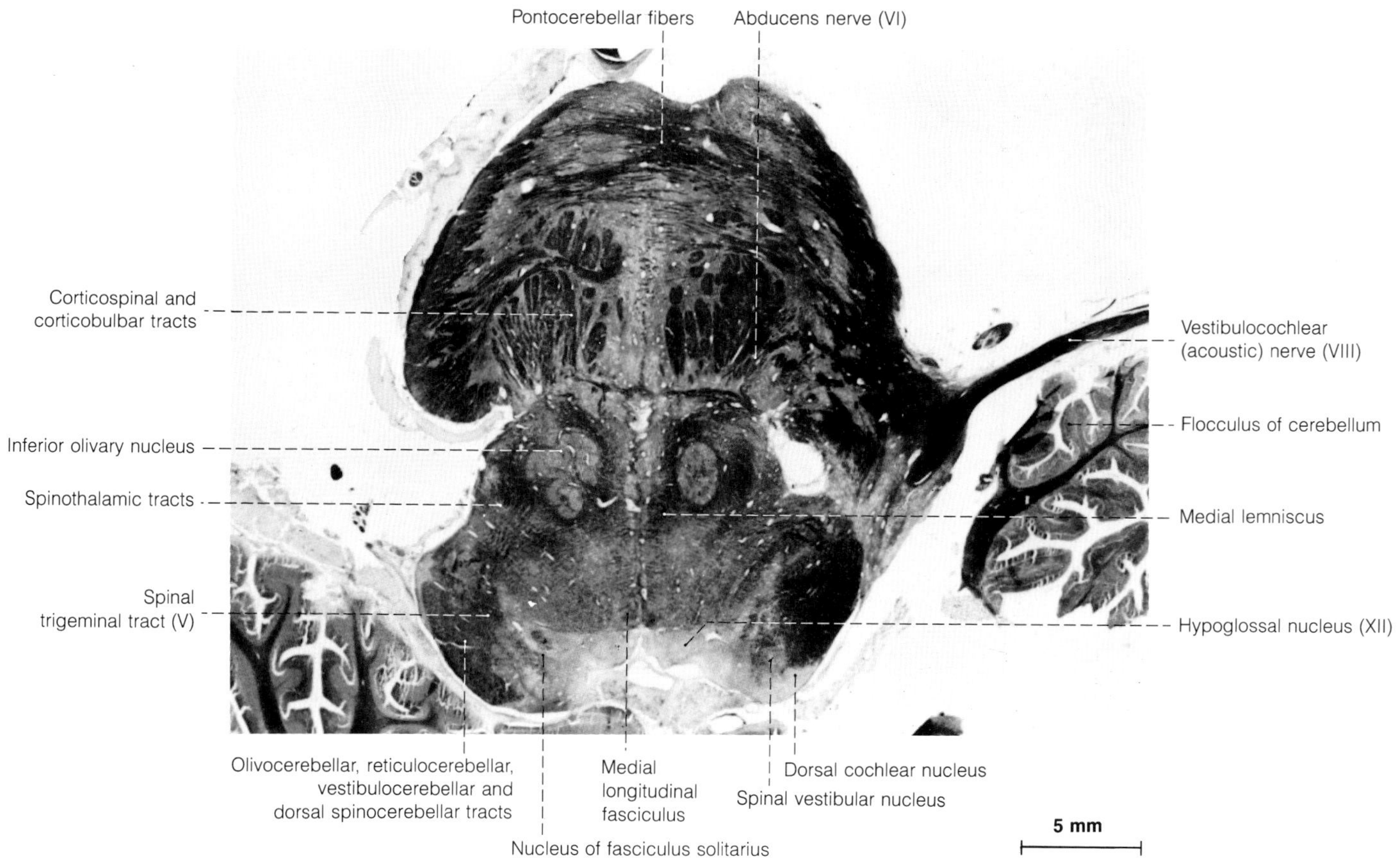
Pontocerebellar fibers
Abducens nerve (VI)
Corticospinal and corticobulbar tracts
Vestibulocochlear (acoustic) nerve (VIII)
Flocculus of cerebellum
Inferior olivary nucleus
Spinothalamic tracts
Medial lemniscus
Spinal trigeminal tract (V)
Hypoglossal nucleus (XII)
Olivocerebellar, reticulocerebellar, vestibulocerebellar and dorsal spinocerebellar tracts
Medial longitudinal fasciculus
Dorsal cochlear nucleus
Spinal vestibular nucleus
Nucleus of fasciculus solitarius
5 mm

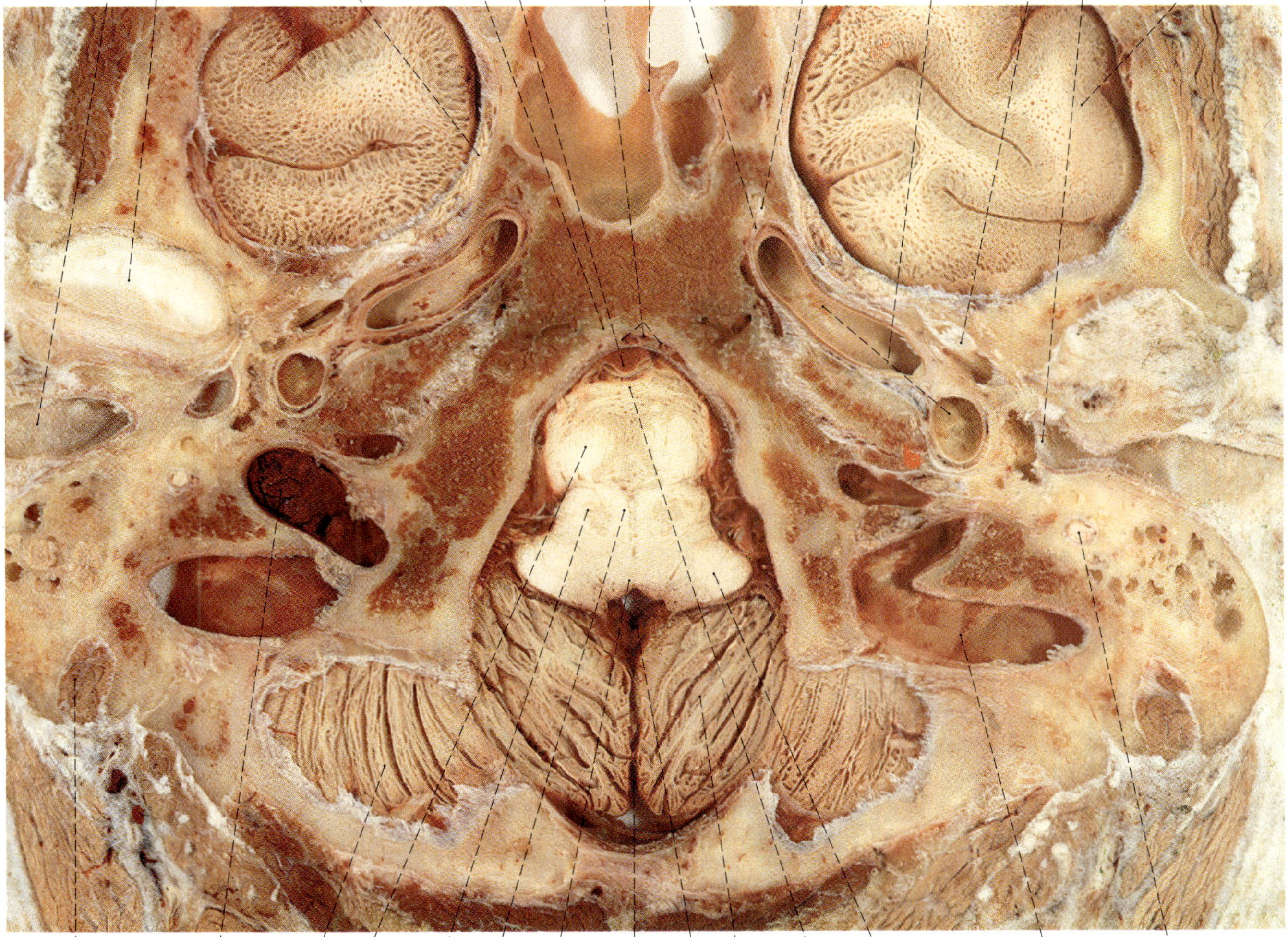

The photographs of the two sections illustrated are at approximately the same magnification. Although the border between the pons and medulla is distinctly delineated ventrally by the caudal limit of the transverse pontine fibers, the more dorsal tegmental region is essentially continuous throughout the brainstem. The emergence of the abducens (VI), facial (VII) and auditory (VIII) nerves at this junction emphasizes its importance diagnostically, as mass lesions in the cerebellopontine angle can often involve all of these nerves clinically.

The medial lemniscus changes from a flat transversely oriented bundle in the upper brainstem to a pair of adjacent vertically oriented bundles in the medulla. This change is the result, in part, of the inferior olivary nuclei of the medulla positioning the lemnisci medially and the massive basilar pons flattening the bundle dorsoventrally. The lateral lemnisci and spinothalamic tracts (spinal lemnisci) maintain their lateral position throughout their course in the brain stem.

Patient CT Scan

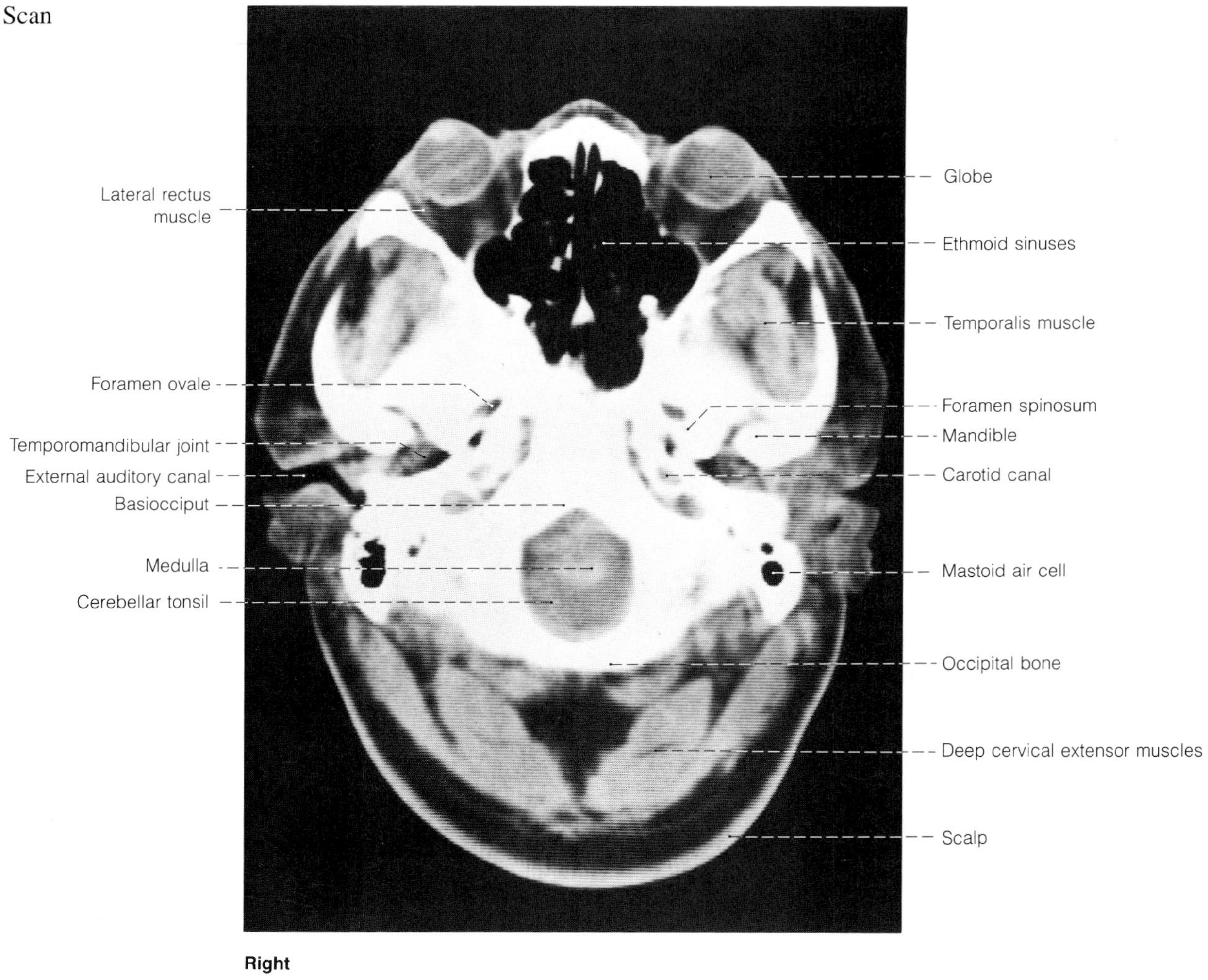

Patient MRI Scan

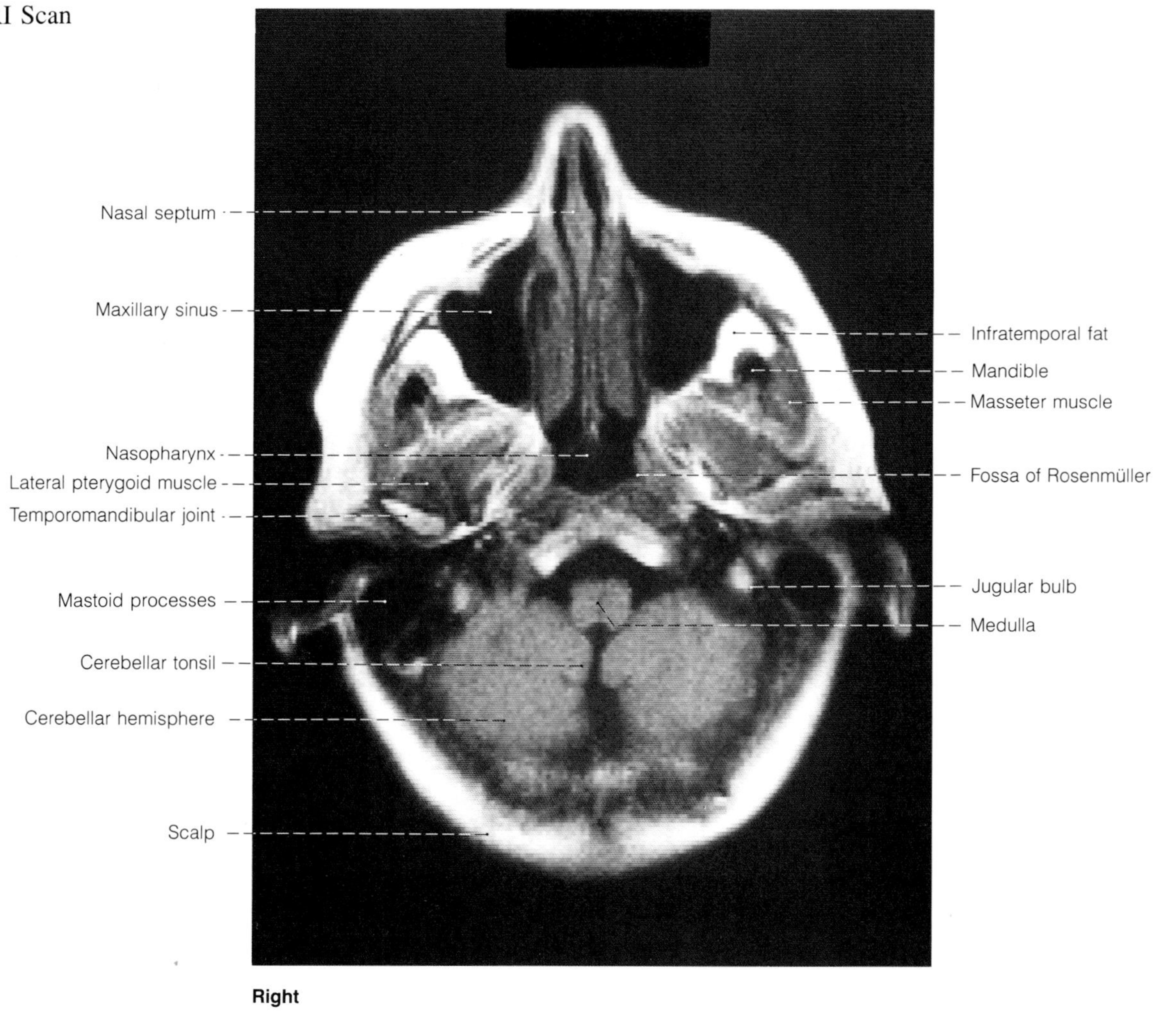

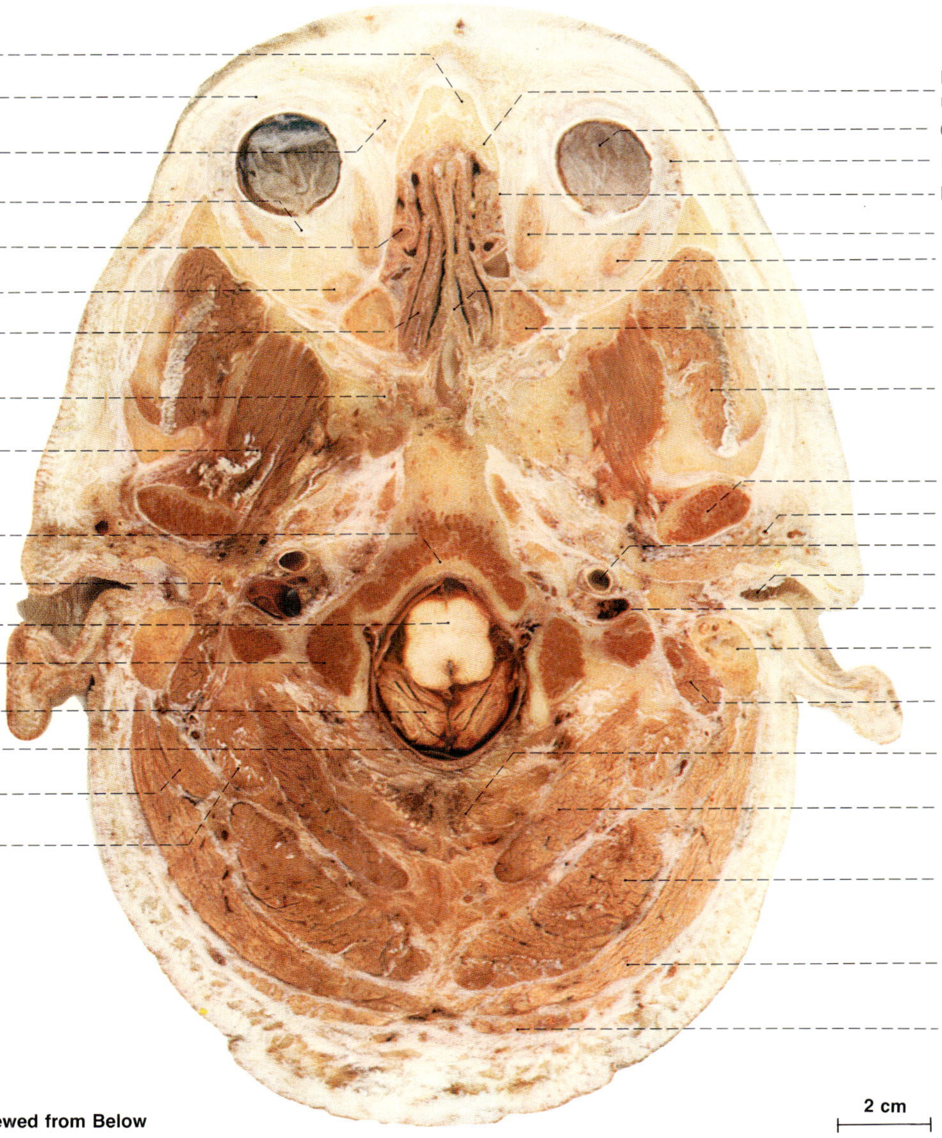

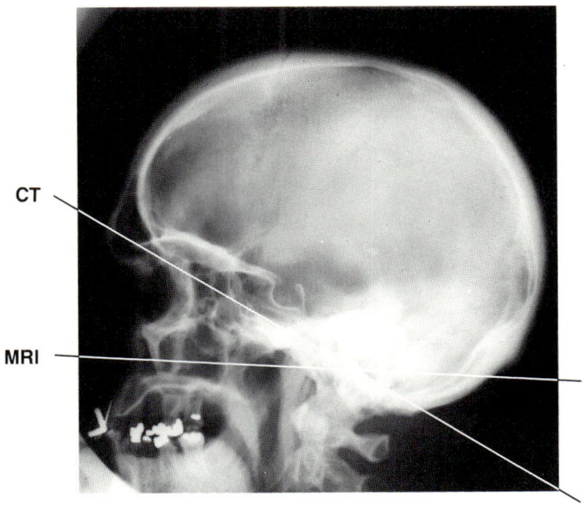

Planes of Sections

The gross anatomical and CT illustrations are in a 15° plane above the IOM line passing through the foramen magnum. The medulla is transected below the obex and above the decussation of the pyramids. The MRI scan is more horizontal and transects the jugular bulb which appears less totally black because of the turbulent blood flow.

CT scans of 10 mm through this region do not usually display with clarity the relationships of the cervical neurovascular structures, i.e. the internal carotid artery, the jugular vein, the glossopharyngeal (IX), vagus (X), spinal accessory (XI) and hypoglossal (XII) nerves or their nuclei within the medulla. A more horizontal plane and thinner cuts are necessary for optimal viewing by CT of these structures at the base of the skull. MRI with increased resolution shows this anatomy to better advantage.

The pterygopalatine fossa is in the plane of the gross section. The contiguity of this space with the nasal cavity, infratemporal fossa, and orbit is well shown with this axial-anatomy.

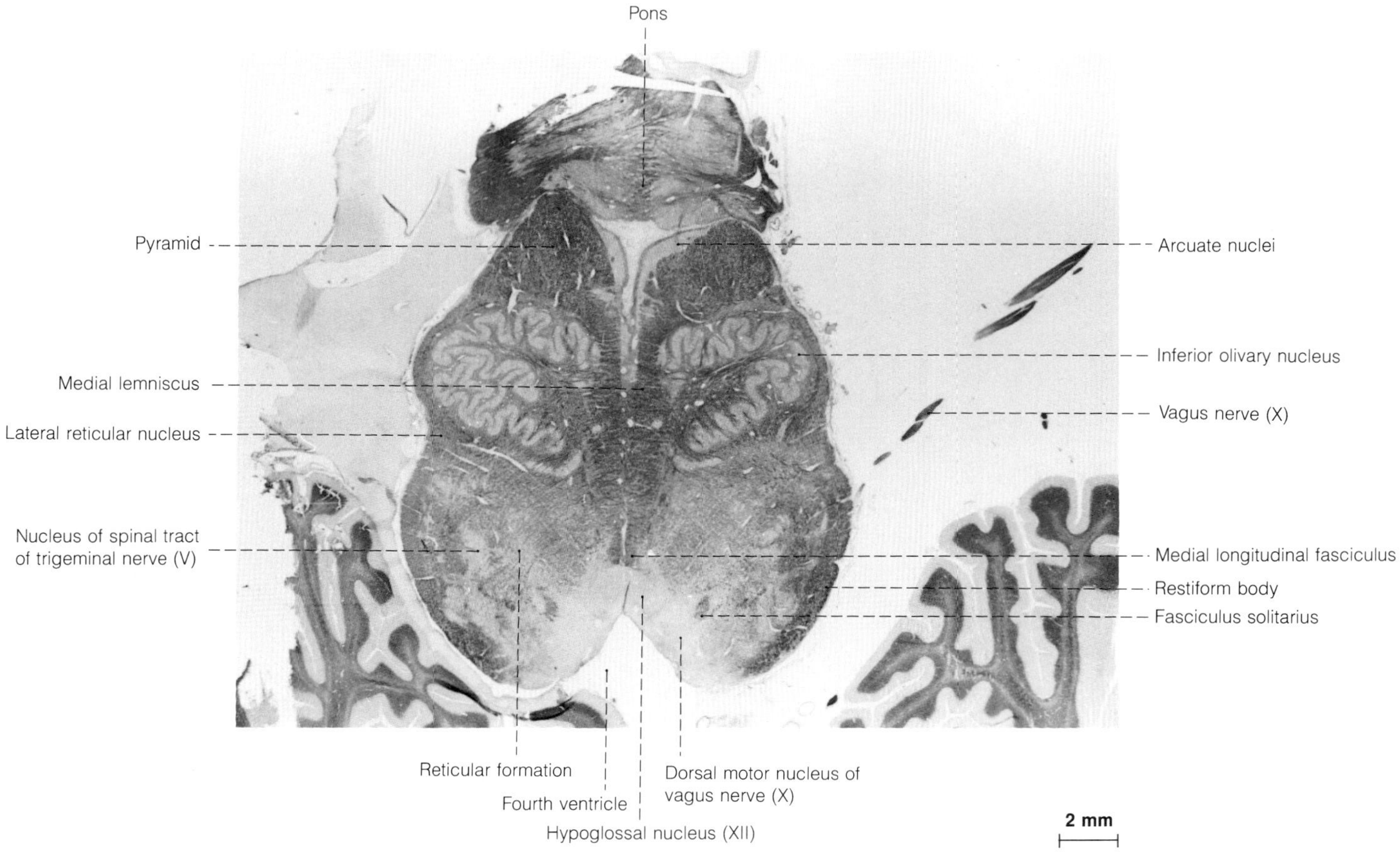
Pons
Pyramid
Arcuate nuclei
Inferior olivary nucleus
Medial lemniscus
Vagus nerve (X)
Lateral reticular nucleus
Nucleus of spinal tract of trigeminal nerve (V)
Medial longitudinal fasciculus
Restiform body
Fasciculus solitarius
Reticular formation
Dorsal motor nucleus of vagus nerve (X)
Fourth ventricle
Hypoglossal nucleus (XII)
2 mm

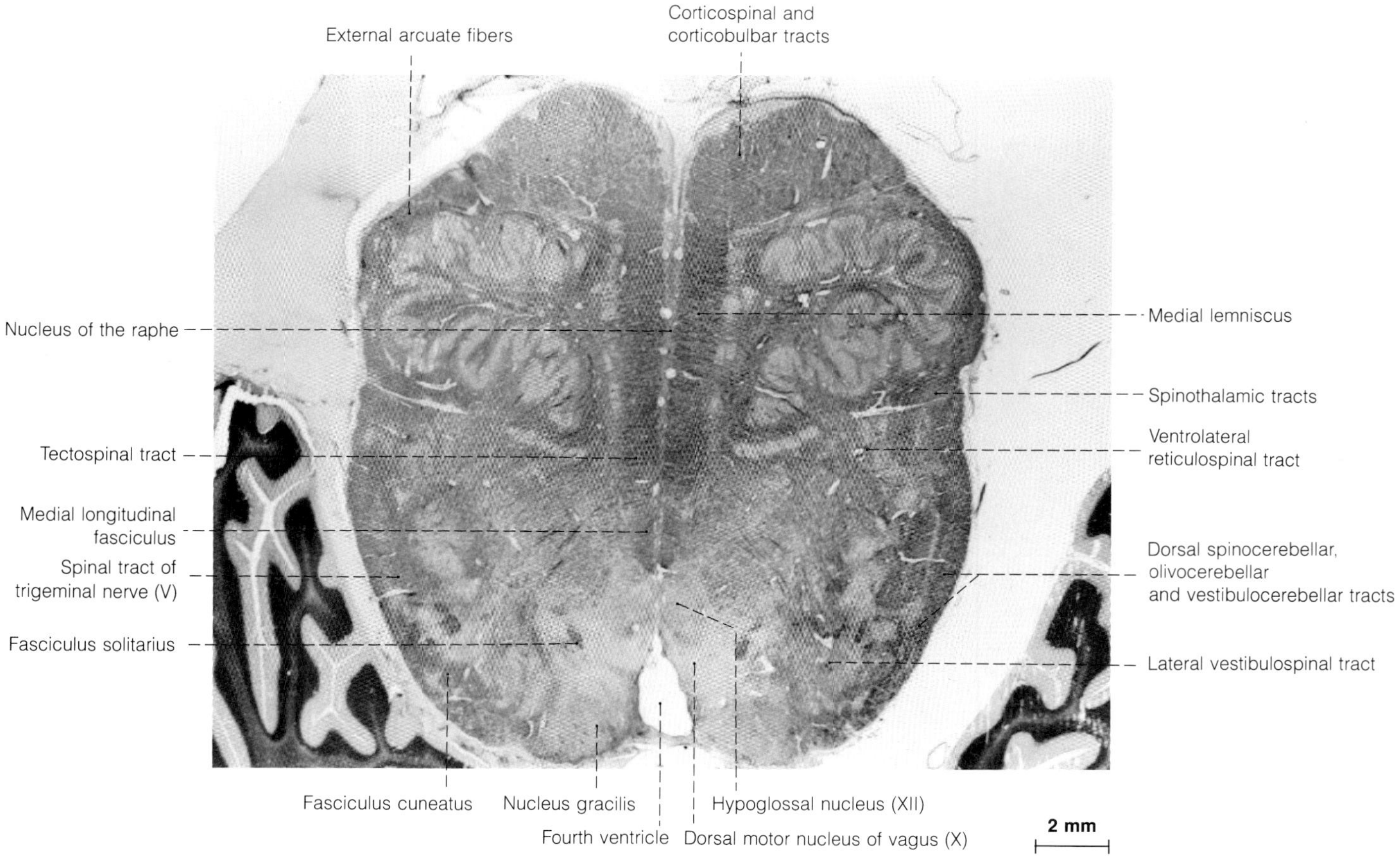
External arcuate fibers
Corticospinal and corticobulbar tracts
Medial lemniscus
Nucleus of the raphe
Spinothalamic tracts
Ventrolateral reticulospinal tract
Tectospinal tract
Medial longitudinal fasciculus
Dorsal spinocerebellar, olivocerebellar and vestibulocerebellar tracts
Spinal tract of trigeminal nerve (V)
Fasciculus solitarius
Lateral vestibulospinal tract
Fasciculus cuneatus
Nucleus gracilis
Hypoglossal nucleus (XII)
Fourth ventricle
Dorsal motor nucleus of vagus (X)
2 mm

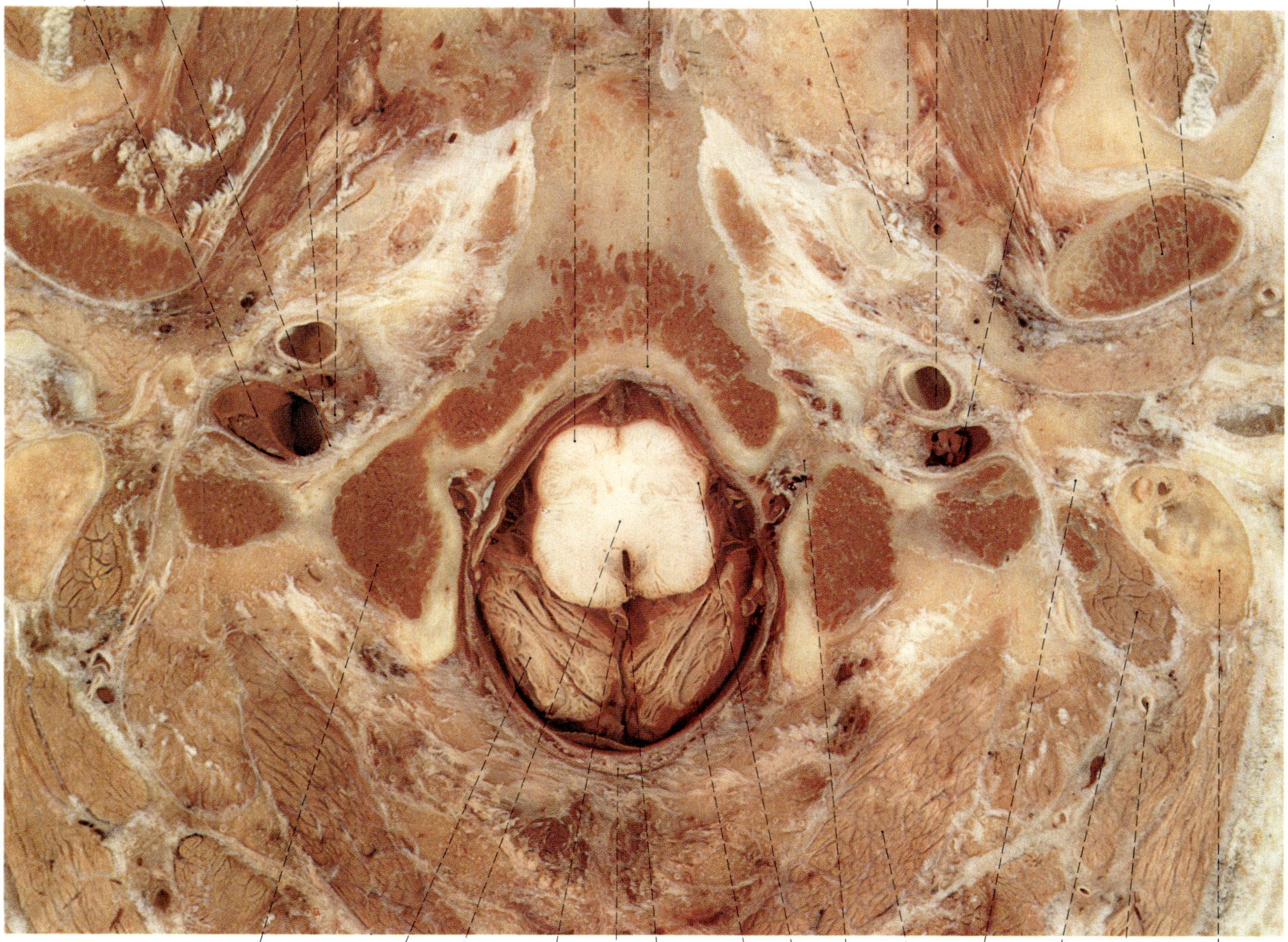

The photograph on the left is at a lower magnification than the more inferior cut illustrated on the right. The angle of the CT anatomy through the posterior fossa results in a plane differing from the usual textbook cross section. This may be easily resolved in the mind of the viewer if the caudal 4th ventricle and cisterna magna are visualized and the plane reconstructed. The medulla is usually only approximately 2.5 cm long and will appear only in 2 or 3 10.0 mm CT displays.

The fibers contributing to the restiform body are lateral to the spinal tract of the trigeminal nerve at this and higher medullary levels but not in lower planes. The nuclei of the inferior olives are prominent structures in these upper medullary levels and it is in this region that vital respiratory and cardiovascular centers reside. The glossopharyngeal (IX), vagus (X), and hypoglossal (XII) nerves also arise from this portion of the medulla.

Patient CT Scan

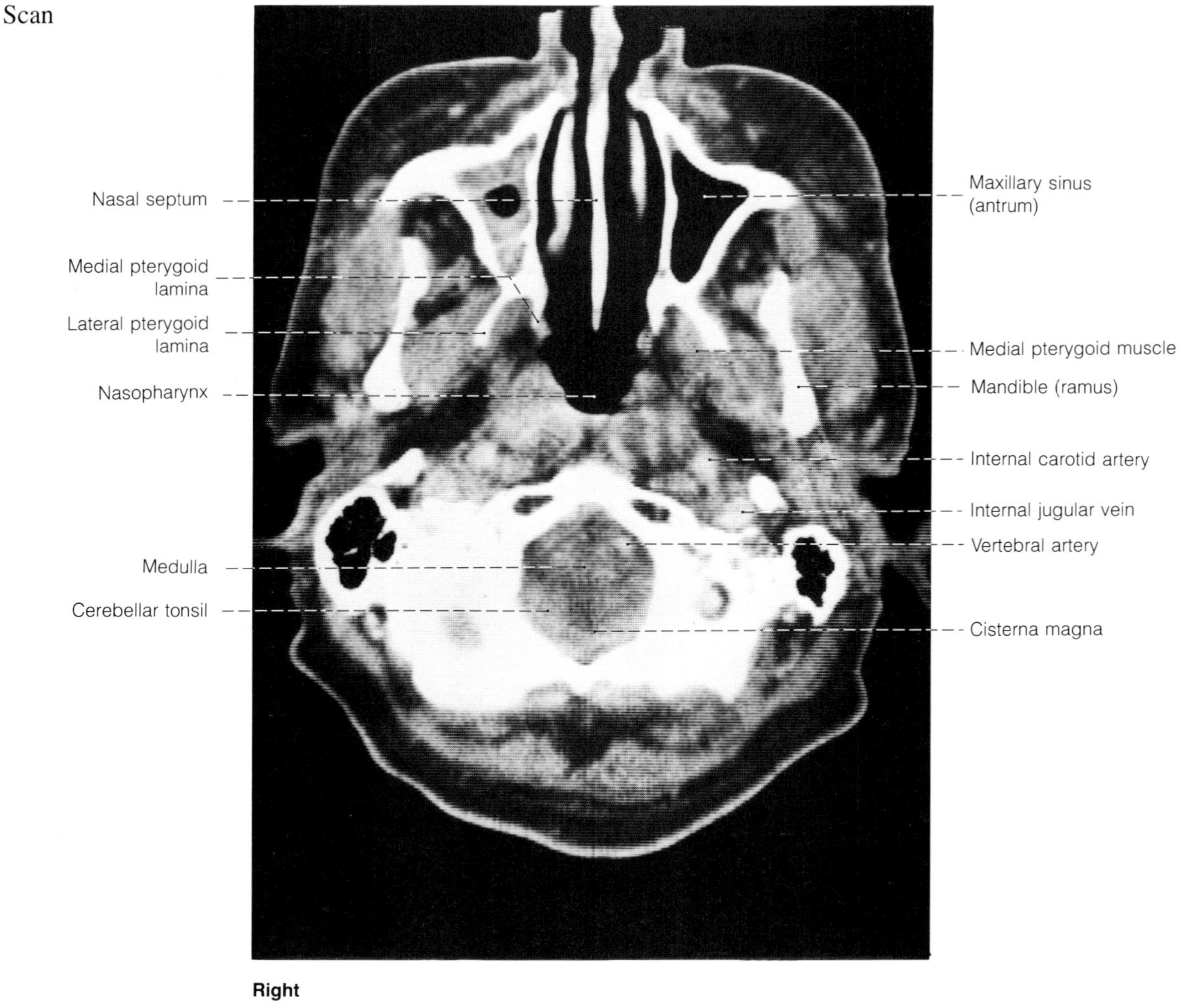

Patient MRI Scan

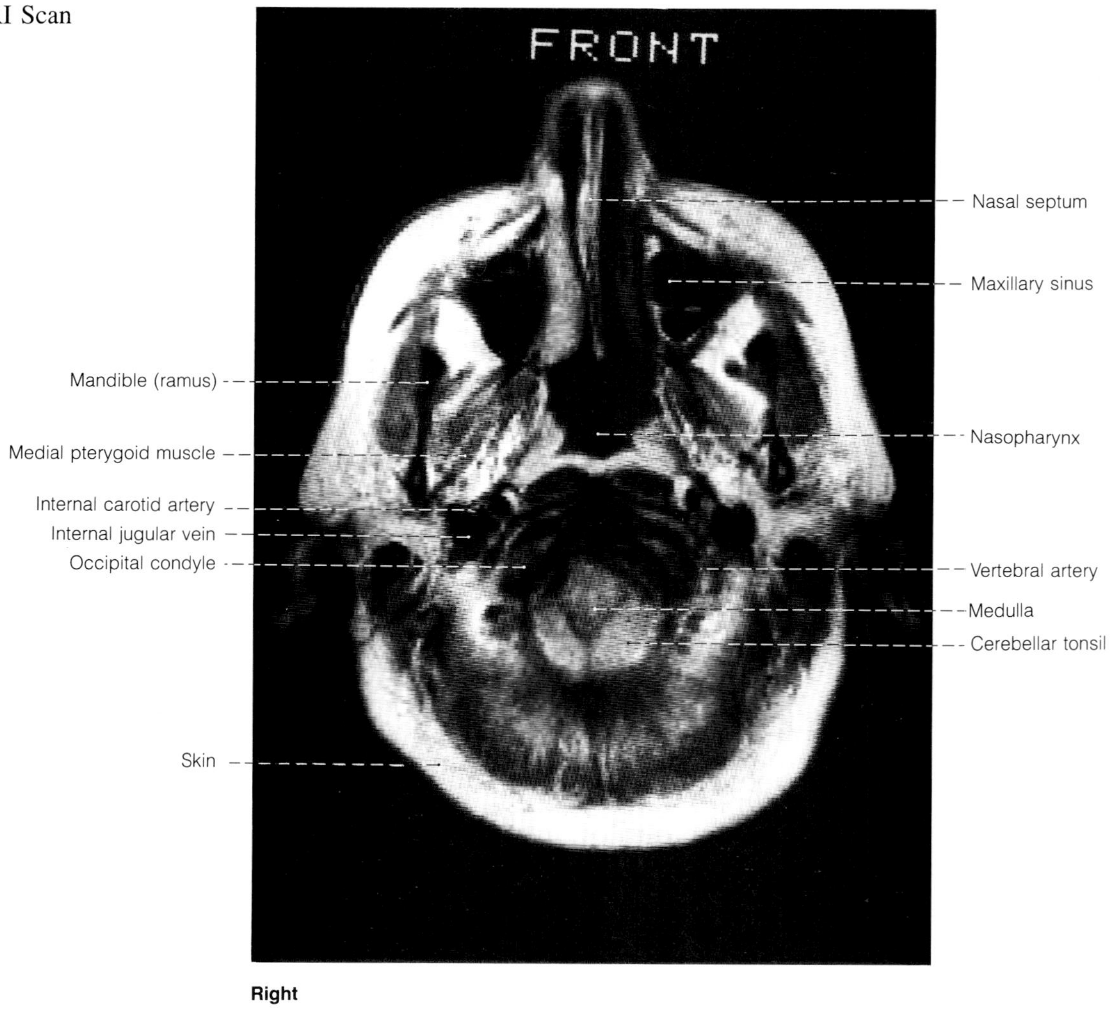

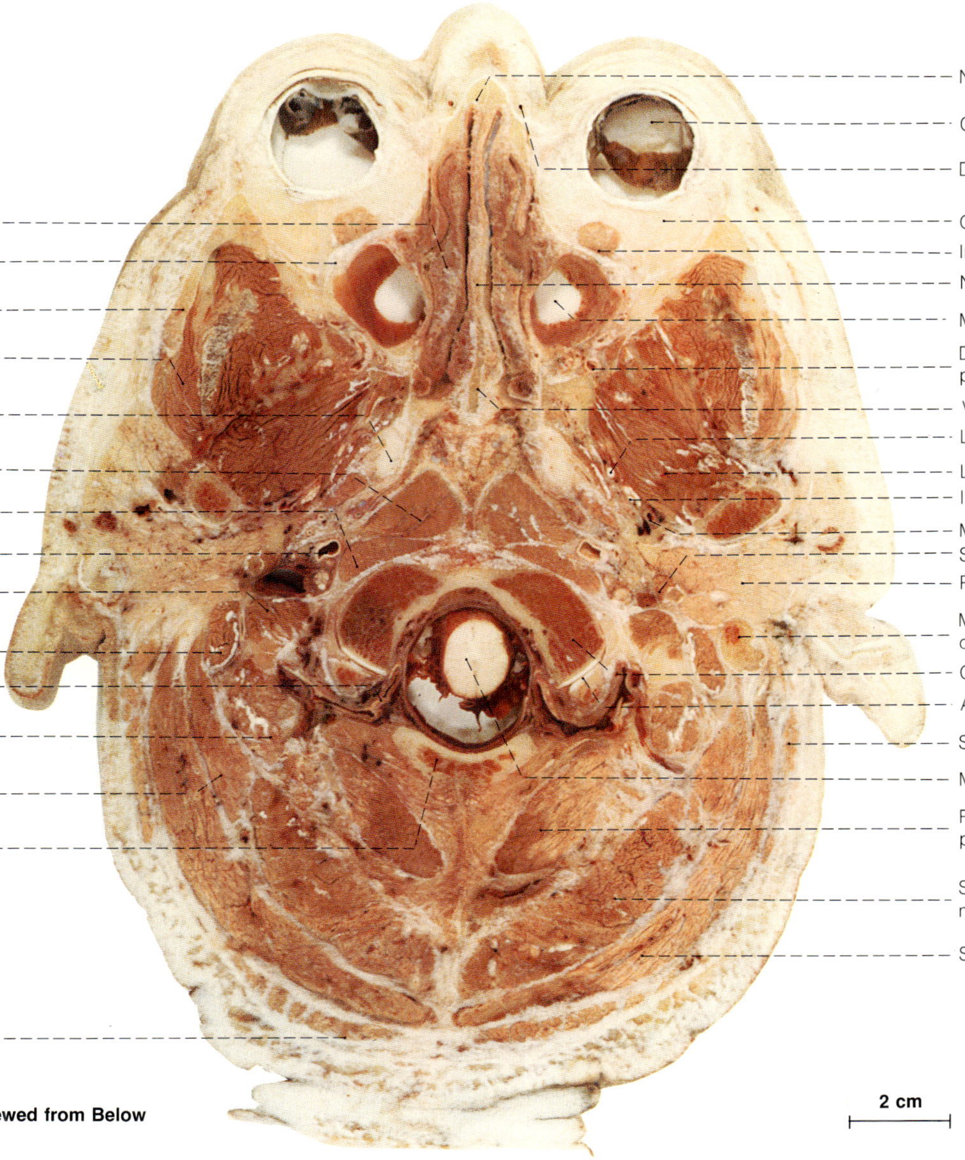

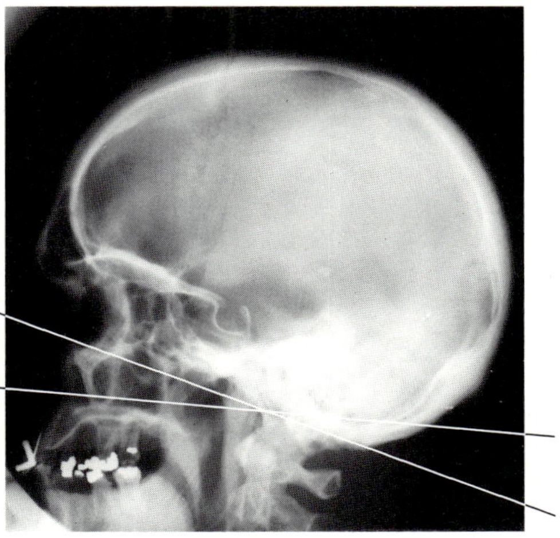

Planes of Sections

The plane of these sections, 7 mm below those on pages 52-54, is through the atlantooccipital joint and foramen magnum. The hypoglossal (anterior condylar) foramina are especially well displayed on the CT image. The size of these canals is a reflection especially of the venous channels (rete hypoglossi) they transmit in addition to the hypoglossal nerves (XII).

The cartilagenous pharyngotympanic (auditory or Eustachian) tube serves as a potential aerated channel between the pharynx and mastoid antrum and as an attachment for the tensor palatini and salpingopharyngeus muscles. It is closed except during swallowing when these opposing muscles pull it open. The pharyngeal opening of the tube is higher in children and the potential for communication of bacterial processes between the pharynx and mastoid air cells is greater.

The atlantooccipital joint is both curved and angled from below supero-medially. The computer averaging of thick CT slices through the joint does not allow the joint to be well imaged. The joint may never be as well visualized with MRI as with CT due to bone imaging problems. The relatively large subarachnoid space (cisterna magna) may be occupied by the cerebellar tonsils in addition to the lower medulla.

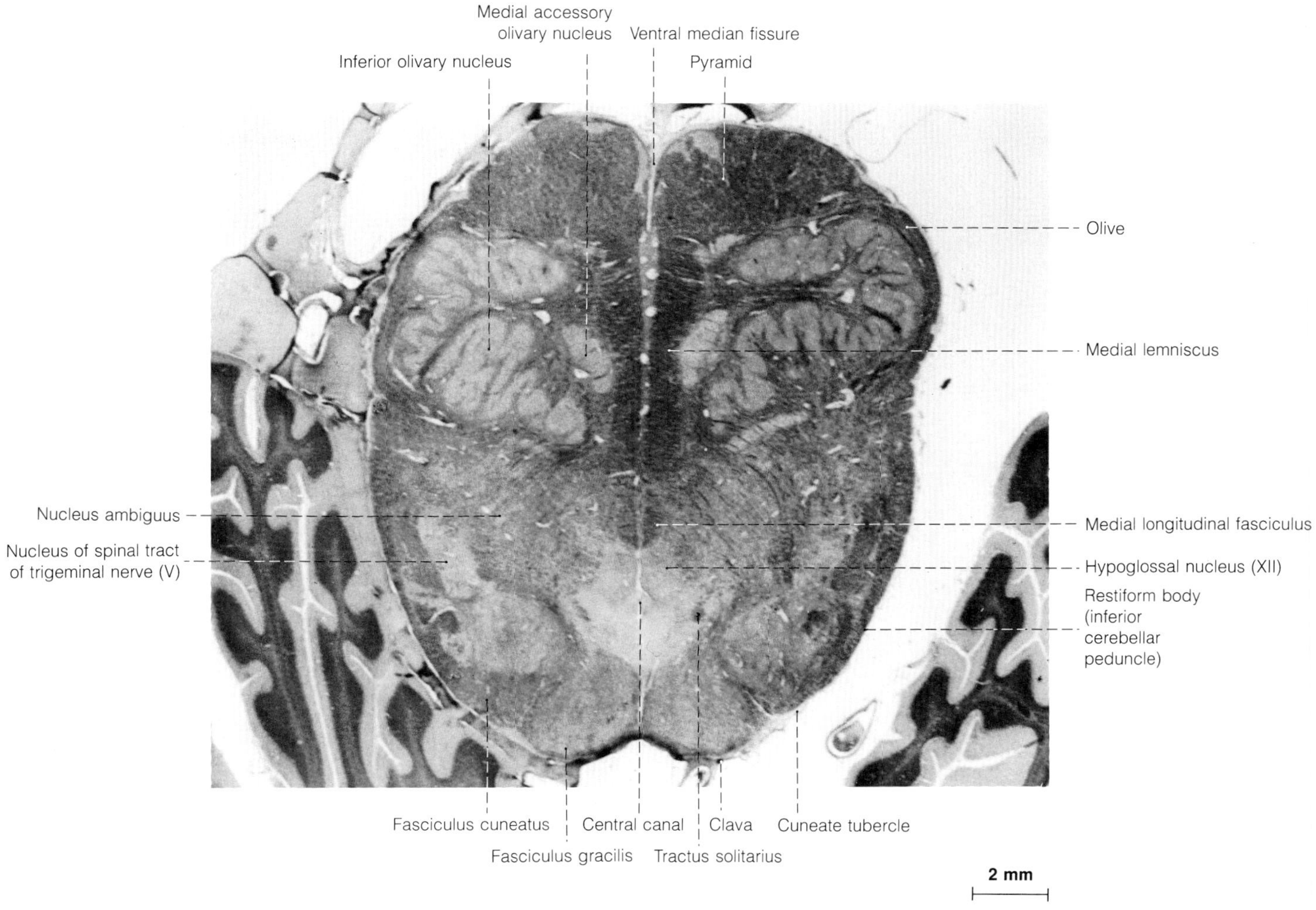
Medial accessory olivary nucleus
Ventral median fissure
Inferior olivary nucleus
Pyramid
Olive
Medial lemniscus
Nucleus ambiguus
Medial longitudinal fasciculus
Nucleus of spinal tract of trigeminal nerve (V)
Hypoglossal nucleus (XII)
Restiform body (inferior cerebellar peduncle)
Fasciculus cuneatus
Central canal
Clava
Cuneate tubercle
Fasciculus gracilis
Tractus solitarius
2 mm

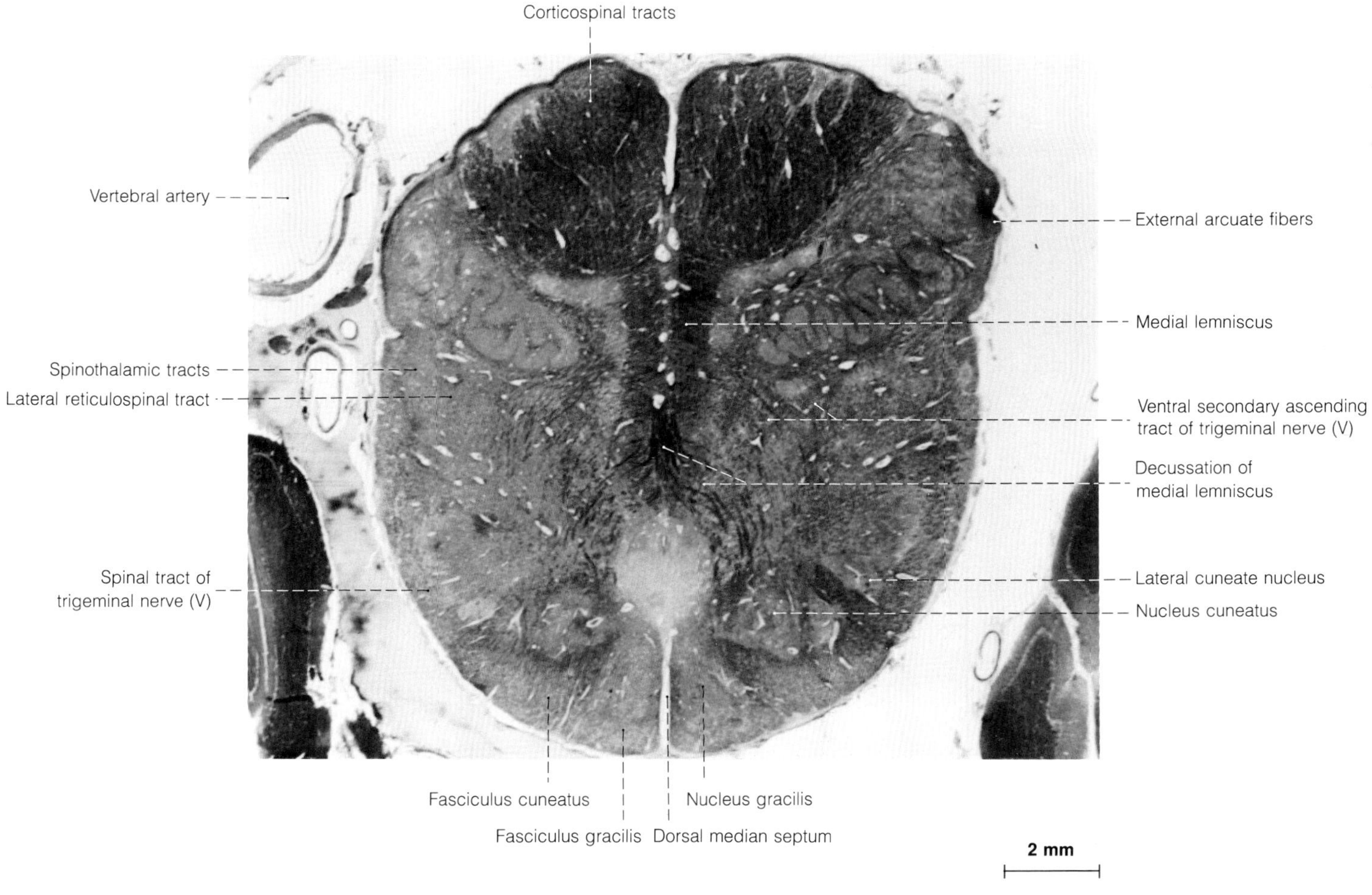
Corticospinal tracts
Vertebral artery
External arcuate fibers
Medial lemniscus
Spinothalamic tracts
Lateral reticulospinal tract
Ventral secondary ascending tract of trigeminal nerve (V)
Decussation of medial lemniscus
Spinal tract of trigeminal nerve (V)
Lateral cuneate nucleus
Nucleus cuneatus
Fasciculus cuneatus
Nucleus gracilis
Fasciculus gracilis
Dorsal median septum
2 mm

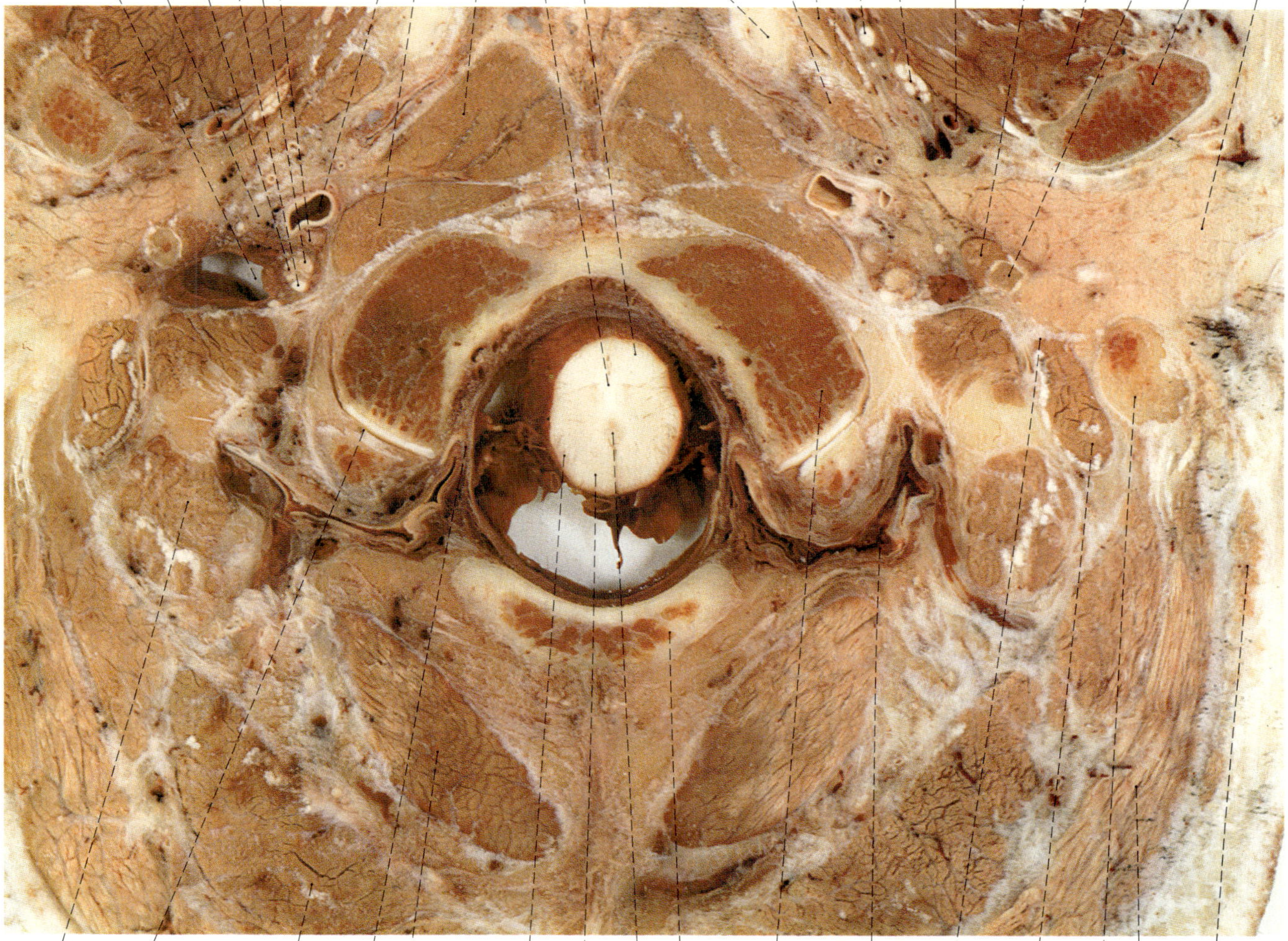

The plane of these microscopic sections is 15° above the IOM line. Within the upper medulla the pyramidal (motor) tracts and olives anteriorly are superior (cephalic) to the posterior (sensory) gracile and cuneate tracts and nuclei. The paths transmitting pain and extremes of temperature and many of the descending visceral paths are laterally located at these levels of the medulla. The plane is also oblique to the decussating medial lemnisci.

Patient CT Scan

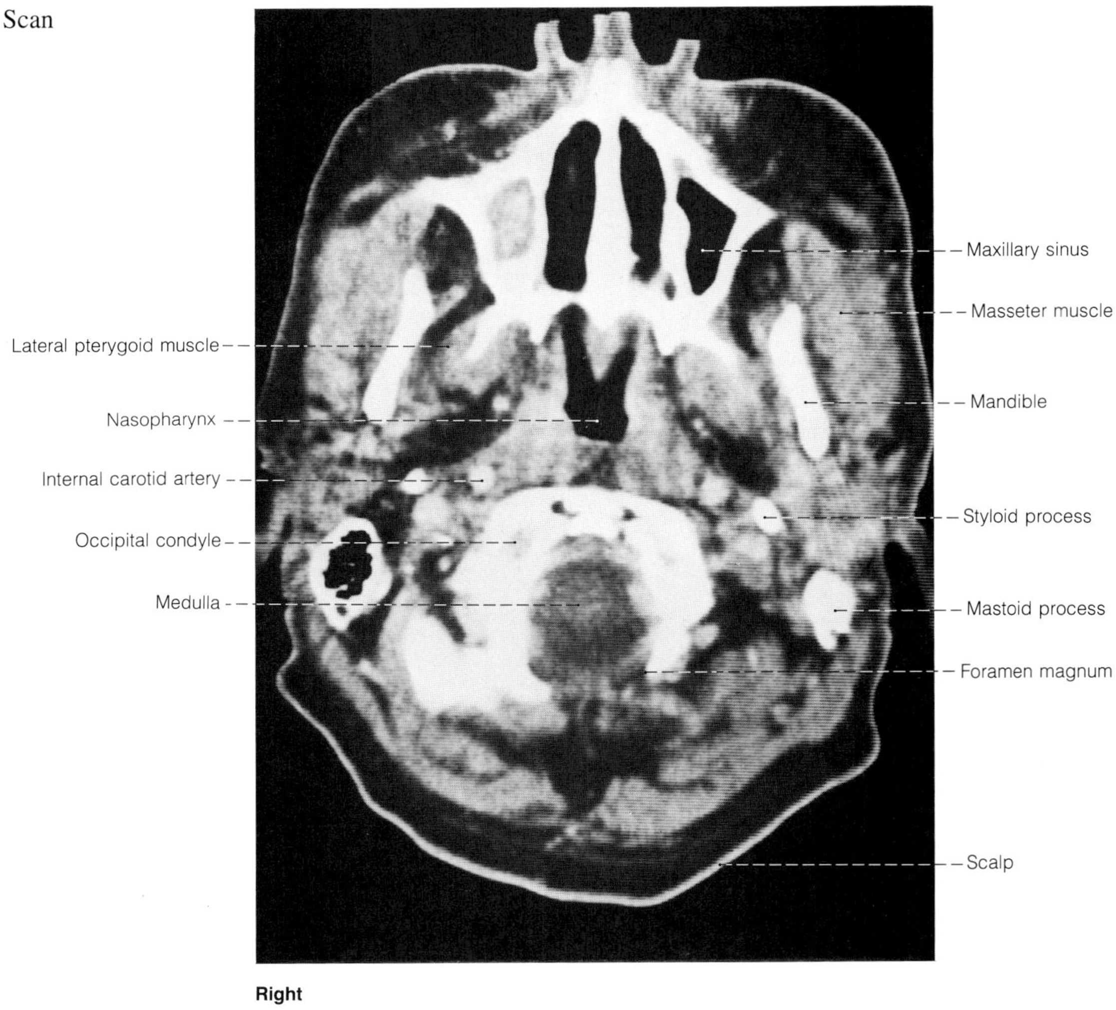

Patient MRI Scan

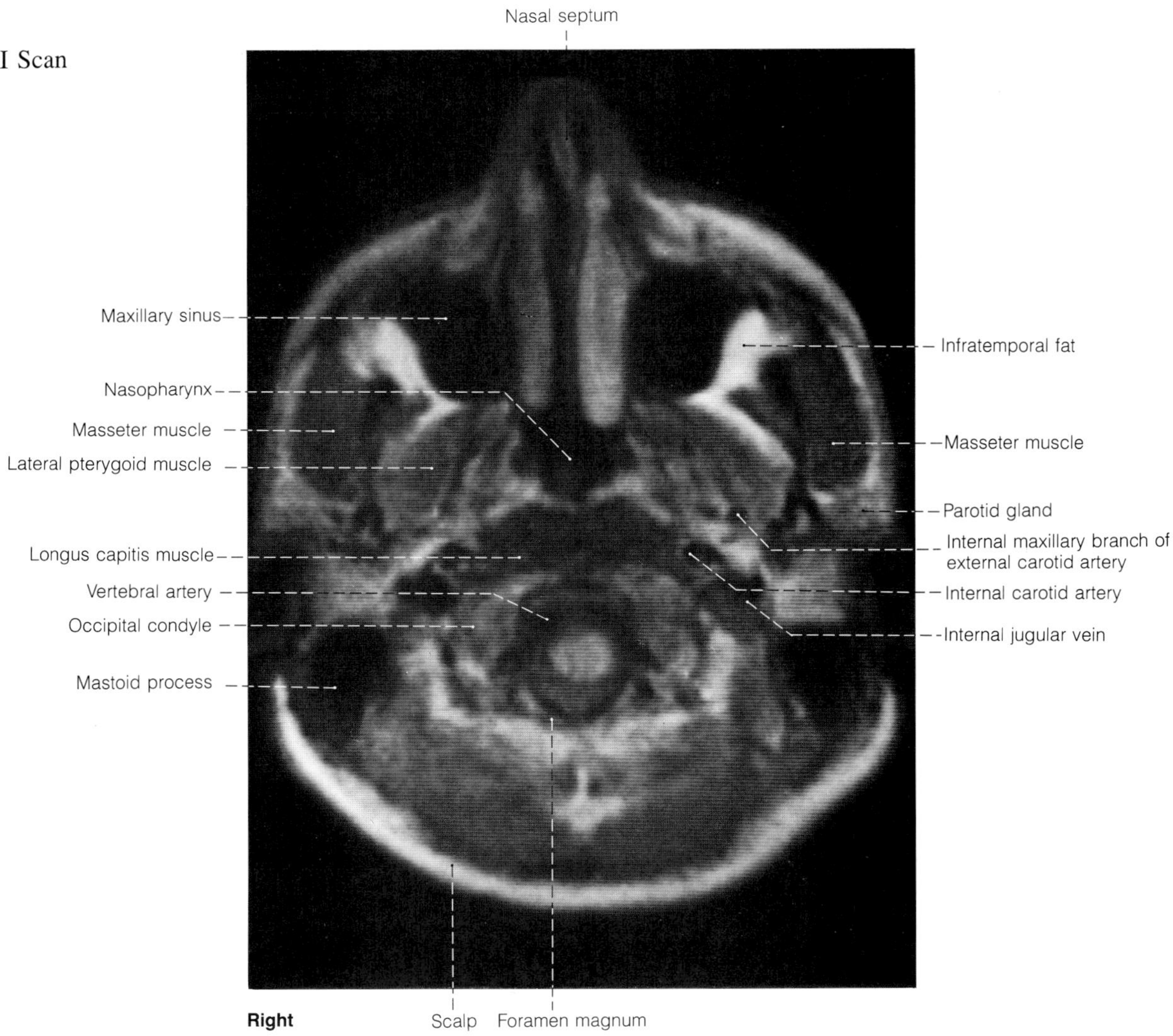

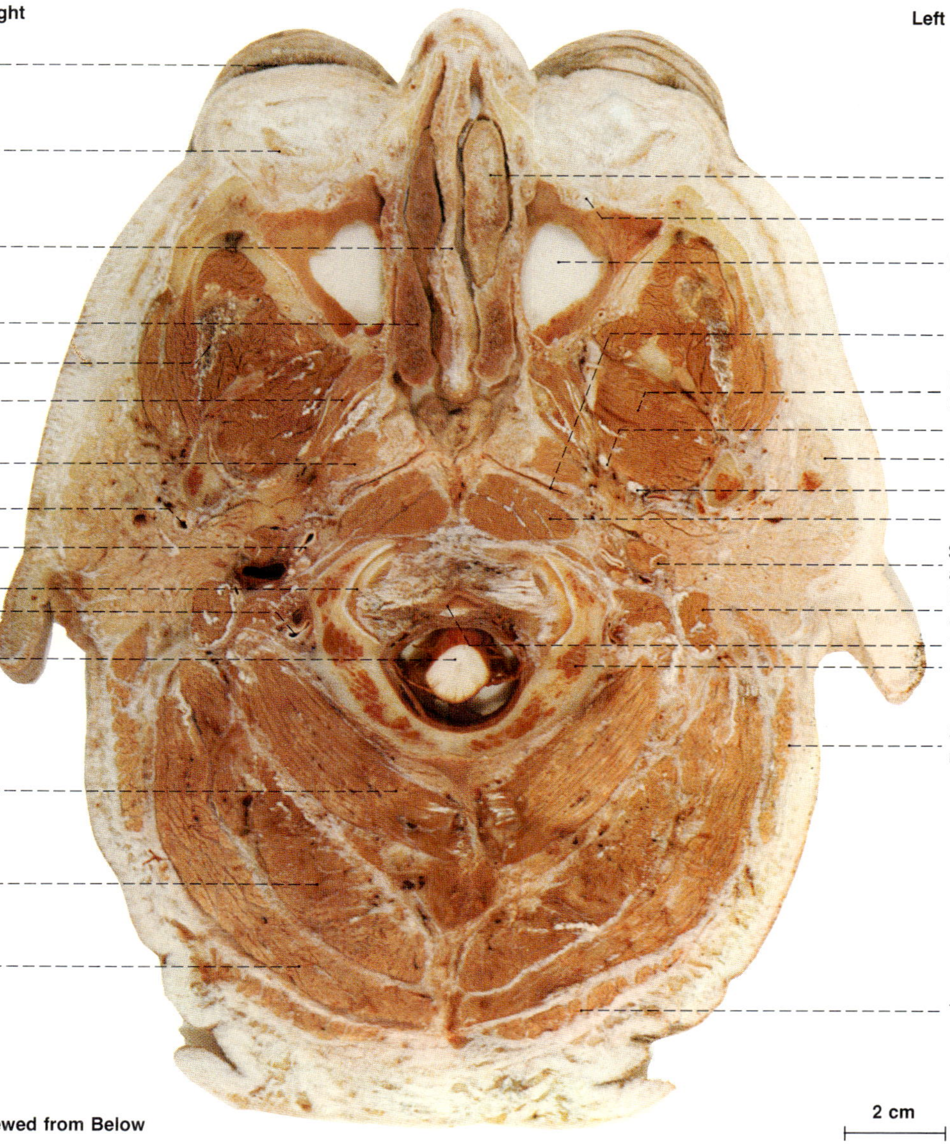

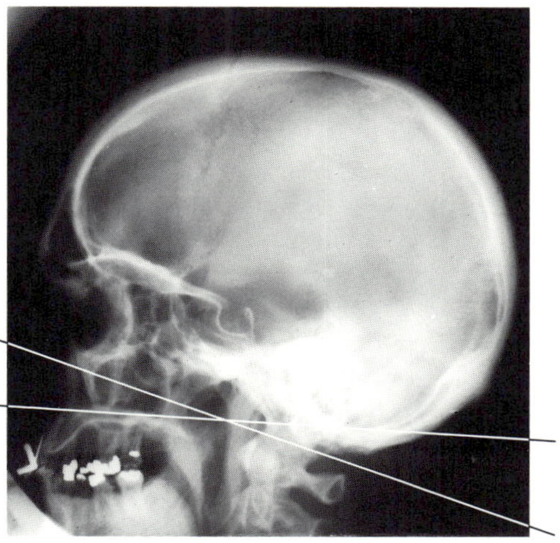

Planes of Sections

The gross anatomical and the CT and MRI sections pass just above the upper tip of the odontoid process (dens) as it articulates with the base of the skull and with the atlas. Such a plane passes through the decussation of the pyramids (motor decussation) at the junction of the medulla and spinal cord.

The parotid gland surrounds the posterior margin of the ramus and neck of the mandible. Visualization of the gland and of the styloid and mastoid processes permits localization of the facial nerve in the region of its pes.

The proximity of the internal carotid artery to the lateral pharyngeal recess (fossa of Rosenmüller) illustrates its precarious position in cases of posterior pharyngeal trauma. It may also be noted that the vertebral artery is less than 2 cm from the internal carotid artery and both are largely antero-lateral to the spinal canal.

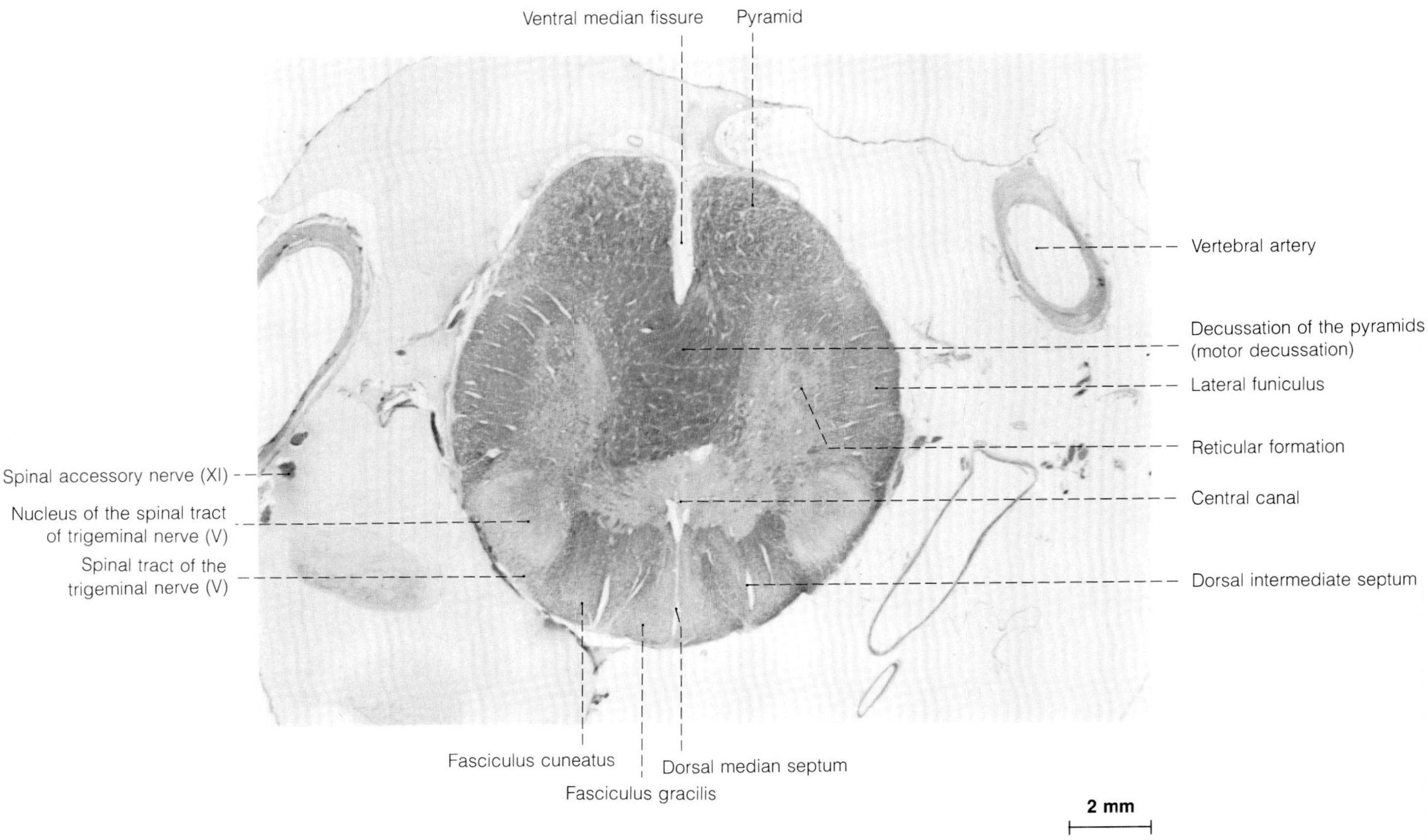
Ventral median fissure
Pyramid
Vertebral artery
Decussation of the pyramids (motor decussation)
Lateral funiculus
Reticular formation
Central canal
Dorsal intermediate septum
Spinal accessory nerve (XI)
Nucleus of the spinal tract of trigeminal nerve (V)
Spinal tract of the trigeminal nerve (V)
Fasciculus cuneatus
Dorsal median septum
Fasciculus gracilis
2 mm

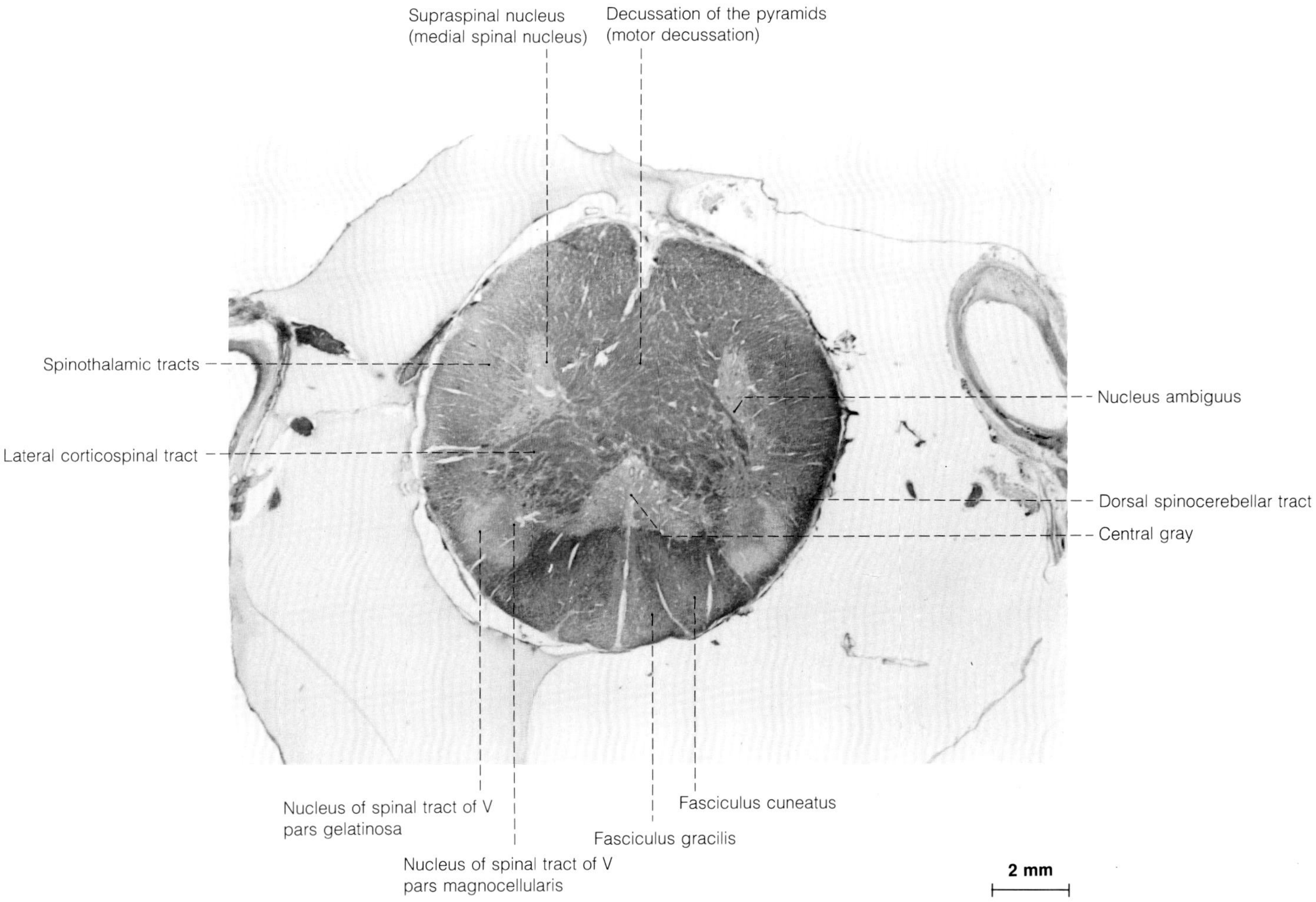
Supraspinal nucleus (medial spinal nucleus)
Decussation of the pyramids (motor decussation)
Spinothalamic tracts
Lateral corticospinal tract
Nucleus ambiguus
Dorsal spinocerebellar tract
Central gray
Nucleus of spinal tract of V pars gelatinosa
Fasciculus cuneatus
Fasciculus gracilis
Nucleus of spinal tract of V pars magnocellularis
2 mm

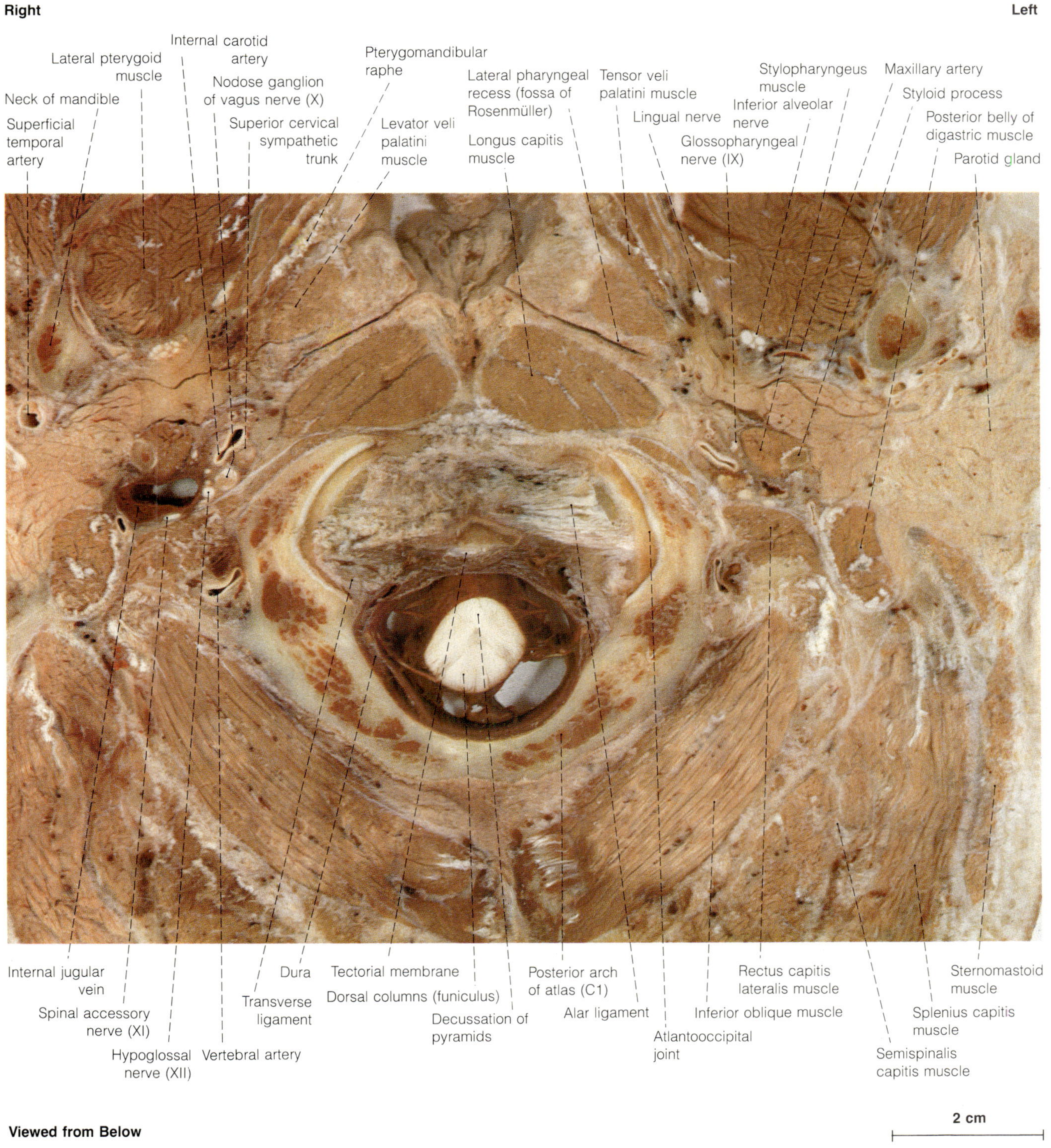

These sections are through the highest part of the pyramidal (motor) decussation and are mostly within the posterior fossa. The uppermost crossing axons of the lateral corticospinal tract are destined for the cervical enlargement for relay to the brachial plexus (upper extremity).

The nucleus of the spinal tract of the trigeminal nerve (V) is relatively large at these levels and is just deep to the superficial spinal tract. Although they are not differentiated on CT, their location can be determined on a silhouette of the cord. The ventral supraspinal nucleus contains motor neurons whose axons enter the C1 spinal nerve, but a dorsal root may be absent from the first cervical nerve. The axons of the nucleus ambiguus at these levels are distributed via the pharyngeal and laryngeal branches of the vagus nerve (X). Since these roots are sometimes considered to be a part of the bulbar accessory nerve (XI), their peripheral distribution may then be described as via branches of the accessory nerve – an academic distinction.

Odontoid

Patient CT Scan

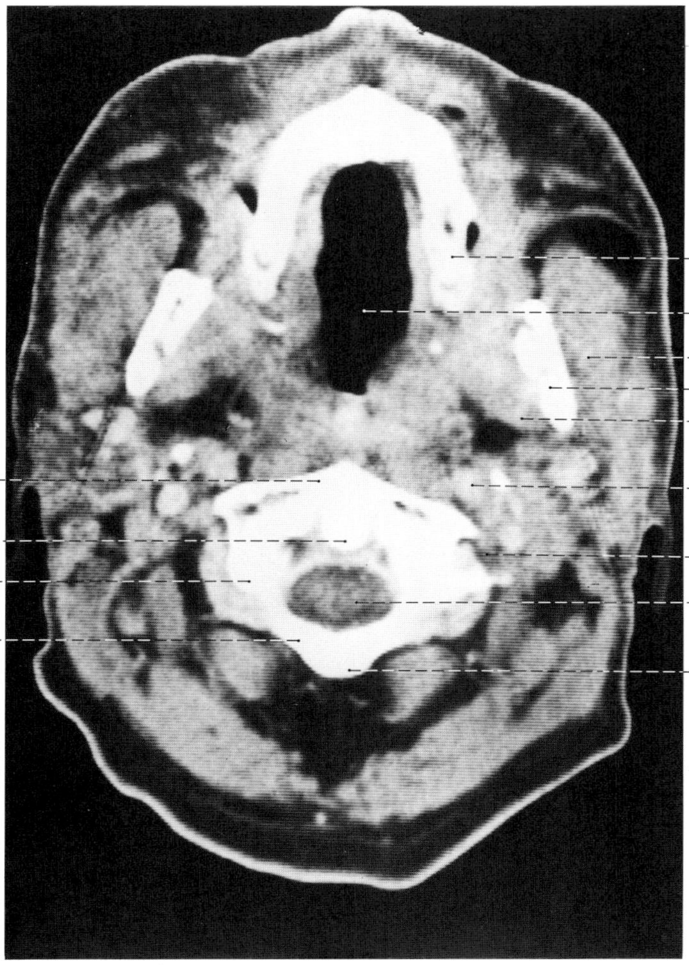

Patient CT Scan

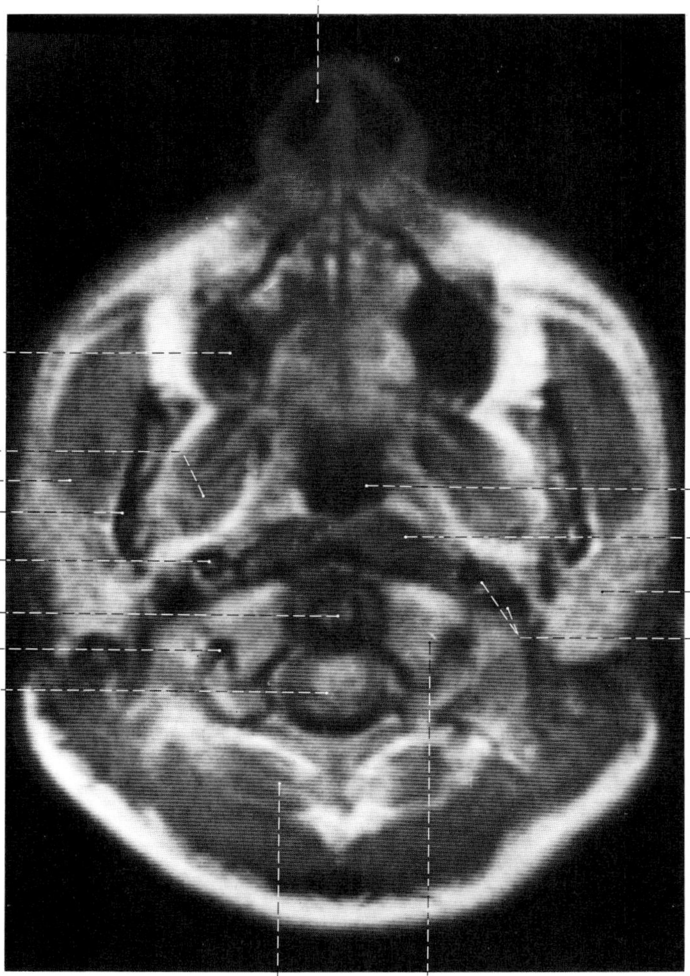

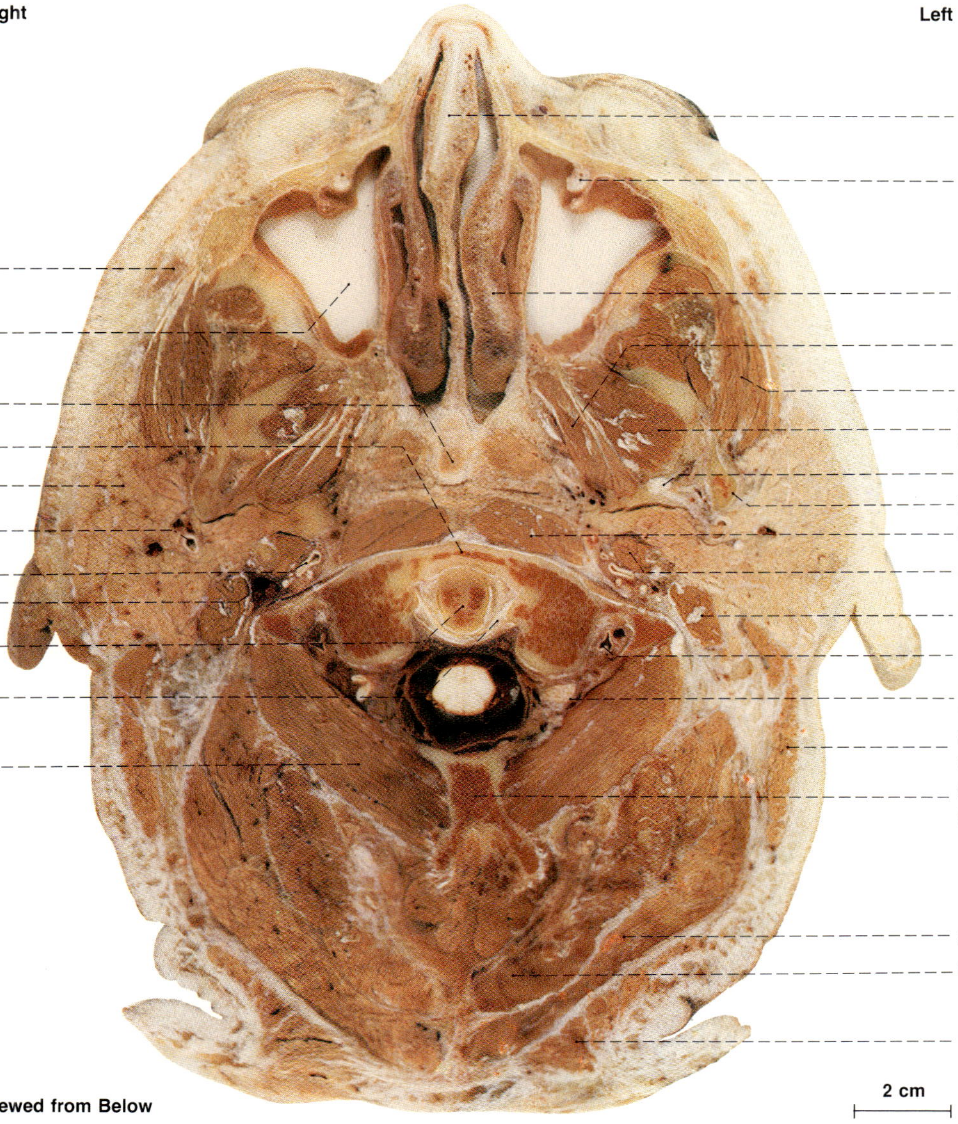

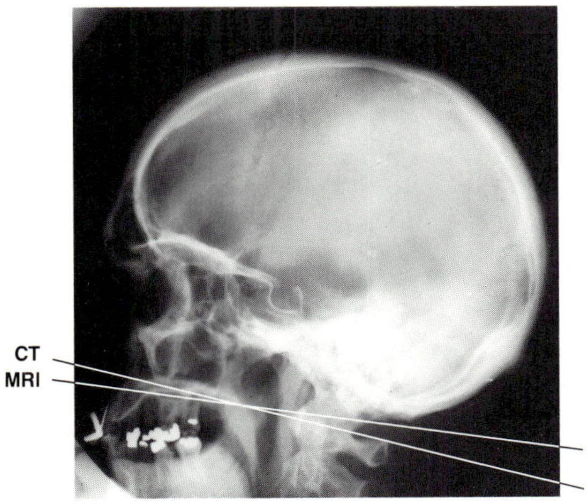

Planes of Sections

The relatively large subarachnoid space in the cervical region is well illustrated at this level. The lower medulla occupies only about ½ to ⅔ of the subarachnoid space and is largely ventrally located. C1-2 punctures are performed at this level in a transverse (lateral) approach and the tip of the needle introduced into the dorsal portion of the subarachnoid space.

In the facial region, the medial and lateral pterygoid plates are noted with their attaching muscles. The infraorbital nerve is seen exiting the roof of the maxillary sinus to provide cutaneous innervation over the maxilla; an artery, a terminal branch of the internal maxillary, accompanies the nerve.

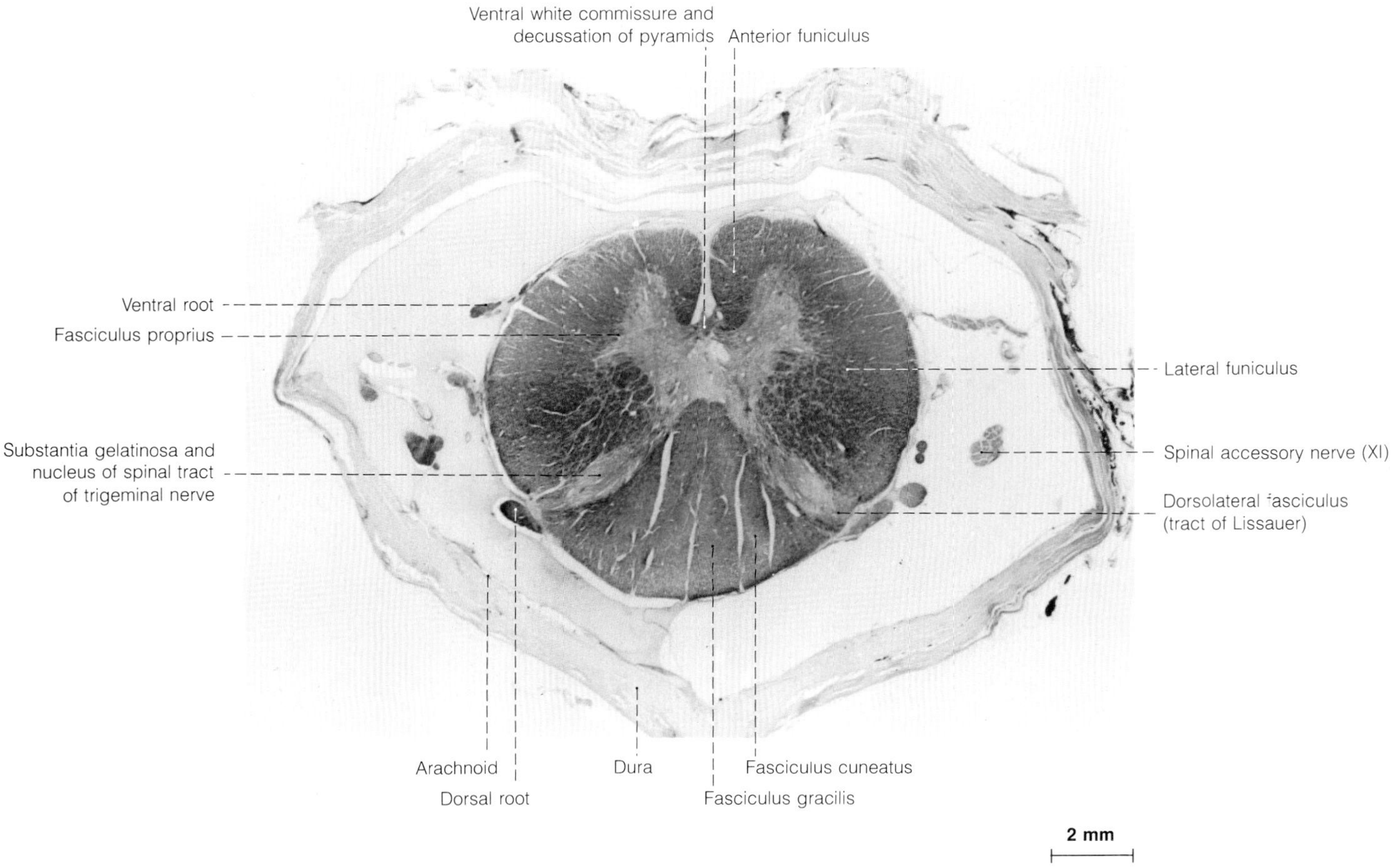
Ventral white commissure and decussation of pyramids
Anterior funiculus
Ventral root
Fasciculus proprius
Substantia gelatinosa and nucleus of spinal tract of trigeminal nerve
Lateral funiculus
Spinal accessory nerve (XI)
Dorsolateral fasciculus (tract of Lissauer)
Arachnoid
Dorsal root
Dura
Fasciculus cuneatus
Fasciculus gracilis
2 mm

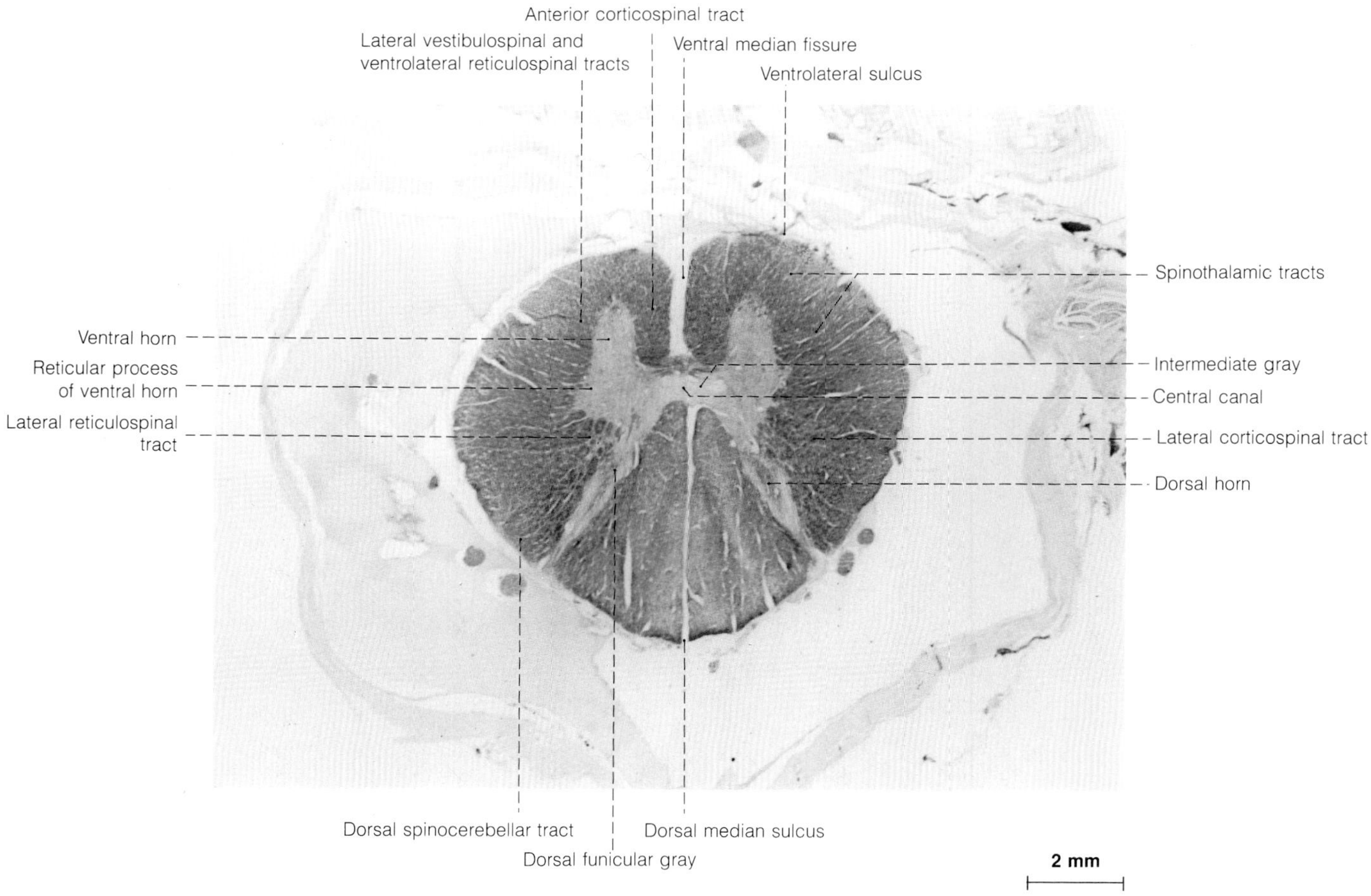
Anterior corticospinal tract
Lateral vestibulospinal and ventrolateral reticulospinal tracts
Ventral median fissure
Ventrolateral sulcus
Spinothalamic tracts
Ventral horn
Reticular process of ventral horn
Lateral reticulospinal tract
Intermediate gray
Central canal
Lateral corticospinal tract
Dorsal horn
Dorsal spinocerebellar tract
Dorsal median sulcus
Dorsal funicular gray
2 mm

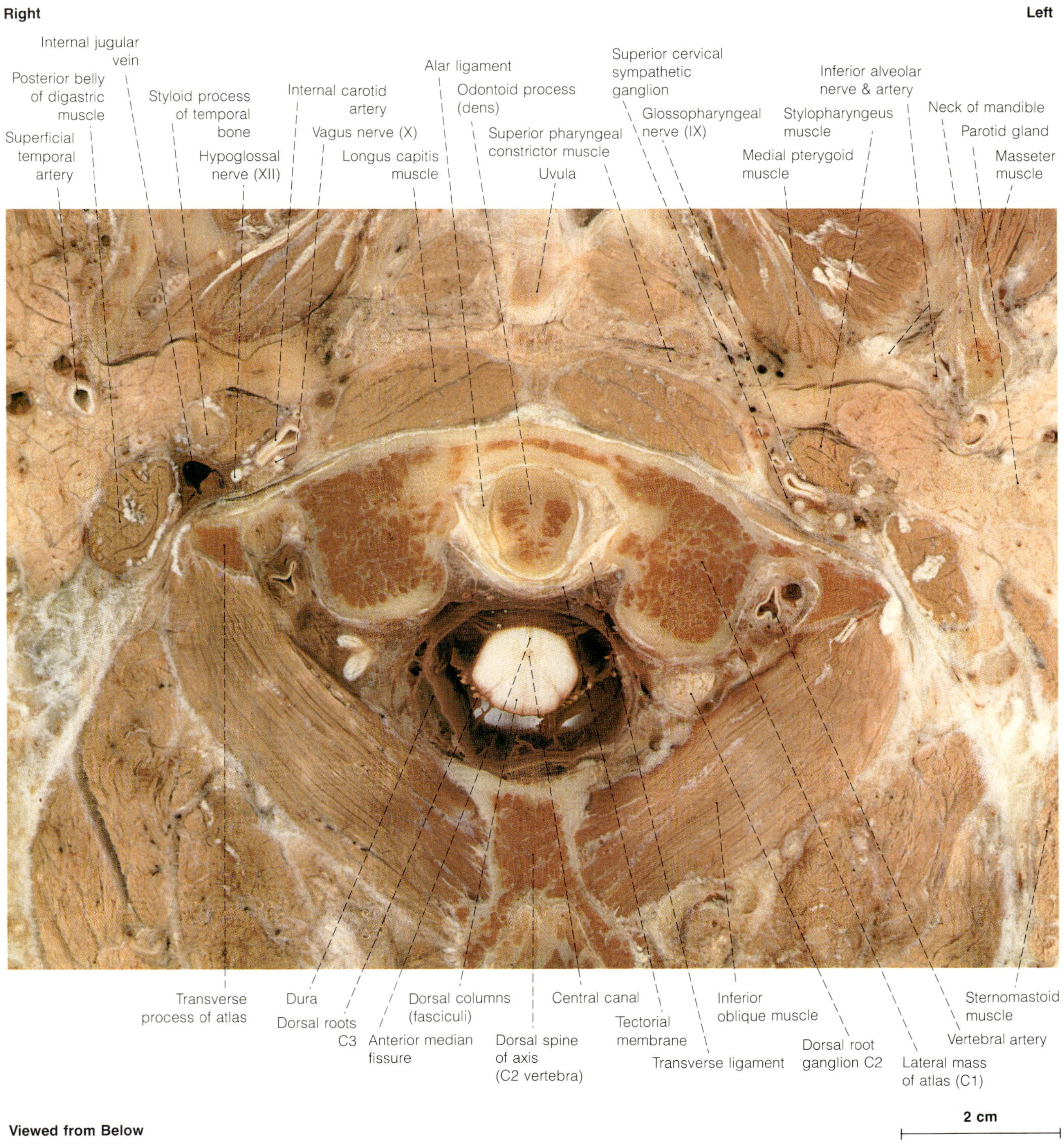

Microscopic sections through the C1-C2 spinal cord are somewhat similar to upper thoracic sections. These cervical sections differ in: (1) lack of the nucleus dorsalis; (2) greater size of the substantia gelatinosa and dorsal funicular gray (nucleus of the spinal tract of the trigeminal); and (3) presence of the lateral reticular nucleus (spinal accessory) instead of a lateral horn (autonomic intermediolateral nucleus).

The lowest descending pyramidal tract decussation involves those axons destined for the lumbosacral cord to influence the lower extremity. As these fibers decussate, they lie first anterior to and then lateral to those axons which decussated higher.

Patient CT Scan

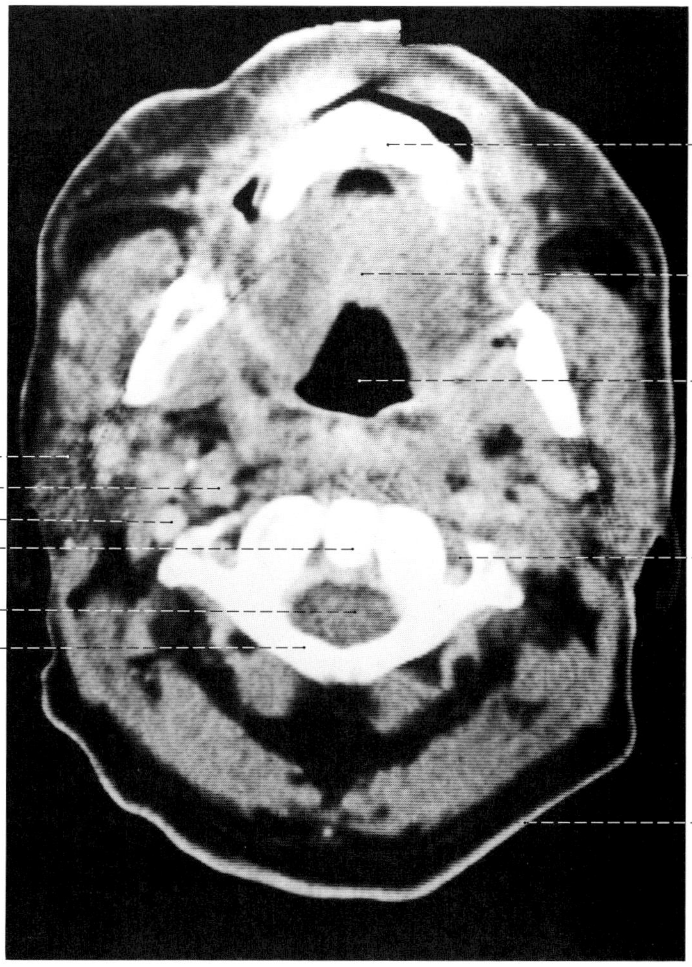

Patient MRI Scan

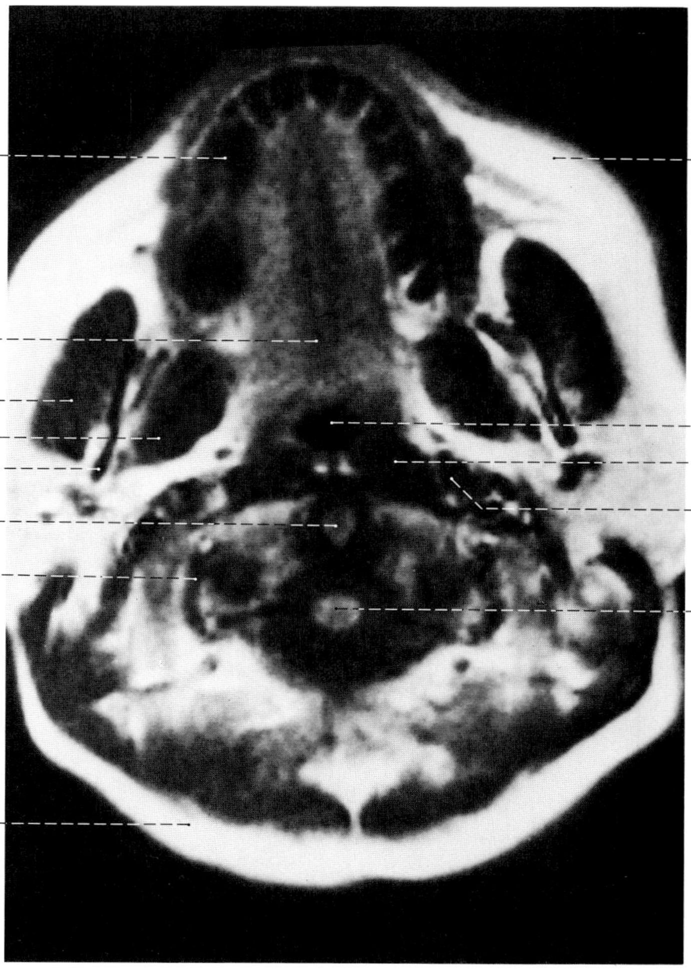

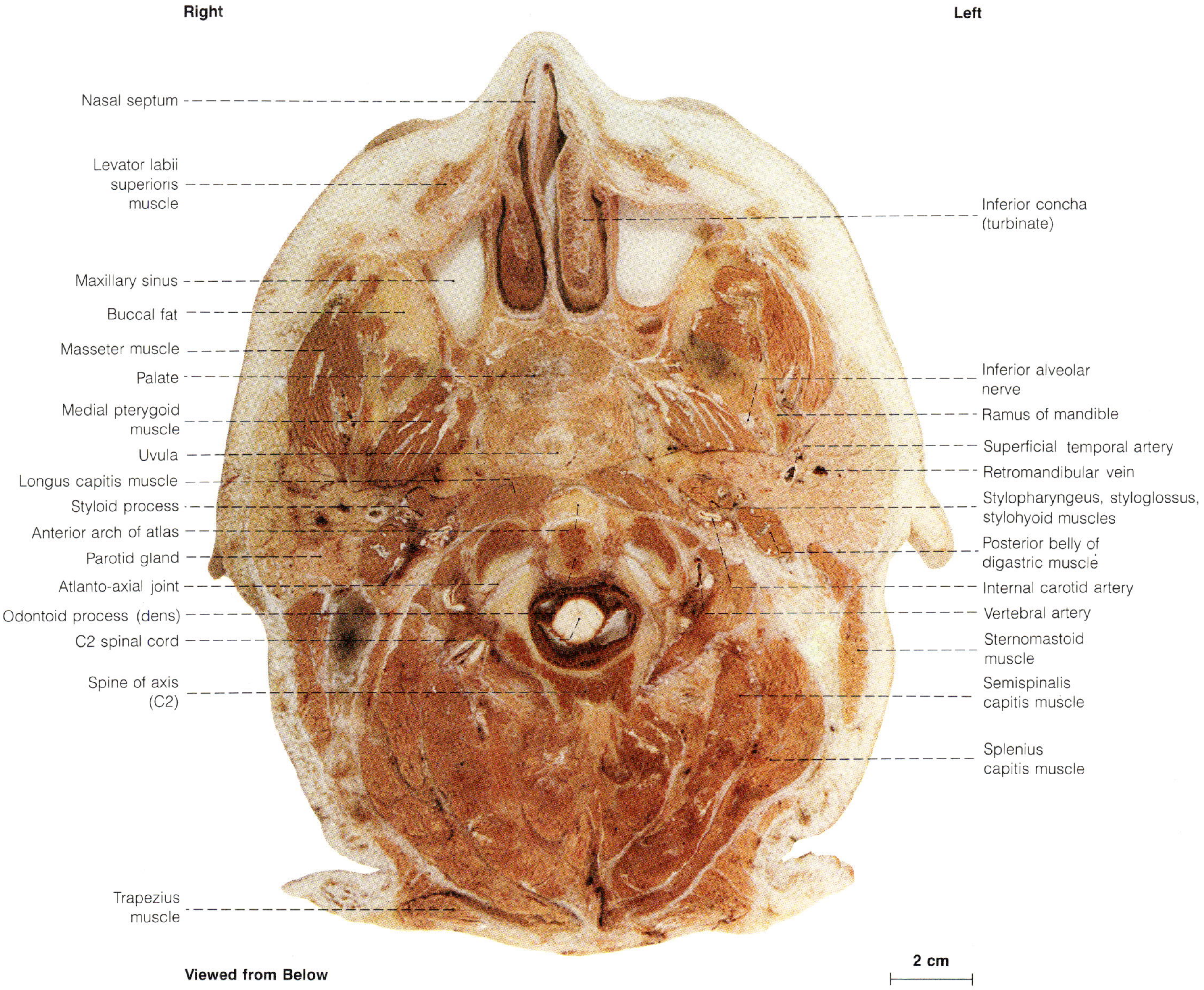

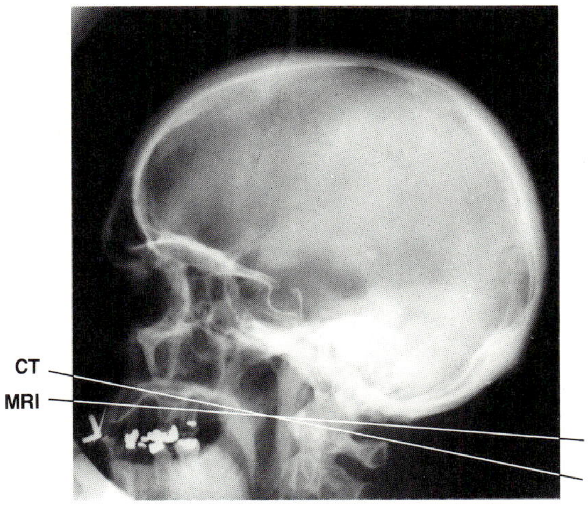

Planes of Sections

The odontoid process of C2 vertebra is evident at this level along with soft tissue structures such as the uvula, parotid gland and palate. In the cord at the C2 level, the characteristic pattern of central grey and white matter pathways is evident on the MRI scan but is seen more clearly in the subsequent stained histological sections.

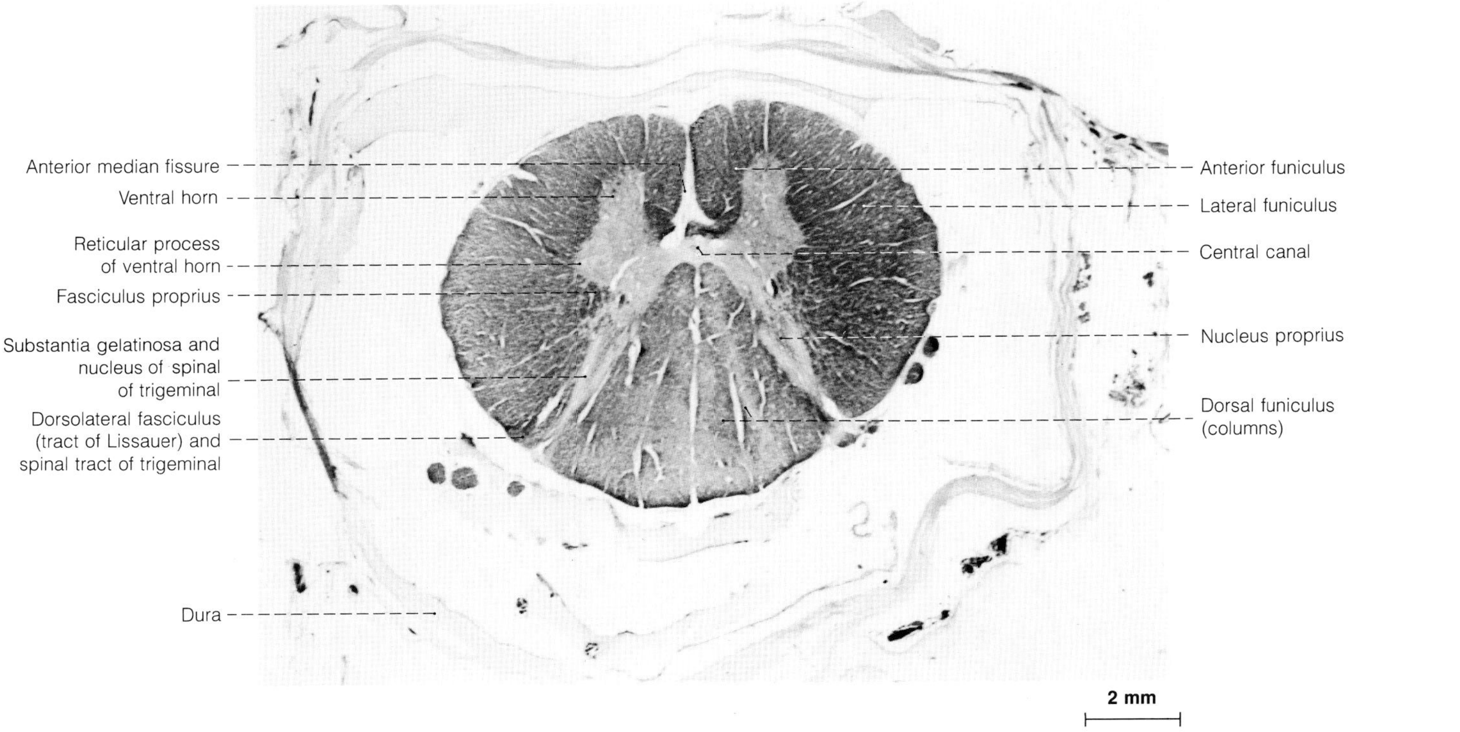
Anterior median fissure
Ventral horn
Reticular process
of ventral horn
Fasciculus proprius
Substantia gelatinosa and
nucleus of spinal
of trigeminal
Dorsolateral fasciculus
(tract of Lissauer) and
spinal tract of trigeminal
Dura
Anterior funiculus
Lateral funiculus
Central canal
Nucleus proprius
Dorsal funiculus
(columns)
2 mm

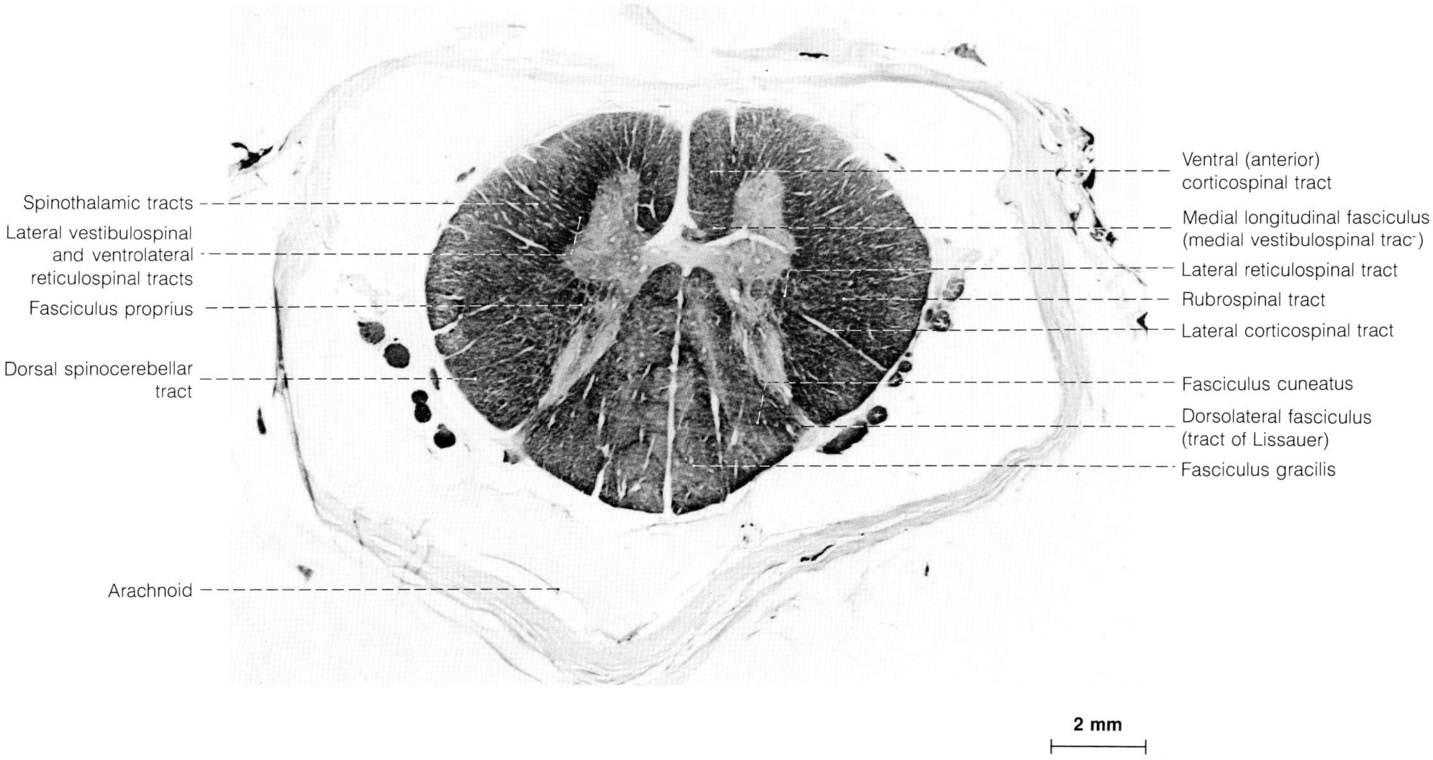
Spinothalamic tracts
Lateral vestibulospinal
and ventrolateral
reticulospinal tracts
Fasciculus proprius
Dorsal spinocerebellar
tract
Arachnoid
Ventral (anterior)
corticospinal tract
Medial longitudinal fasciculus
(medial vestibulospinal trac-)
Lateral reticulospinal tract
Rubrospinal tract
Lateral corticospinal tract
Fasciculus cuneatus
Dorsolateral fasciculus
(tract of Lissauer)
Fasciculus gracilis
2 mm

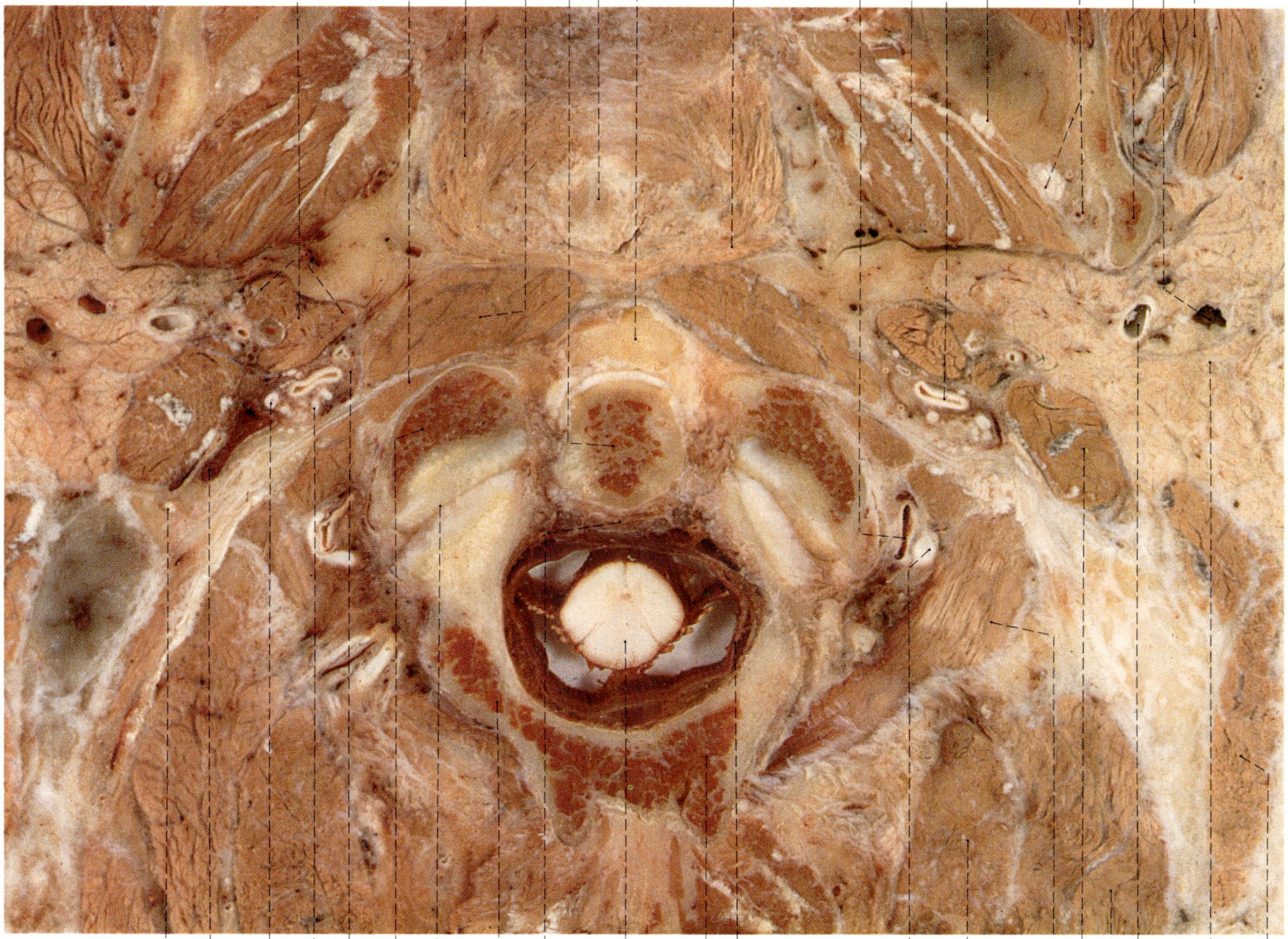

The sensory component of the C2 spinal nerve is distributed largely to the back of the head. These peripheral axons are contiguous with the cutaneous branches of the trigeminal nerve on the anterior scalp. Likewise, the tract of Lissauer and spinal tract of the trigeminal and their related nuclei overlap at these levels centrally.

Visceral sensory impulses ascend bilaterally as well as contralaterally in the lateral spinothalamic tracts. The lateral spinothalamic tract is located in the lateral funiculus ventral to the dentate ligament and is intermingled at these levels with the ventrolateral reticulospinal tract which regulates respiration during sleep.

Patient CT Scan

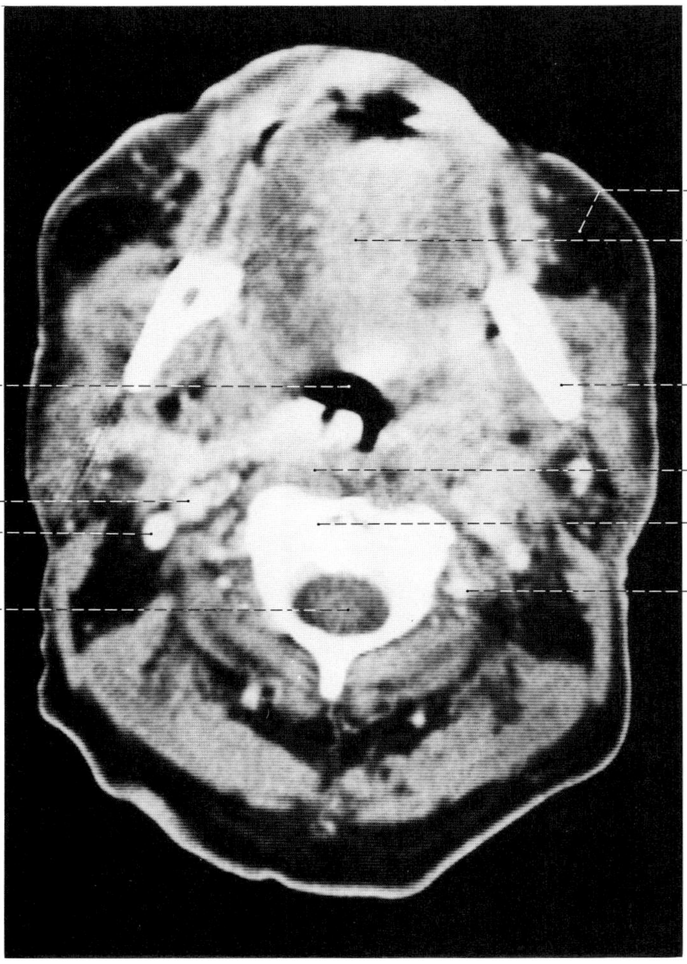

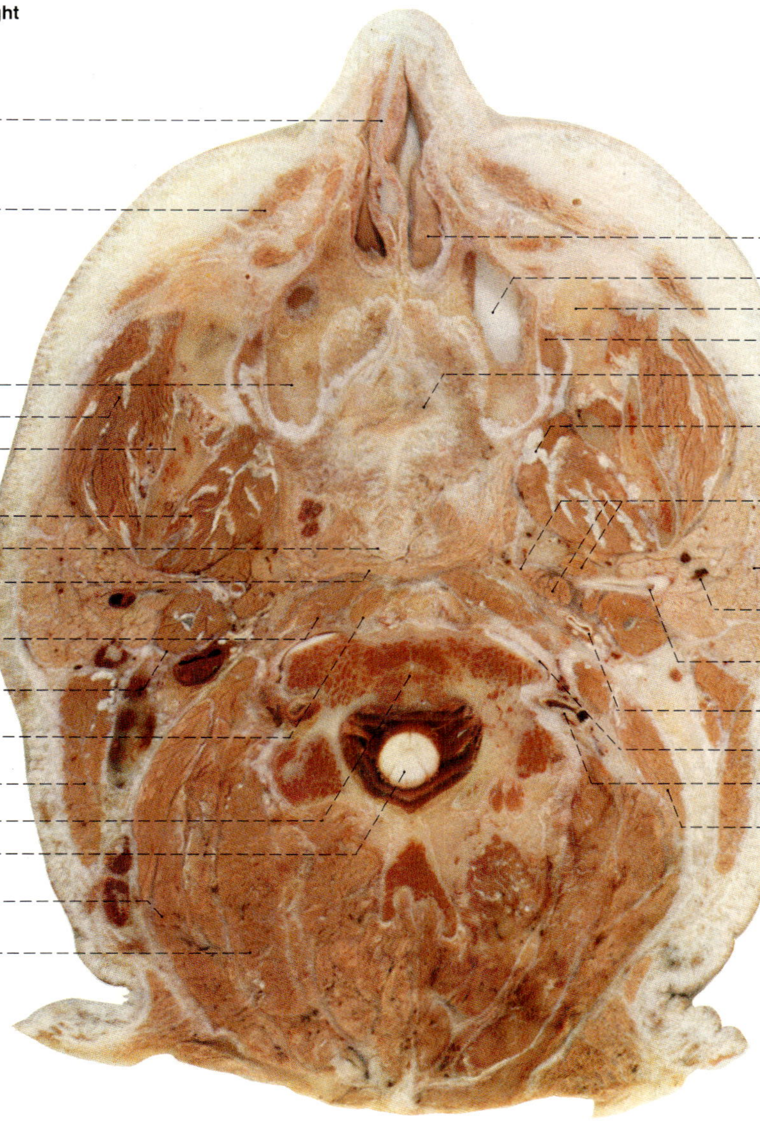

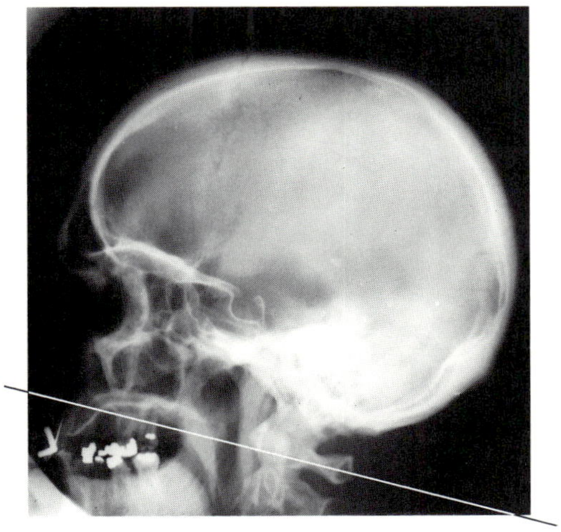

Plane of Sections

At the level of the C3 cord, the C2–3 facet joint is well visualized on either side of the spinal canal in a posterolateral position on the anatomical preparation. The posterior belly of the digastric muscle lies at this level, an important landmark since a digastric lymph node in this area might be an important clue to metastases from head and neck carcinoma.

The current method of MRI scanning does not usually include axial images of the mid-cervical spine with studies of the head. The CT image may be compared with the gross anatomical specimen; however, the more common CT procedure for examination of the spine is a horizontal section such as illustrated in the section on the cervical spine (pages 255-288).

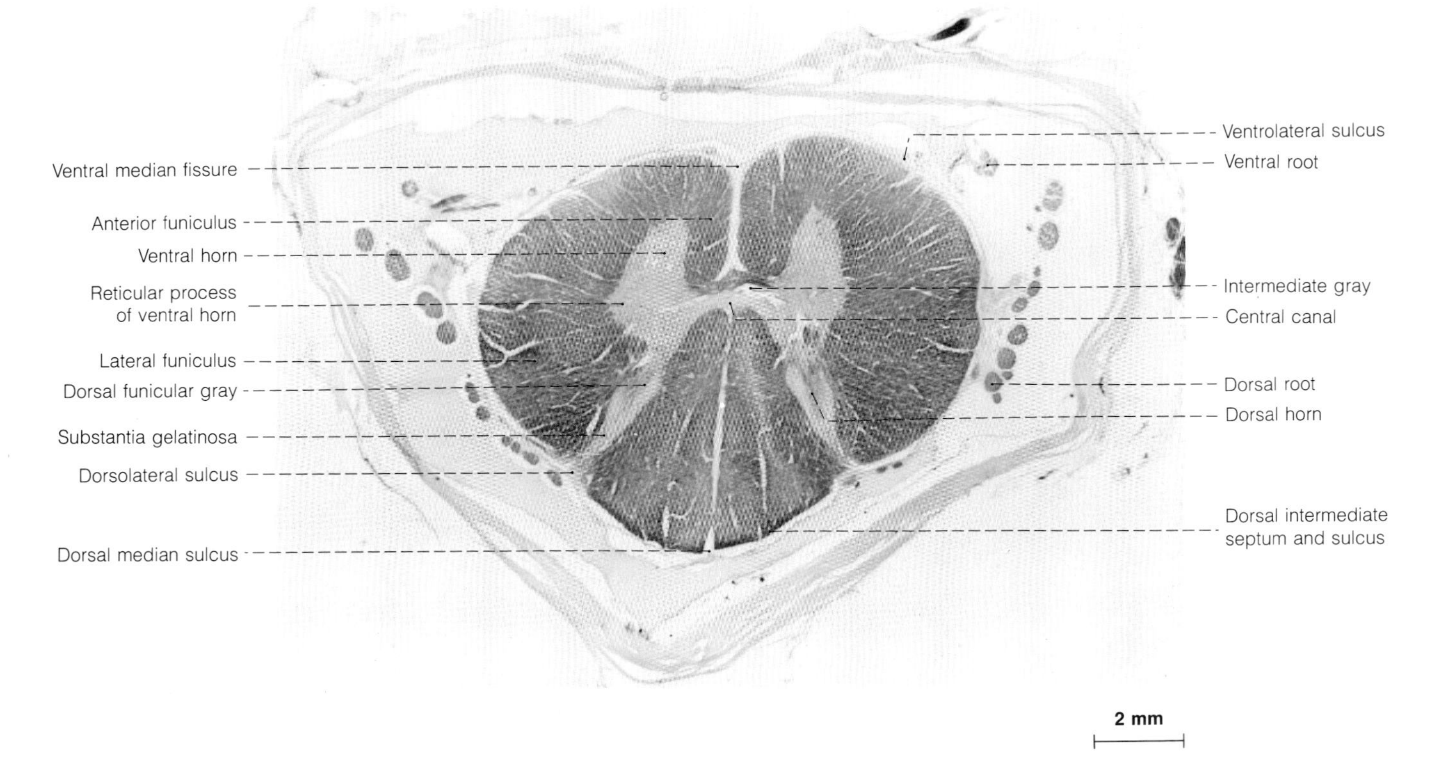
Ventral median fissure
Anterior funiculus
Ventral horn
Reticular process of ventral horn
Lateral funiculus
Dorsal funicular gray
Substantia gelatinosa
Dorsolateral sulcus
Dorsal median sulcus
Ventrolateral sulcus
Ventral root
Intermediate gray
Central canal
Dorsal root
Dorsal horn
Dorsal intermediate septum and sulcus
2 mm

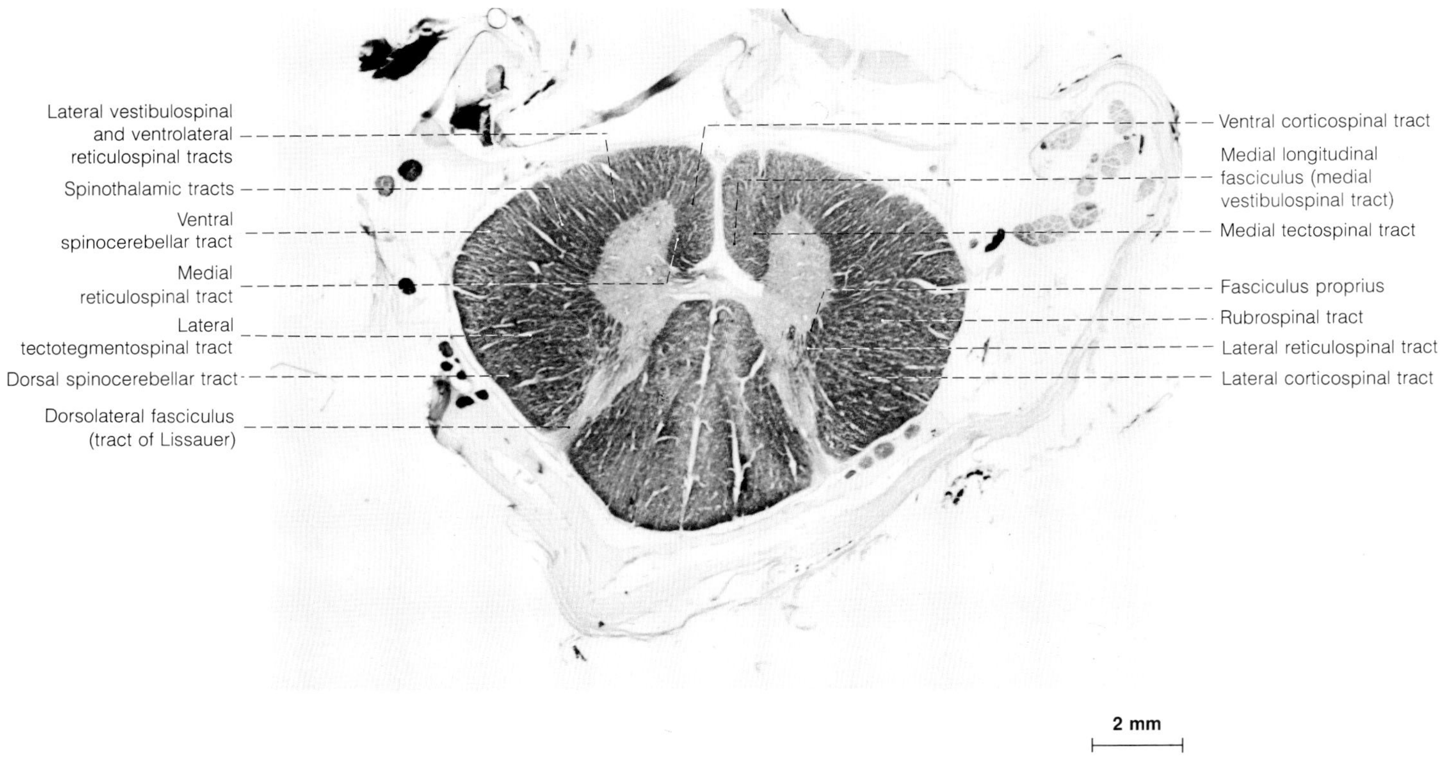
Lateral vestibulospinal and ventrolateral reticulospinal tracts
Spinothalamic tracts
Ventral spinocerebellar tract
Medial reticulospinal tract
Lateral tectotegmentospinal tract
Dorsal spinocerebellar tract
Dorsolateral fasciculus (tract of Lissauer)
Ventral corticospinal tract
Medial longitudinal fasciculus (medial vestibulospinal tract)
Medial tectospinal tract
Fasciculus proprius
Rubrospinal tract
Lateral reticulospinal tract
Lateral corticospinal tract
2 mm

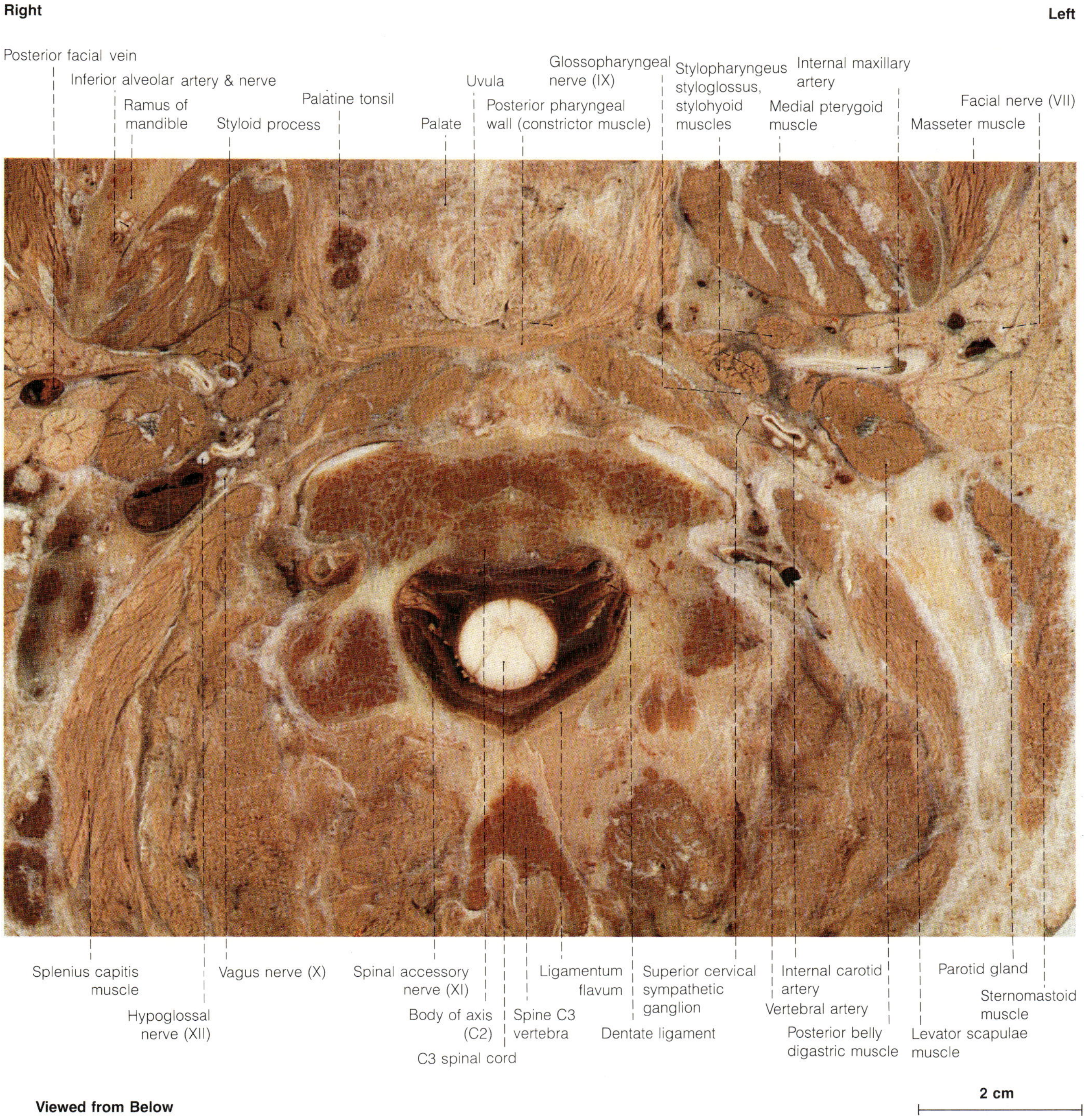

The peripheral fibers of the C3 nerve are distributed in part to the diaphragm via the phrenic nerve. The increase in size in the ventral horn over C1-C2 levels is a reflection of this larger peripheral contribution. The sensory fibers entering these dorsal roots are the processes of neurons distributed in part through the supraclavicular nerves. The ventral white commissure contains decussating spinothalamic projections. Few (if any) axons decussate dorsal to the central canal.

In the anatomical section, the muscles arising from the styloid process are indicated. The intimate relationship of the glossopharyngeal nerve and stylopharyngeus muscle (which it innervates) to the pharyngeal wall and tonsils illustrates the precarious position of the nerve during tonsillectomy.

Patient CT Scan

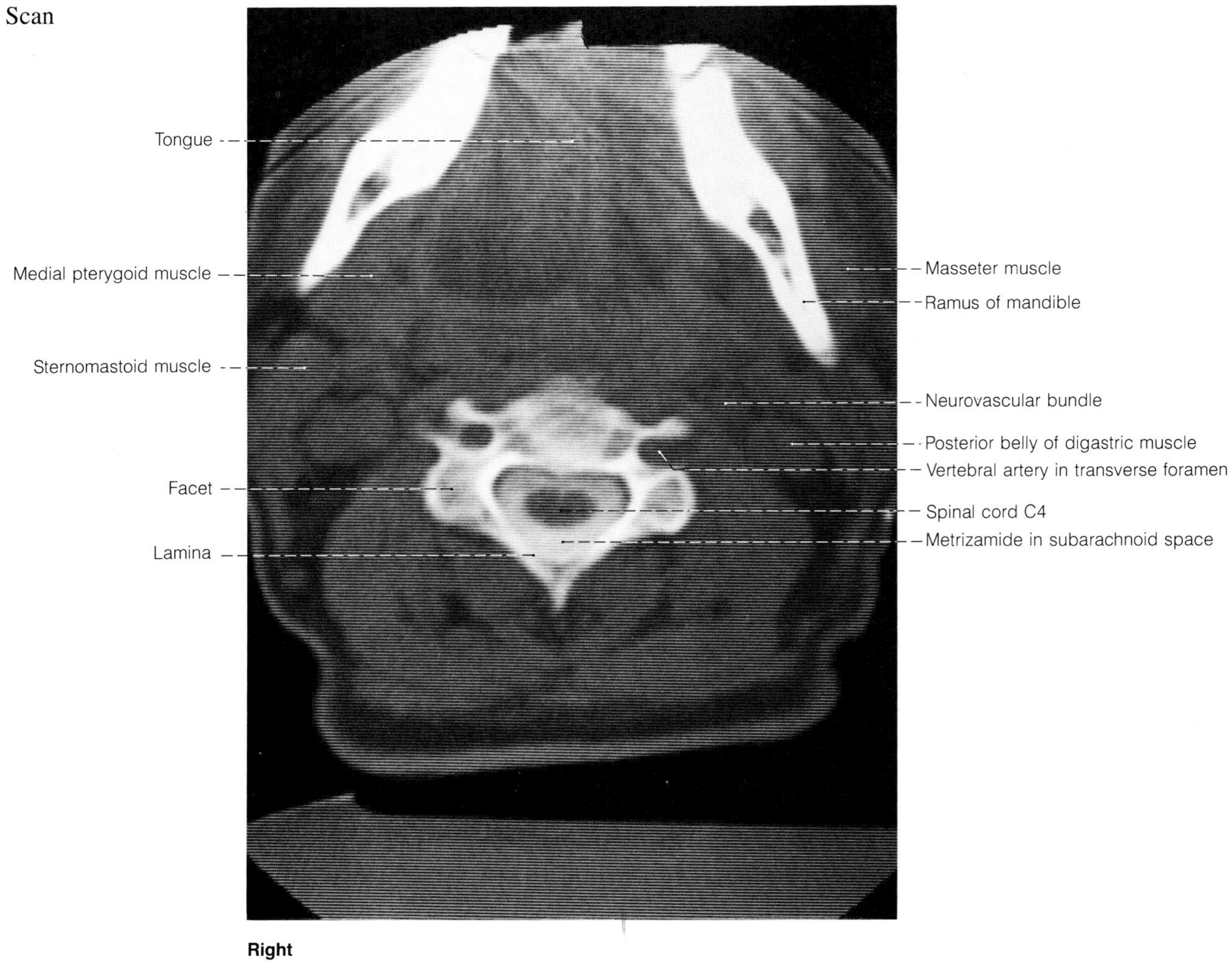

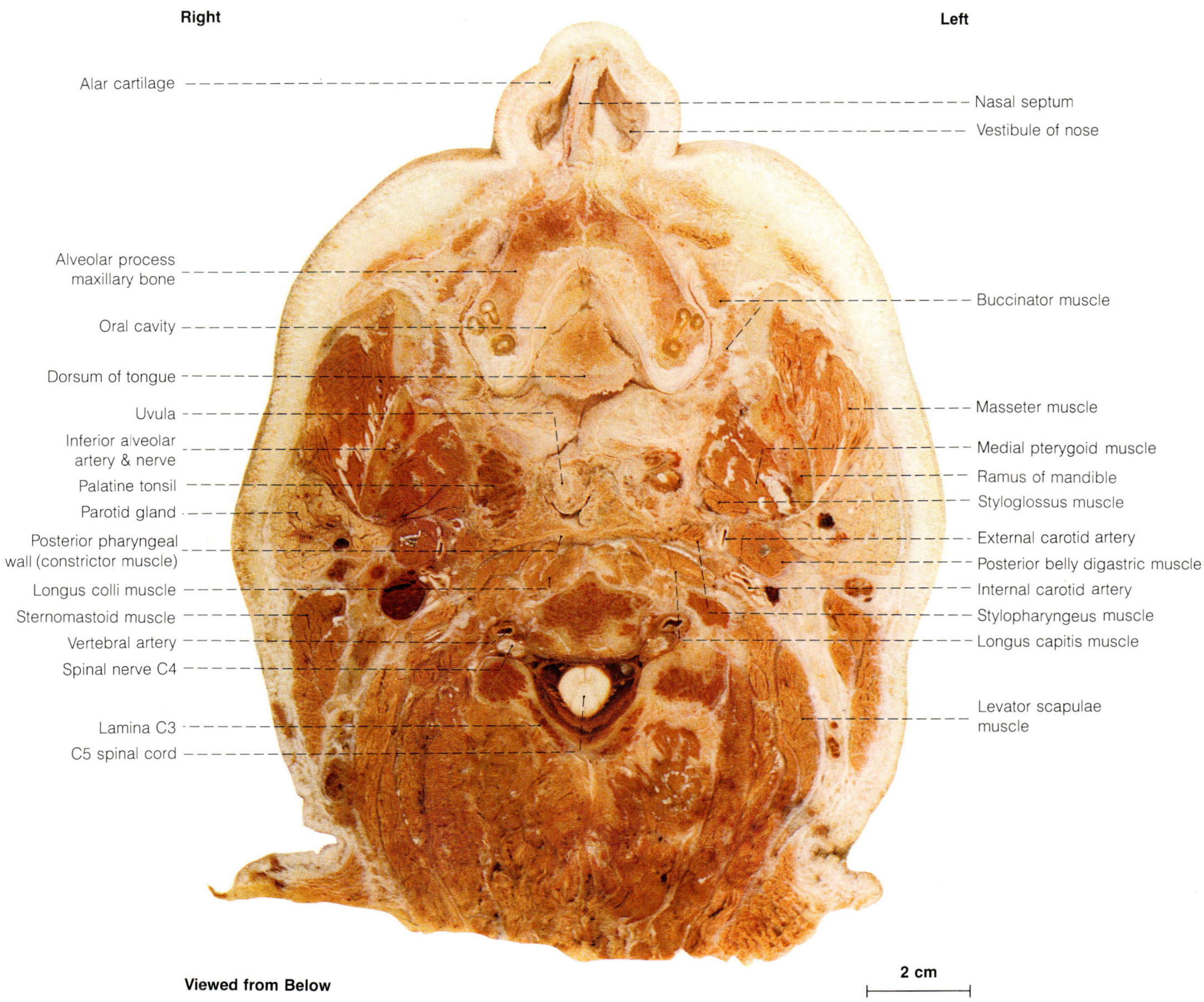

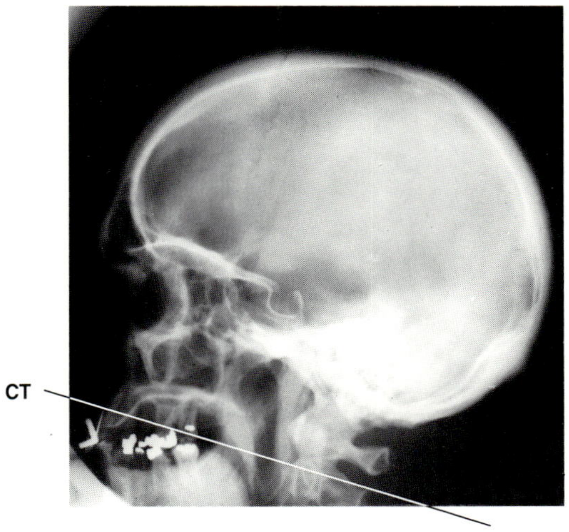

Plane of Section

In this axial section, the body of the mandible dominates the anterior anatomy. Beneath the sternocleidomastoids lie the neurovascular bundles, bilaterally consisting of the internal jugular veins and carotid arteries, sometimes better seen on CT with contrast drip. On the CT slice, metrizamide is present in the subarachnoid space and nicely outlines the cervical cord of about the C4-C5 level. A ventral median fissure is noted in the cord.

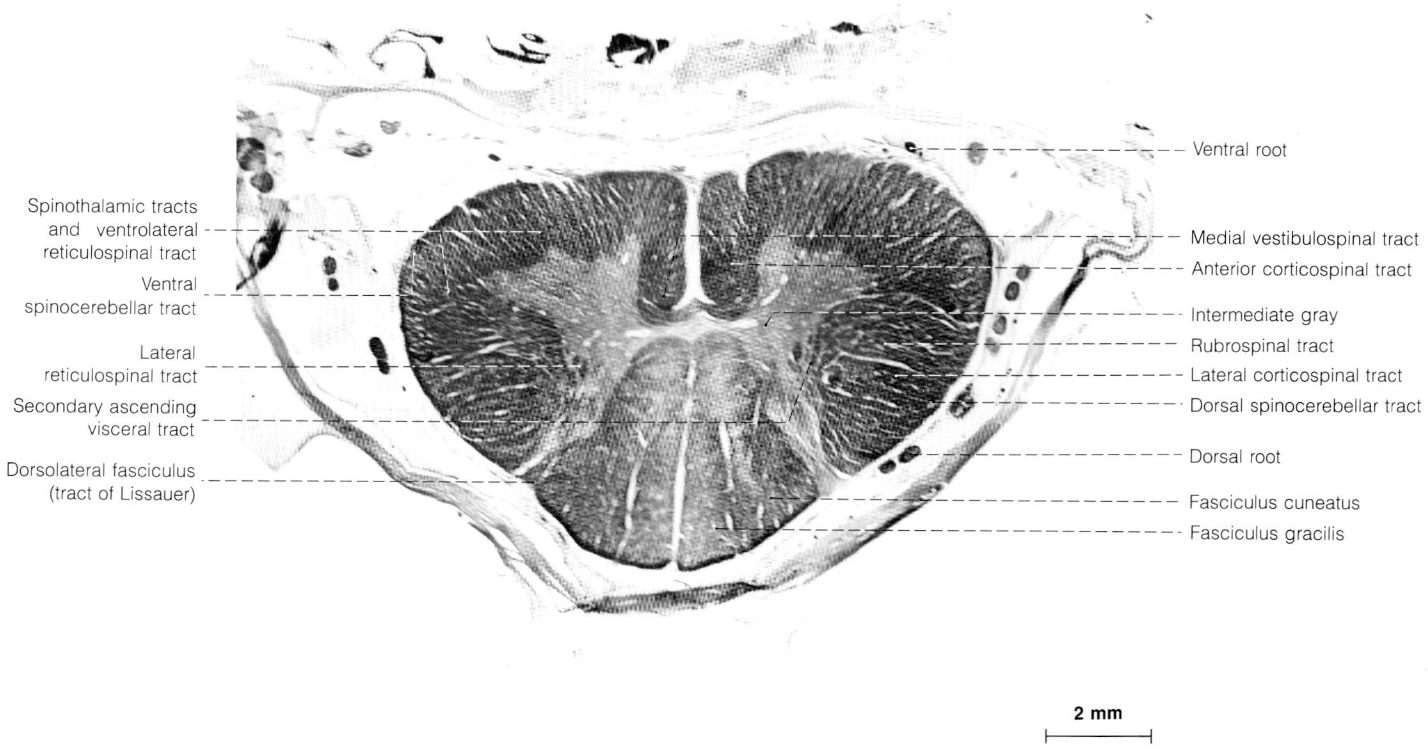
Ventral root
Spinothalamic tracts and ventrolateral reticulospinal tract
Medial vestibulospinal tract
Anterior corticospinal tract
Ventral spinocerebellar tract
Intermediate gray
Rubrospinal tract
Lateral reticulospinal tract
Lateral corticospinal tract
Secondary ascending visceral tract
Dorsal spinocerebellar tract
Dorsal root
Dorsolateral fasciculus (tract of Lissauer)
Fasciculus cuneatus
Fasciculus gracilis
2 mm

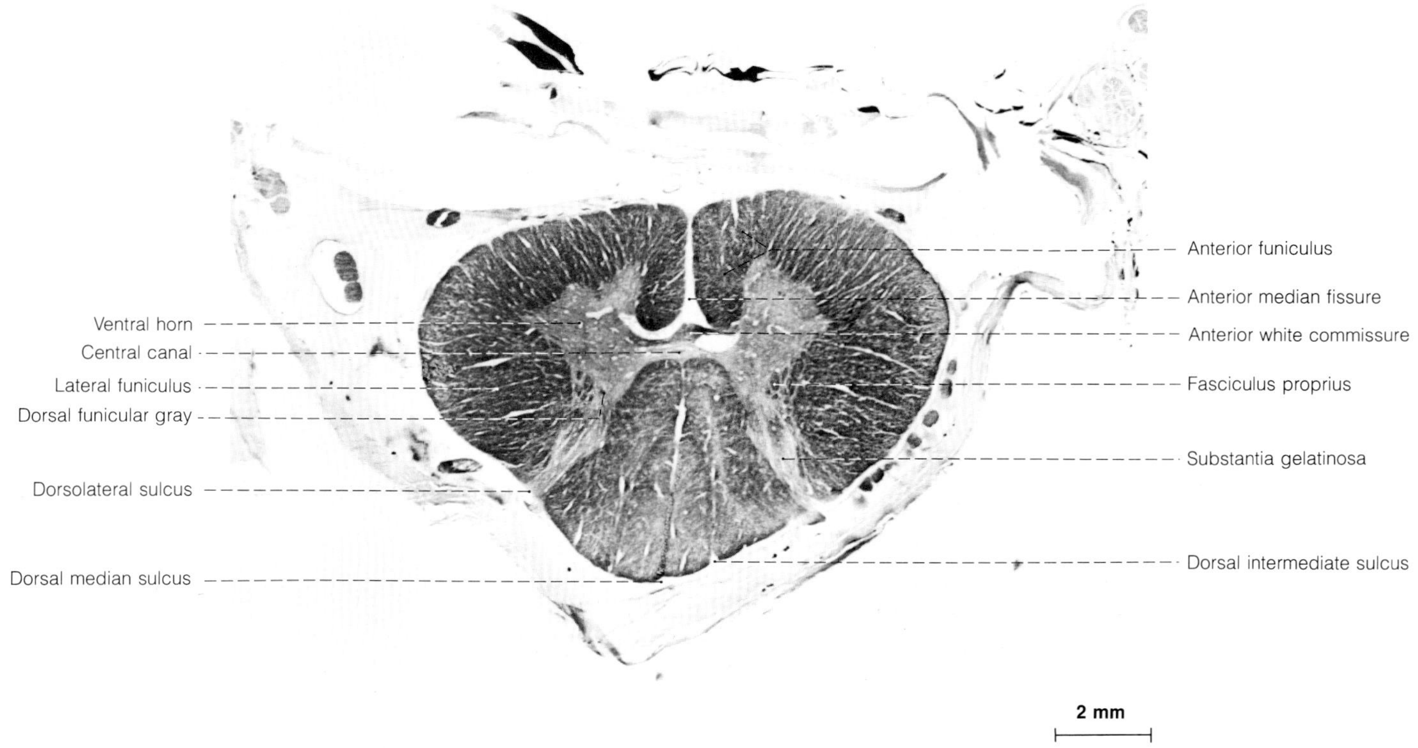
Anterior funiculus
Anterior median fissure
Ventral horn
Anterior white commissure
Central canal
Lateral funiculus
Fasciculus proprius
Dorsal funicular gray
Substantia gelatinosa
Dorsolateral sulcus
Dorsal intermediate sulcus
Dorsal median sulcus
2 mm

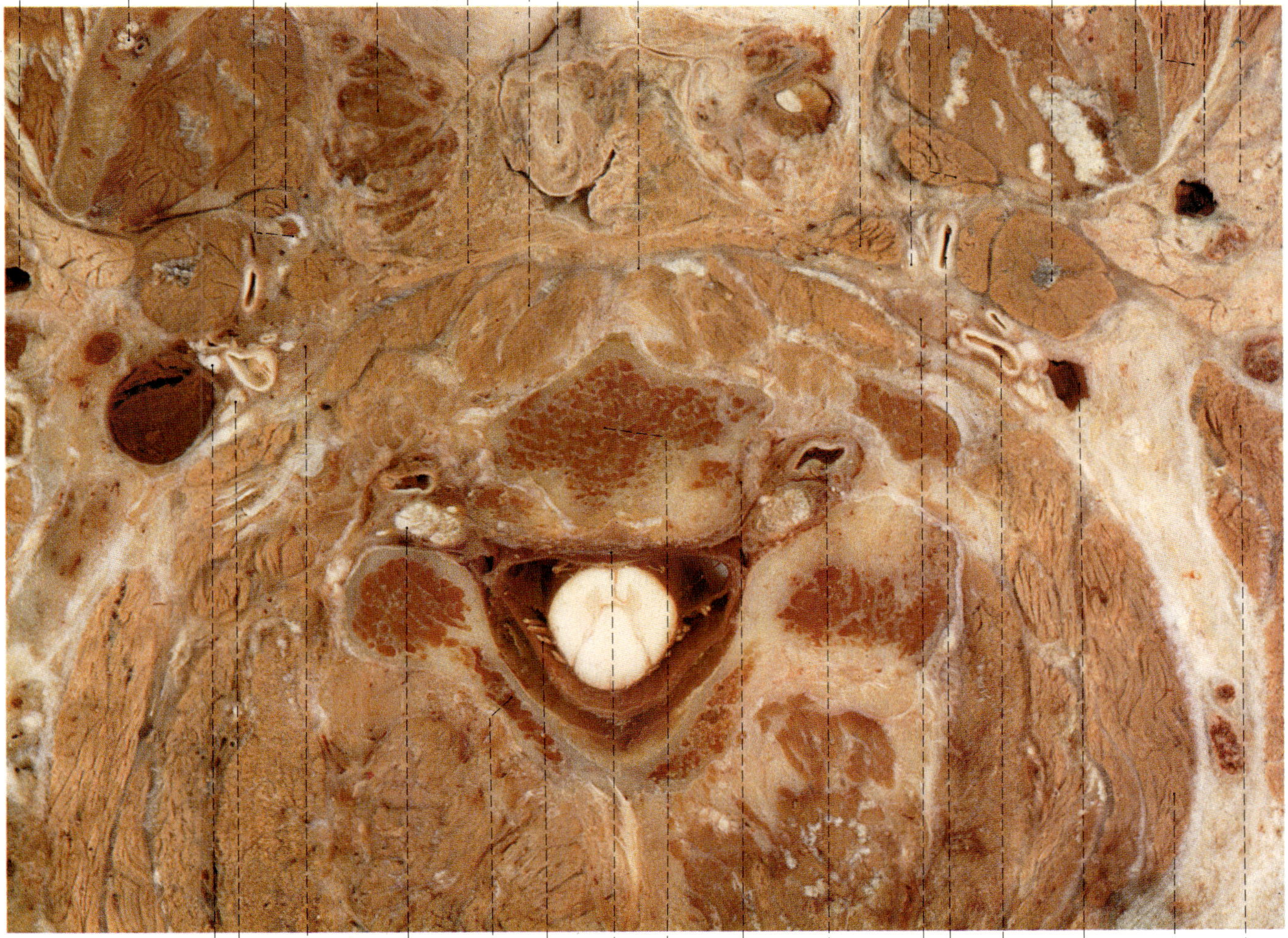

The C4 spinal cord is obviously larger in its lateral diameter than it is at higher levels. The increase in the ventral horn is quite apparent. This increase in size of the cord is accompanied by a concomitant decrease in the size of the subarachnoid space and a greater vulnerability of the cord to any displacement of the related vertebrae.

The fibers of the lateral corticospinal tract terminating at cervical levels are deep (medial) to those which continue down to the lumbosacral enlargement. The crossed spinothalamic fibers in the ventral part of the lateral funiculus are oriented in the tract so that those from the sacral cord are dorsal (dorsolateral) to those arising at succeeding higher levels with the cervical contributions most ventral (ventromedial).

Patient CT Scan

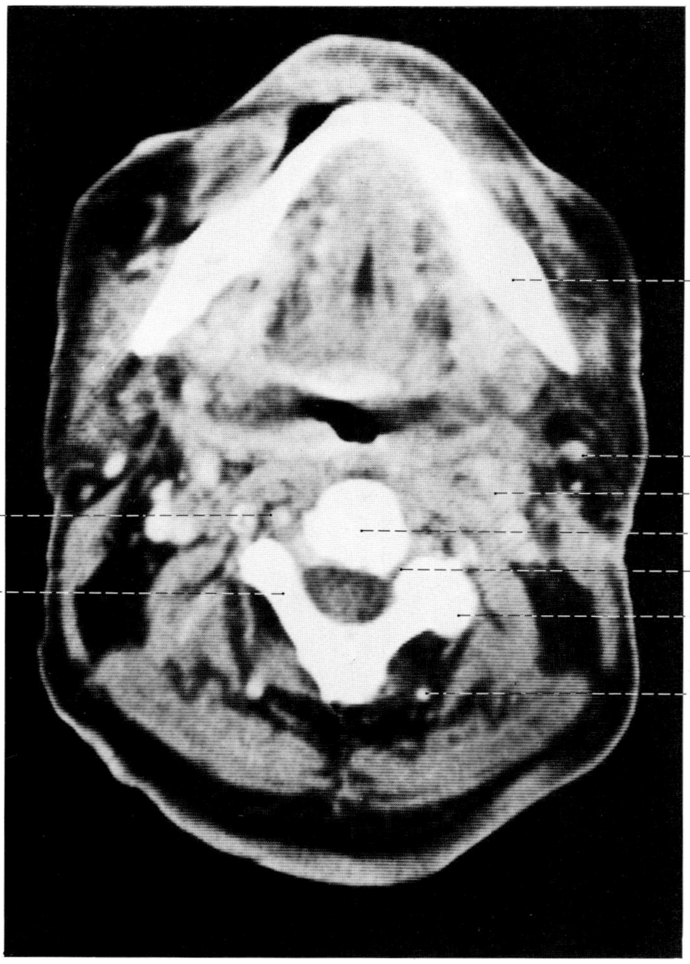

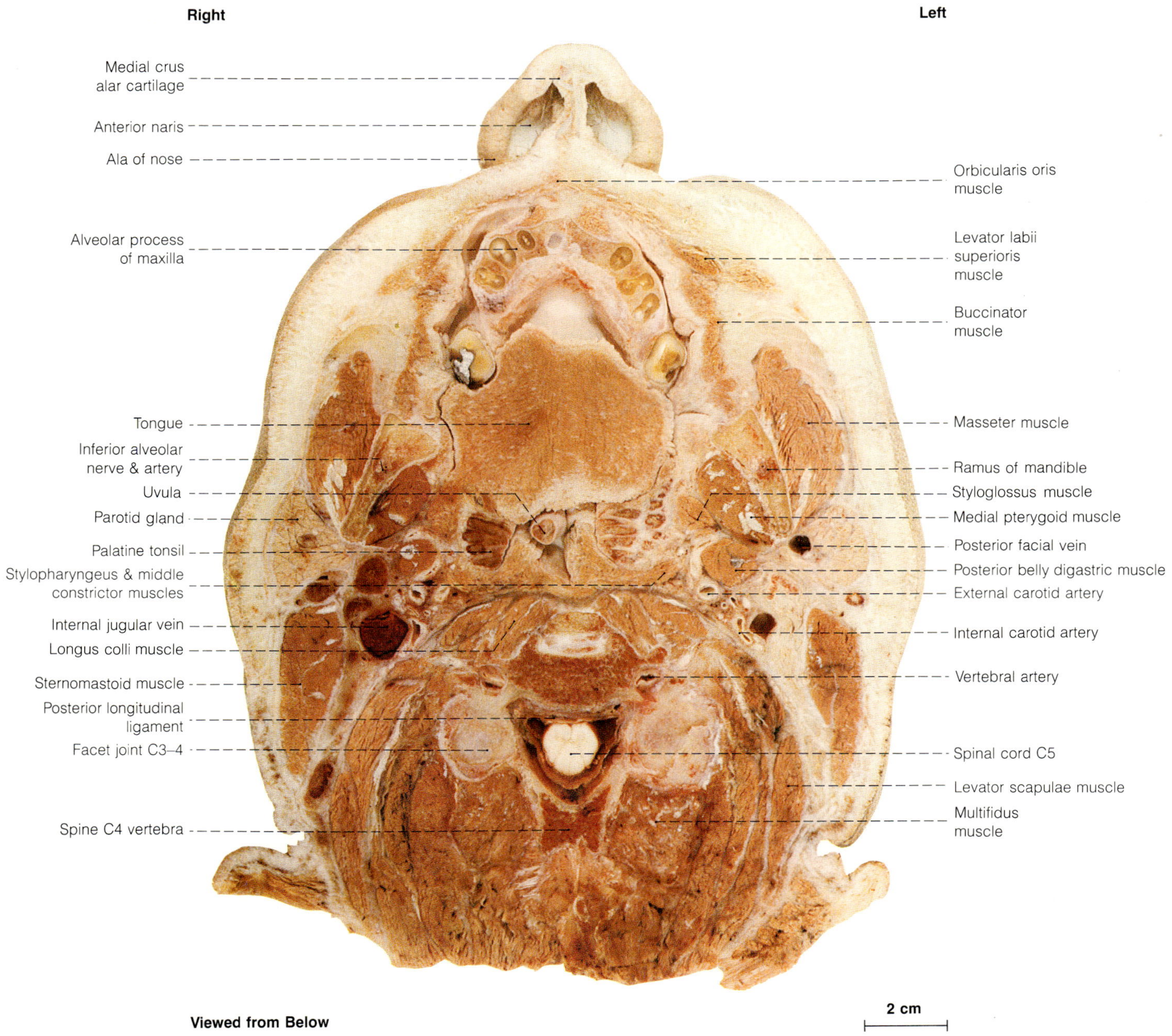

Plane of Section

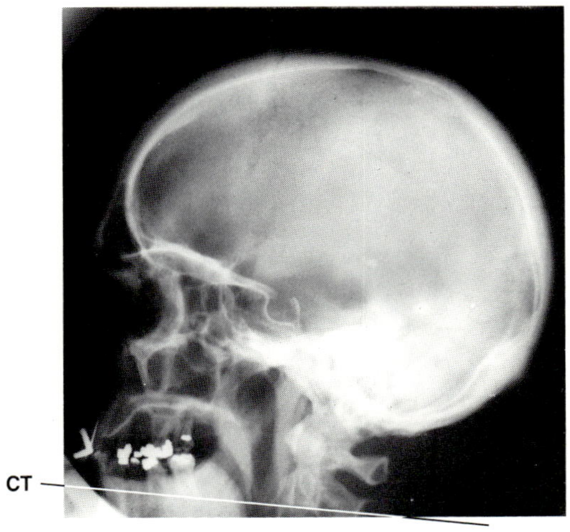

At this level, through the lower pharynx, the oral cavity is partially visualized and the palatine tonsil can be noted laterally on the gross specimen. The semispinalis muscle group dominates the posterior anatomy with the large muscle bands of the sternocleidomastoids seen laterally. Contrast in the vascular channels of the CT image not only enhances the vessels but may permit better localization of adjacent structures.

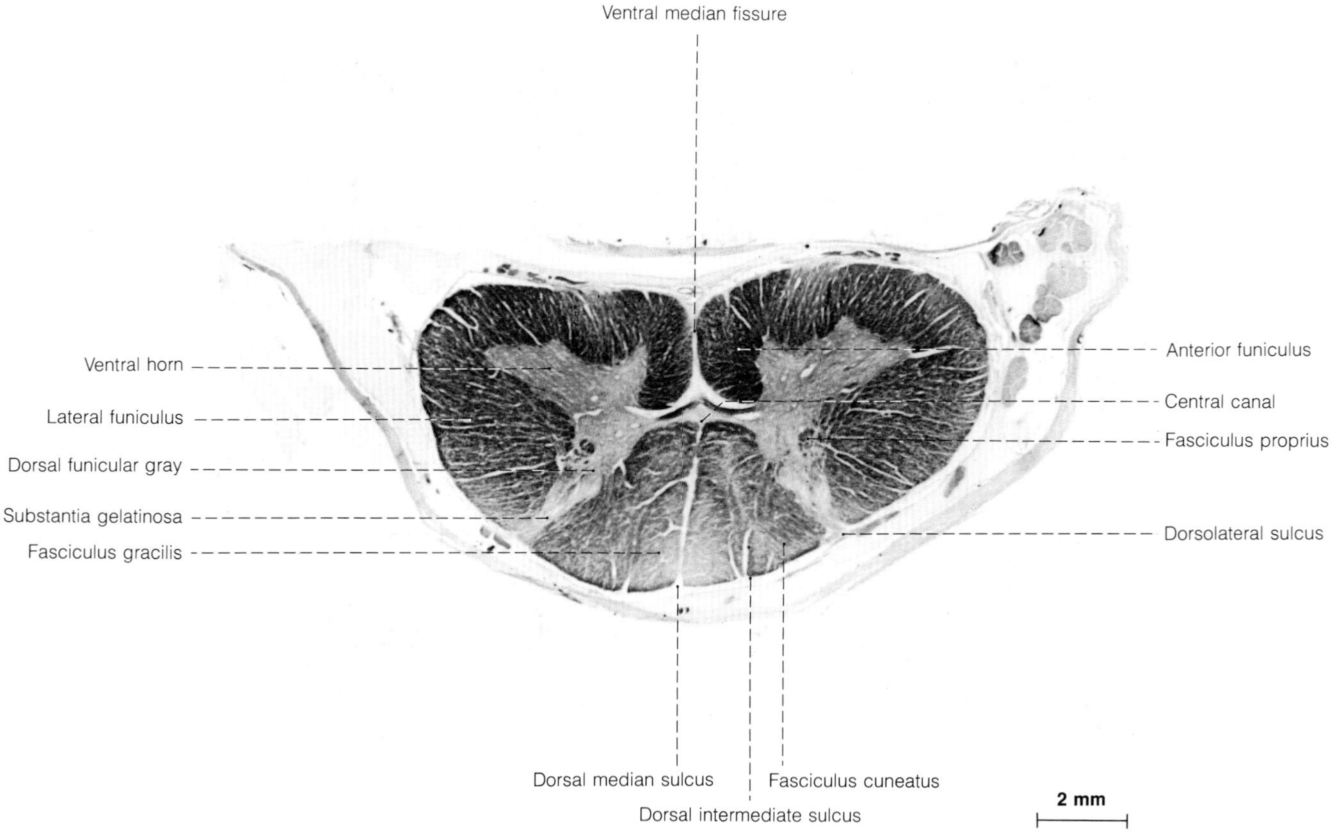
Ventral median fissure
Ventral horn
Lateral funiculus
Dorsal funicular gray
Substantia gelatinosa
Fasciculus gracilis
Anterior funiculus
Central canal
Fasciculus proprius
Dorsolateral sulcus
Dorsal median sulcus
Fasciculus cuneatus
Dorsal intermediate sulcus
2 mm

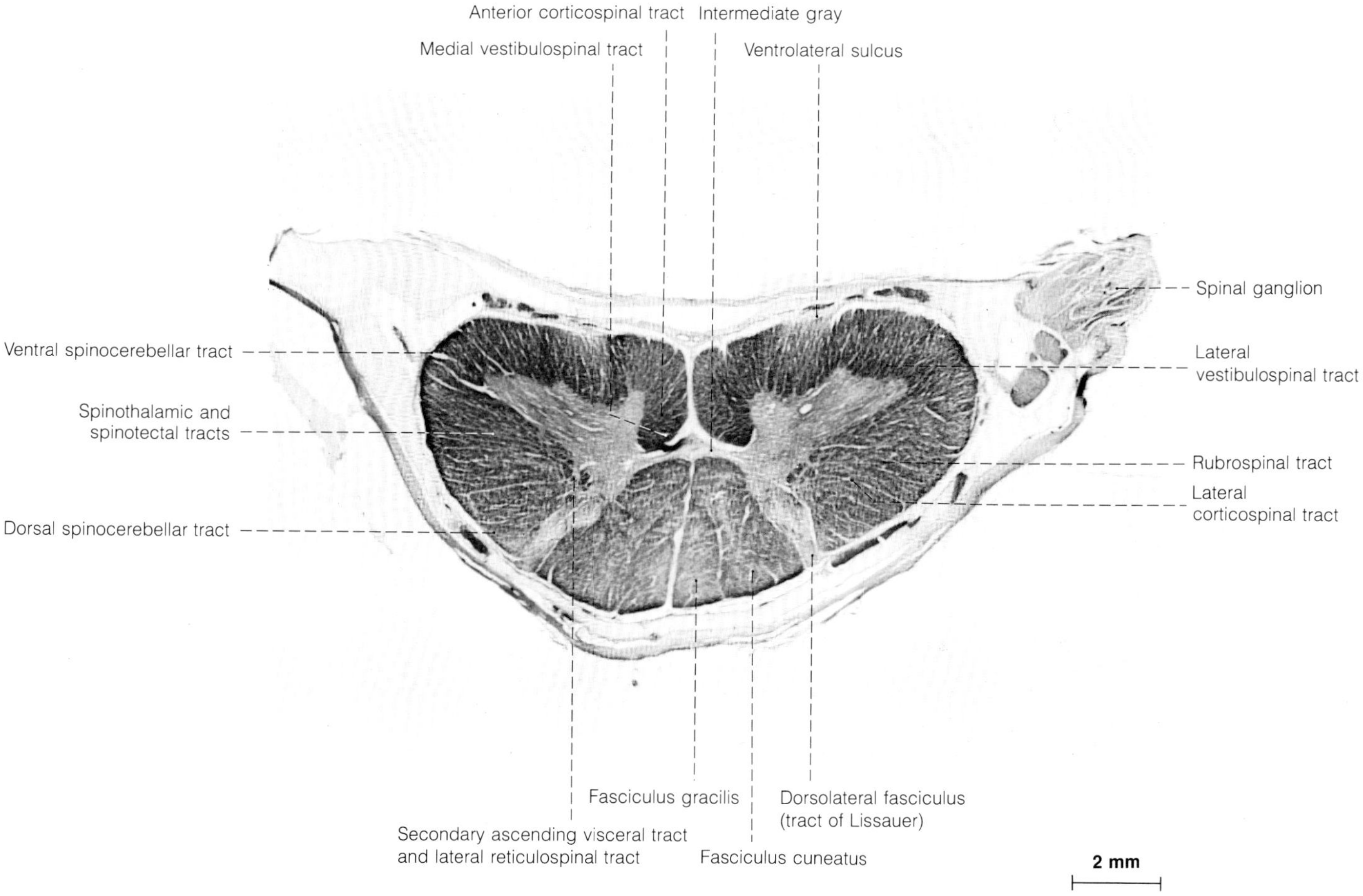
Anterior corticospinal tract
Intermediate gray
Medial vestibulospinal tract
Ventrolateral sulcus
Spinal ganglion
Ventral spinocerebellar tract
Lateral vestibulospinal tract
Spinothalamic and spinotectal tracts
Rubrospinal tract
Lateral corticospinal tract
Dorsal spinocerebellar tract
Fasciculus gracilis
Dorsolateral fasciculus (tract of Lissauer)
Secondary ascending visceral tract and lateral reticulospinal tract
Fasciculus cuneatus
2 mm

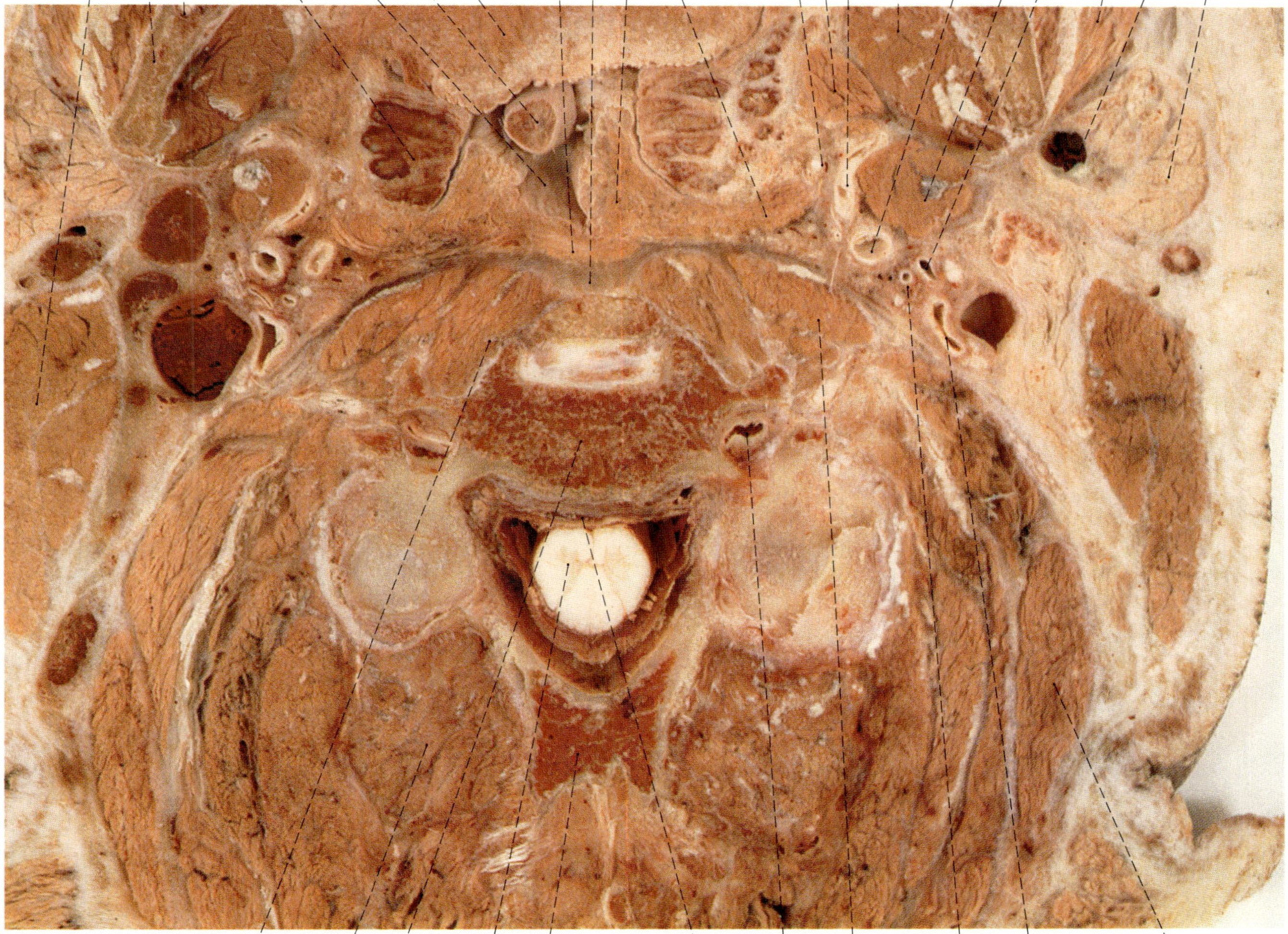

These sections through the C4-C5 spinal cord contain neurons of the upper brachial plexus and may provide some of the lowest contributions of the spinal accessory nerve. The oval shape of the section is typical of the cervical cord and, since the plane is not a true transverse, the cord is even more flattened antero-posteriorly than illustrated. The cervical enlargement occupies most of the dural (arachnoid) sac at this level. Additional cervical relations are shown in Section VII (pages 255-288).

Selected Bibliography

Bo, W. J., I. Meschan, and W. A. Krueger. *Basic Atlas of Cross-Sectional Anatomy.* W. B. Saunders Co., Philadelphia, London, and Toronto, 1980

Brodal, A. *The Cranial Nerves: Anatomical and Anatomico-clinical Correlations.* Blackwell Scientific Publications, Oxford, 1965.

Burrows, E. H., and N. E. Leeds. *Neuroradiology, Vol. 1.* Churchill Livingstone, N. Y., 1981.

Carpenter, M. B., and J. Sutin. *Human Neuroanatomy, 8th ed.* Williams & Wilkins, Baltimore, 1983.

Carter, B. L., J. Morehead, S. M. Wolpert, S. B. Hammerschlag, H. J. Griffiths, and P. C. Kahn. *Cross-sectional Anatomy, Computed Tomography and Ultrasound Correlation.* Appleton-Century-Crofts, New York, 1977.

Clemente, C. D. *Anatomy, A Regional Atlas of the Human Body, 2nd ed.* Urban & Schwarzenberg, Baltimore and Munich, 1981.

Crosby, E. C., T. Humphrey, and E. W. Lauer. *Correlative Anatomy of the Nervous System.* The Macmillan Co., New York, 1962.

Ferner, H. *Eduard Pernkopf Atlas of Topographical and Applied Human Anatomy, 2nd Revised ed. Vol. I, Head and Neck.* Urban & Schwarzenberg, Baltimore and Munich, 1980.

Ferner, H., and J. Staubesand. *Sobotta Atlas of Human Anatomy, 10th English ed.,* Translated by W. Hild. Urban & Schwarzenberg, Baltimore and Munich, 1983.

Haines, D. E. *Neuroanatomy, An Atlas of Structures, Sections, and Systems.* Urban & Schwarzenberg, Baltimore and Munich, 1983.

Lang, J. *Clinical Anatomy of the Head, Neurocranium, Orbit, Craniocervical Regions.* Trans. by R. R. Wilson and D. P. Winstanley. Springer-Verlag, Berlin, Heidelberg, N. Y., 1983.

Ledley, R. S., H. K. Huang, and J. C. Mazziotta. *Cross Sectional Anatomy – An Atlas for Computerized Tomography.* Williams & Wilkins Co., Baltimore, 1977.

Matsui, T., and A. Hirano. *An Atlas of the Human Brain for Computerized Tomography.* Igaku-Shoin, Tokyo, 1978.

Merritt, H. H. *A Textbook of Neurology.* Lea and Febiger, Philadelphia, 1979.

Meschan, I. *An Atlas of Anatomy Basic to Radiology.* W. B.Saunders Co., Philadelphia, 1975.

New, P. F. J., and W. R. Scott. *Computed Tomography of the Brain and Orbit.* William & Wilkins Co., Baltimore, 1975

Newton, T. H., and D. G. Potts, eds. *Radiology of the Skull and Brain: Vol. 3: Anatomy and Pathology* (1975); *Vol. 4: Ventricles and Cisterns* (1978); *Vol. 5: Technical Aspects of Computed Tomography* (1981). C. V. Mosby Co., St. Louis.

Newton, T. H., and D. G. Potts. *Advanced Imaging Techniques, Modern Neuroradiology, Vol. 2.* Clavadel Press, San Anselmo, Calif., 1983.

Oldendorf, W. F. *The Quest for an Image of Brain. Computerized Tomography in the Perspective of Past and Future Imaging Methods.* Raven Press, New York, 1980.

Peterson, R. R. *A Cross-Sectional Approach to Anatomy.* Yearbook Medical Publishers, Inc., 1980.

Peyster, R. G., and E. D. Hoover. CT in head trauma. *J. Trauma* 22: 25-38, 1982.

Plum, F., and J. B. Posner. *The Diagnosis of Stupor and Coma.* F. A. Davis, Philadelphia, 1980.

Romanes, G. J. *Cunningham's Manual of Practical Anatomy. Vol. III: Head and Neck and Brain.* Oxford University Press, New York, 1966.

Schaltenbrand, G., and P. Bailey. *Introduction to Stereotaxis with an Atlas of the Human Brain.* Grune & Stratton, New York, 1959.

Steele, J. R., and J. C. Hoffman. Brainstem evaluation with CT cisternography. *AJNR* 1: 521–526, 1980.

Taveras, J., and E. H. Wood. *Diagnostic Neuroradiology, 2nd ed.* Williams & Wilkins Co., Baltimore, 1976.

Truex, R. C., and C. E. Kellner. *Detailed Atlas of the Head and Neck.* Oxford University Press, New York, 1948.

Wagner, M., and T. L. Lawson. *Segmental Anatomy, Applications to Clinical Medicine.* The Macmillan Co., New York, 1982.

Walton, J. N. *Brain's Diseases of the Nervous System.* Oxford University Press, New York, 1977.

Warwick, R., and P. L. Williams, eds. *The Gray's Anatomy.* W. B. Saunders Co., Philadelphia, 1981.

Coronal Planes

Coronal planes are especially useful in examining the orbit, the paranasal sinuses, especially the ethmoid region, and the cribriform plate, and for localization within the frontal and temporal lobes. The sella turcica and parasellar region, including the cavernous sinus and pentagonal cistern, may also be displayed to great advantage in the coronal plane. Although the clarity of most coronal CT images through the posterior fossa is limited, MRI scans may be very useful.

Coronal images differ anatomically between CT and MRI. In CT, the patient needs to hyperextend his head and coronal slices are then obtained directly for the best images (coronal reconstruction of axial information is also available but is not as fine as direct coronals). Fillings in teeth often cause insurmountable artifacts, and coronal CT images are usually in anything but a true coronal plane. MRI images, however, are generated directly and are coronal throughout matching the true coronal anatomical slices.

The anatomical specimen illustrated was orientated in a true coronal plane in a CT scanner and marked for future sectioning. These cadaver CT scans and the scout film of the cadaver are included for comparison with the MRI images of patients. Although cadaver CT is not the same as CT of a living patient, they do provide great assistance in interpreting the newer modes of display with MRI. An additional photograph of each section at greater magnification is included to illustrate the detailed anatomy not so evident on the entire slice of the head.

Cadaver CT Scan

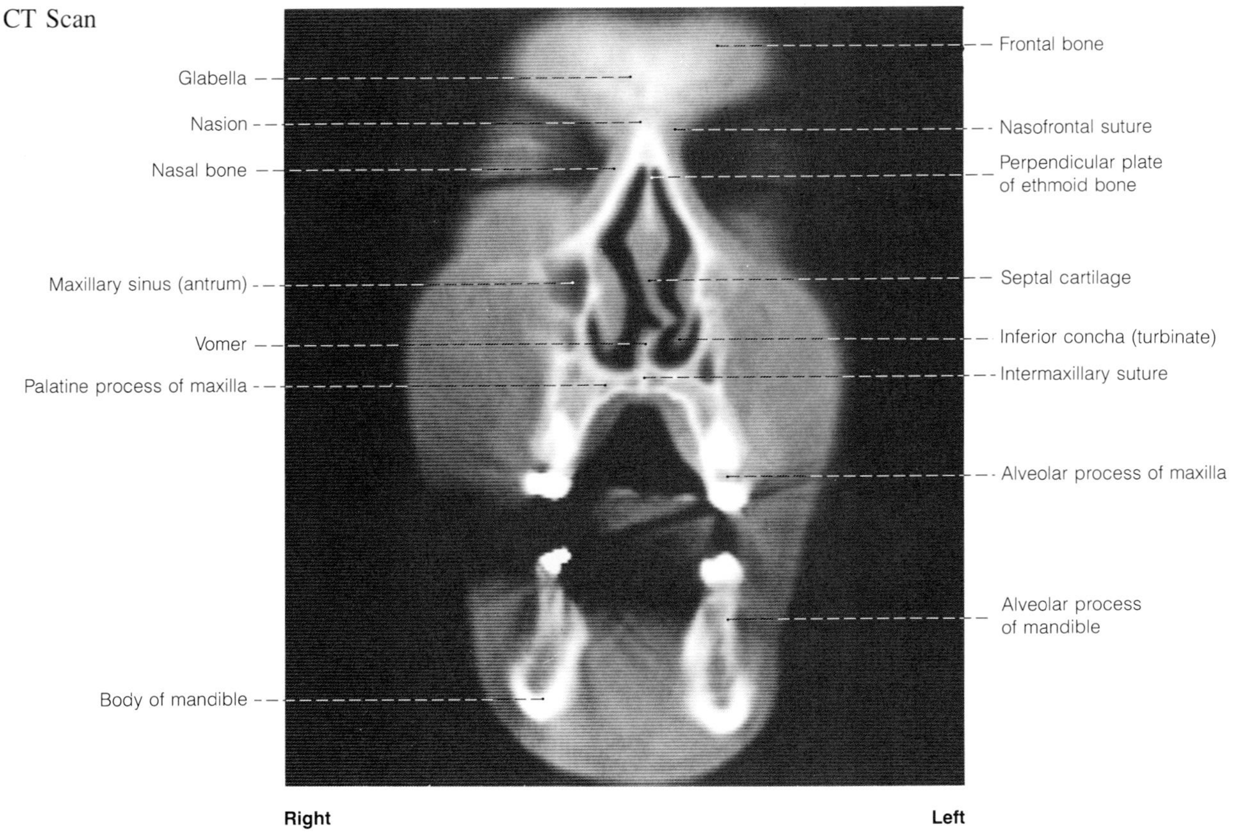

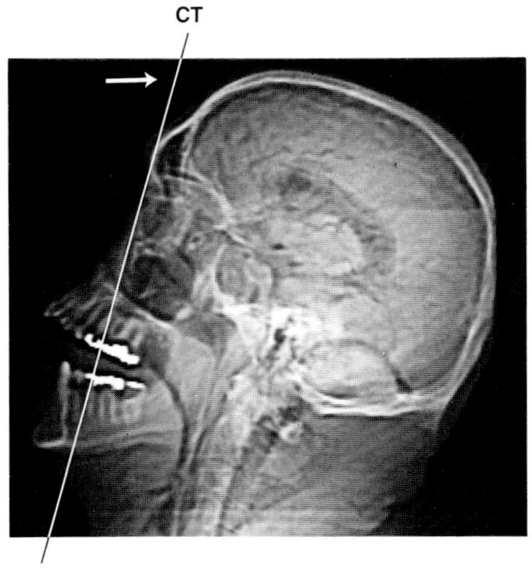

Plane of Section

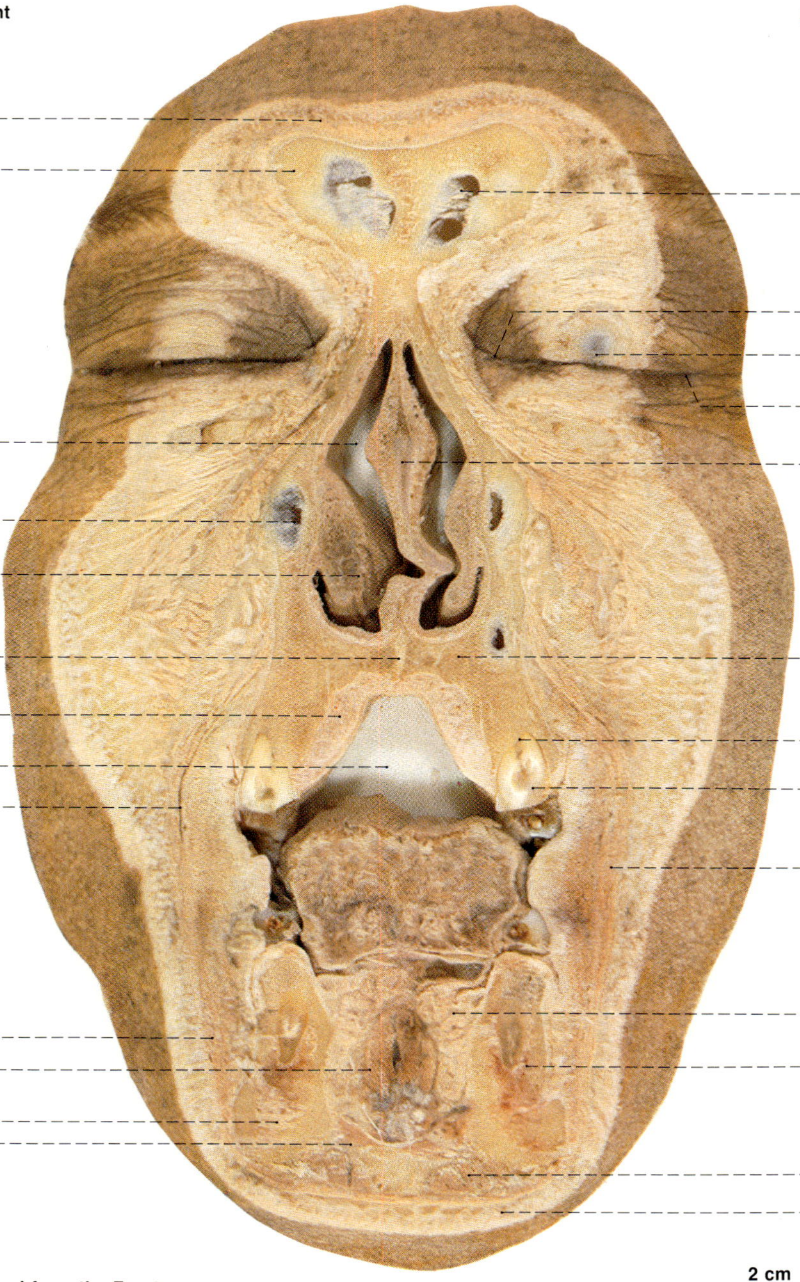

Coronal planes through the anterior face illustrated are of somewhat limited clinical value in diagnosis by CT or MRI since most structures can be visualized or palpated with superficial examination. They may, however, be useful in demonstrating the nasal fossa, turbinates, anterior maxilla and oral structures. The cadaver specimen has a nasal septum sharply deviated to the left at the junction of the palatine process of the maxilla with the nasal septal cartilage.

In this plane and in more posterior sections through the mouth, the teeth and especially their metallic fillings and crowns may cause extensive artifact in CT imaging. MRI displays do not have such interference.

Coronal sections performed on CT are not true coronal due to the fact that the patient must extend his neck rather severely to fit into the CT gantry so that a true coronal is impossible even in the most cooperative patient. Sections are then often angled more or less than the ideal to avoid artifacts from fillings in teeth. MRI scans, on the other hand, are generated directly and do not depend upon patient repositioning to achieve coronal planes. A coronal scan on MRI will be a true coronal cut and should match the specimen scan much better than the "coronal" CT scan. This will be seen to be true throughout this section.

Cadaver CT Scan

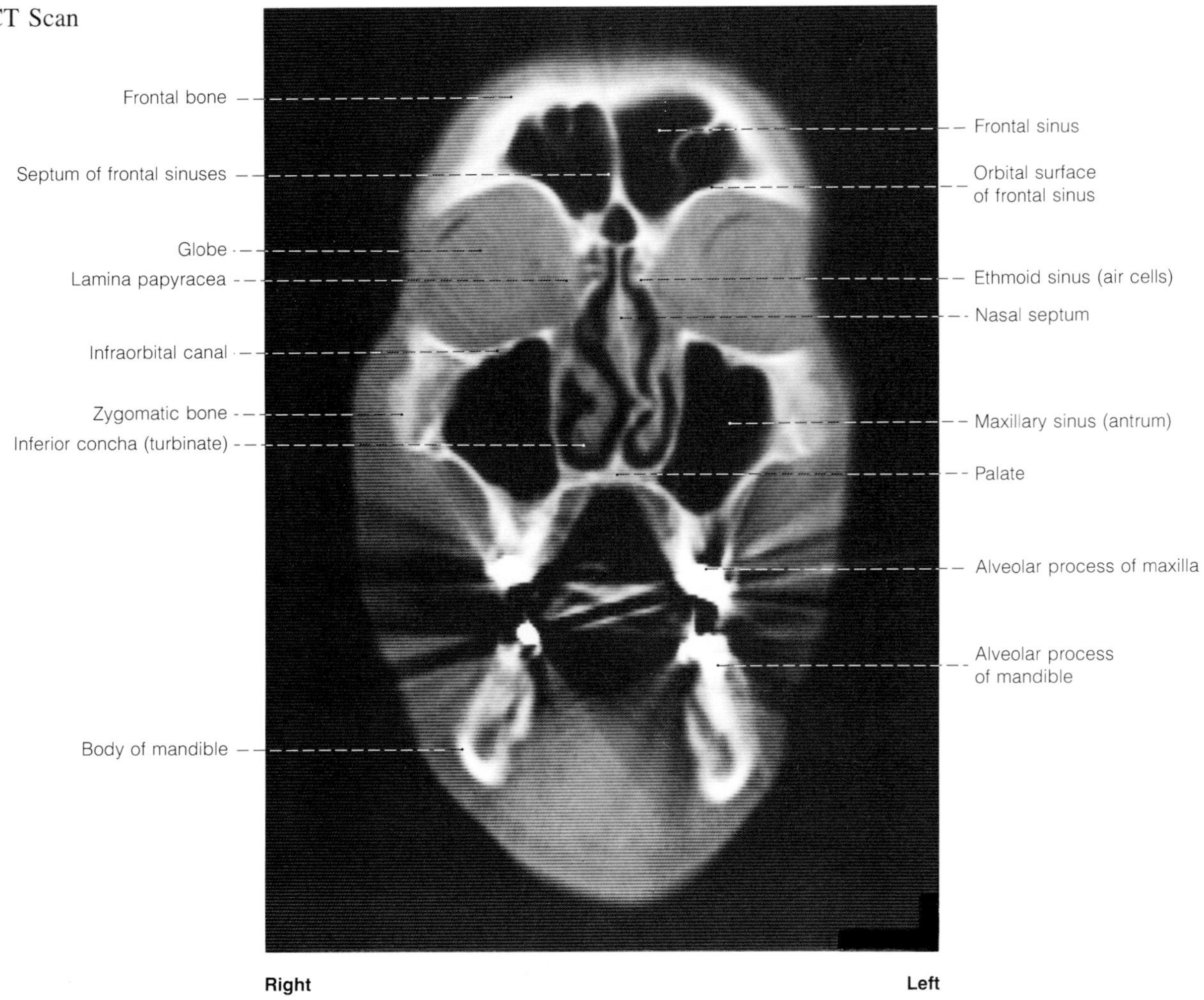

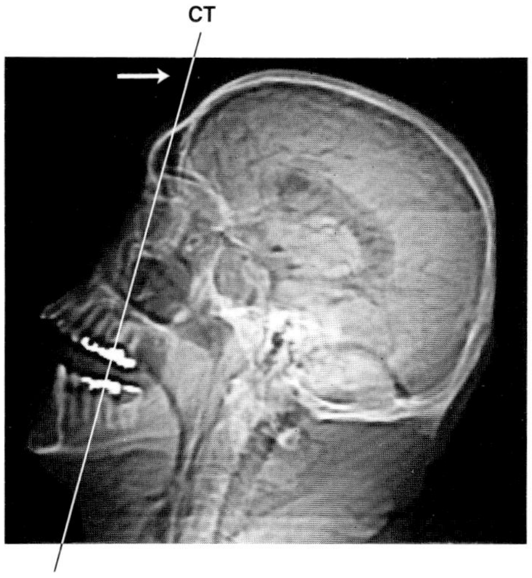

Plane of Section

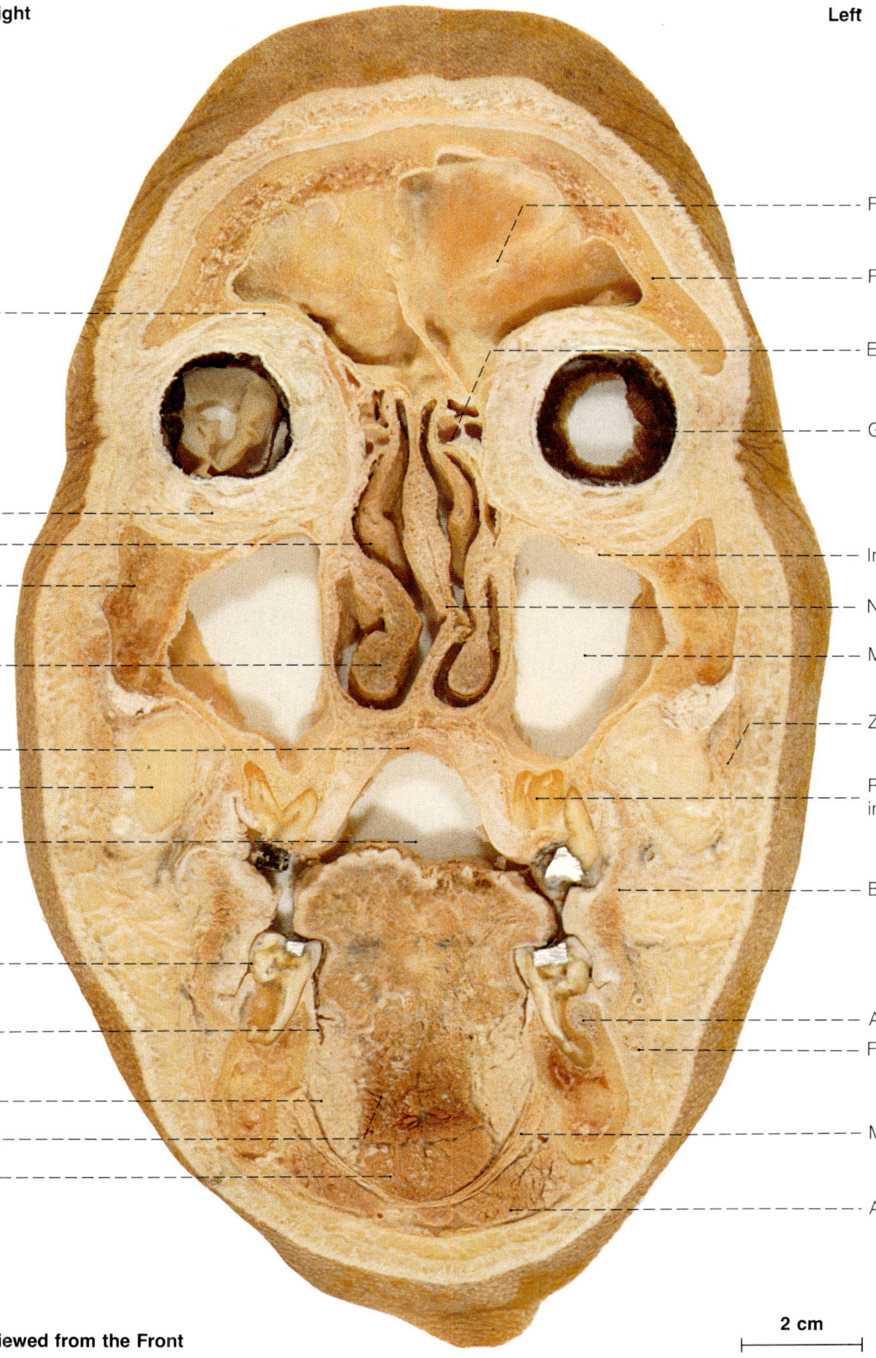

A coronal section passing through the anterior orbits illustrates the globes, mid-portions of the frontal sinuses, anterior ethmoidal sinuses, and anterior maxillary sinuses. In this cadaver, the frontal sinuses are especially large and irregular, and, as is usual, the intervening frontal septum is displaced to one side causing some asymmetry. These sinuses are frequently divided into several incomplete compartments and their size has no relationship to the superciliary of frontal eminences. When small, these sinuses may be confined to the pars orbitalis of the frontal bone or may be absent on one side. The nasofrontal duct usually drains into the middle meatus of the nasal cavity; however, variations of relationships with the ethmoidal sinuses are not uncommon.

Inflammatory and neoplastic conditions involving the paranasal sinuses are routinely imaged in the coronal plane to evaluate the extent of involvement.

Traumatic injuries causing facial fractures are also visualized well in coronal images. In both of these instances, one is primarily interested in bone detail which is not available with MRI because of its inability to image protons tightly bound in the matrix of bone. Thus, coronal CT images will continue to be of primary diagnostic importance in diagnosis of facial fractures and evaluation of bone involvement by tumors.

Patient CT Scan

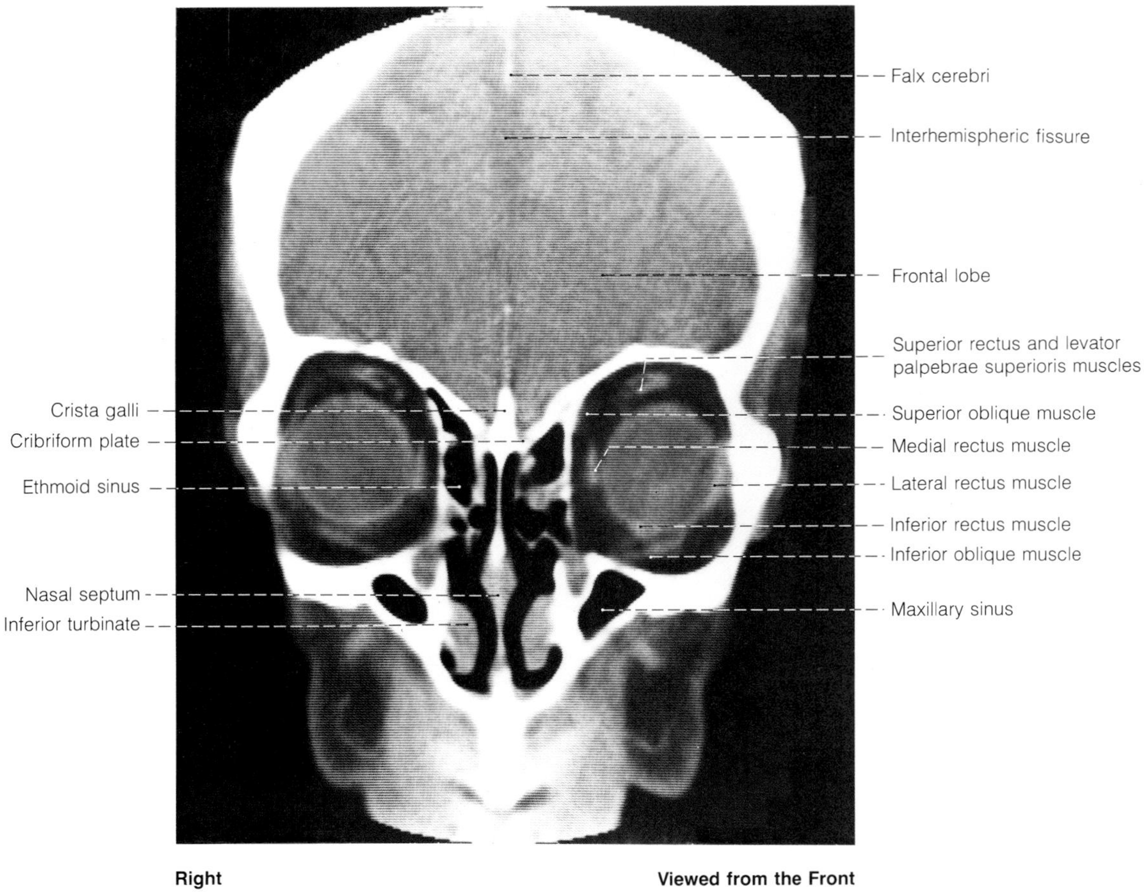

Patient MRI Scan

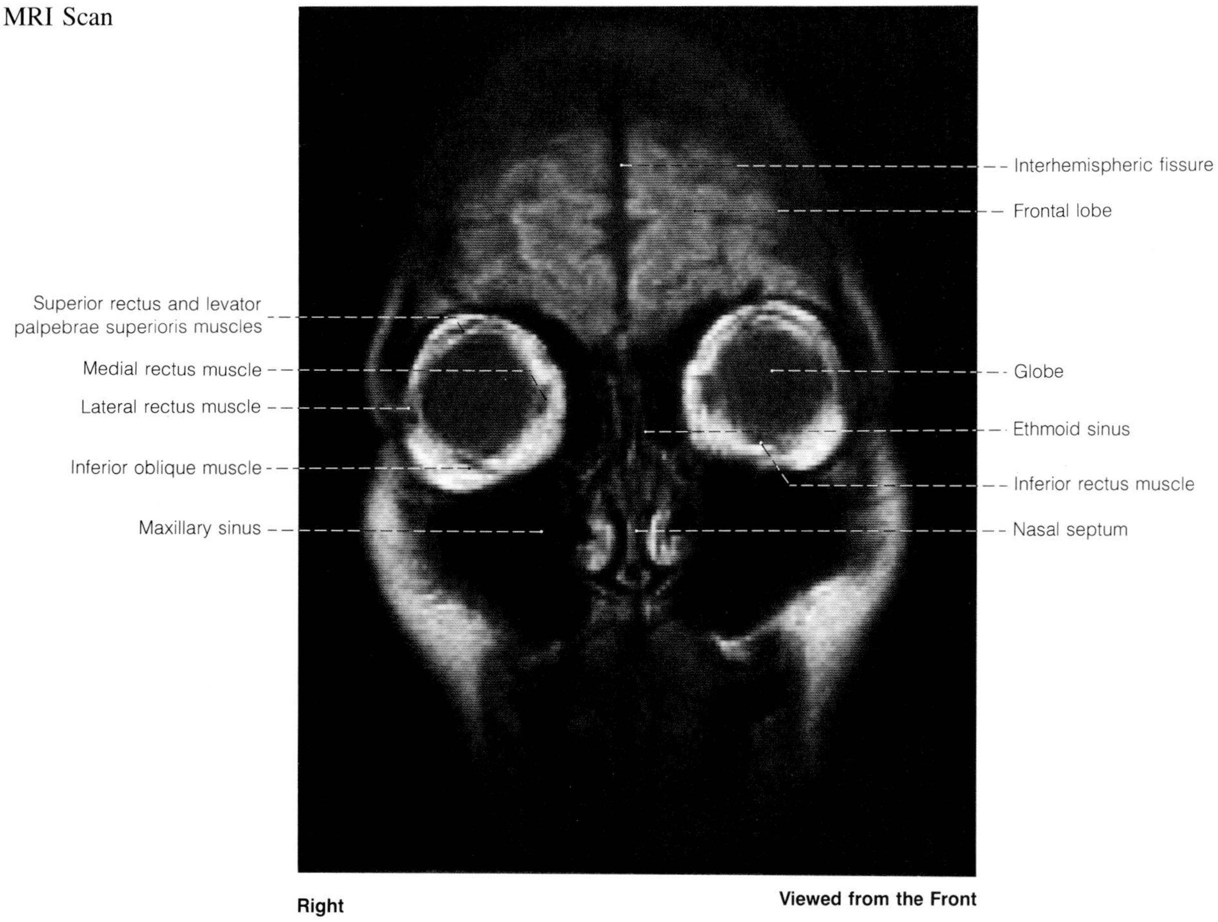

The anterior orbits, nasal cavities, and anterior maxillary sinuses are all well visualized in CT and MRI images because of their contrasting fat or air content, and their well-defined margins of bone. Extensions of pathological processes from the orbits and frontal or ethmoidal sinuses into the frontal lobes may be advantageously displayed in coronal planes, and their close proximity is well-illustrated here.

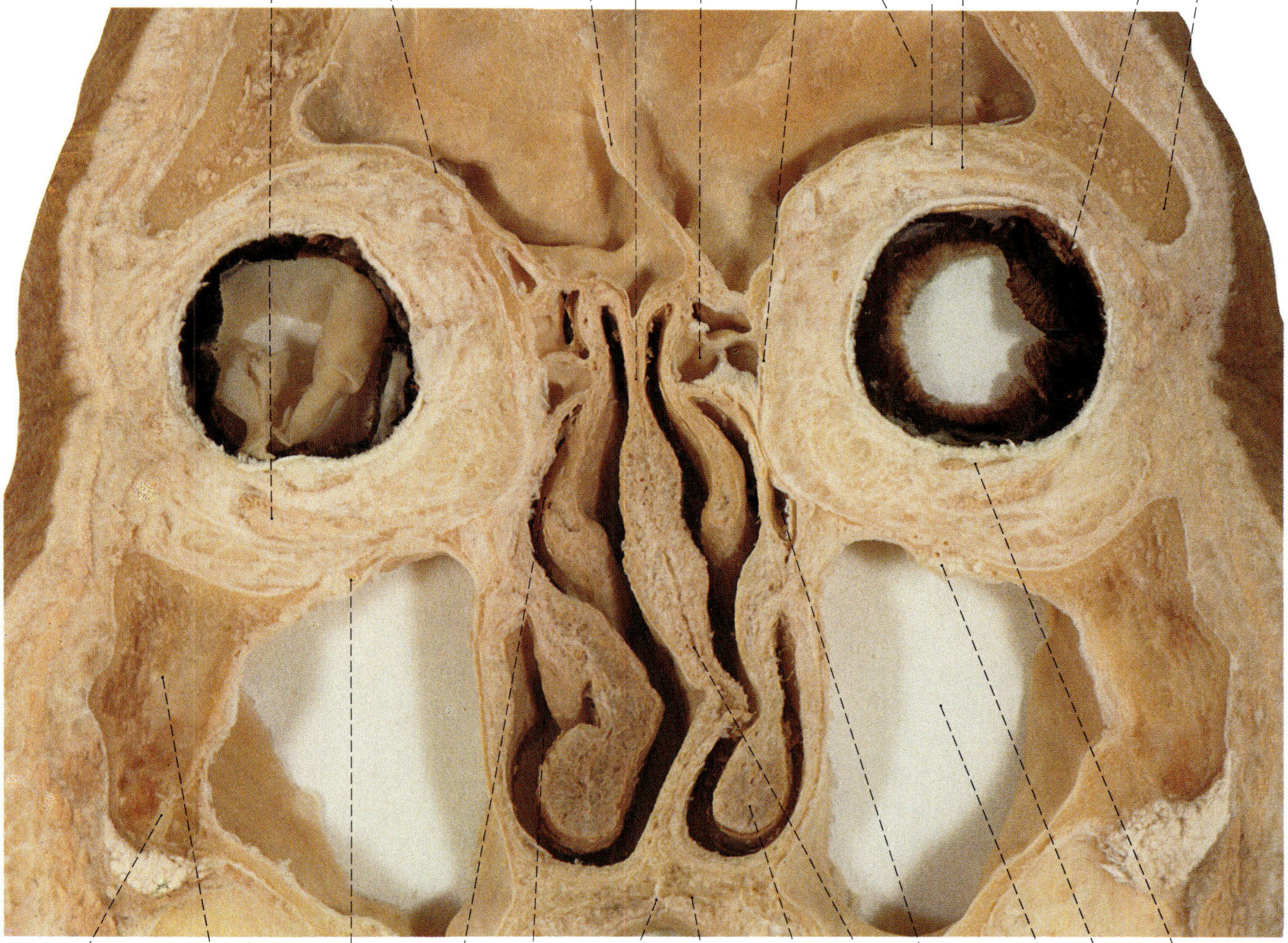

Viewed from the Front

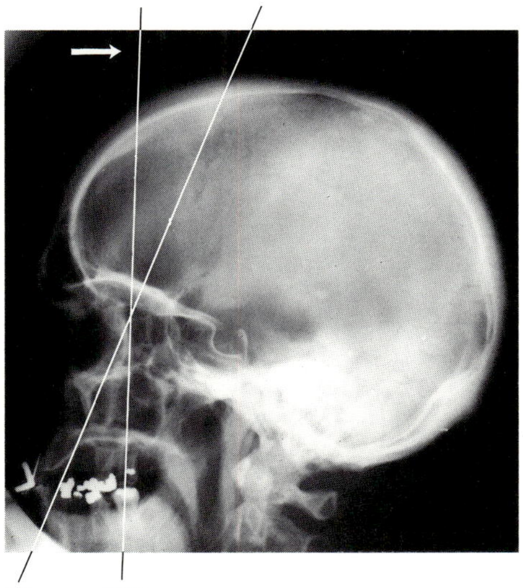

Planes of Sections

This section directly through the globe distinctly shows the attachments of periorbital muscles, as does the corresponding CT and MRI images. As mentioned above, abundant fat in the orbit, with its black appearance on CT and its bright white appearance on MRI contrasts with other soft tissue contents of the orbit.

Differences in angulation from the true coronal plane will account for the different amounts of maxillary sinus represented in any particular scan. The sinus is not represented as well in the CT scan shown here as on the true coronal anatomical section and the MRI scan.

Cadaver CT Scan

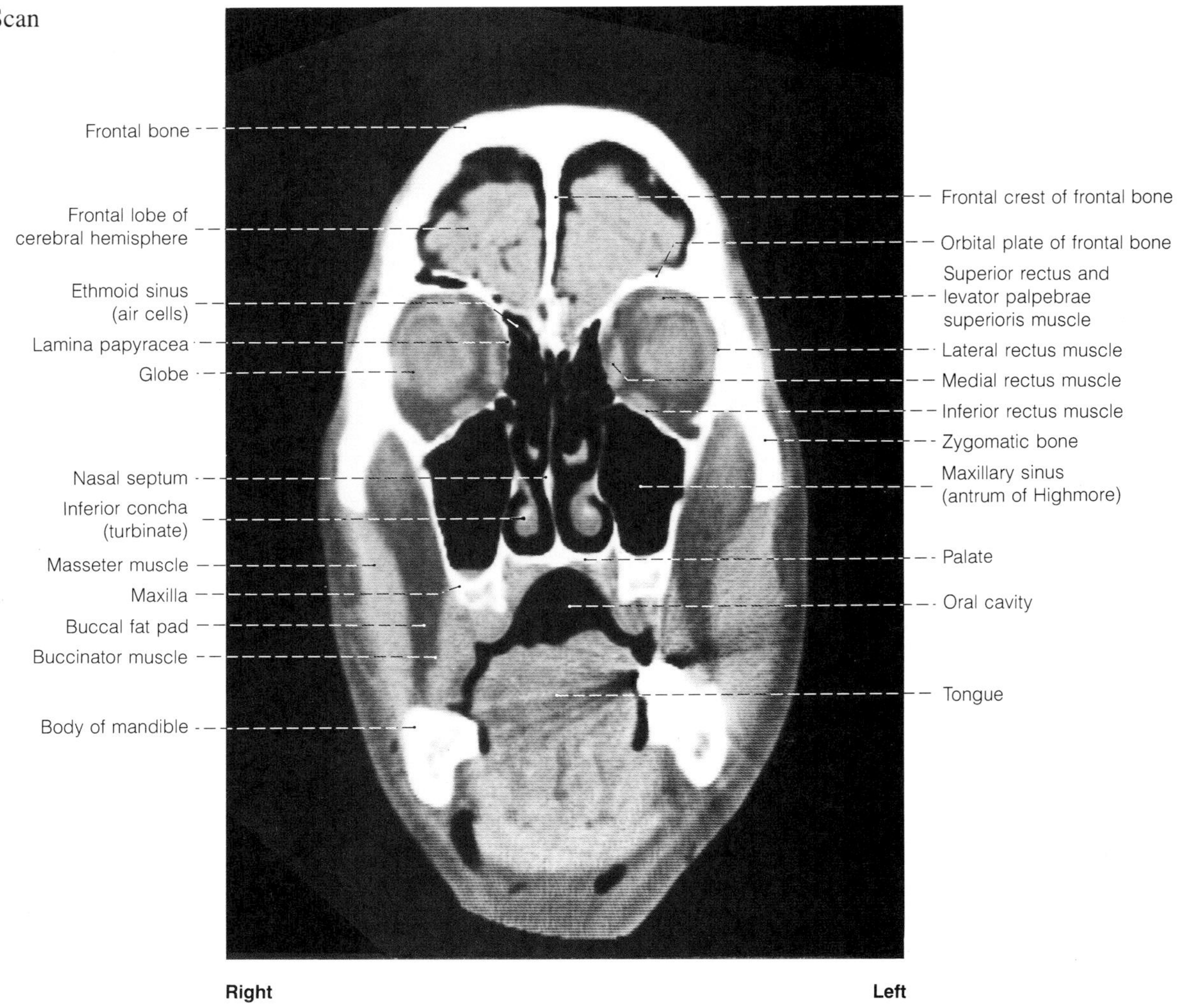

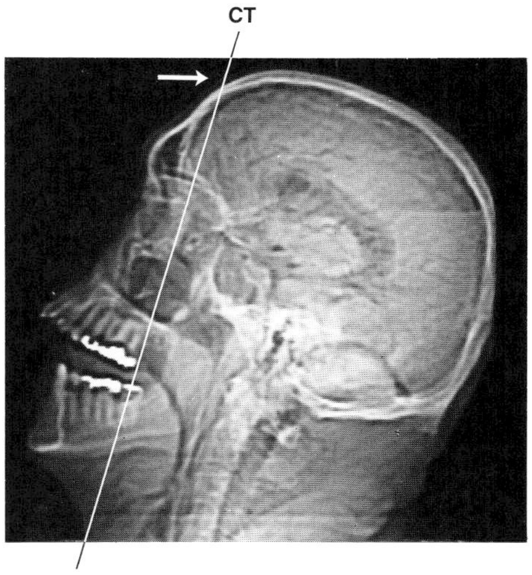

Plane of Section

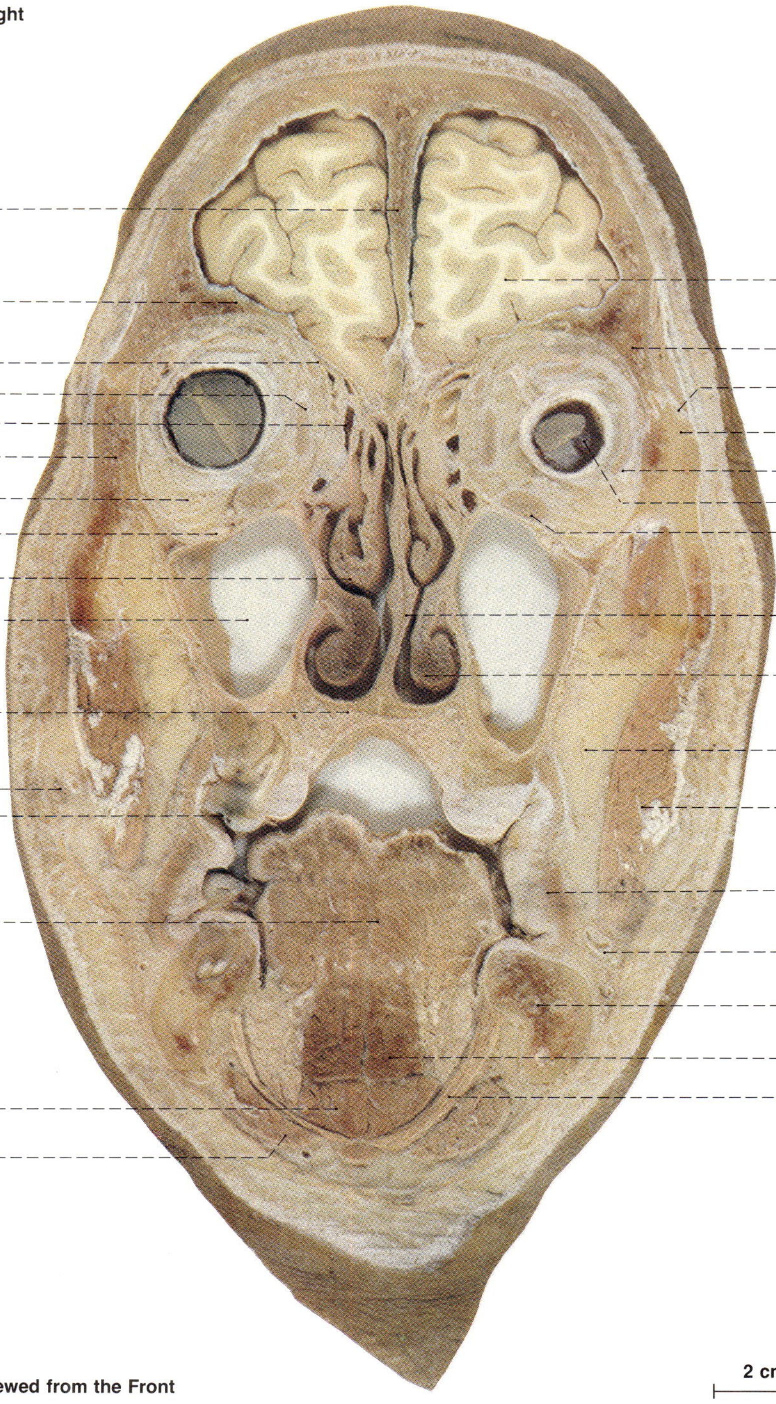

This coronal plane through the middle of the orbit and posterior portion of the globe illustrates the walls of the orbits and extraocular muscles. The lateral walls, which angle medially, are formed by relatively heavy bony processes of the frontal, maxillary, and zygomatic bones, but the parallel medial walls and the sloping superior and the inferior boundaries consist of relatively thin bone. The ethmoidal air cells are separated from the orbital contents only by the lamina papyracea and its thin periosteum and mucosa. The roof of the maxillary sinus is also rather thin bone and is prone to fracture especially with a direct blow to the orbit which may cause a so-called "blow-out" fracture. In such a fracture, the entrapment of the inferior rectus muscle, and rarely the inferior division of the oculomotor nerve in the fracture fragments, is easily understood from the section illustrating the close approximation of the muscle to the inferior orbital wall. The infratemporal fossa is well-demonstrated in the coronal views, and as more posterior slices are examined, it becomes apparent that the great size of this area is often not appreciated on axial CT.

The downward slope of the orbital roofs and the floor of the anterior fossa is shown at this level. Also of note is how the medial portion of each frontal lobe lies inferior to the lateral portion. The crista galli and cribriform plate are noted in the midline.

Patient CT Scan

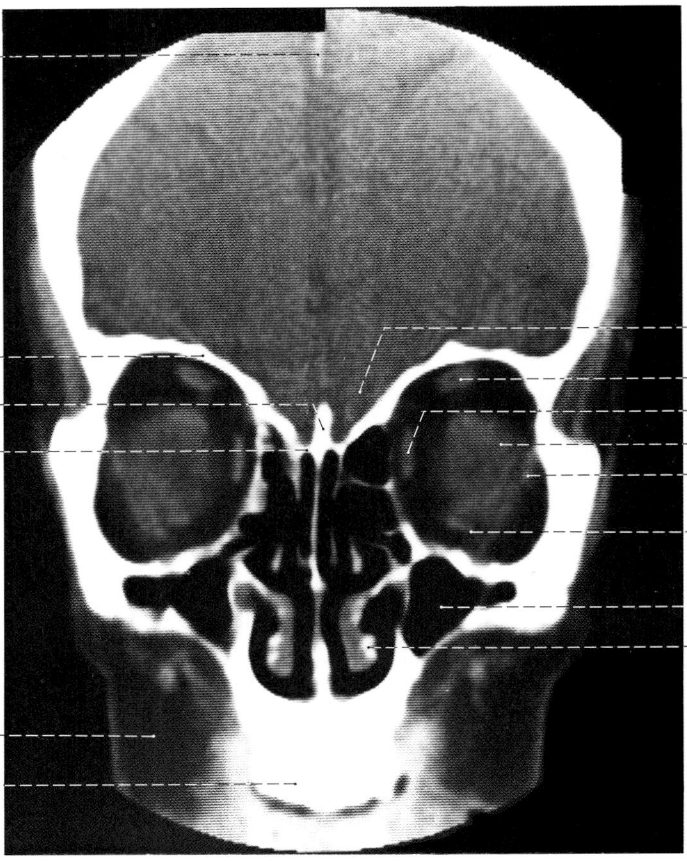

Patient MRI Scan

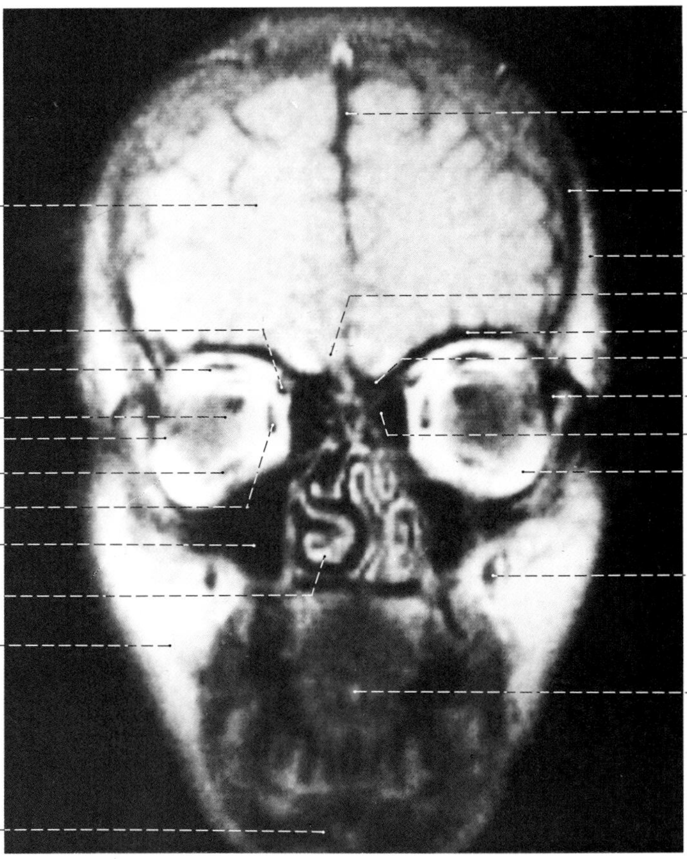

The anatomical section is a plane through the olfactory bulb as it rests on the cribriform plate. Pathology anterior to this plane may spare olfaction but may involve large portions of the frontal lobes. The scleral coat of the globe is well-defined and a portion of the lacrimal gland may be observed on the right of the anatomical specimen. This gland is poorly encapsulated although attached to the lacrimal fossa by fibrous bands. The lacrimal gland drains into the conjunctival sac by several small lacrimal ducts. Tumors in the lacrimal gland may erode adjacent bony structures.

Intracranial tumors commonly occurring in this area such as planum (jugum) sphenoidale meningiomas or anterior falx meningiomas are routinely imaged by CT in the coronal plane to determine their extent. Nasopharyngeal tumors or orbital pathological processes may erode upward through the cribriform plate and coronal imaging may also detect this.

The MRI sequence does not emphasize grey-white matter differences but the signal difference between brain and CSF is appreciated giving excellent visualization of sulci and gyri. The MRI is

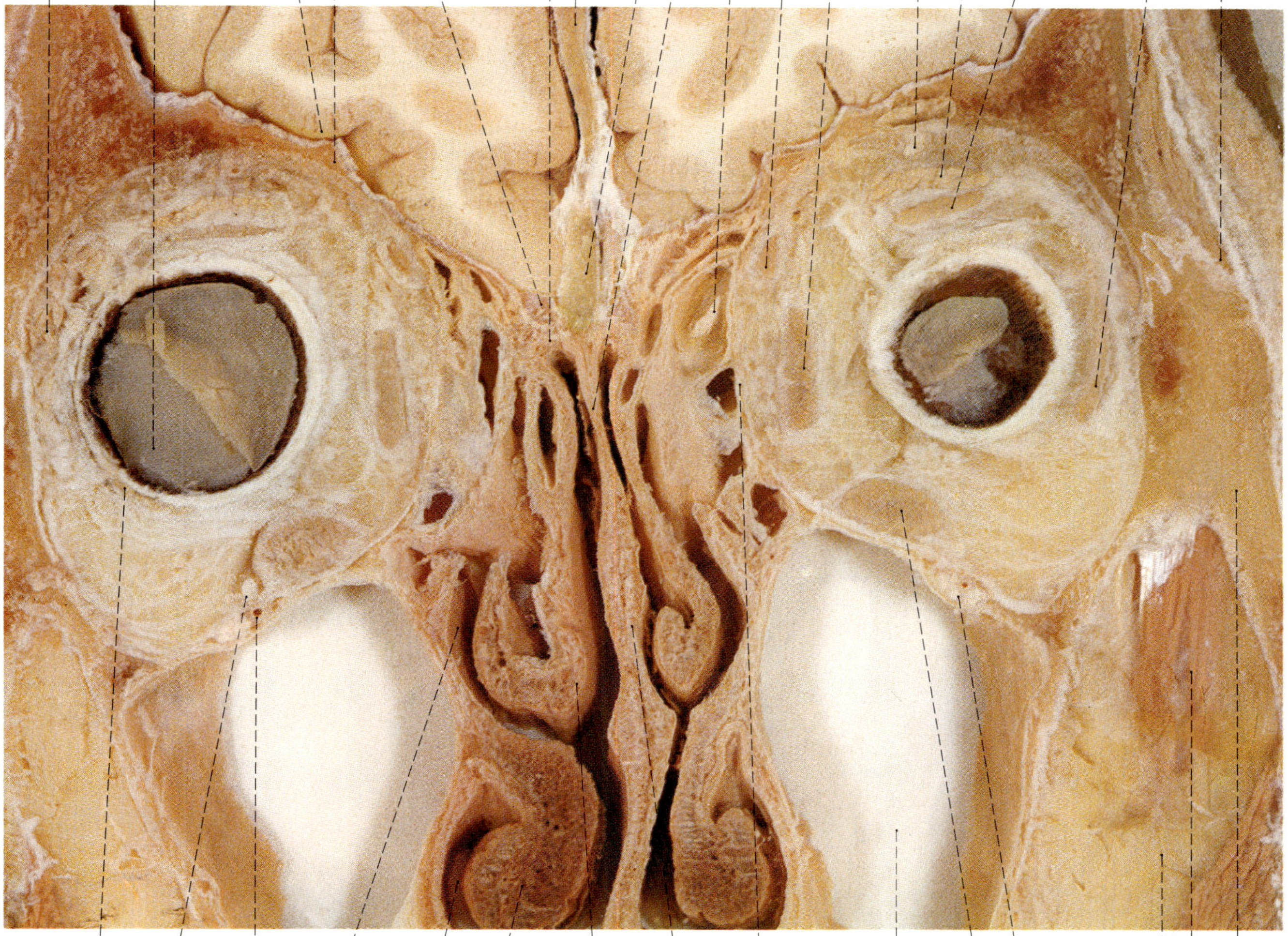

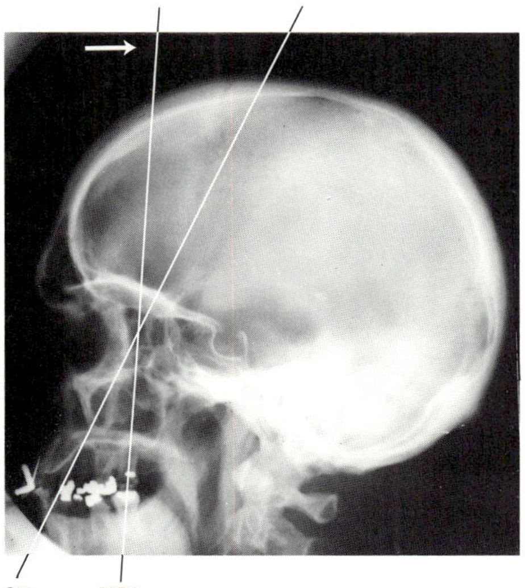

Planes of Sections

true coronal but still shows the medially placed portions of the frontal lobes in inferior locations (gyrus rectus), a relationship perhaps better appreciated on the angulated coronal CT slice.

In the MRI figure, the black triangles under the globes represent composite lack-of-signal from the maxillary sinus air and the envelope of maxillary sinus bone. The same is true of the ethmoidal sinuses.

The plane of the CT and MRI slices both pass through the posterior globe. On CT, the globe is of uniform density but on MRI a pure black spot at the supero-medial globe probably represents lack of signal from blood flowing in the central artery of the retina. Two densely black structures surrounded by high-signal (white) fat in the buccal areas just below the maxillary sinuses are probably due to blood flowing in the anterior facial veins.

Cadaver CT Scan

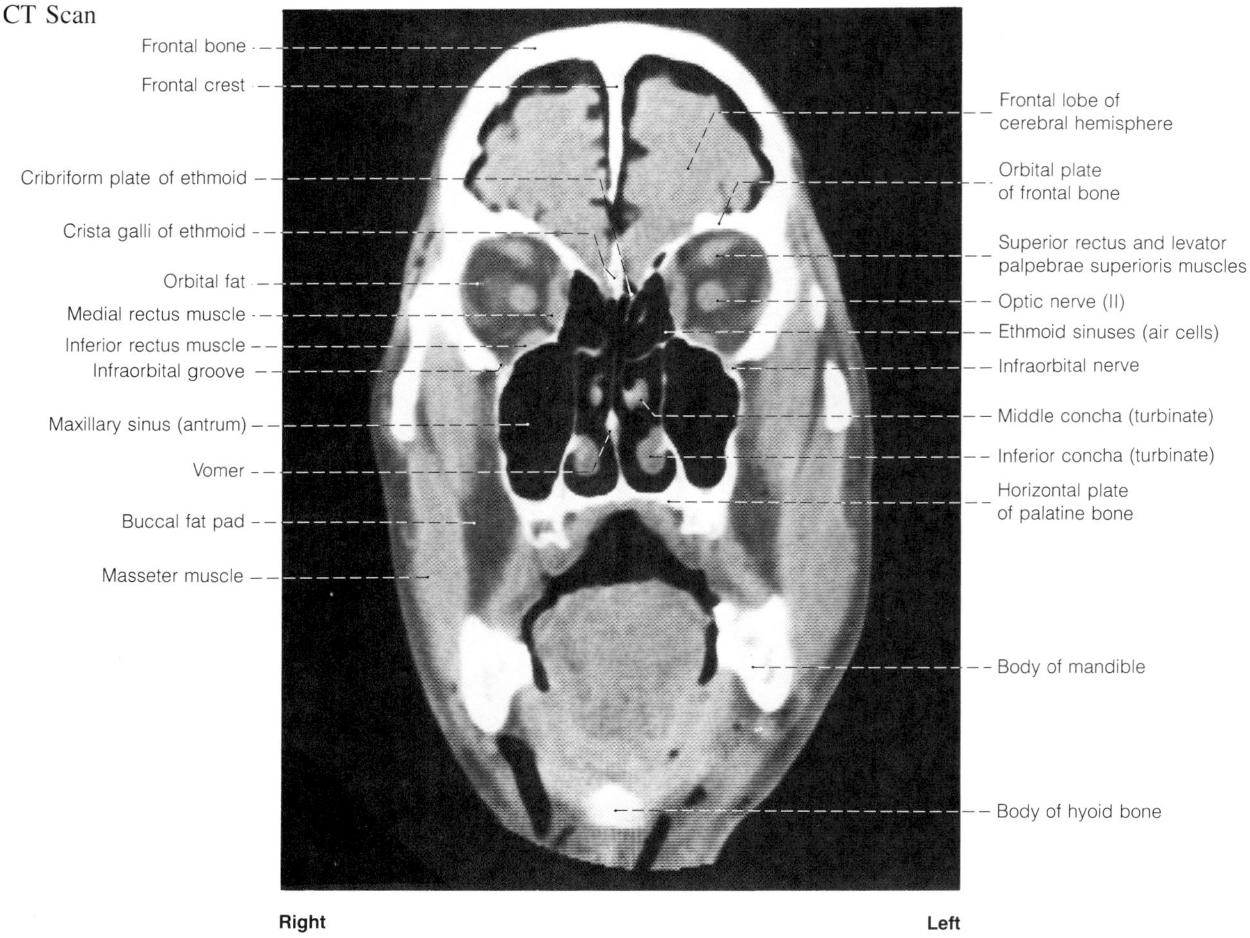

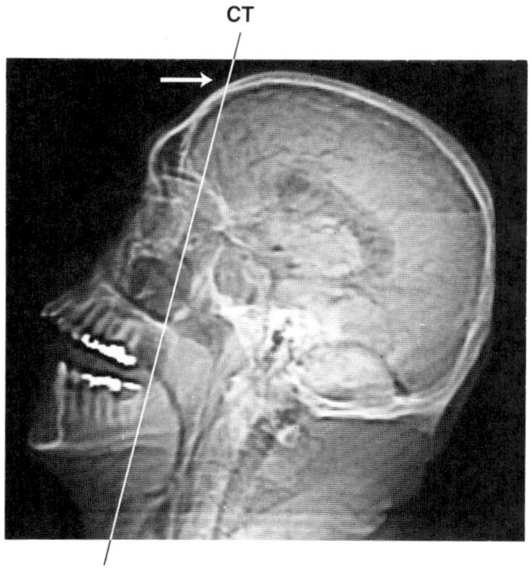

Plane of Section

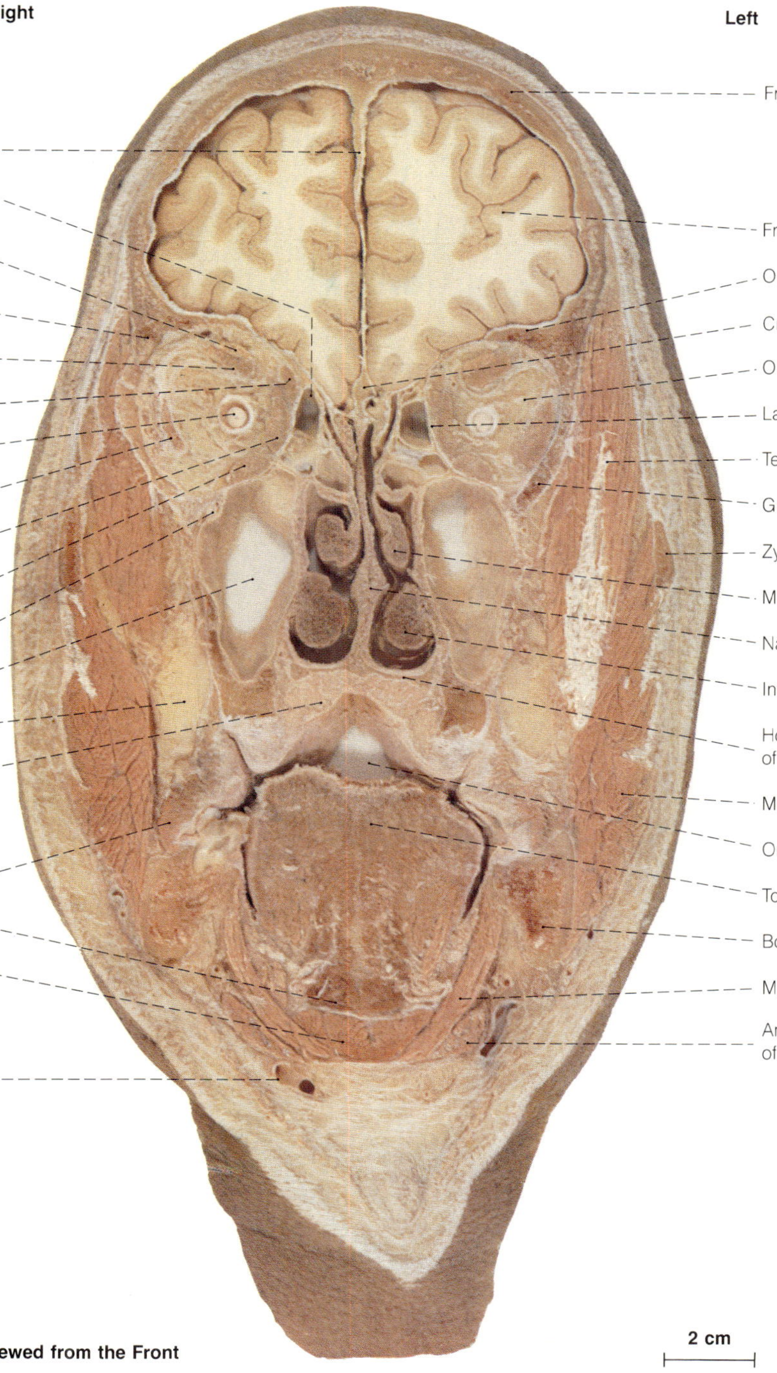

In this coronal section through the orbit just posterior to the globe, the optic nerve is seen in cross section with the cone of muscles delineated by the orbital fat. The contrast between the heavier lateral and the thin superior, medial, and inferior walls of the orbit is quite apparent.

Adjacent to the frontal lobes of the cerebral hemispheres one notes the crista galli and cribriform plate along with the characteristic medial slope to the orbital roof (floor of anterior cranial fossa). The frontal crest forming the anterior attachment of the falx cerebri is especially evident in the cadaver illustrated. Most CSF leaks will occur in this region.

The superior and middle turbinates (nasal conchae) are processes of the ethmoid bone; however, the inferior turbinate is a separate bone articulating largely with the maxilla. The inferior turbinate is a relatively large bone at birth.

The relationships of the muscles of the floor of the oral cavity are especially well visualized in this coronal section. These muscles form an anatomical boundary between some pathological processes within the mouth and those more superficial in the face and neck.

Patient CT Scan

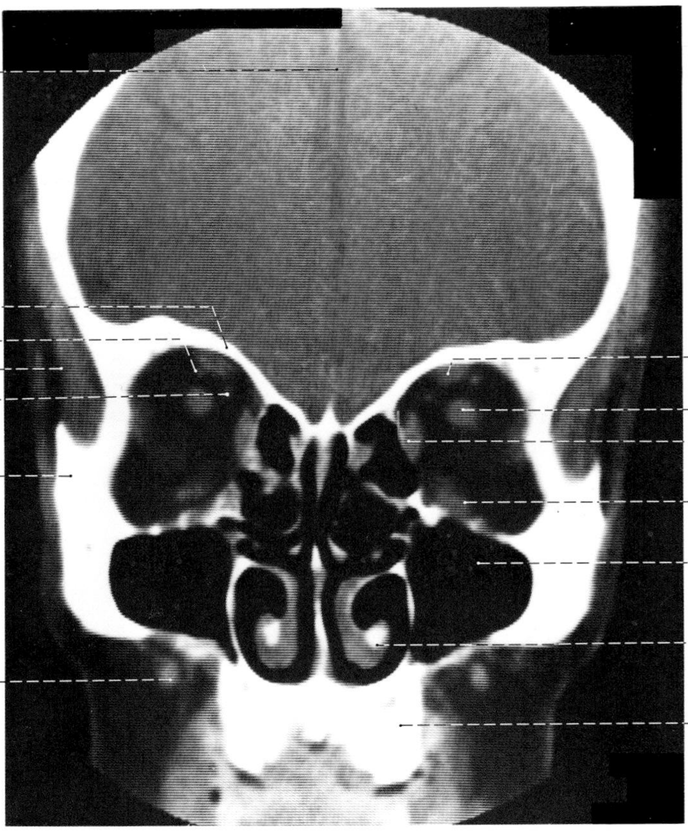

Patient MRI Scan

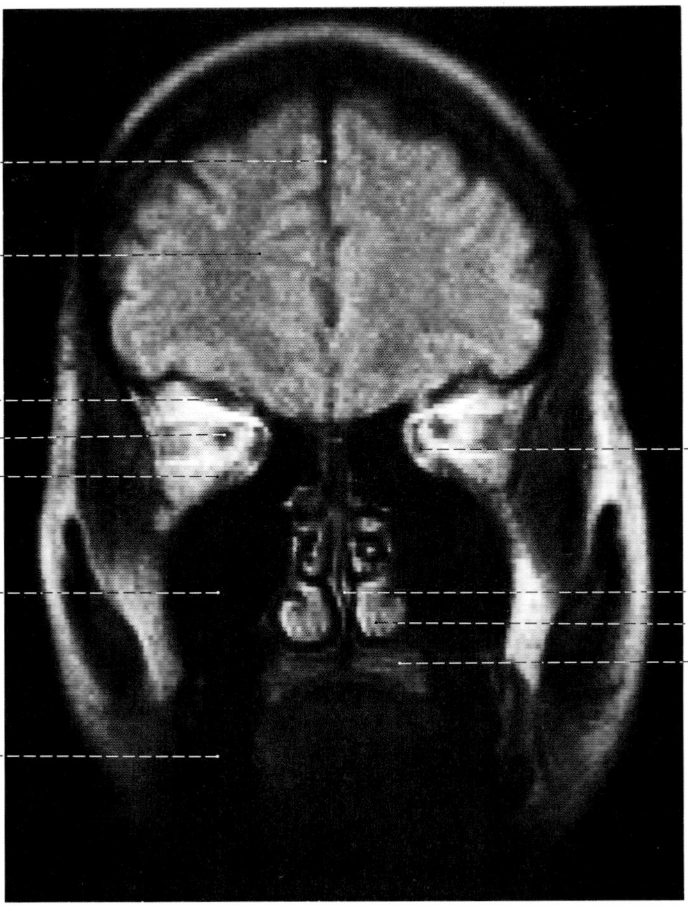

This coronal section is near the orbital apex where the cone of extraocular muscles is narrowing still further. The ophthalmic artery at this level is supero-medial to the optic nerve, but may course either medial or lateral to the nerve more anteriorly. Its lacrimal and supraorbital terminal branches anastomose over the face with the internal maxillary branch of the external carotid.

In this coronal section through the posterior orbit (nearing the apex), the optic nerve (CN II) is seen in cross-section revealing its dural coat and extension of the intracranial subarachnoid space. The central artery of the retina, a branch of the ophthalmic artery, is clearly illustrated on the gross anatomical photograph. The ophthalmic artery supplies not only the orbital contents, but through its ethmoidal branches supplies the ethmoidal sinuses and the anterior falx. Anastomotic branches with the facial artery may provide the globe with retrograde flow which, in cases of occlusion of the internal carotid artery, may be sufficient to limit retinal loss.

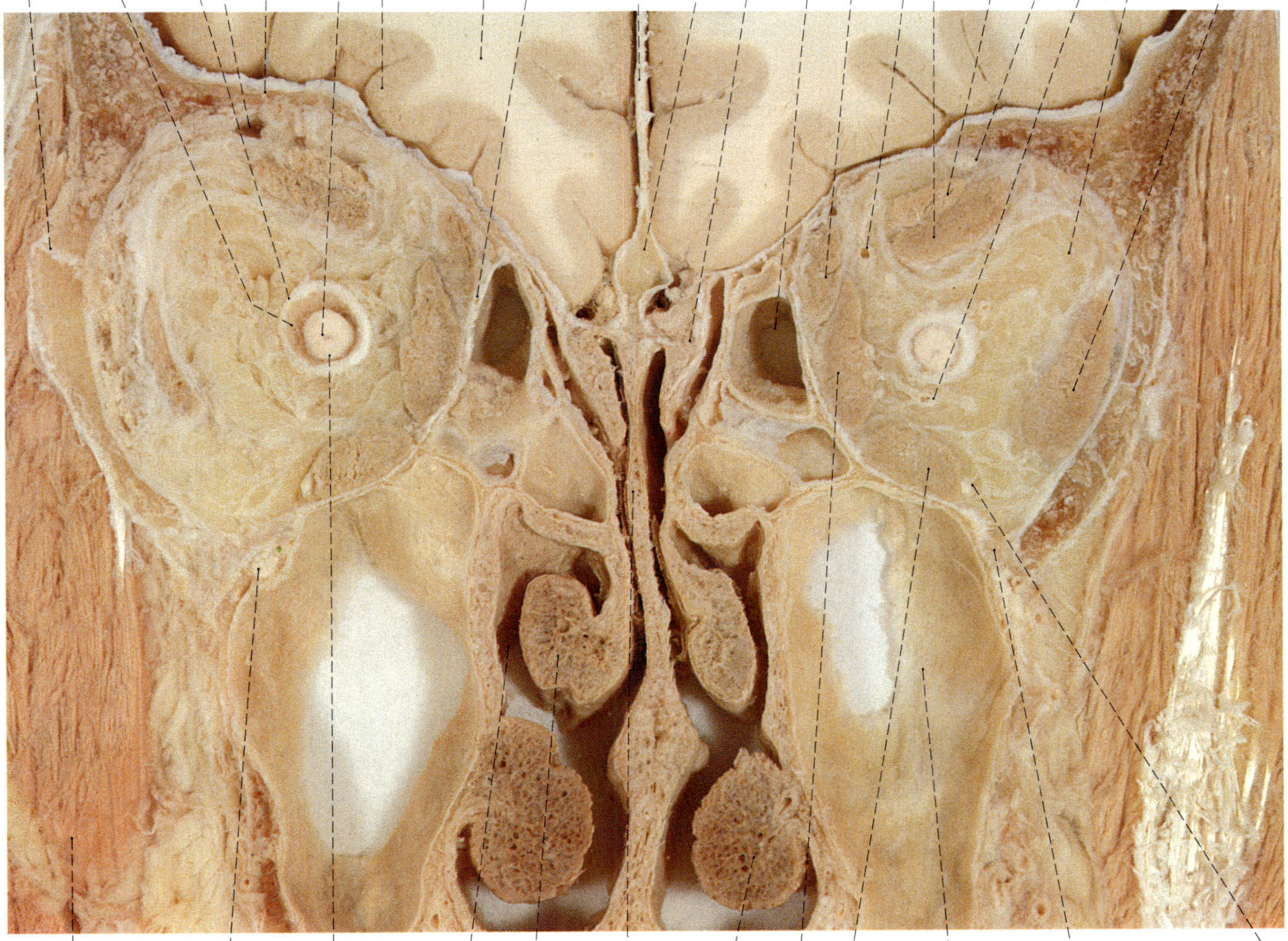

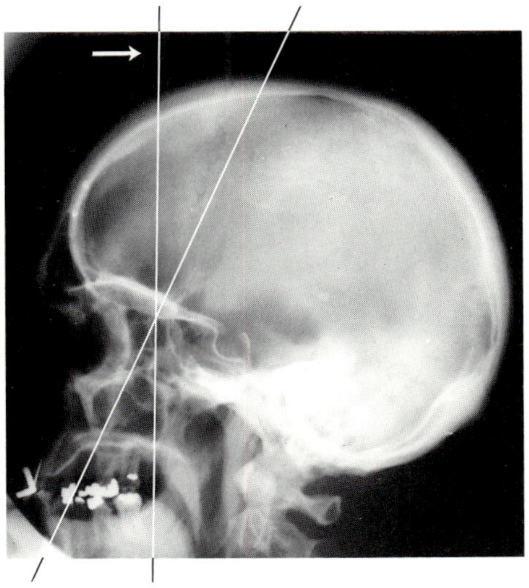

Planes of Sections

Emphasized in this anatomical section are the extremely thin bony plates of the orbital roof – floor of anterior fossa.

On CT, the extraocular muscles are well seen as they approach each other in the apex of the orbit, forming the muscle cone. The optic nerves can be appreciated and checked for symmetry. If metrizamide is placed intrathecally, the subarachnoid space surrounding the optic nerve may be clearly appreciated. On MRI, the white fat of the orbit provides excellent contrast for delineation of orbital structures including the vascular structures which appear densely black because of the lack of an accumulated signal from the blood flowing within them.

Cadaver CT Scan

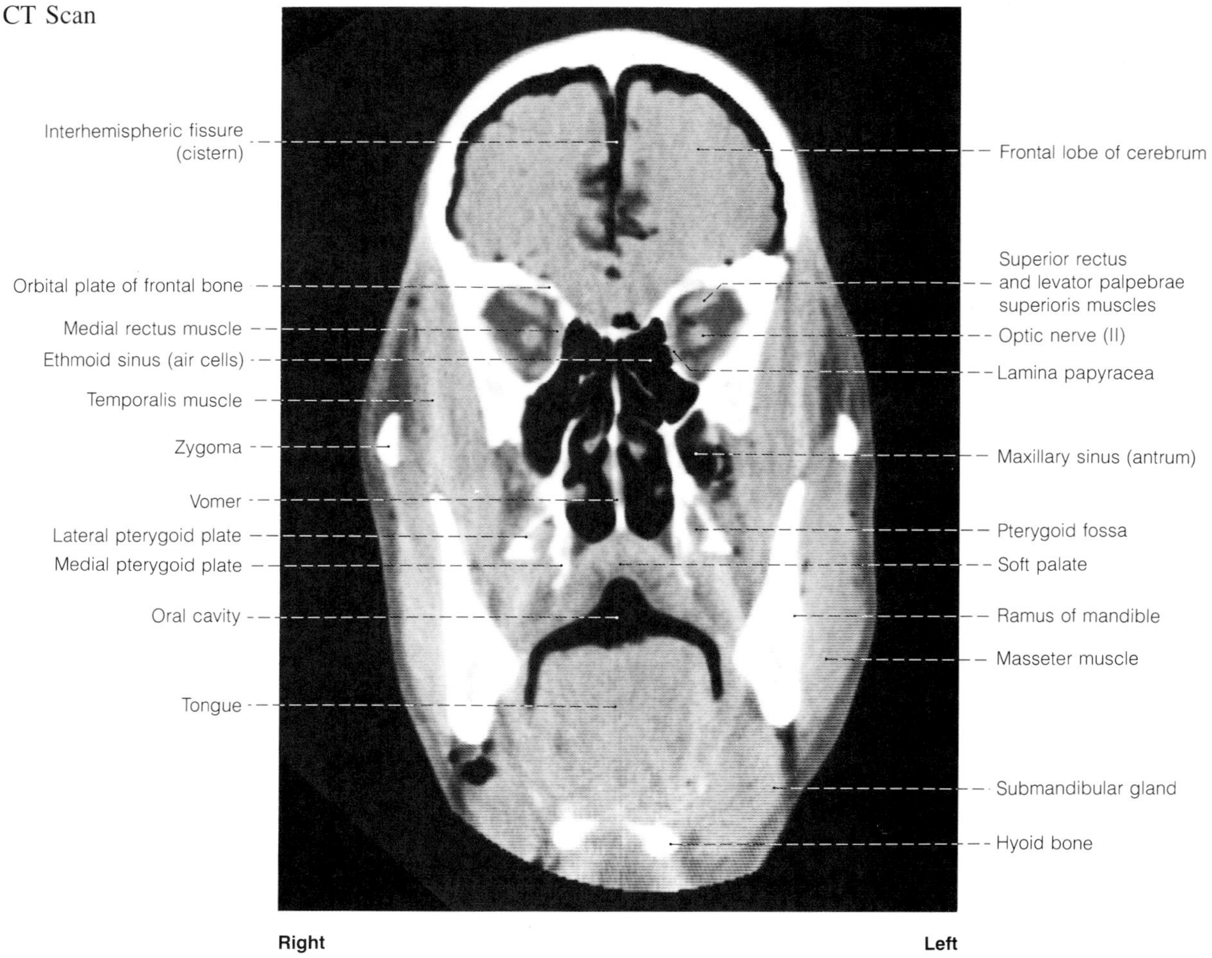

Plane of Section

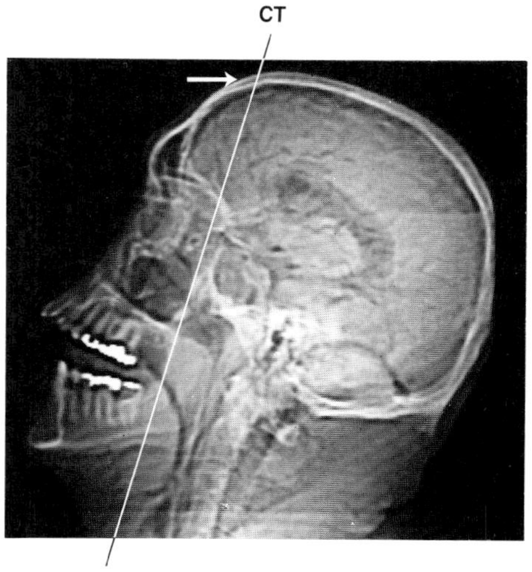

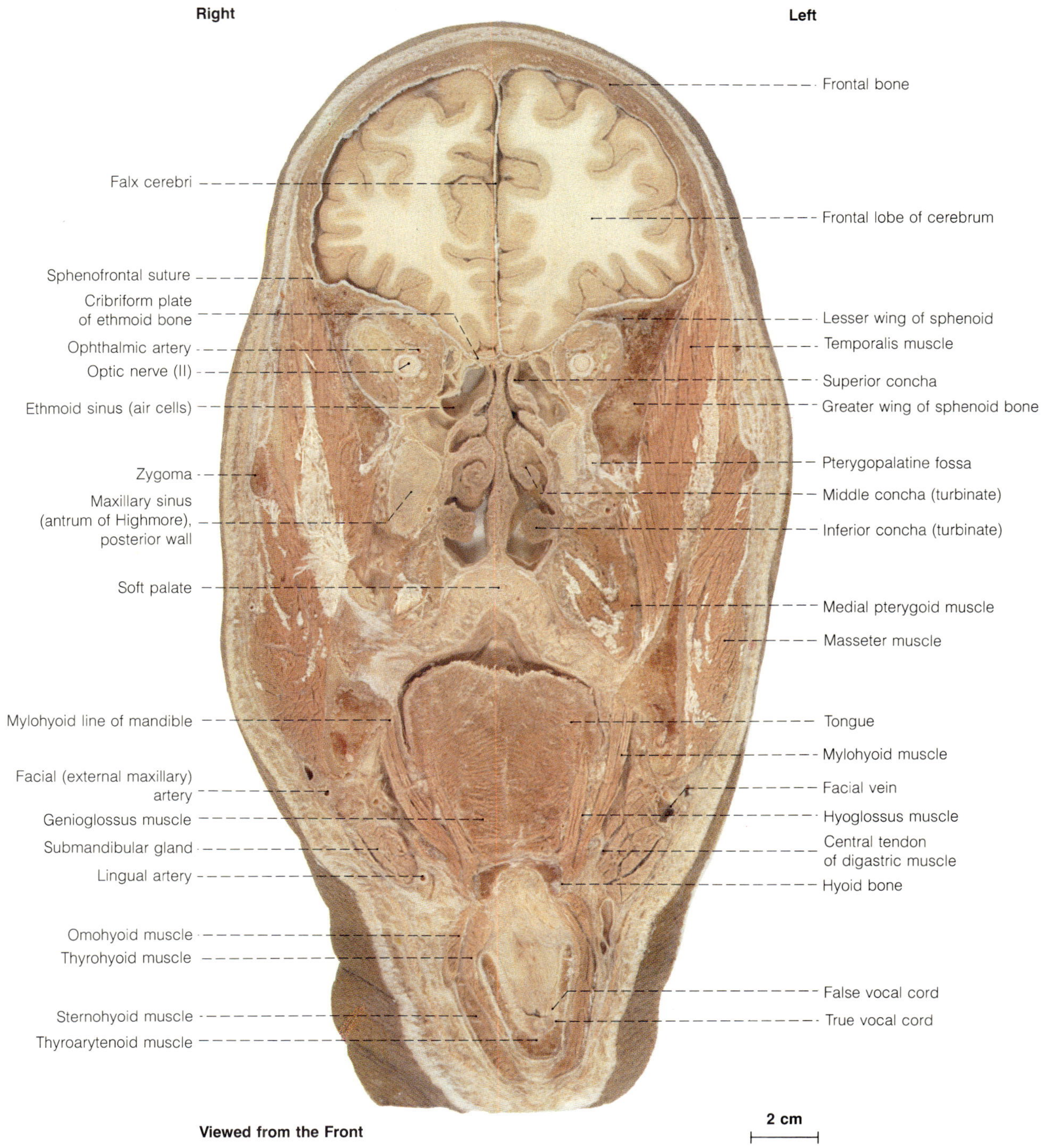

The plane of the section on the left side of the specimen passes through the pterygopalatine fossa and its communication with the orbit through the inferior orbital fissure. This fossa contains the sphenopalatine (pterygopalatine) ganglion and the maxillary division (V_2) of the trigeminal nerve.

One gains an appreciation of the very large amount of space occupied by the facial structures in relation to the remainder of the cranial contents.

Patient CT Scan

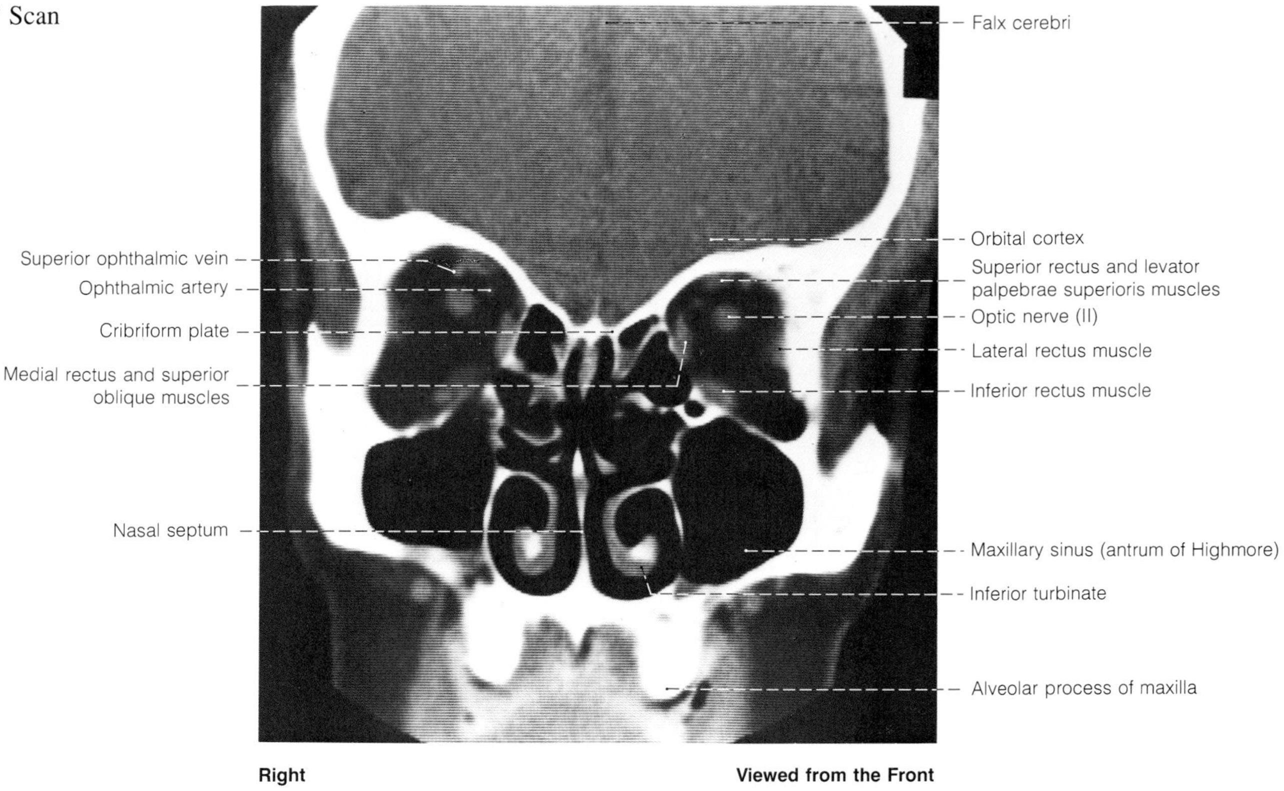

Patient MRI Scan

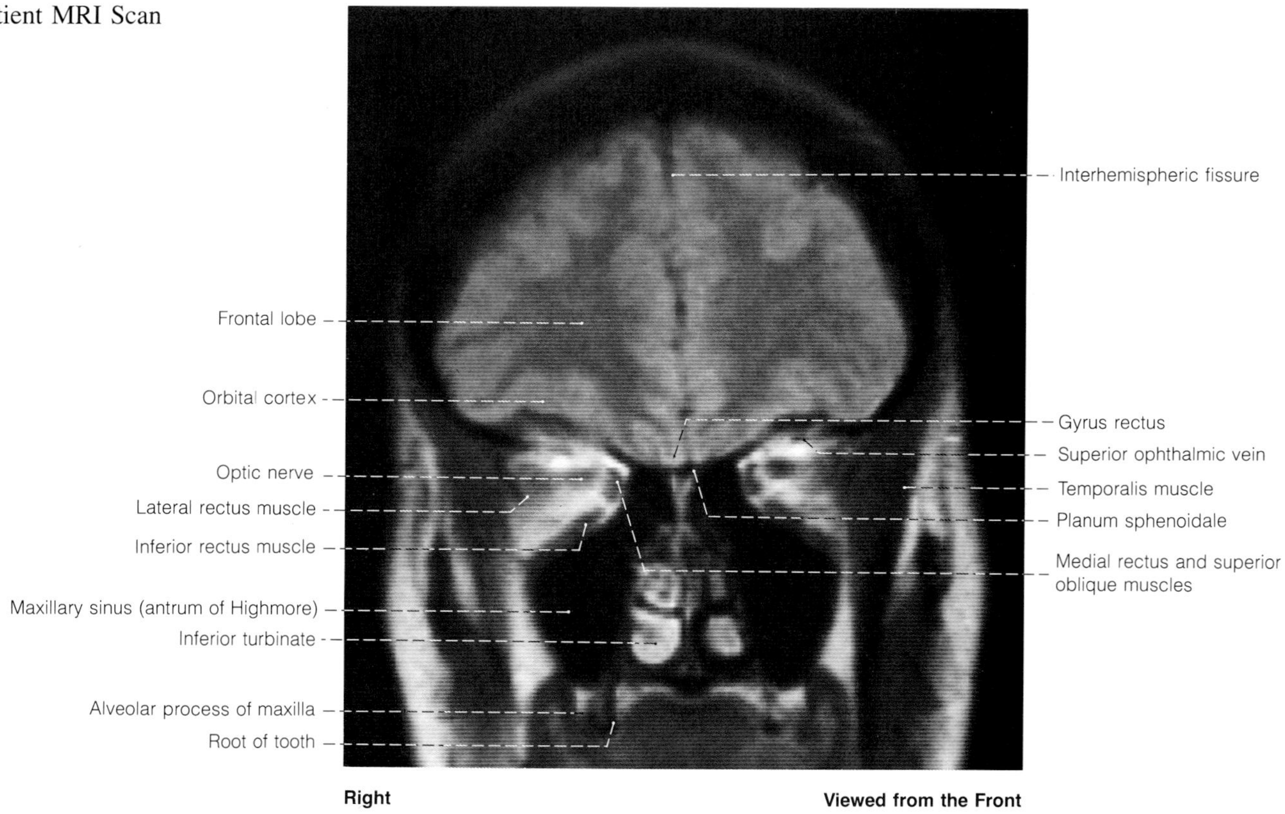

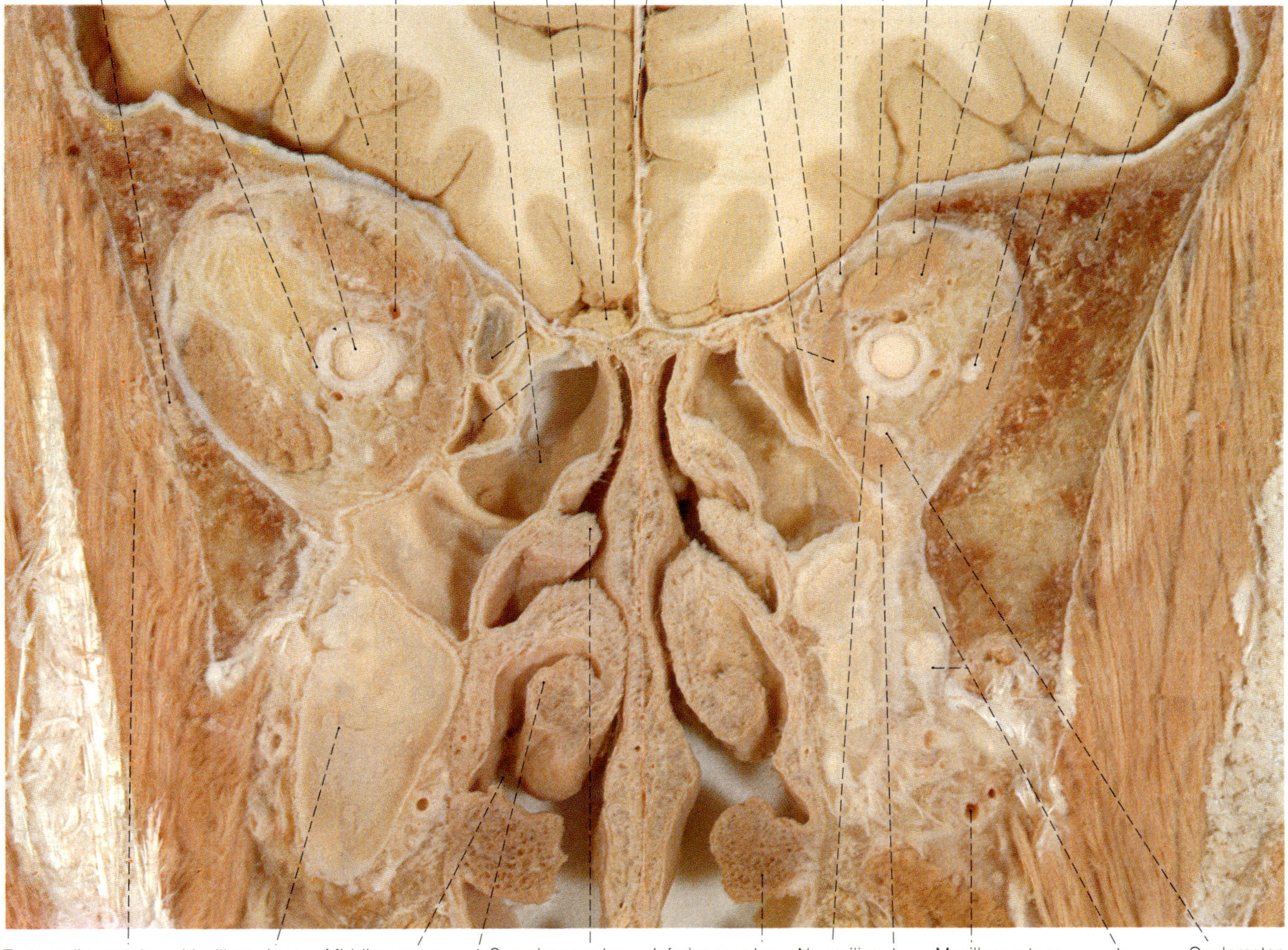

Planes of Sections

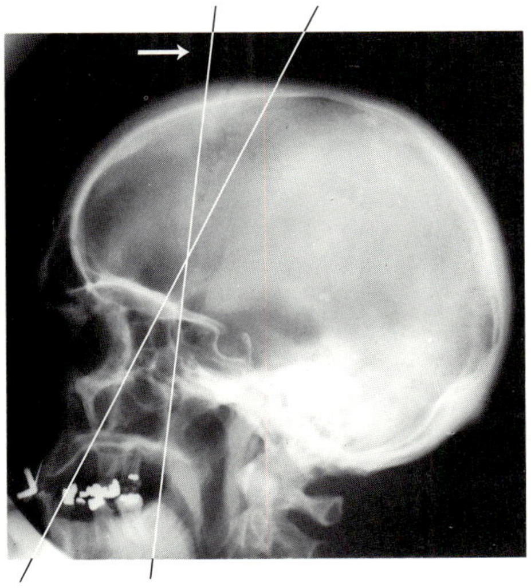

These coronal sections through the posterior orbit also expose the large posterior expanses of the maxillary sinuses and, on the left side of the anatomical section, the pterygopalatine fossa. Pathological processes in this region may expand into the ethmoidal sinuses, orbits, or posteriorly into the middle cranial fossa.

The superior ophthalmic vein is visualized on the CT scan with the use of contrast medium but is evident on MRI because of the low signal of moving blood. This vein communicates posteriorly with the cavernous sinus and anteriorly with the anterior facial vein. With slightly higher resolution the dense black of the ophthalmic artery might be separable from the grey of the optic nerve.

This MRI sequence emphasizes grey-white matter differences to a slight extent with the frontal association fibers in the frontal lobe clearly shown along with adjacent cortical grey areas.

Cadaver CT Scan

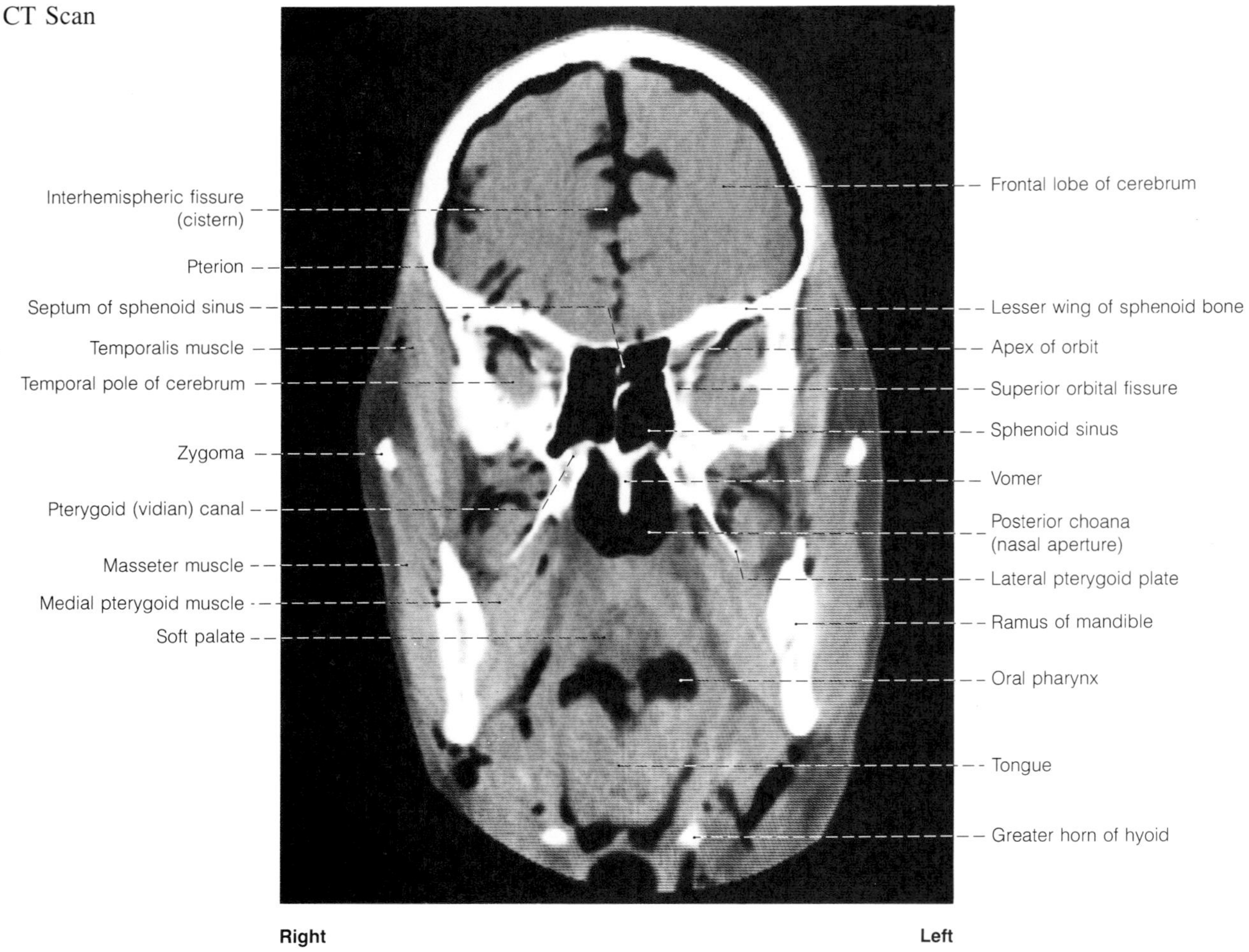

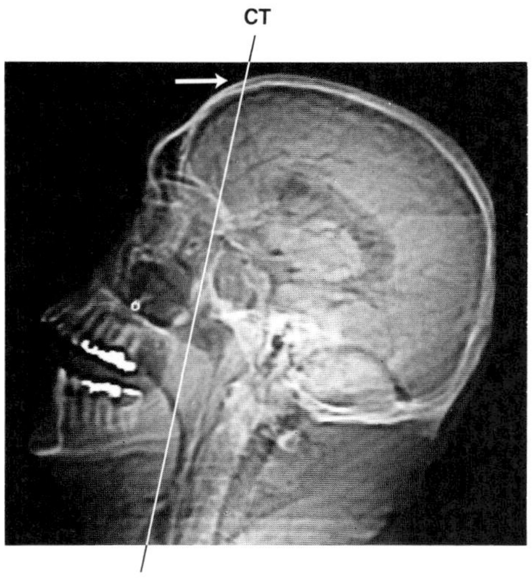

Plane of Section

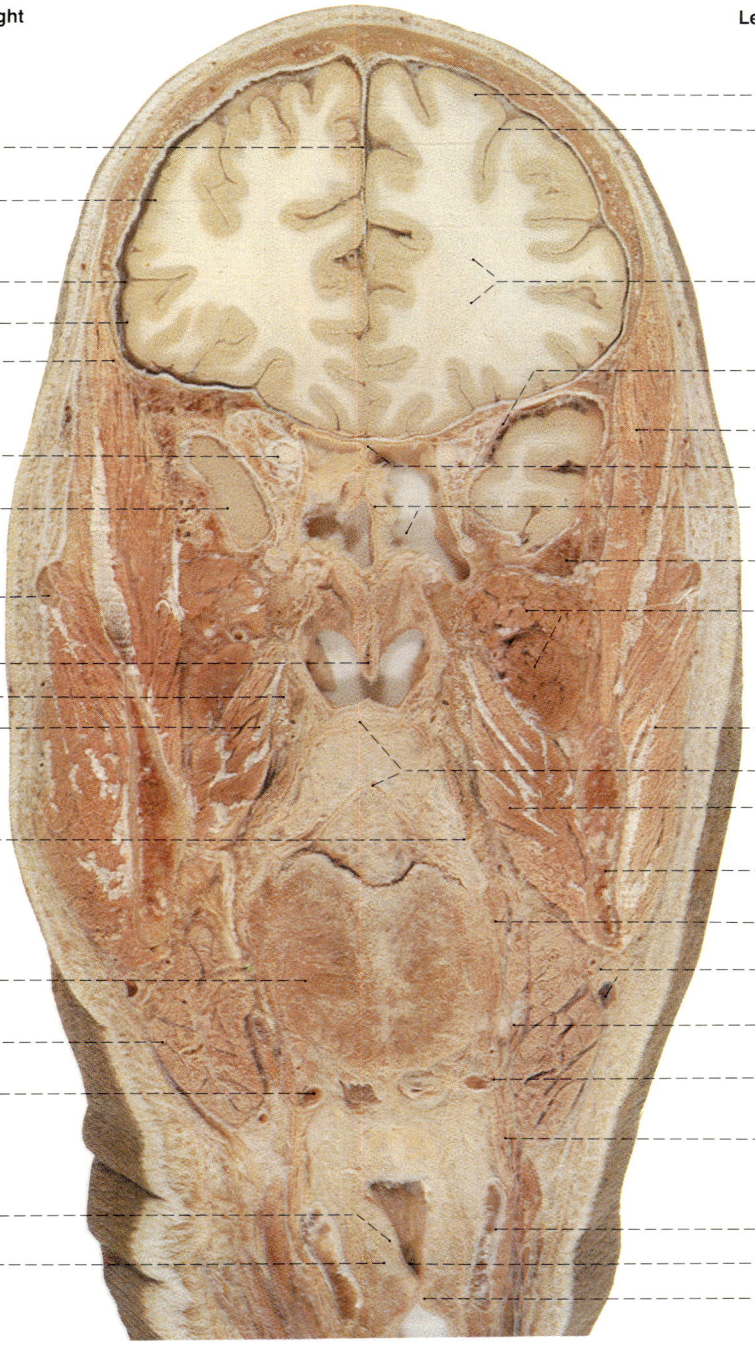

At the apex of the orbit, the dura surrounding the optic nerve is continuous with intracranial dura. A portion is condensed to form the anulus of Zinn (common tendinous ring) to which the extraocular muscles (except the inferior oblique) attach. The sphenoid sinus comes into view (with highly variable septation), as does the tip of the temporal lobe in the anterior portion of the middle fossa. The anterior and middle fossa are divided by the lesser wing of the sphenoid bone. The subcortical white matter of the frontal lobe contains the very important interconnections with the diencephalon and with other cortical areas as well as projections to the pons. The interhemispheric fissure (cistern) contains the relatively short anterior portion of the falx (and branches of the anterior cerebral arteries) and may appear larger than in planes through the posterior hemispheres. Within the posterior portion of the oral cavity, approaching the nasopharynx, the cut passes through the soft palate.

The opposing actions of the medial (internal) and lateral (external) pterygoid muscles of elevating and lowering the mandible and the chewing or grinding actions of the masseter and medial pterygoids are easily visualized in this section. With the temporalis, these muscles form an impressive mass acting on the mandible.

Patient CT Scan

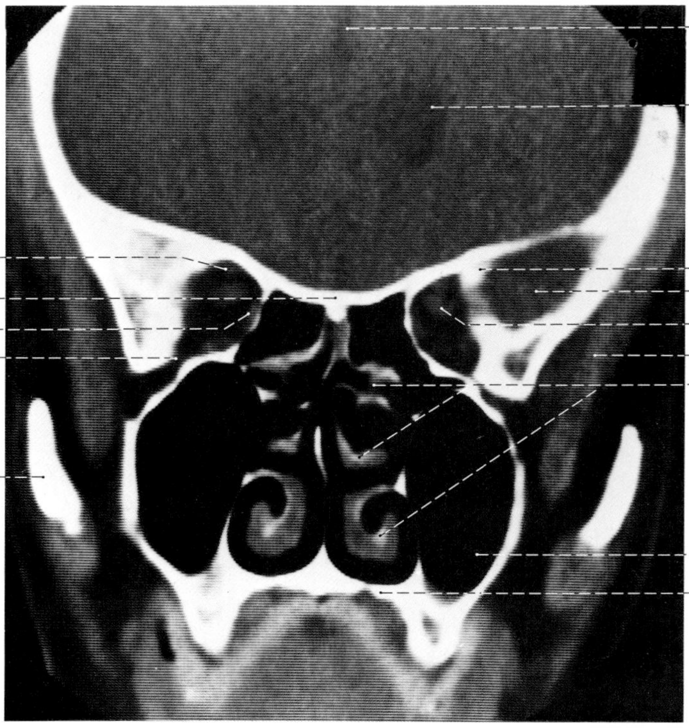

Patient MRI Scan

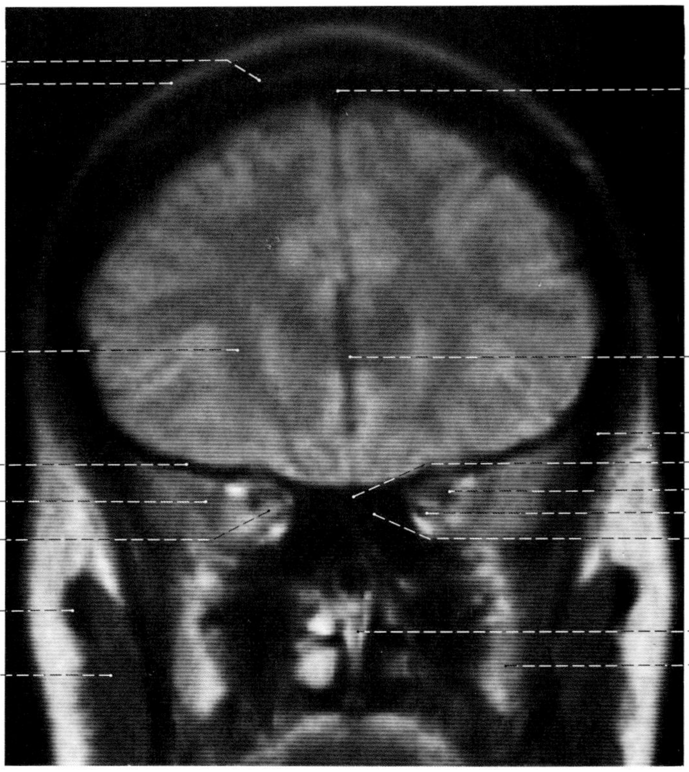

The vertical coronal sections through the posterior orbit and jugum (planum) sphenoidale in the anatomical section and MRI scan pass through the pterygoid plates and sphenoid sinus, but, because of the different angle, only intersect the maxillary sinus in the CT image. At the apex of the orbit, the frontal branch of the 1st division (ophthalmic, V_1) of the trigeminal nerve (V) is superior and the inferior division of the oculomotor nerve (III) is inferior to the optic nerve. The 2nd division (maxillary, V_2) of the trigeminal nerve (V) is viewed entering the foramen rotundum. The olfactory tracts, true tracts of the CNS, terminate in the telencephalon and are enclosed within the subarachnoid space in the olfactory sulcus.

The differentiation between the grey matter of the cerebral cortex and the subcortical white matter is nicely demonstrated on the MRI scan. The orbital and medial gyri of the frontal lobes have

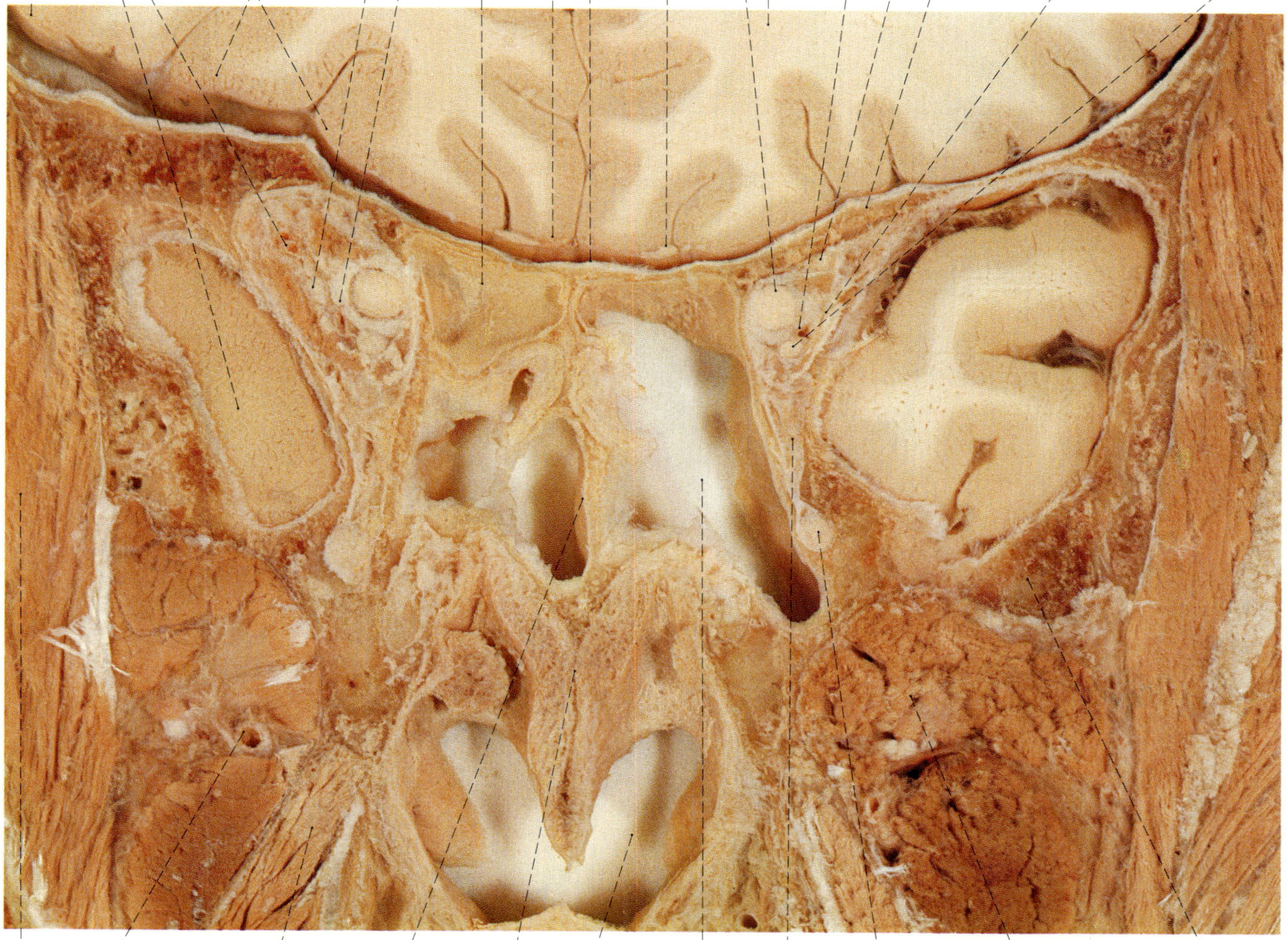

Viewed from the Front

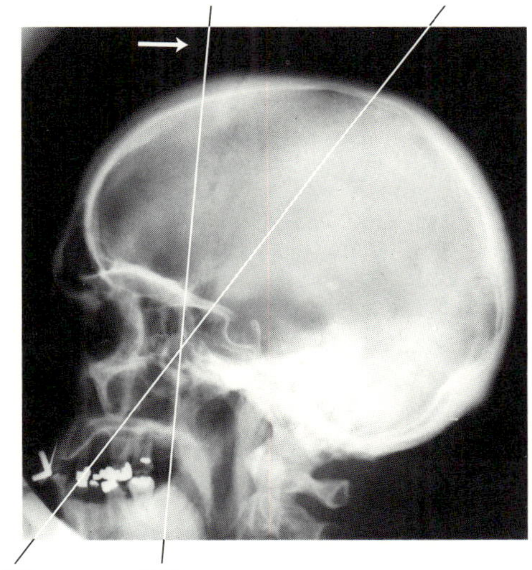

Planes of Sections

interconnections with limbic areas of the brain, and consequently, visceral and behavioral alterations may accompany lesions in these areas.

A dense black curvilinear midline structure may represent the genu of the pericallosal branch of the anterior cerebral artery. Fibers crossing between hemispheres at the same level are probably callosal fibers in the genu of the corpus callosum. The state of the art for MRI scans at the time of this printing displays slices approximately 1 cm thick which will include several structures that overlie each other in a volume-averaging effect.

Another interesting anatomical feature well represented on both the MRI and the CT slices is the proximity of temporal lobe tip to the orbital apex and lesser wing of the sphenoid.

Cadaver CT Scan

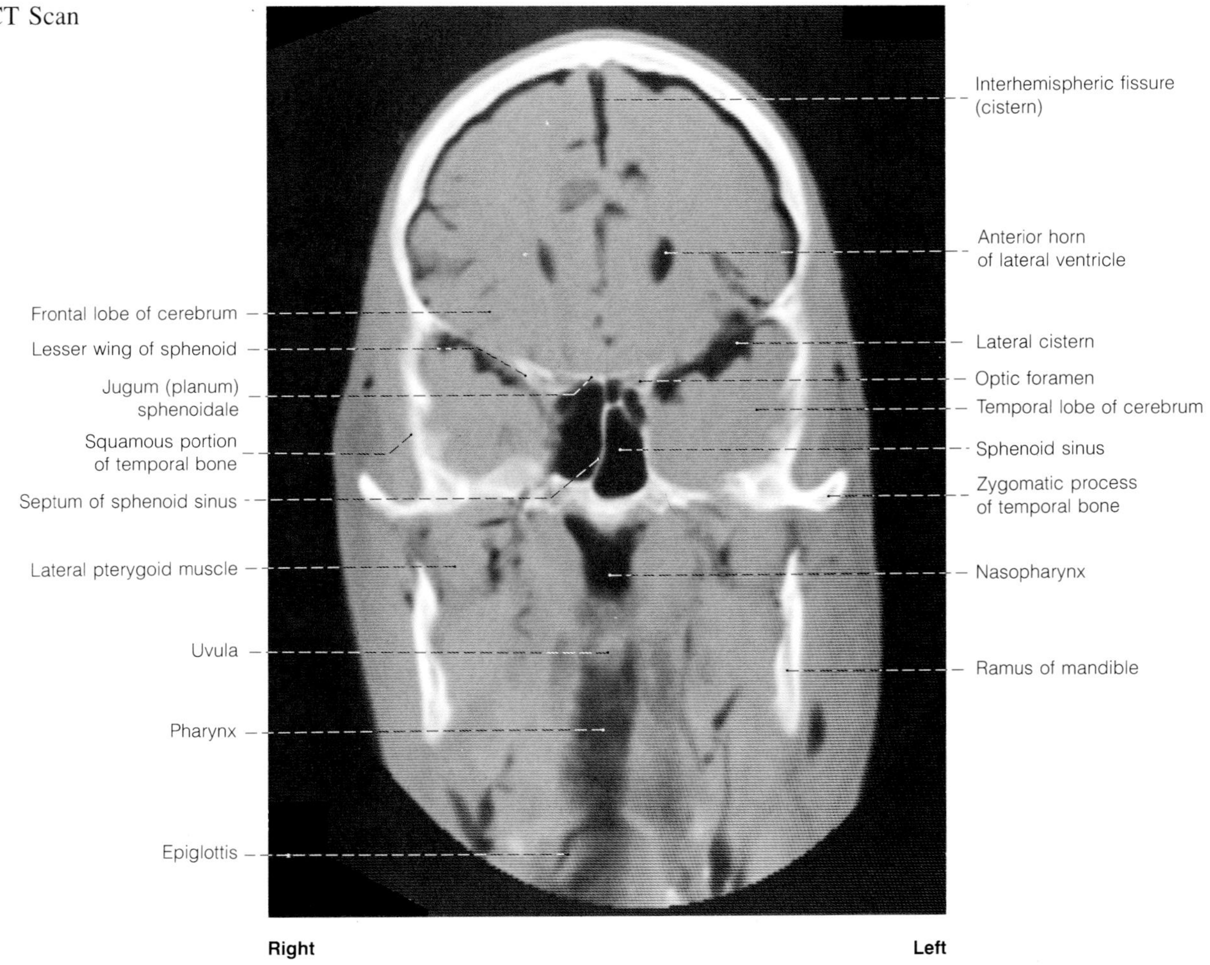

Plane of Section

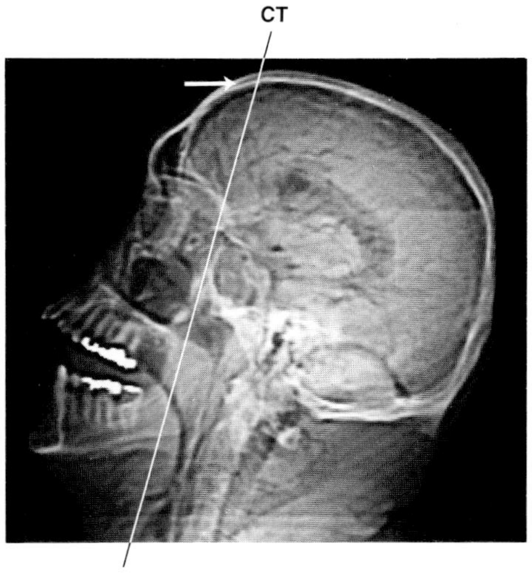

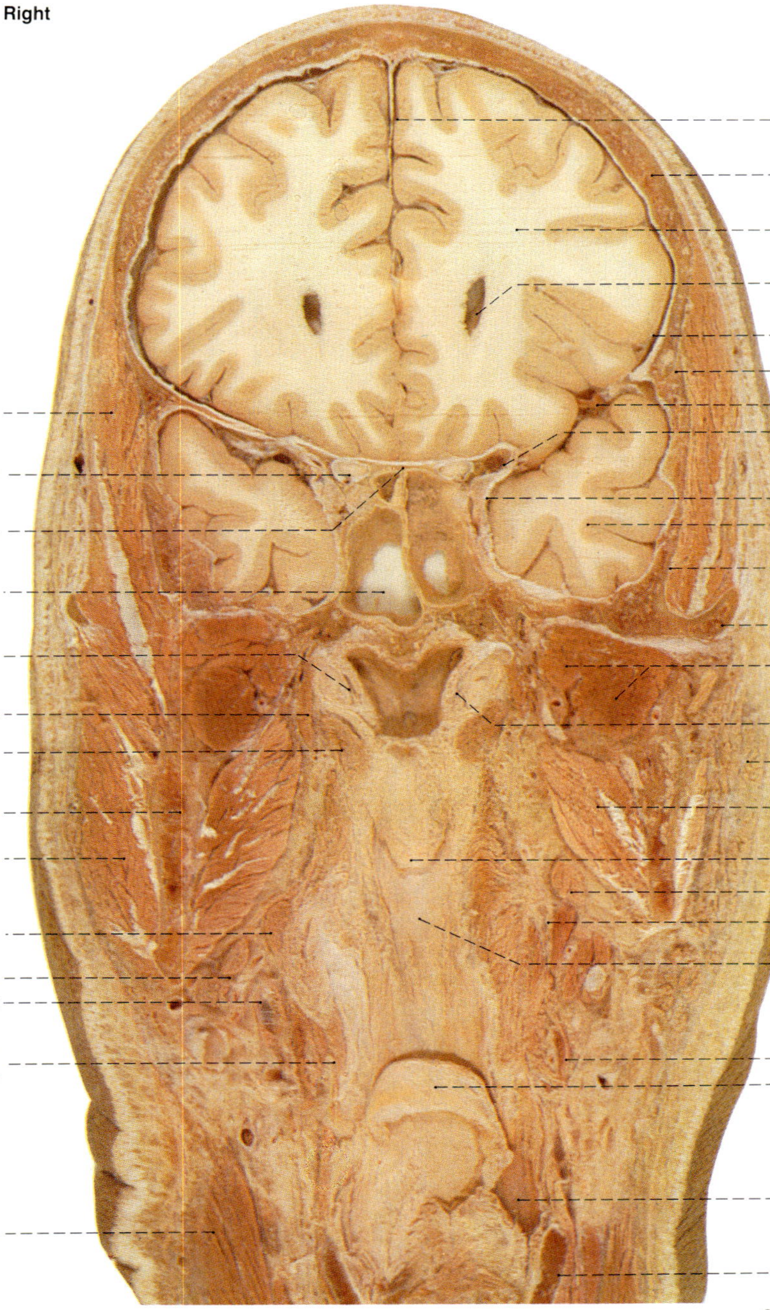

Viewed from the Front

In this coronal section through the middle of the sphenoid sinus, the optic nerve (II) passes intracranially, medial to the anterior clinoids. The posterior pharyngeal wall, uvula, pterygoid muscles, and epiglottis are also visualized in this plane. The pharyngeal opening of the Eustachian (auditory or pharyngo-tympanic) tube, communicating with the middle ear and mastoid air cells, is just anterior to the plane of the section. In infants, lymphoid tissue surrounds this pharyngeal orifice and may be quite extensive.

The most anterior extent of the frontal horns of the lateral ventricles is located in this coronal section which also passes through the posterior margin of the lesser wing of the sphenoid. Variations in the size of the ventricles or in the angle of the cut will obviously alter this relationship.

Optic Nerve in Optic Canal (Foramen)

Patient CT Scan

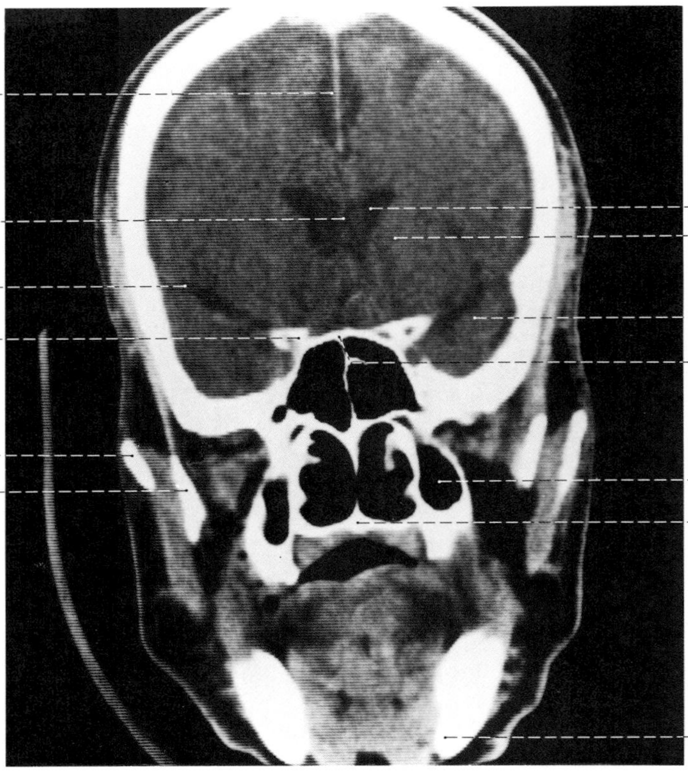

Patient MRI Scan

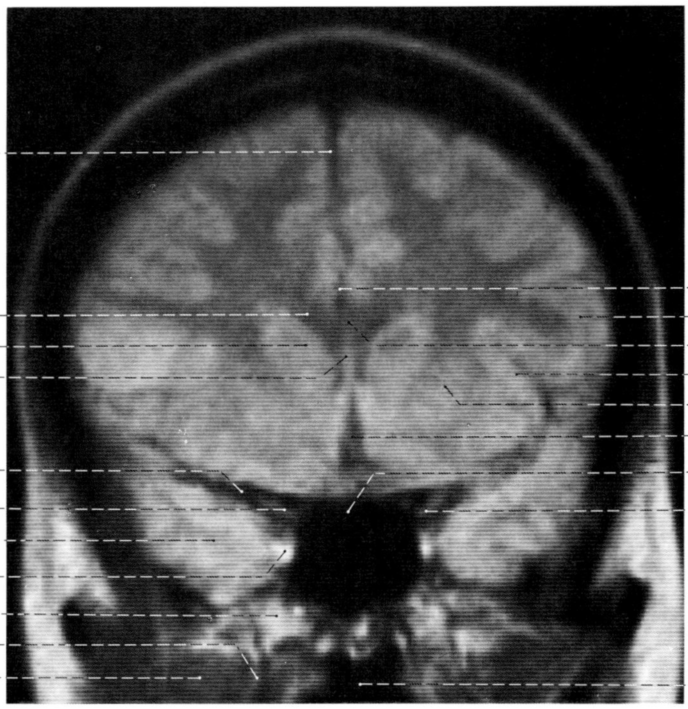

In this coronal section through the anterior clinoids, the ophthalmic artery is seen inferiolateral to the optic nerve. More inferior, the vidian nerve (nerve of the pterygoid canal) is exposed as it courses toward the pterygopalatine fossa.

Although the ventricular surface of the caudate nucleus can be visualized on the CT scan because of the low impedance of the ventricular cerebrospinal fluid (CSF) to x-rays, it is entirely visible in the MRI image as is the anterior limb of the internal capsule and putamen. The continuity of the frontal and temporal lobes with the insula is also clearly shown because this MRI sequence of imaging emphasizes grey-white matter differences. These areas are intimately interconnected by the uncinate fasciculus providing an anatomical substrate for the clinical problems frequently encountered in localization of lesions here. There is clearly more information available on MRI with relation to fiber tracts and nuclei due to the ability to differentiate grey and white matter than there is on CT which depends in large part upon interfaces in brain parenchyma and CSF for its differentiation.

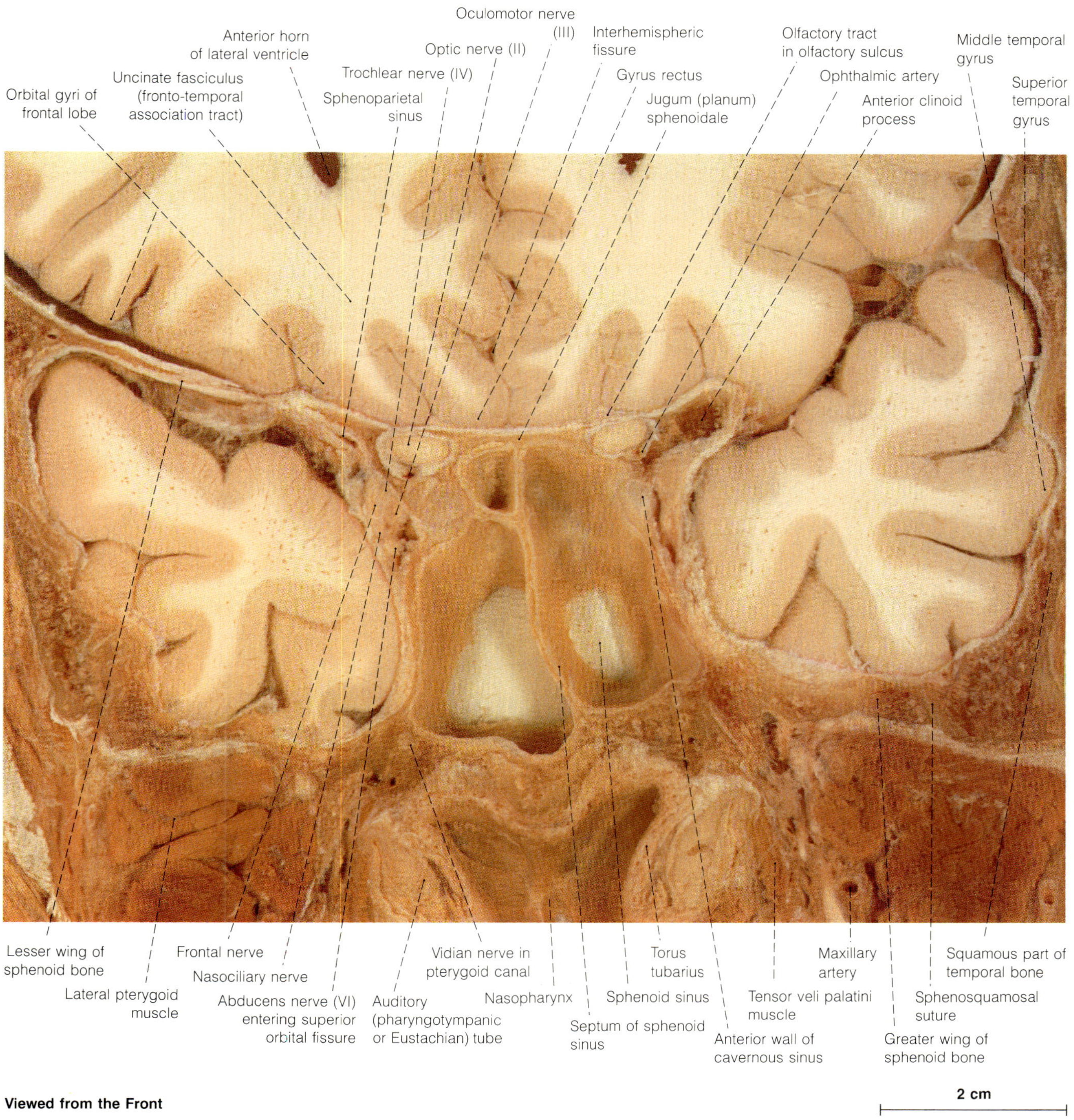

Viewed from the Front

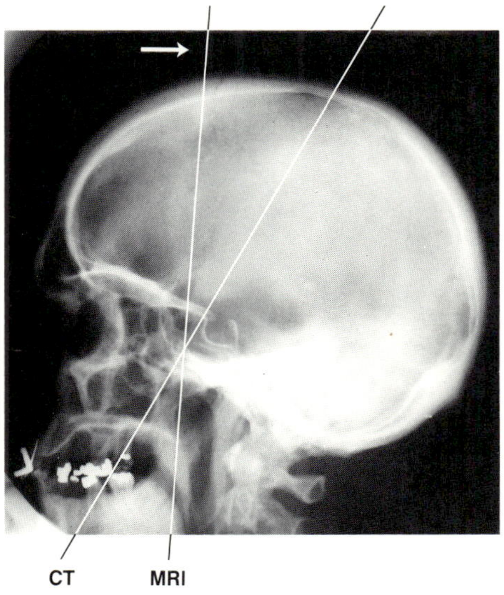

Planes of Sections

Cadaver CT Scan

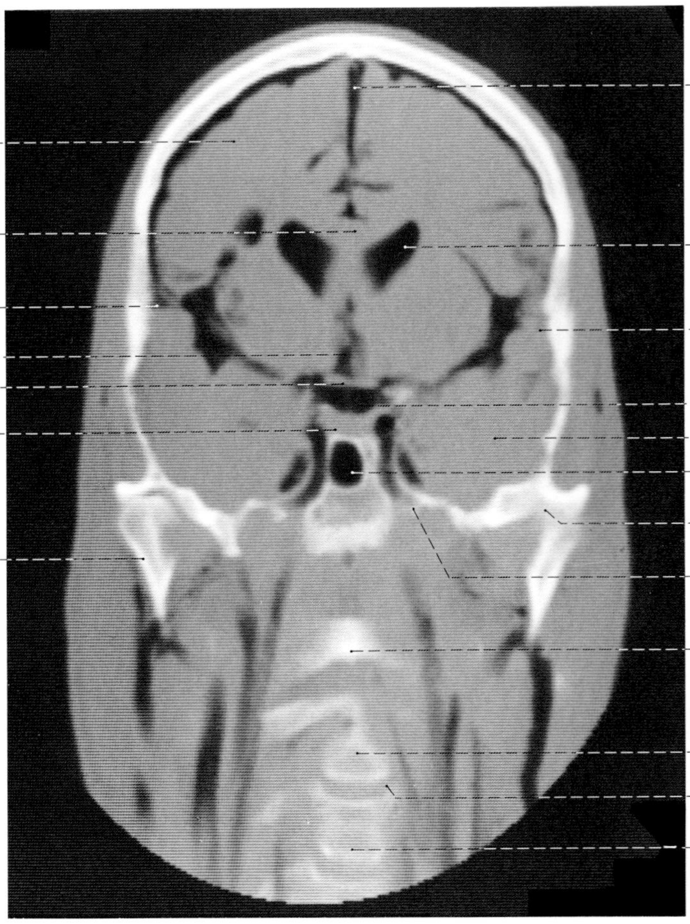

This coronal slice passes through the pituitary fossa where the pituitary gland is well visualized (normal superior-inferior dimensions 7-9 mm). Depending upon amount of pneumatization, the posterior part of the sphenoid sinus extends to this plane. An excellent view of the parasellar relationships of the optic nerve just anterior to the chiasm (superio-medially), and the internal carotid artery (inferio-medially) is obtained. The inferior part of the cavernous carotid (the carotid siphon) is seen in cross-section within the cavernous sinus. The lateral confines of the sella are clearly shown as limited to a dural envelope which is all that separates the pituitary from the internal carotid artery. Pituitary neoplasms may grow superiorly enough to obliterate the cistern and may impinge upward to involve hypothalamic structures or anteriorly to involve the optic chiasm.

The bulk of parenchyma at this coronal level is the frontal lobe but large amounts of temporal lobe proper and operculum are seen separated from the basal ganglia by the Sylvian and insular cisterns.

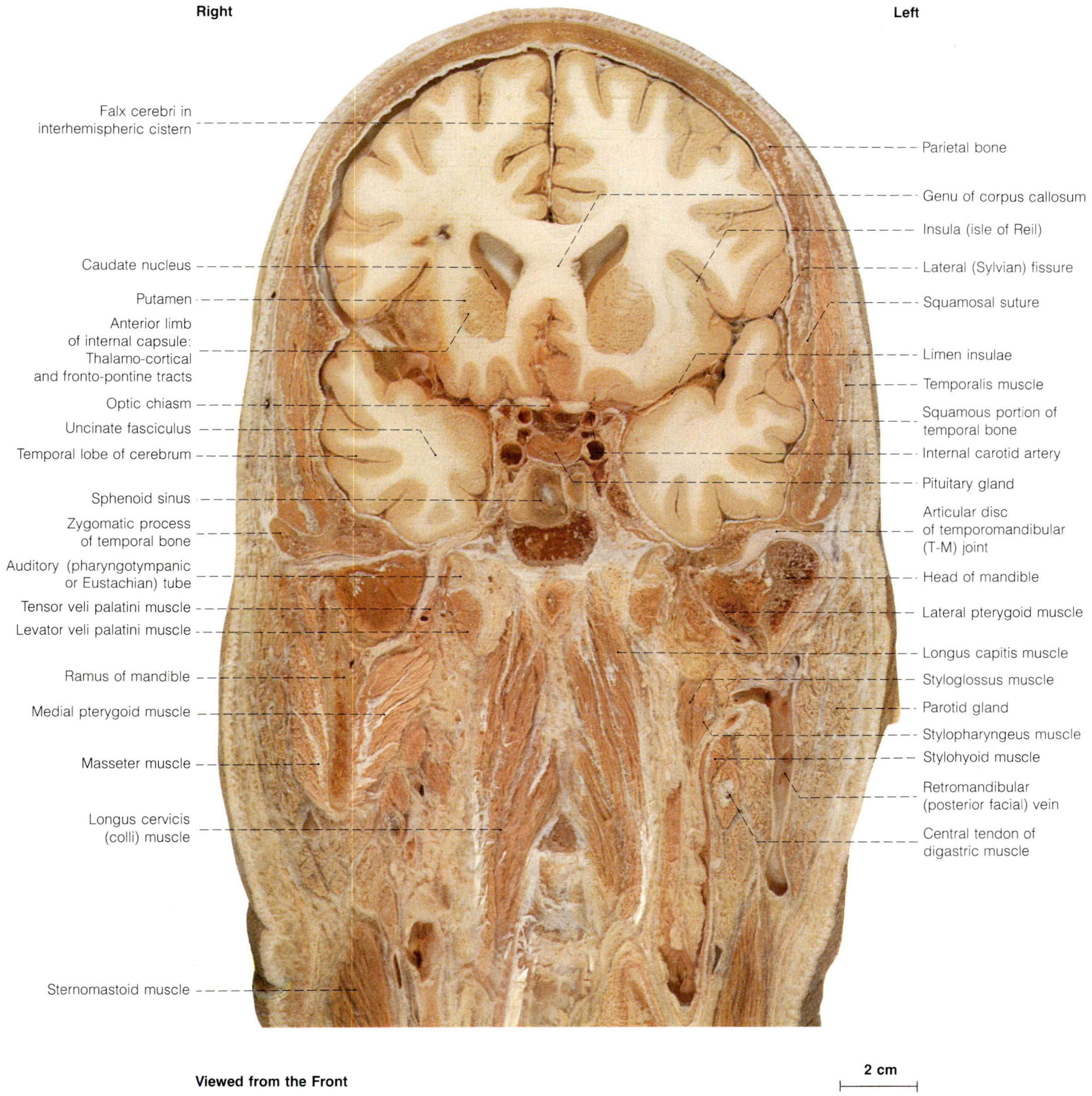

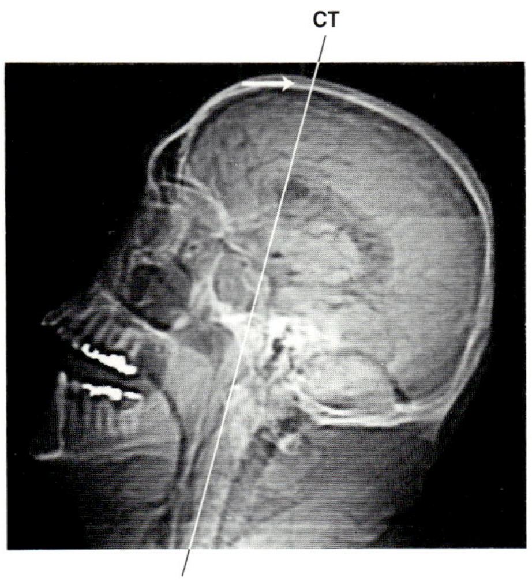

Plane of Section

Patient CT Scan

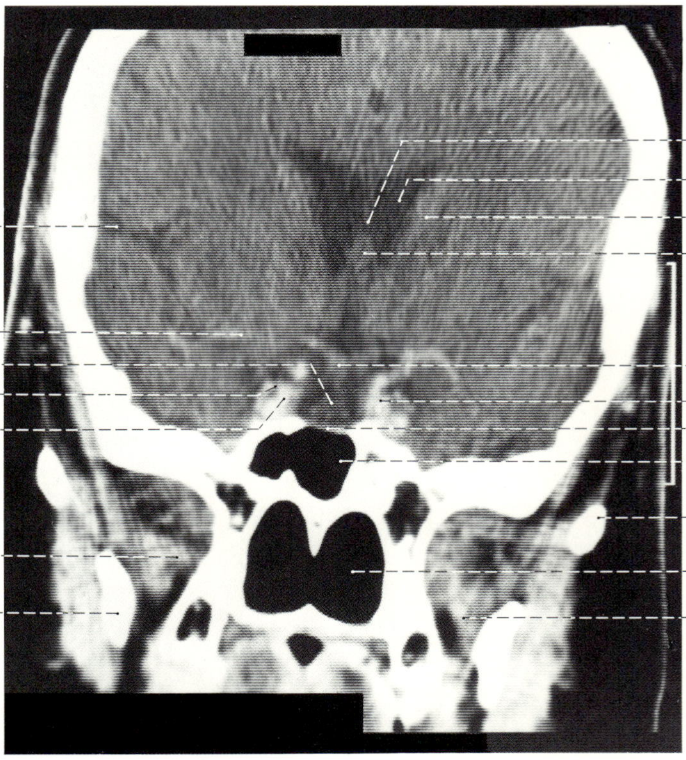

Patient MRI Scan

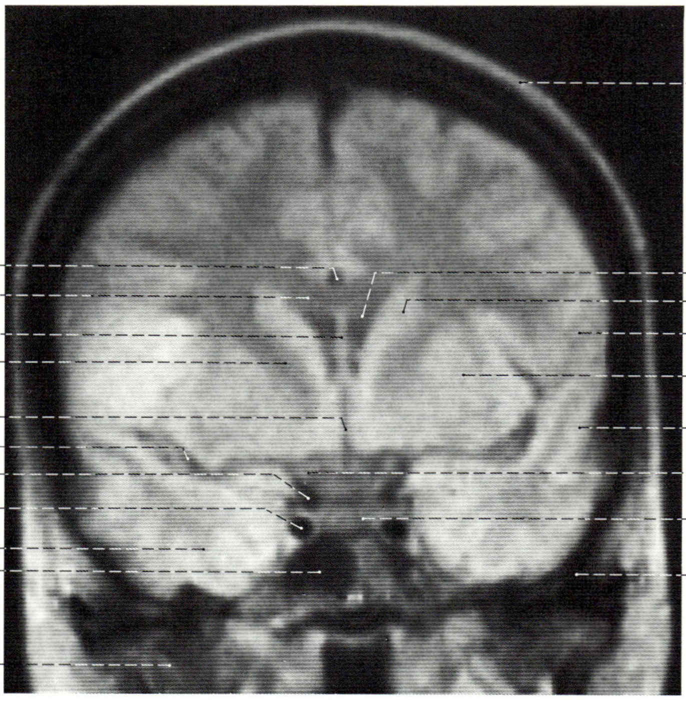

In the coronal slices, the pituitary fossa is bounded superiorly by the diaphragma sellae and laterally by the cavernous sinuses. The oculomotor nerve (III) and trochlear nerve (IV) course just lateral to the cavernous carotid in the wall of the cavernous sinus. The abducens nerve (VI) is within the sinus just inferio-lateral to the internal carotid artery at this level. On the right, an excellent longitudinal view of the third division (mandibular, V_3) of the trigeminal nerve is seen exiting from the semilunar (Gasserian) ganglion, hugging the floor of the middle fossa, and then exiting the skull via the foramen ovale. Because of the slight obliquity of the cut on the left, the middle meningeal artery is seen entering the skull through the foramen spinosum which is postero-lateral to the foramen ovale.

The lateral (Sylvian) fissure and adjacent uncus are immediately lateral to the parasellar structures. The initial segment of the middle cerebral artery is well demonstrated on the CT (with contrast) and on the MRI scans. The slit-like third ventricle may be easily confused in sectional images with the anterior interhemispheric fissure and it is useful to remember that the anterior (preoptic) extent of the third ventricle usually extends only as far anteriorly as the optic chiasm.

The caudate nucleus head forms the lateral wall of the anterior horn of the lateral ventricle and is well demonstrated on both CT and MRI. In addition, the MRI sequence presented here shows clear delineations of the anterior limb of the internal capsule which is made up of myelinated fiber tracts and is contiguous with the subcortical white matter in the frontoparietal region.

Flowing blood within the Sylvian branches of the middle cerebral artery is difficult to separate from the CSF in the Sylvian fissure which gives about the same signal. The same vessels are slightly better seen on the contrast enhanced CT.

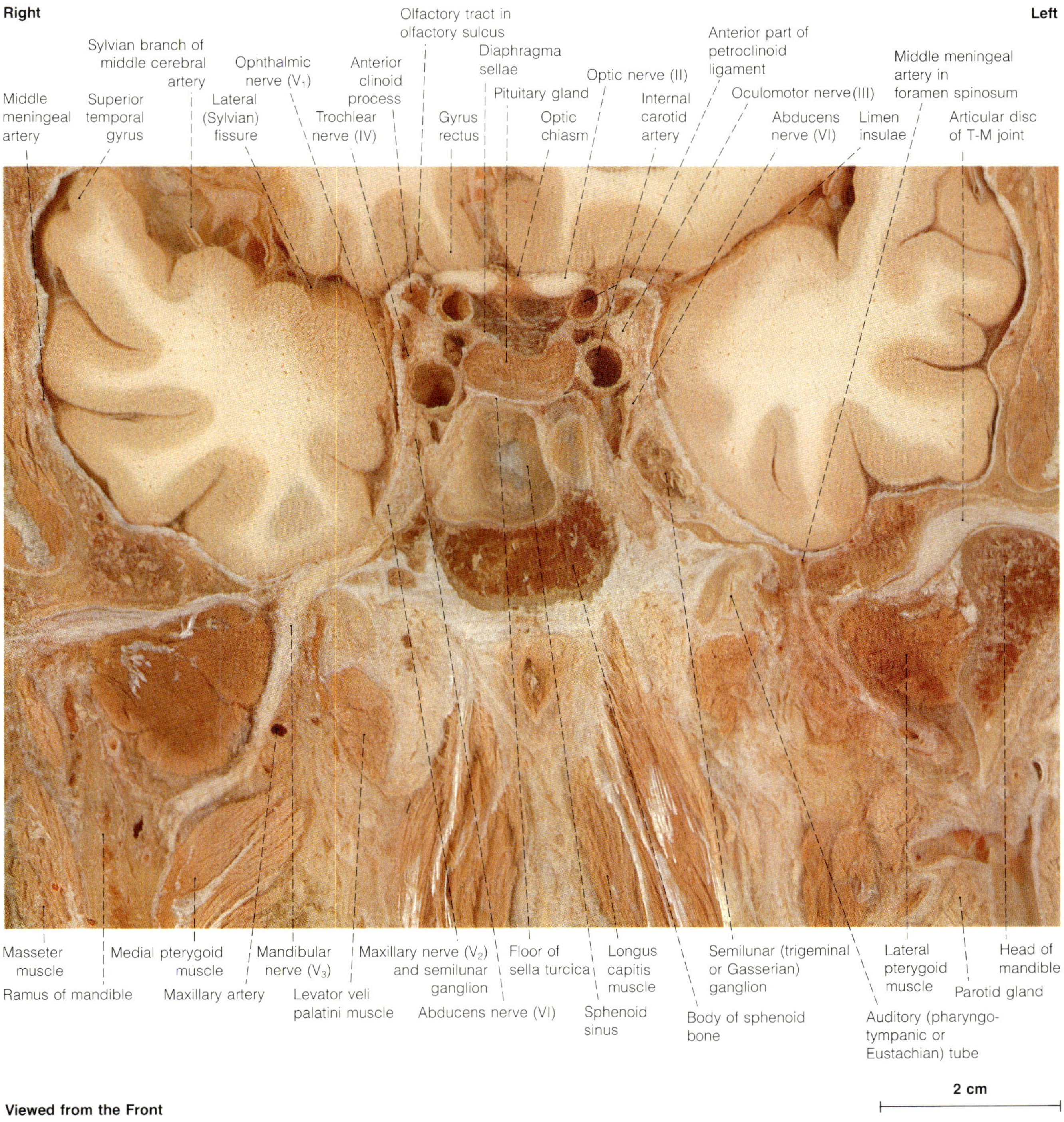

Viewed from the Front

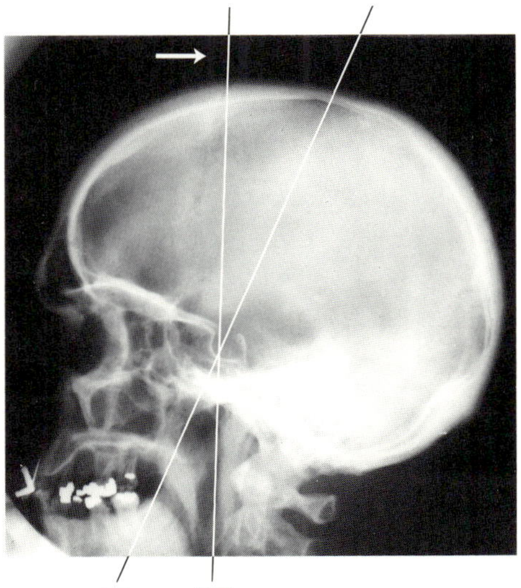

Planes of Sections

Cadaver CT Scan

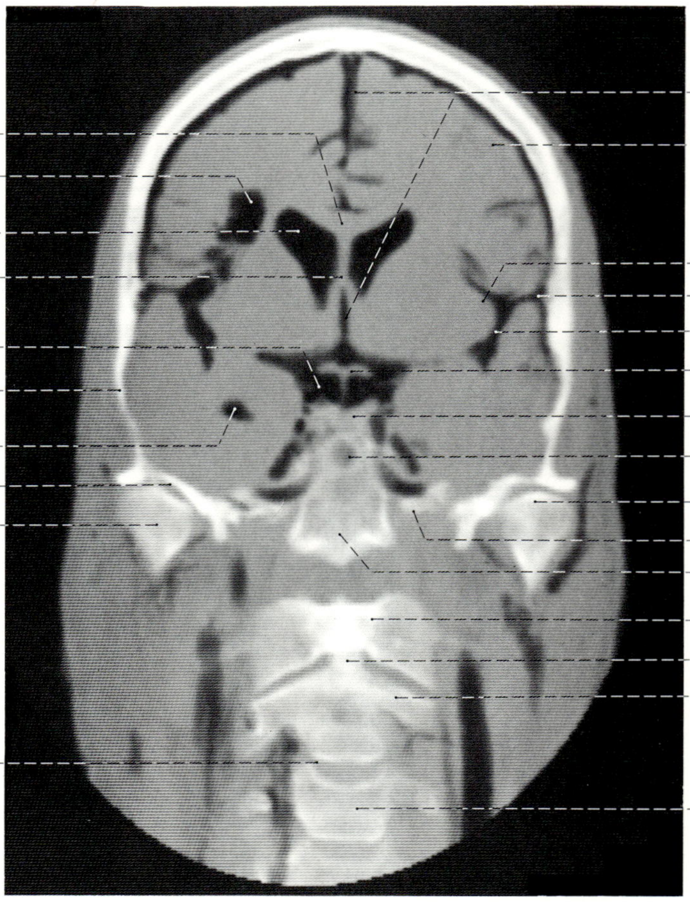

Full coronal views of the temporal lobes are afforded here with tiny slits representing the anterior tips of the temporal (inferior) horns of the lateral ventricles. The anterior (frontal) horns of the lateral ventricles have their characteristic appearance with the lateral walls formed by the caudate nuclei (head). The lateral wall of the suprasellar cistern is the uncus and amygdala (and adjacent oculomotor nerve) which can herniate medially and inferiorly in response to temporal or parietal masses. Good anatomical relationships of the insular cortex, Sylvian fissure, and operculum can be seen in this slice.

In the cervical spine, coronal anatomy of the odontoid (dens)-base of C2 complex along with the lateral masses of the atlas is demonstrated. The disc spaces, uncovertebral (Luschka) joints, and cancellous bone of vertebral bodies are well seen.

The temporomandibular joint and parotid gland are lateral and inferior to the temporal lobes. Their relationship to the middle fossa and the petrous bone (just posterior) is often important clinically as is the course of the facial nerve and its branches (not possible to distinctly identify since they are transversely sectioned) through the parotid gland.

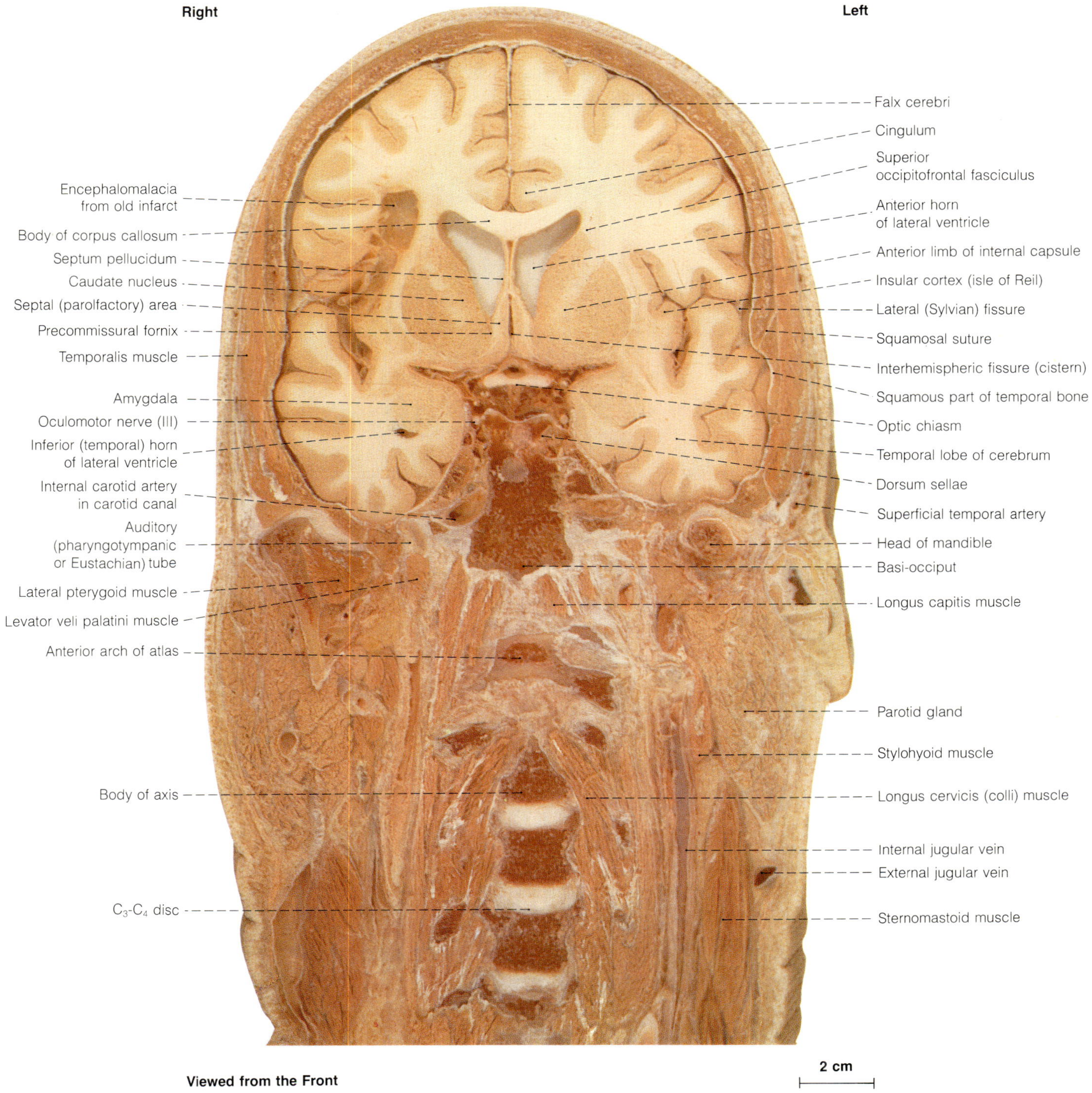

Viewed from the Front

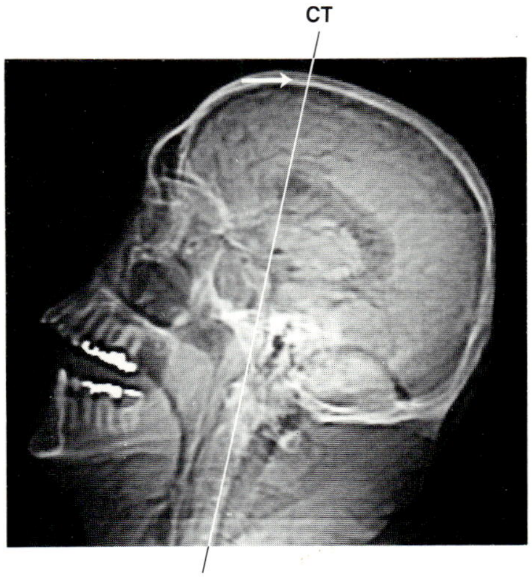

Plane of Section

Patient CT Scan

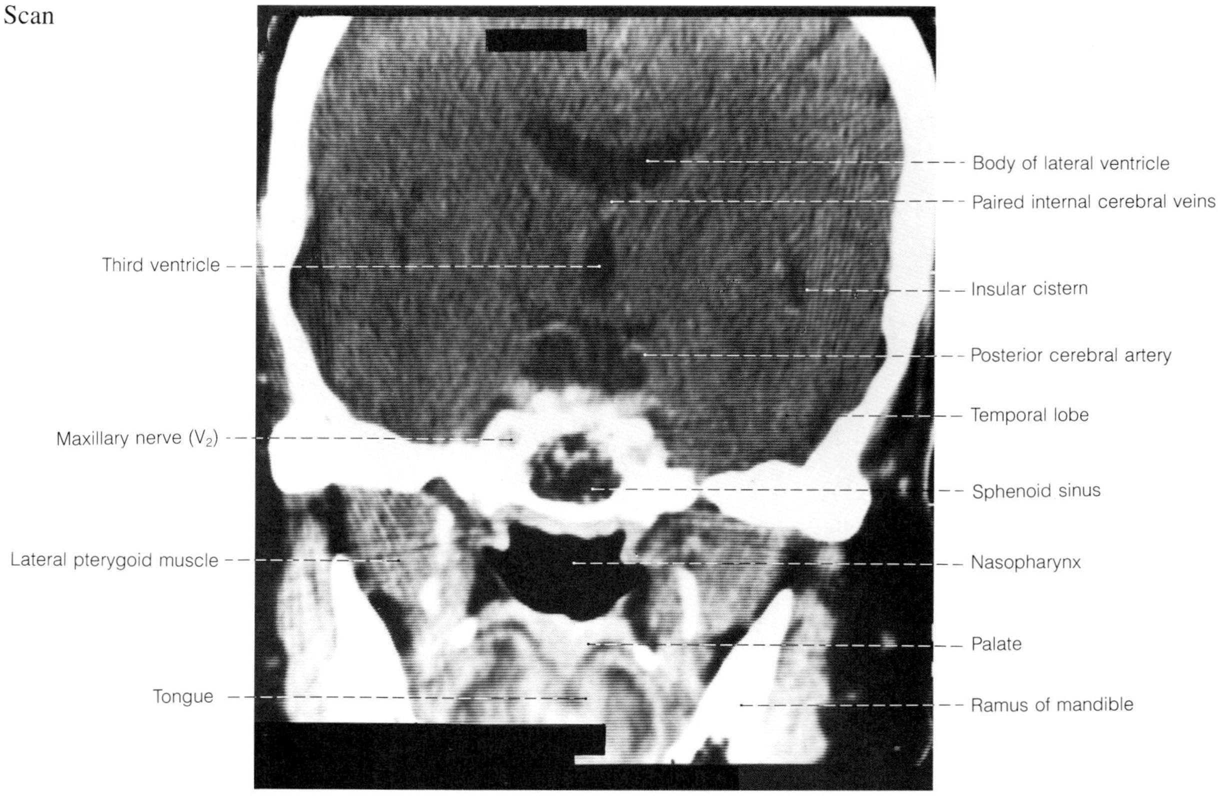

Right **Viewed from the Front**

Patient MRI Scan

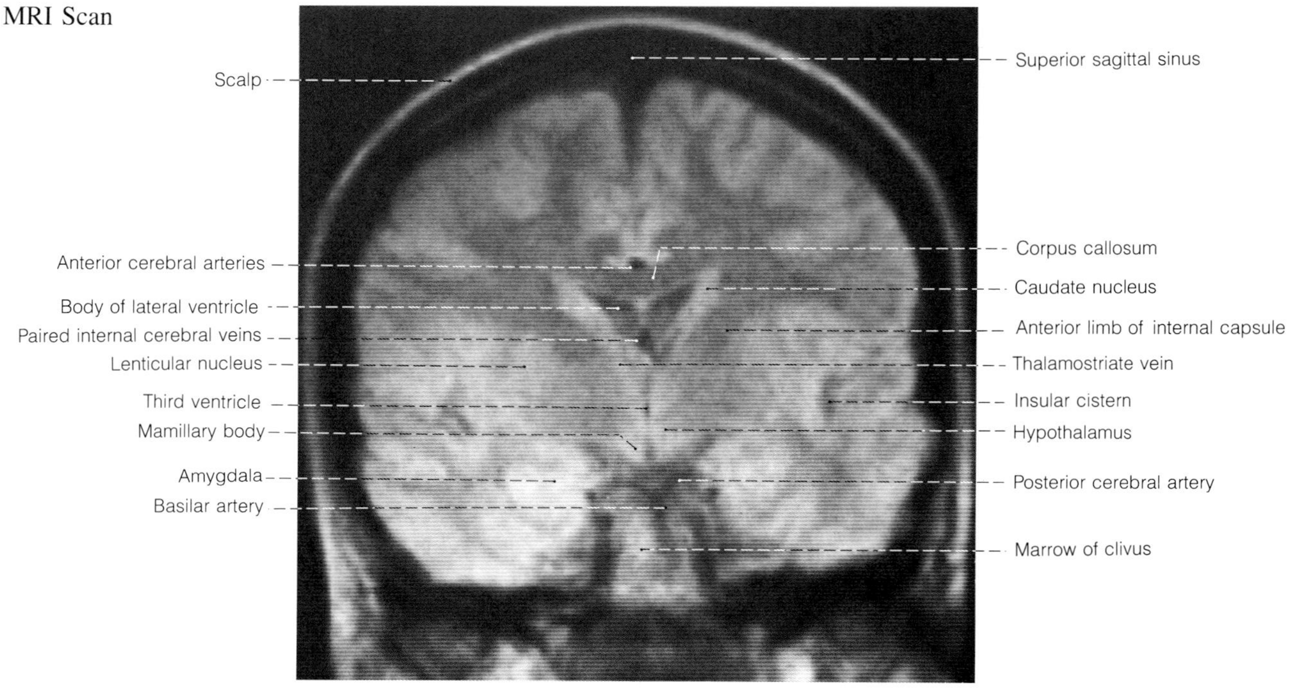

Right **Viewed from the Front**

On the left of the anatomical specimen (right of viewer), the temporo-mandibular joint (TMJ) anatomy is well-delineated. The fibrocartilage meniscus of the TMJ is seen along with the mandibular condyle and the temporal fossa articulation. The plane of the MRI is through the inferior-posterior portion of the clivus, which is actually united basi-sphenoid and basi-occiput. A very interesting feature, shown to advantage here, is the semilunar ganglion of the trigeminal nerve (V) lying in the dural reflection known as Meckel's cave prior to the separation of CN V into its three main divisions.

This particular cut runs through the mid-portion of the temporal lobe on either side, revealing the relationship of the amygdala and adjacent oculomotor nerve (III) to the temporal horn of lateral ventricle. The oculomotor nerve (III) can be seen before entering the cavernous sinus and the abducens nerve (VI) is in Dorello's canal.

The walls of the ventral part of the interhemispheric fissure are the septal or parolfactory nuclei. The nucleus accumbens, adjacent to the ventral border of the frontal horn of the lateral ventricle, is interposed between these nuclei and the head of the caudate nucleus. The tuberculum olfactorium intervenes between the amygdala, ventro-laterally, the septum dorso-medially, and the caudate-putamen complex superiorly. From the close approximation of these limbic areas, it is easy to visualize the anatomical reasons for the alterations in personality commonly noted with pathology in this ventromedial part of the brain.

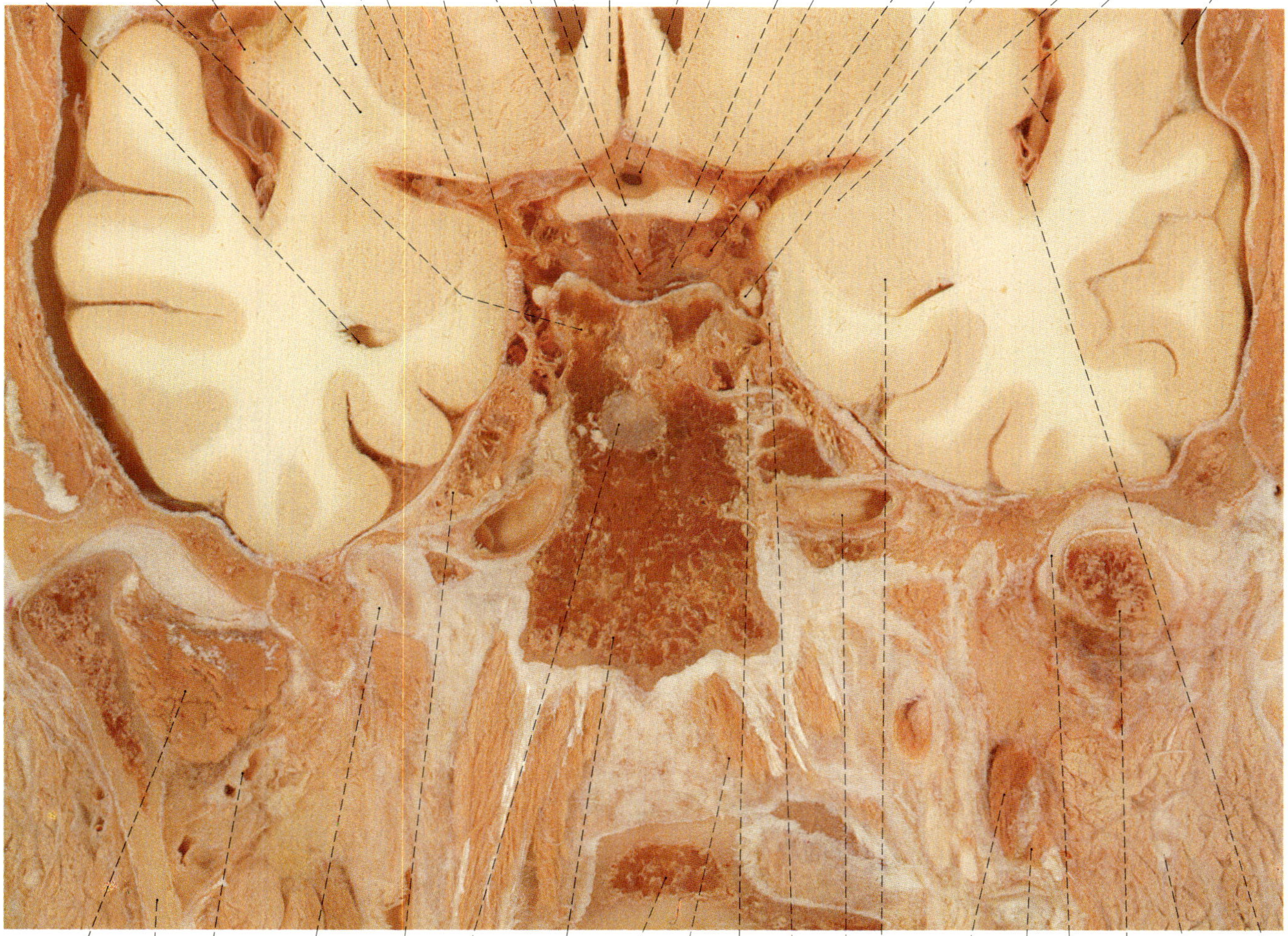

Viewed from the Front

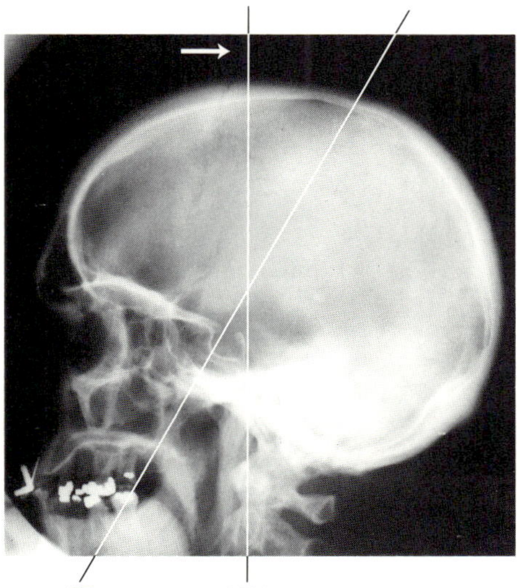

Planes of Sections

Areas of the suprasellar cistern and hypothalamus, which are so well shown here, were not directly visible in any diagnostic modality before the advent of CT, and now, MRI. Landmark vascular channels also seen here are the paired internal cerebral veins (white on contrast enhanced CT and black on MRI) as well as the distal pericallosal branches of the anterior cerebral arteries and the basilar artery on MRI.

Cadaver CT Scan

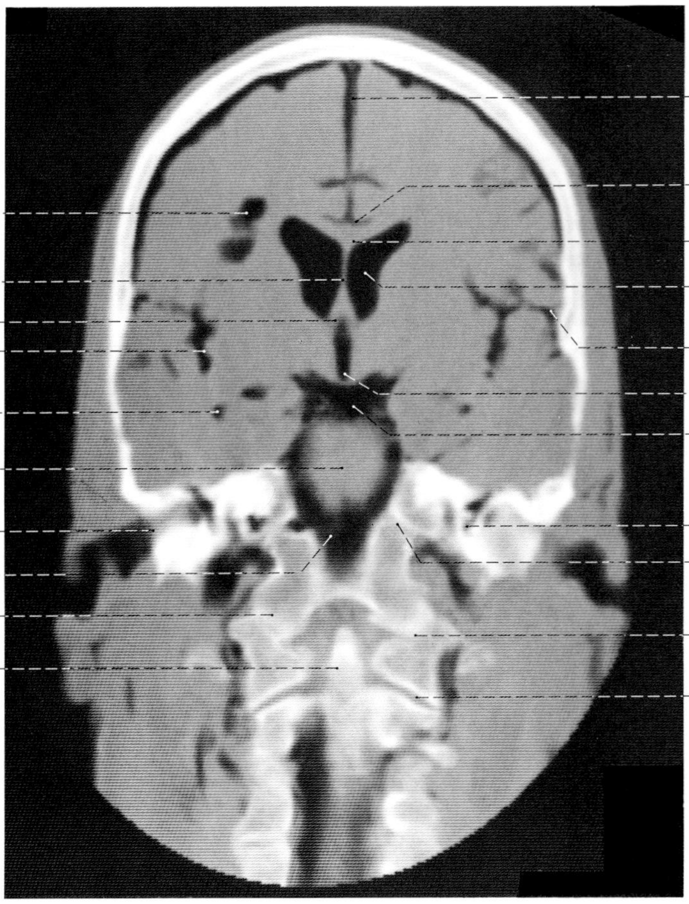

The plane of the slice passes fortuitously through the anterior portion of the base of the pons and above it the interpeduncular cistern. Above this the third ventricle and the bodies of lateral ventricles are visualized.

Because of asymmetry of the plane of this coronal cut and the small size of structures in this region, there are some notable differences between right and left. On the right of the specimen (left of viewer) the temporo-mandibular joint (TMJ) anatomy is well-delineated. The fibro-cartilaginous meniscus of the TMJ is seen along with the mandibular condyle and the temporal fossa articulation. Anterior elements of the petrous bone are seen, in particular the external auditory canal which normally passes 2-3 mm posterior to the TMJ. The plane passing through the inferio-posterior portion of the clivus exposes the occipital condyles in articular relationship to the atlas at the atlanto-occipital joint. Note the cortical bone along both sides of the joint margin here and in the atlanto-axial joints. These are covered with synovia and form the synovial joints. The petro-occipital fissure is normally filled with cartilage.

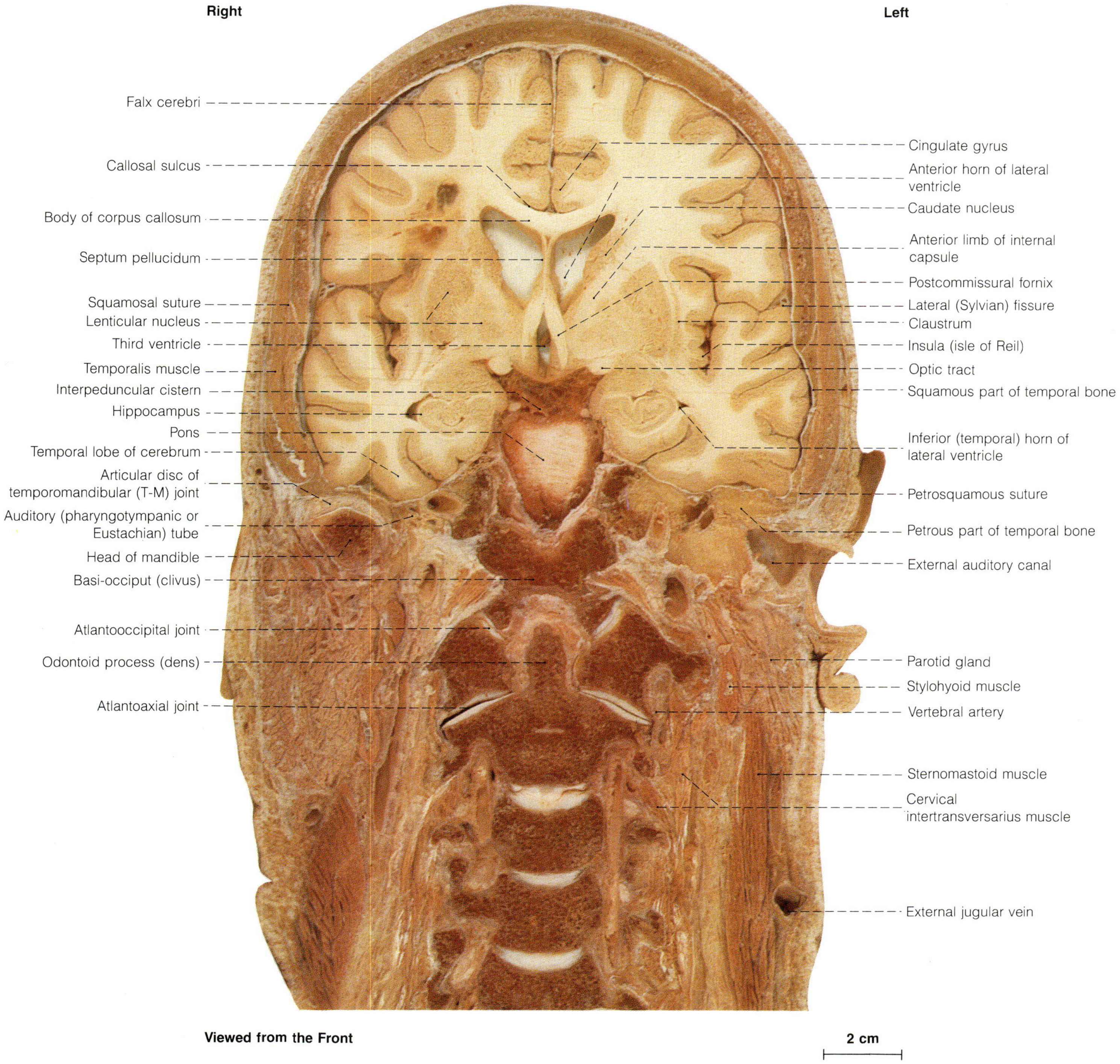

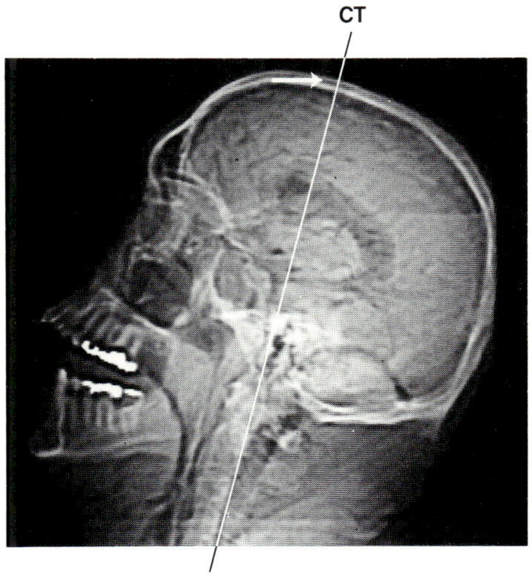

Plane of Section

Interpeduncular Cistern

Patient CT Scan

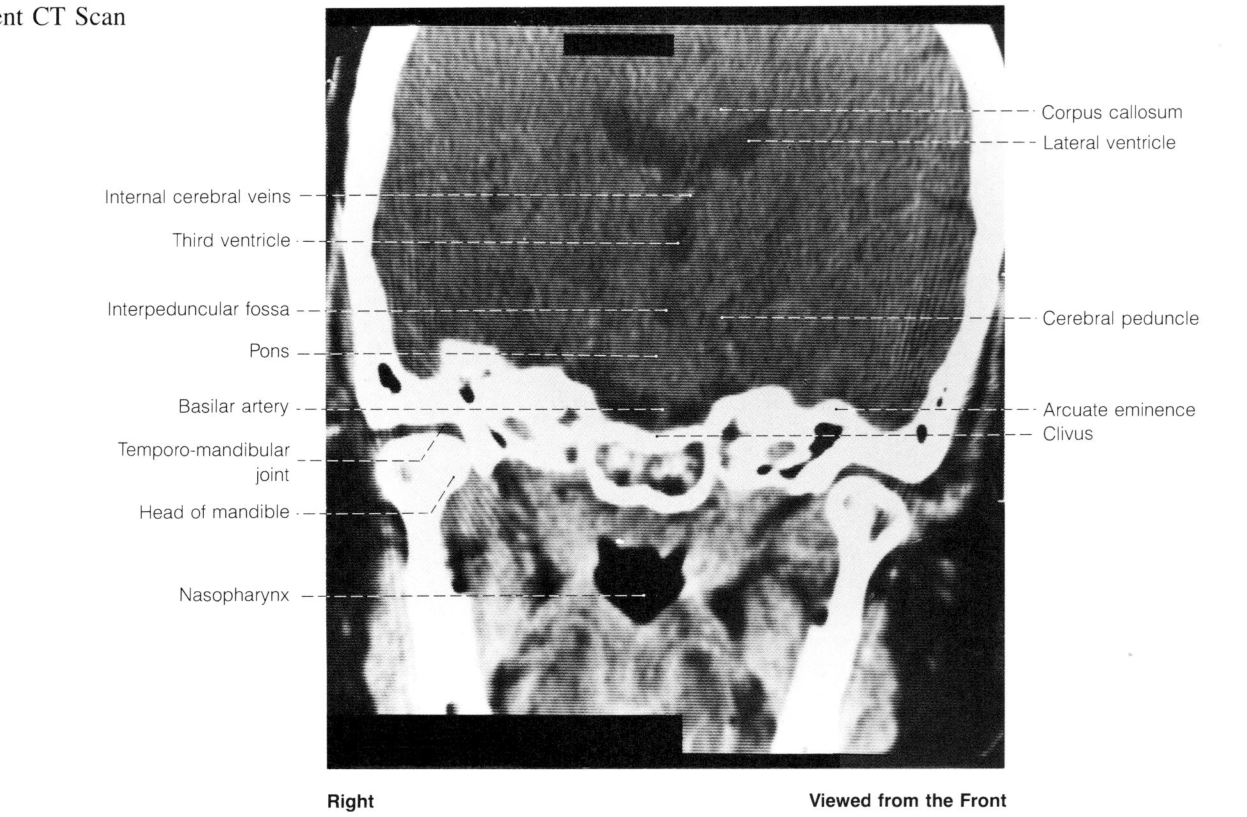

Patient MRI Scan

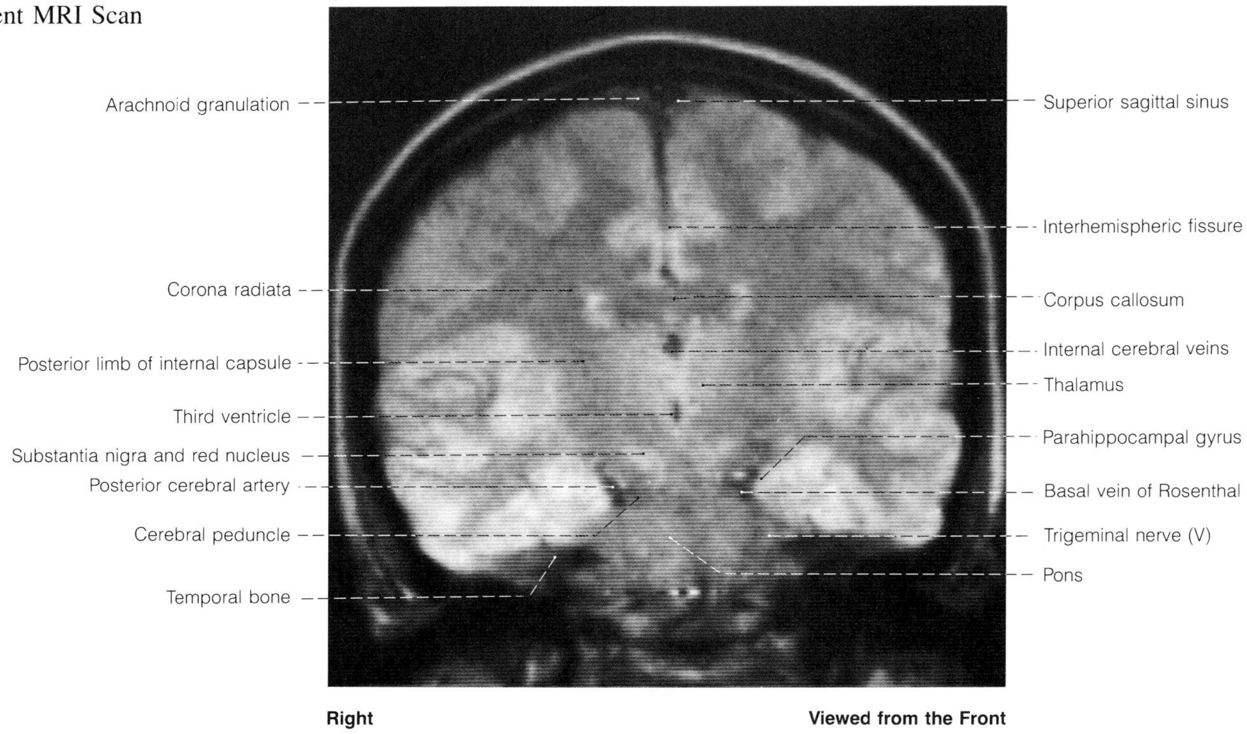

This coronal cut transects the mid-portions of the temporal lobe on either side, revealing the close relationship of the amygdala (and adjacent oculomotor nerve), hippocampus, and temporal horn of the lateral ventricle. Transverse pontocerebellar fibers are noted in the slice through the very anterior (basilar) portion of the pons. The cut also traverses the middle of the third ventricle and the tuber cinereum region. The optic tracts are seen just before entering the lateral geniculates.

The angle of a coronal CT scan will determine whether a cut through the pituitary fossa also passes through the interhemispheric fissure between the frontal lobes (and septal nuclei), or whether it intersects the third ventricle, an obviously important distinction. The anterior cerebral arteries ascend between the hemispheres. The optic chiasm is located in the floor of the most anterior part of the third ventricle; consequently, the third ventricle is situated in this coronal plane caudal to the chiasm. The CT scan plane is really quite different from the pure coronal scan of the MRI, but one must keep in mind the physical limitations placed on the patients in the CT.

The MRI more nearly matches the anatomical slice and a very interesting relationship of the splenium of the corpus callosum and the internal cerebral veins is noted. The latter may be just merging to form the vein of Galen which is one plane posterior. The large thalamic nuclei dominate the midline anatomy at this level, and this, like the cellular regions of cortex and substantia nigra, are depicted by a white signal in this sequence.

Black vascular structures of interest here are the cross-sectioned posterior cerebral arteries and basal veins of Rosenthal which are traveling around the brainstem in the ambient cistern at this level.

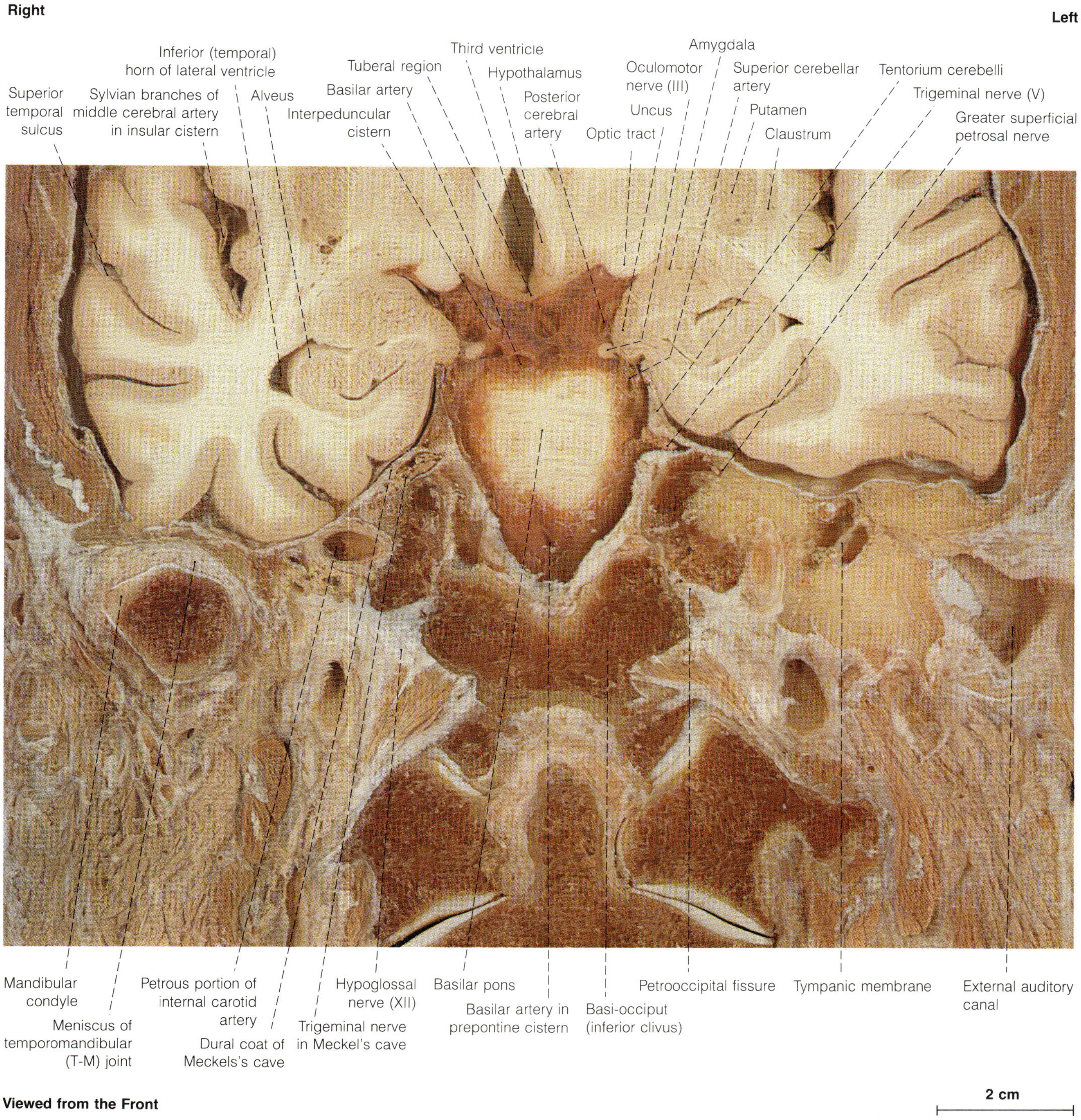

Viewed from the Front

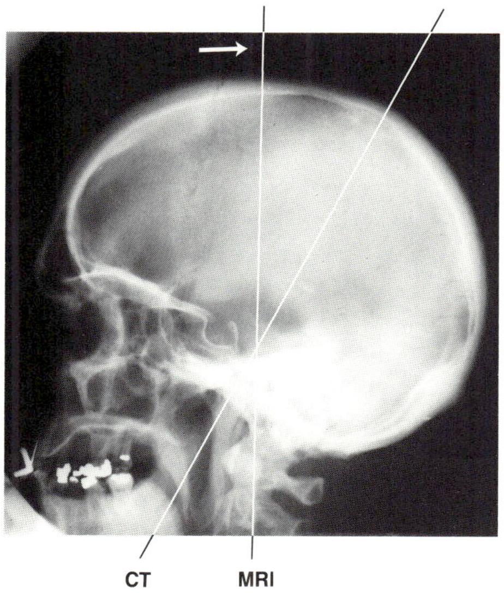

Planes of Sections

Cadaver CT Scan

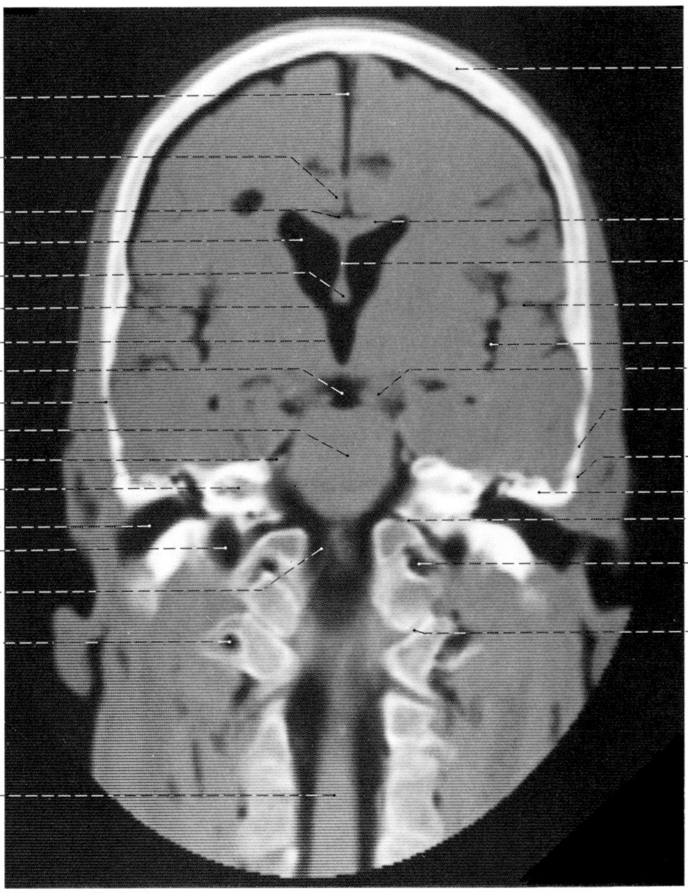

This coronal cut fortuitously passes through the lateral ventricles and their connections to the third ventricle, the interventricular foramen of Monro. It is surprising (but anatomically normal) to find this landmark so far posterior in the brain, i.e., in the same plane as the pons. The fornix, seen in cross-section at the lower extent of the septum pellucidum, forms the superior and anterior boundary of the interventricular foramen.

Many of the fibers in the posterior limb of the internal capsule near the genu descend from the cortex to the pons and spinal cord. This is clearly demonstrated in this cadaver where the subcortical encephalomalacia destroyed these paths on the right side and there is an obvious loss (when compared to the left) in the internal capsule and cerebral peduncle. Since the CT scan is a display of a computed average of a 5 mm slab, it is not so evident in the CT scan. Excellent delineation of the cerebral peduncles is afforded here with the cortico-spinal tracts clearly shown flowing from cerebral cortex, through the corona radiata, into the internal capsule, thence to the cerebral peduncles, and through the pons.

Midline structures including the pillars of the fornix are well noted with the precise delineation of thalamic nuclei forming the third ventricular walls.

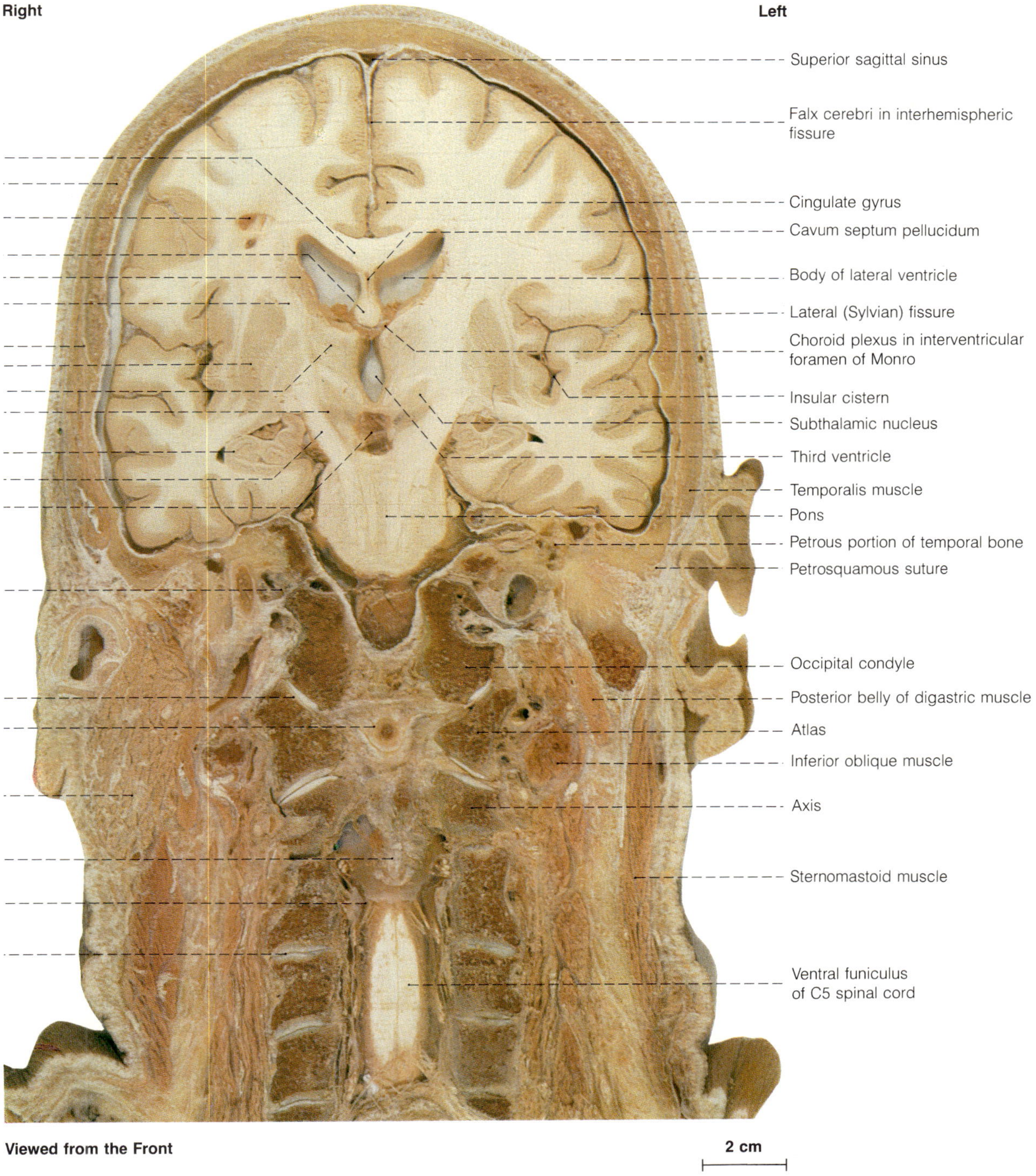

Viewed from the Front

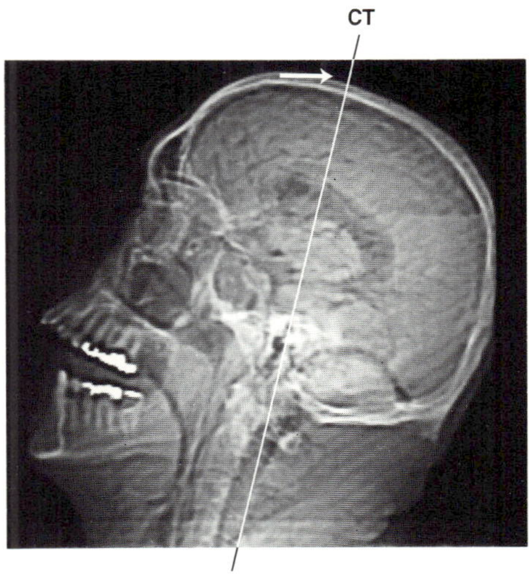

Plane of Section

Patient CT Scan

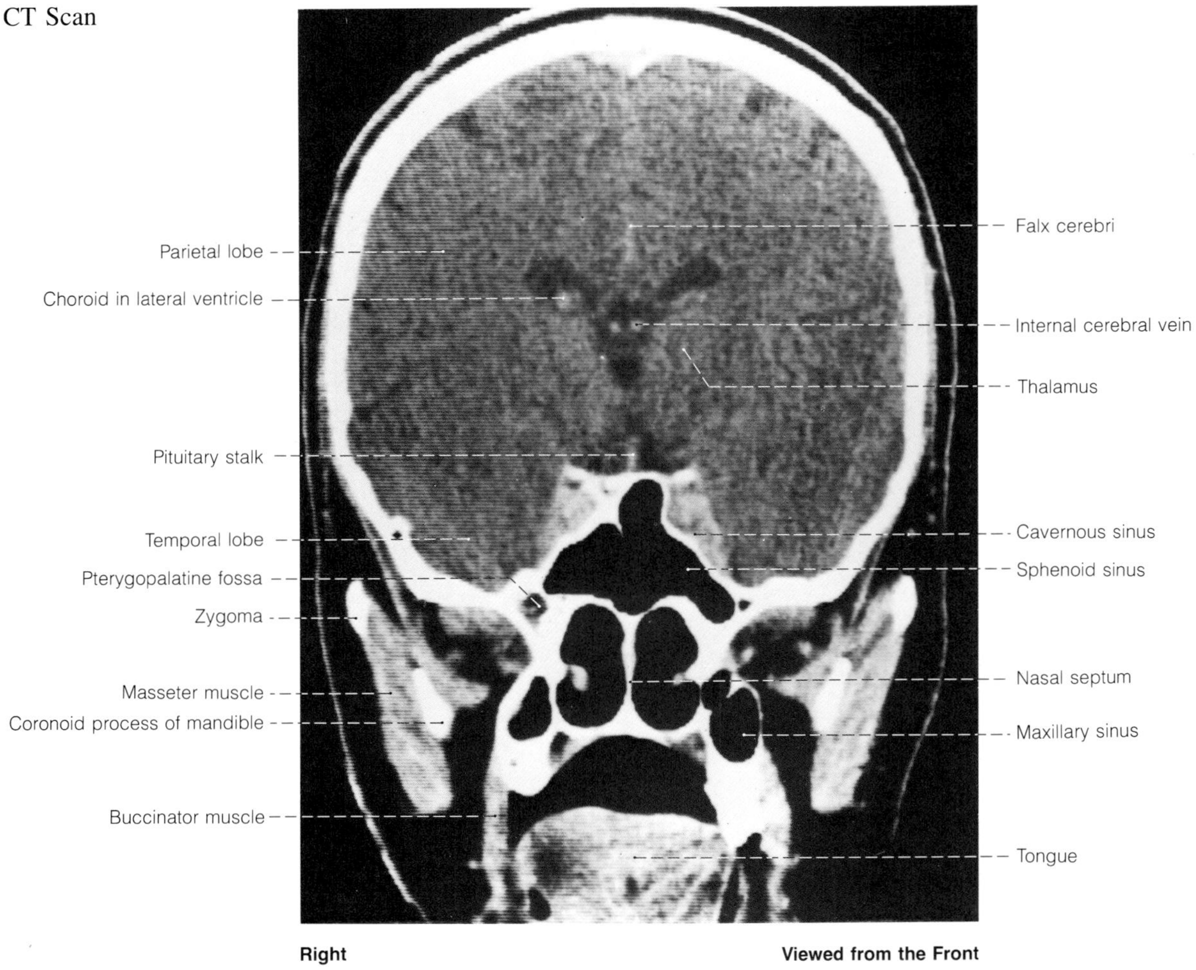

Patient MRI Scan

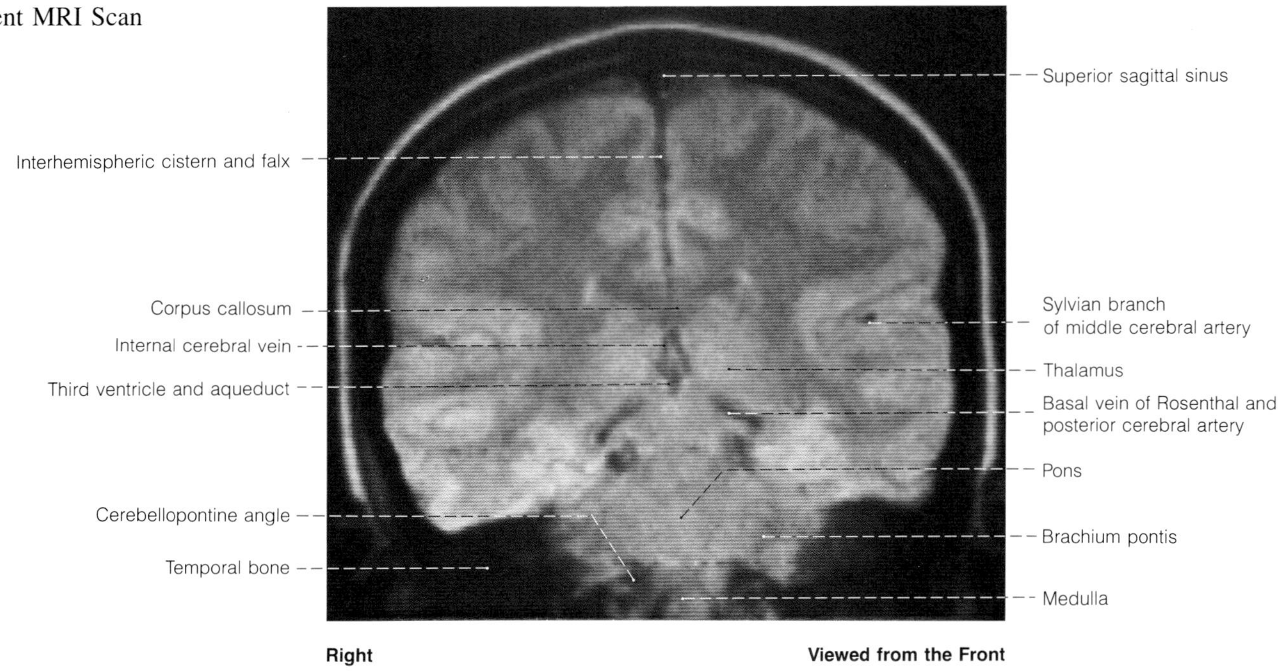

This coronal section passes through the temporal bone on the specimen's left (viewer's right) including the internal auditory canal with the facial nerve (VII) immediately superior to the auditory nerve (VIII). The vagus (X) and glossopharyngeal (IX) are demonstrated in relationship to the jugular bulb portion of the internal jugular vein.

In the pons, both longitudinal and transverse fibers are clearly seen in their relationship to each other. The longitudinal fibers are in continuity with the internal capsule and cerebral peduncle above, and with the medullary pyramids below. The posterior-most portion of the interpeduncular fossa can be noted immediately below the postmamillary decussation (commissure of Forel), and the posterior hypothalamus in the walls of the third ventricle. The juxtaposition of the substantia nigra, subthalamic nucleus, and zona incerta medial to the cerebral peduncles is quite evident as are the intimate relationships of the optic tracts, lenticular nuclei, and medial temporal lobes (including the hippocampus) lateral to the cerebral peduncles and/or internal capsule. An often difficult-to-visualize structure is the choroid fissure seen at this level. Through this fissure courses the anterior choroidal artery, a branch of the supra-clinoid carotid, and the posterior choroidal branches of the posterior cerebral artery.

On the MRI, the level of gray which represents the pons is of note; longitudinal corticospinal fibers interdigitate with transverse cerebellar fibers of the brachium pontis and with the pontine nuclei. The entire complex appears not as dark as cortical white matter and not as white as cortical grey matter.

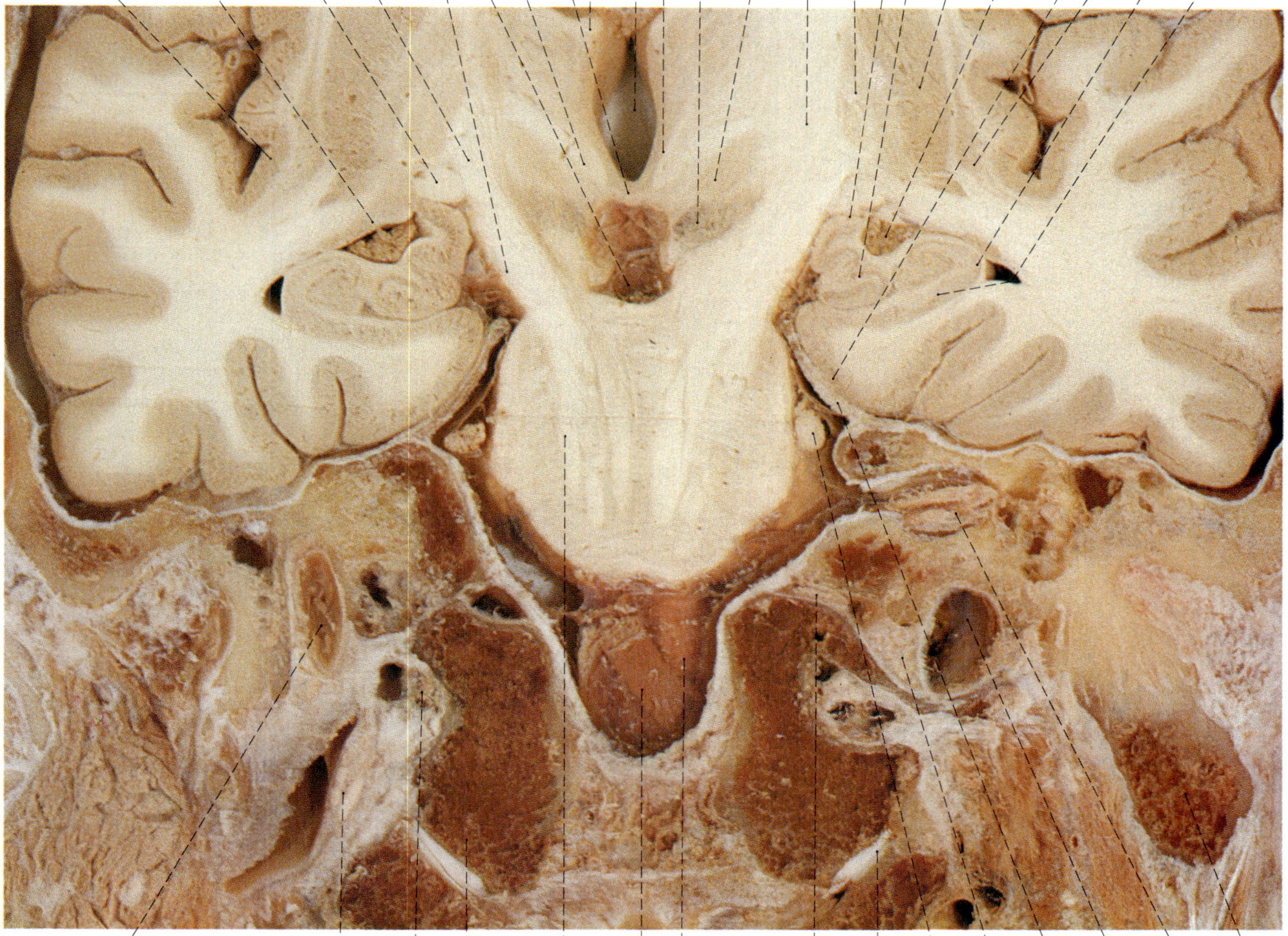

Viewed from the Front

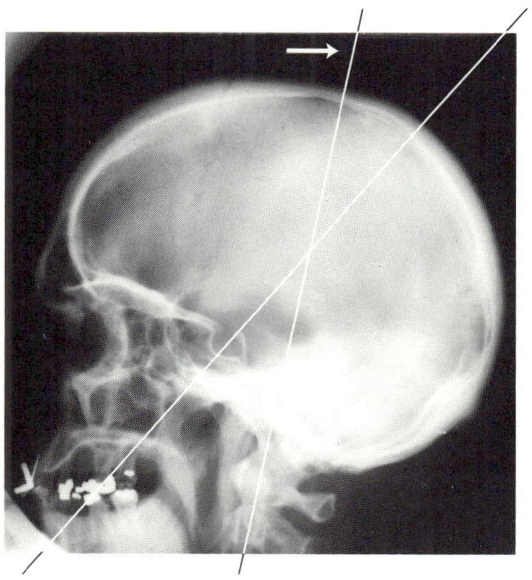

Planes of Sections

Cadaver CT Scan

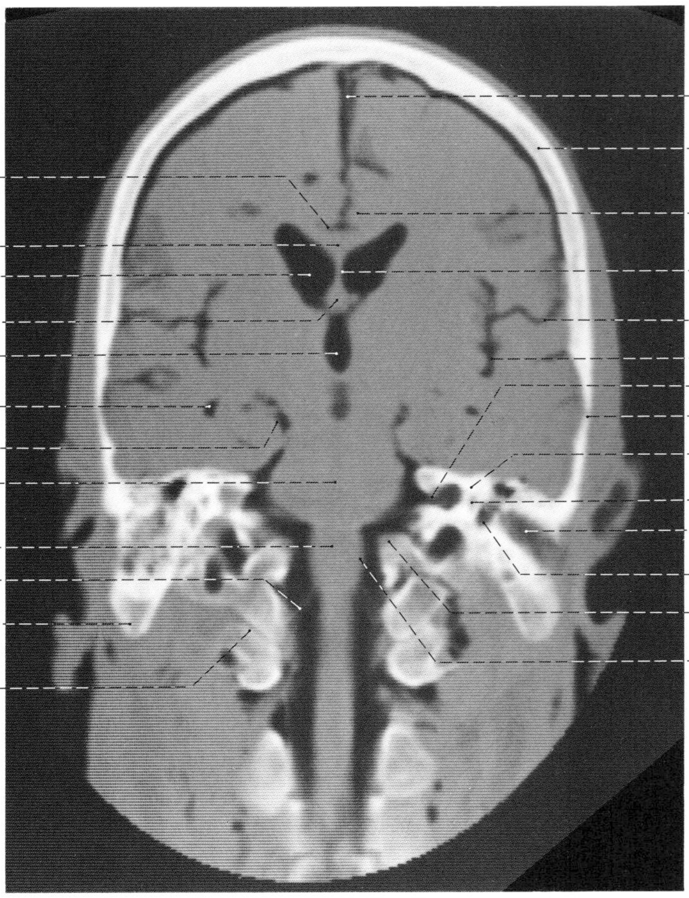

The posterior temporal bone structures are viewed at the same time as the middle of the diencephalon, the ventral mesencephalon, the basilar pons, the medulla, and the upper cervical spinal cord in coronal fullness. The decussation of the pyramids at the foramen magnum extends both above and below this foramen and the attachment of the first cervical nerve (on the specimen's left) is in these same planes. The lateral expanse of the cisterna magna and its caudal subarachnoid prolongation into upper cervical levels are also well visualized in this section. The swelling of the medulla just caudal to the ponto-medullary junction is the inferior olivary nucleus. Just caudal to the olive, the hypoglossal nerve (CN XII) can be seen entering the hypoglossal canal below the bony jugular tubercle. The lateral flaring of the pons represents fibers traveling into the cerebellar hemispheres as the brachium pontis (middle cerebellar peduncle). The free edge of the tentorium (tentorial notch or foramen ovale of Pacchioni) passes directly up to the midbrain in the region of the cerebral peduncles medially, and to the postero-medial-most portions of the temporal lobe laterally.

Above the lateral ventricles one notes crossing interhemispheric fibers of the body of the corpus callosum and below the lateral ventricles and fornix some of the thalamic nuclei are visualized.

The potential subarachnoid space and pia between the fornix and its attached choroid above and the choroid forming the roof of the third ventricle below is the velum interpositum. An enlargement and cavitation of this subarachnoid space is referred to as the cavum of the velum interpositum.

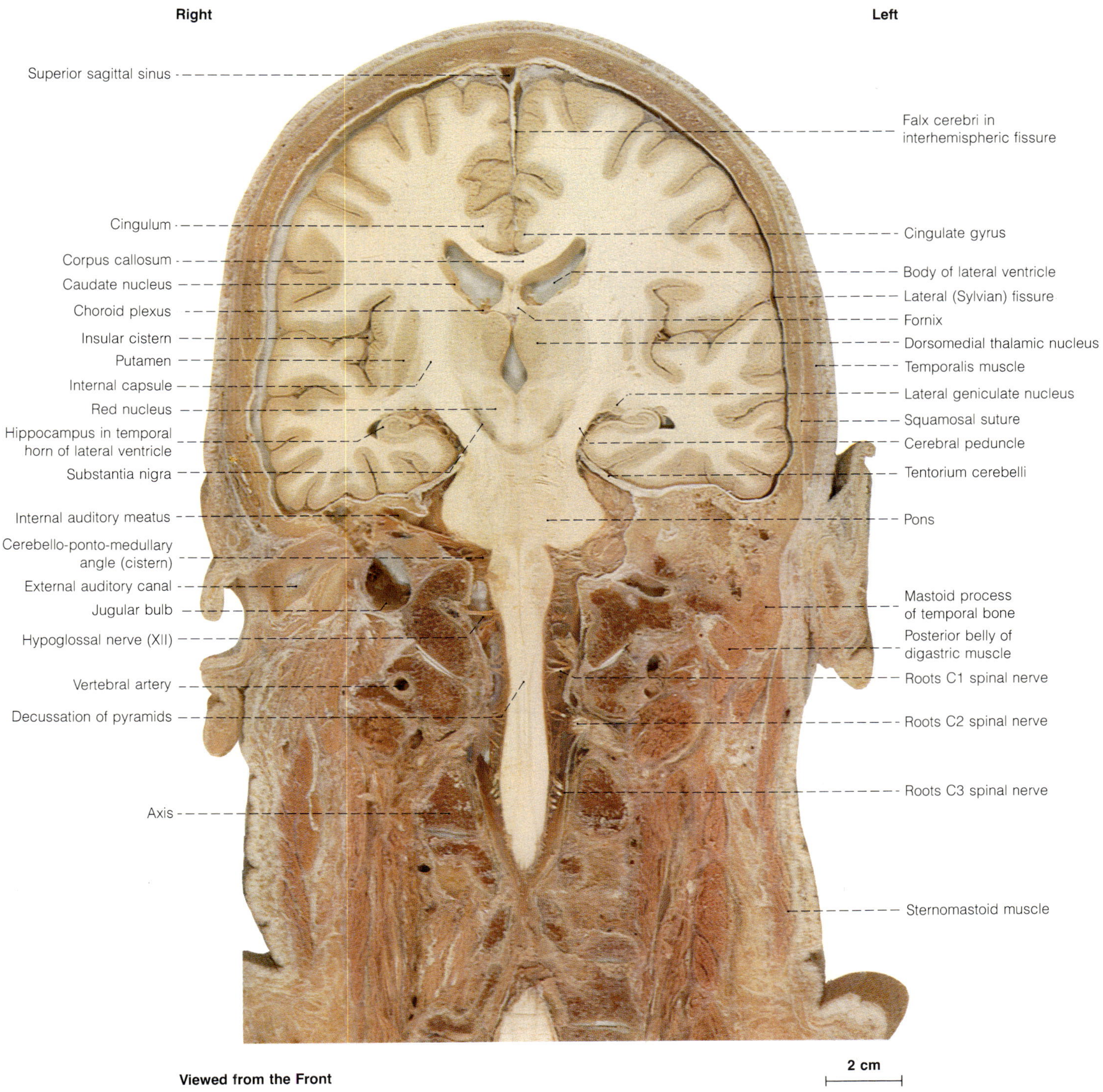

Viewed from the Front

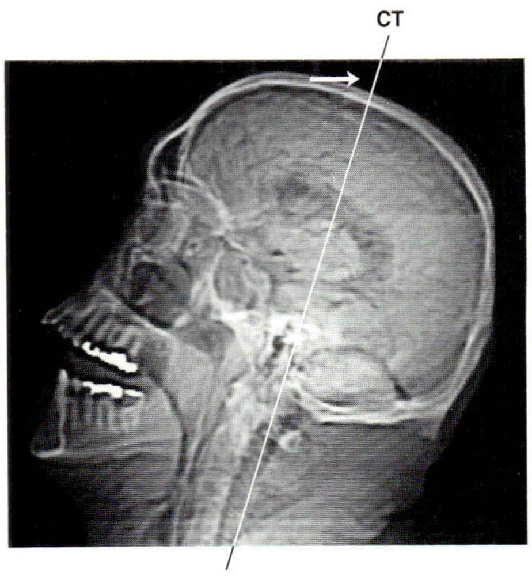

Plane of Section

Patient CT Scan

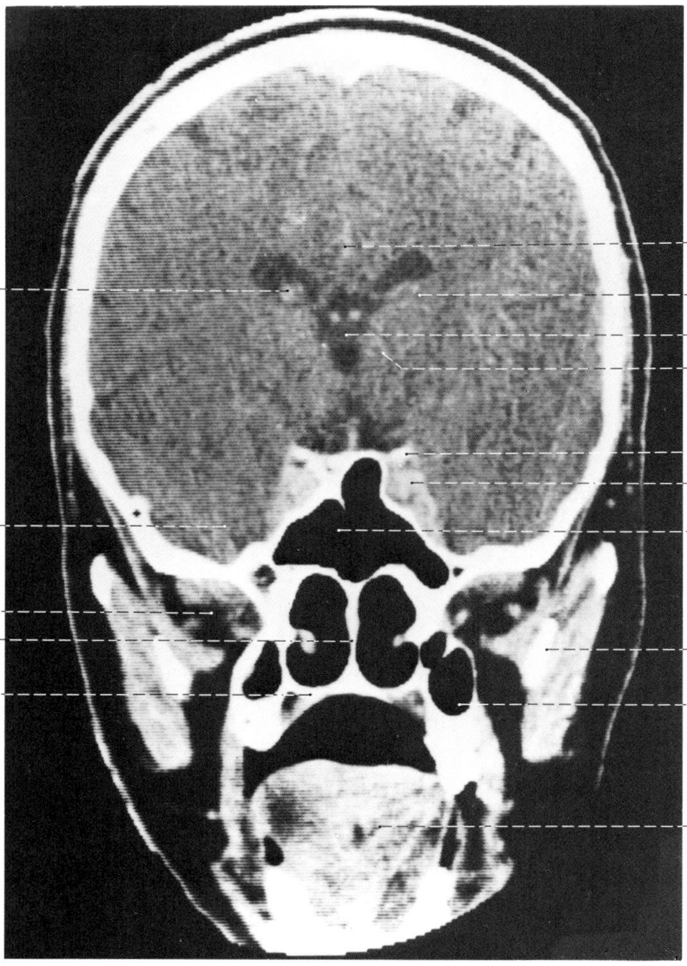

Planes of Sections

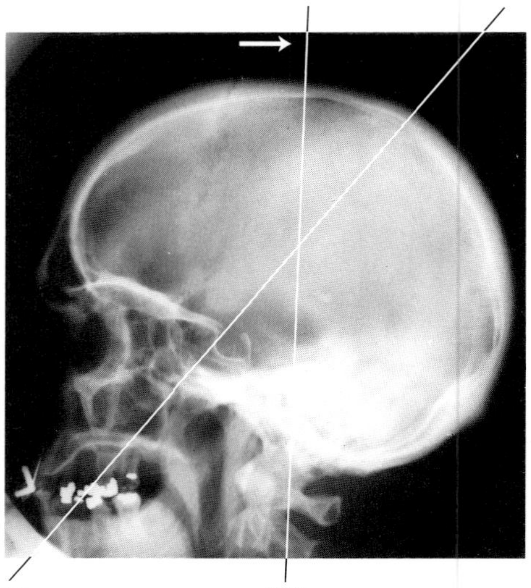

Patient MRI Scan

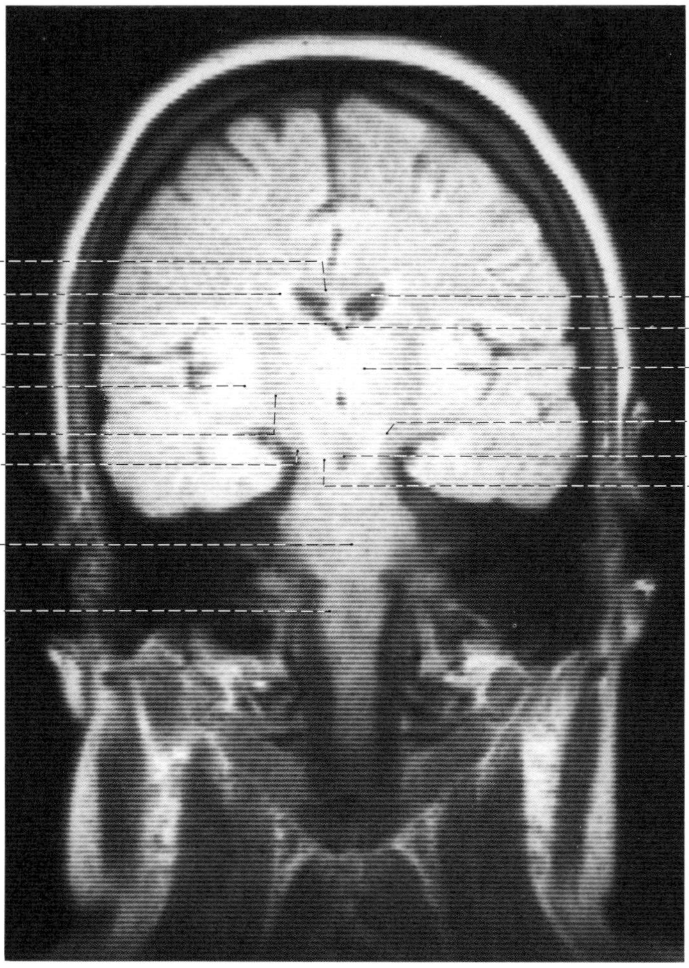

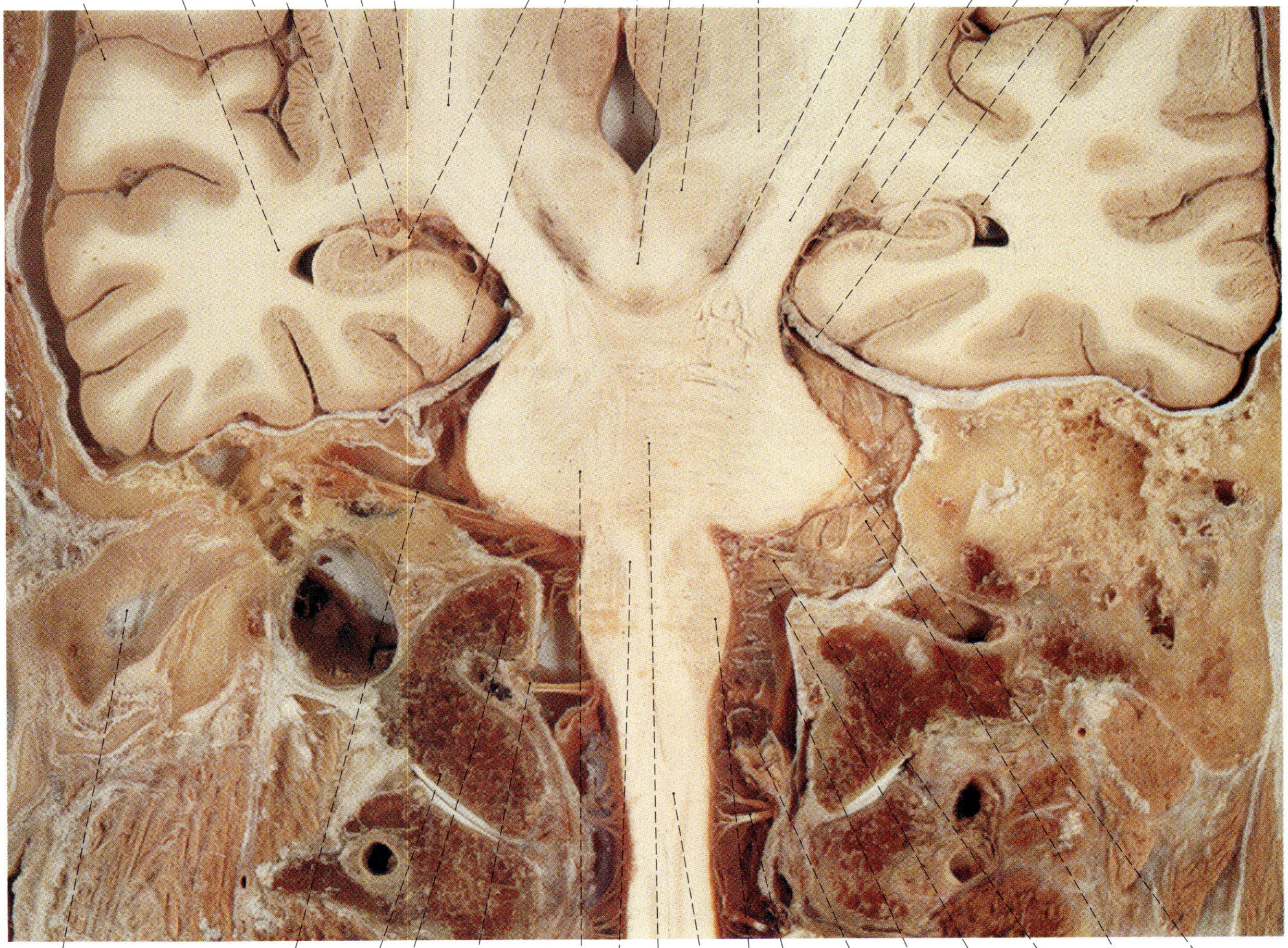

The melanin-containing nuclei in the substantia nigra are just inferio-lateral to the red nuclei and both are inferio-lateral to the posterior third ventricle but medial to the cerebral peduncles. These are not visible on the CT scan but focal infarcts in their vicinity might be. Different pulse sequences on MRI might better demonstrate these nuclei. Lateral to the peduncles, the lateral geniculate nucleus and hippocampal formation are well visualized in this coronal cut.

The vertical plane of the MRI scan not only differentiates the grey and white matter of the brain but also nicely demonstrates cerebral veins such as the inferior cerebral veins and basal vein of Rosenthal as it joins the great cerebral vein of Galen.

The tentorium is visualized only as a thin black line representing dura separating occipito-temporal bone from cerebellum. Of interest are vessels seen in cross section which are closely applied to the tentorium. The anterior temporal branch of the posterior cerebral artery being a case in point as noted here. The inferio-lateral black spot probably represents a cortical vein complex in this slice.

Basal veins of Rosenthal converge on the vein of Galen but are difficult to separate from the CSF in the quadrigeminal plate cistern. The superior colliculi are noted well outlined by the CSF of that cistern.

The CT, being severely angled, passes through the third ventricle. It includes the posteriorly located corpus callosum structures in the same plane as the cavernous sinus (nicely delineated with filling defects representing branches of CN V) and, more anteriorly, the nasopharynx and paranasal sinuses.

Cadaver CT Scan

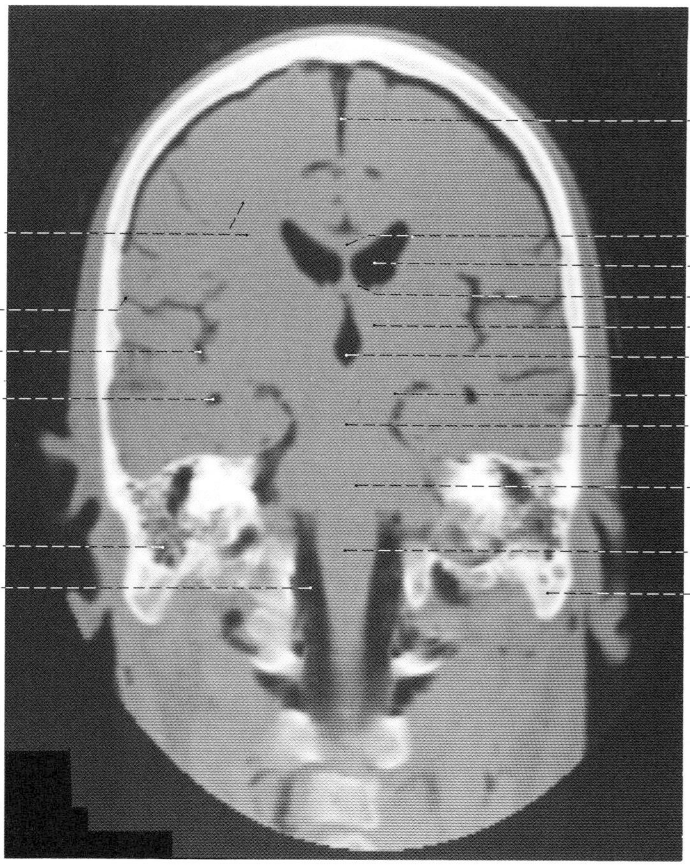

This coronal cut passes through the brainstem and thalamus illustrating the continuity and relationships of this core of nuclei and fiber tracts, including the entire extent of the corticospinal tract. One may also note the fan of the corona radiata fibers in this slice, representing the final (or initial) pathway of fiber tracts making up the thalamo-cortical sensory paths, the cortical projection paths including the cortico-spinal tracts in their course from cortical nuclei to anterior horn cells, and especially the mass of subcortical association fibers.

The "arbor vitae" of the cut surface of the cerebellum is well seen (on the viewer's right) and there is fortuitous visualization of the opened sigmoid sinus on this side as well. The bony confines of the foramen magnum are seen laterally, along with cervical spinal dural attachments to the foramen lip.

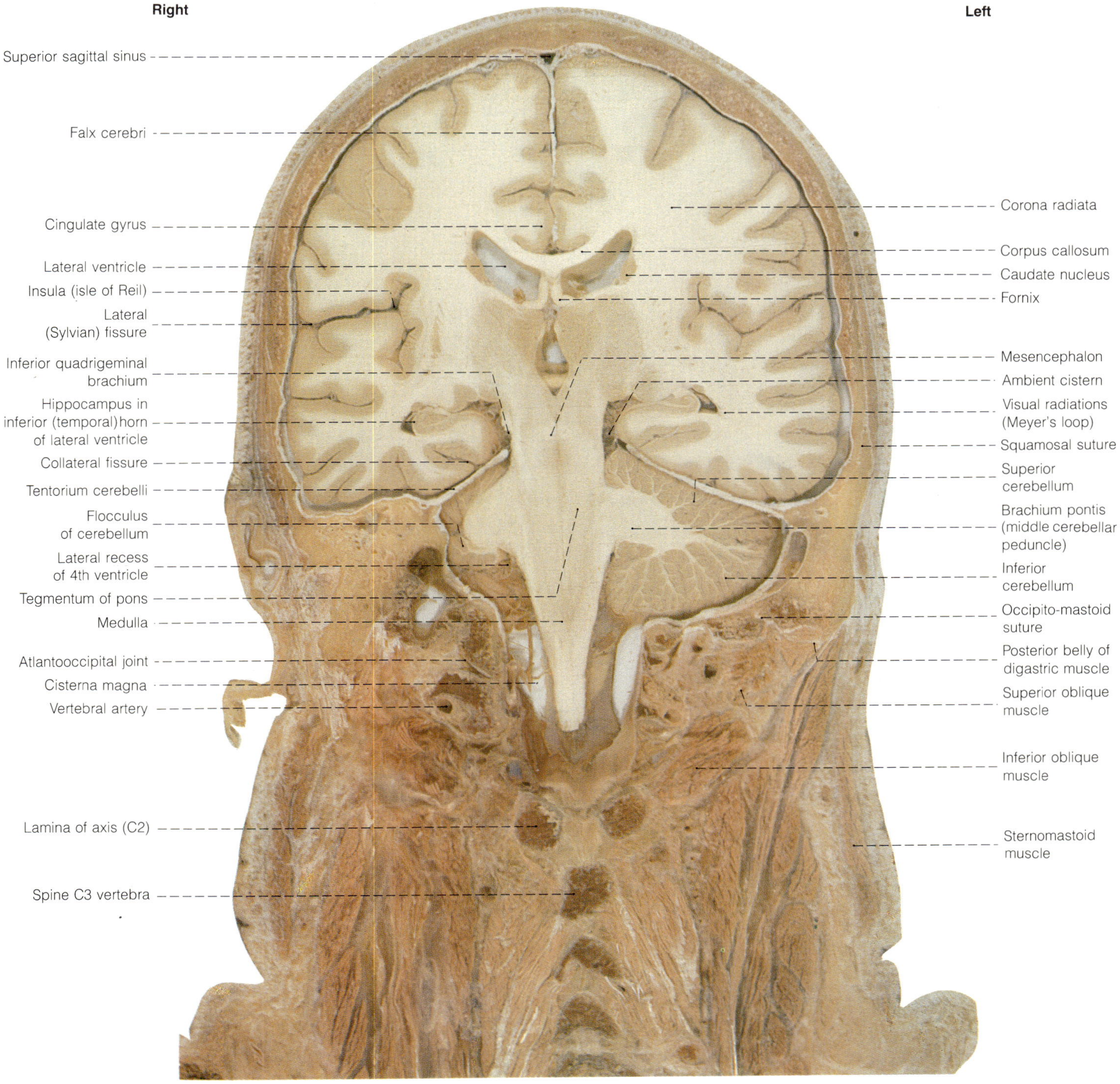

Viewed from the Front

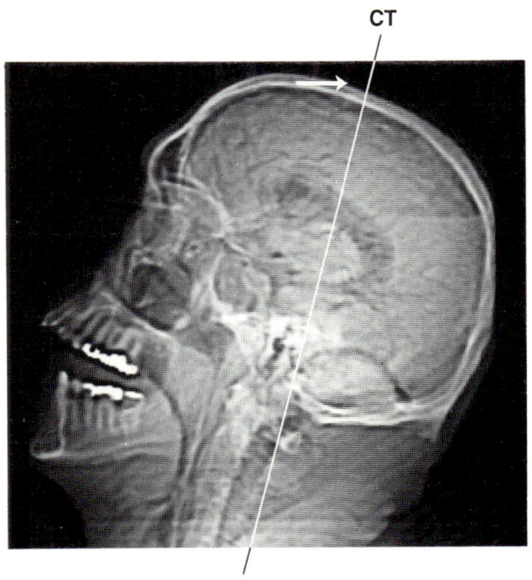

Plane of Section

Patient CT Scan

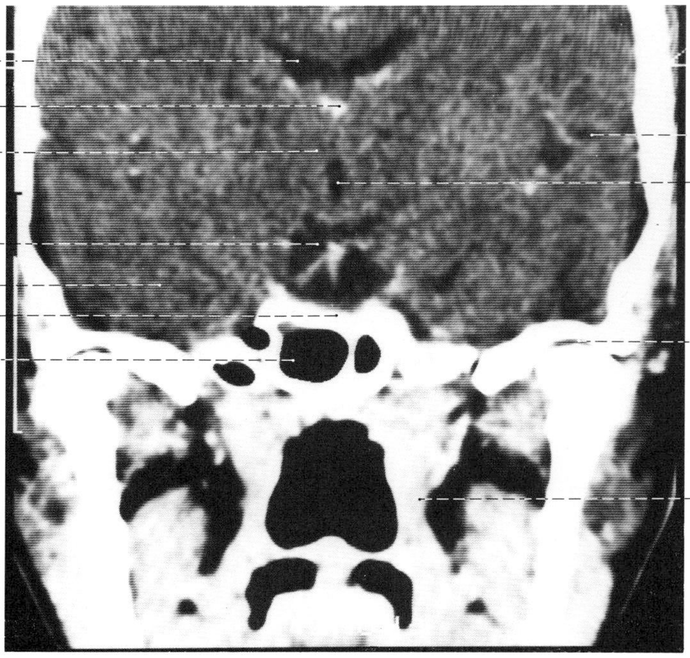

Patient MRI Scan

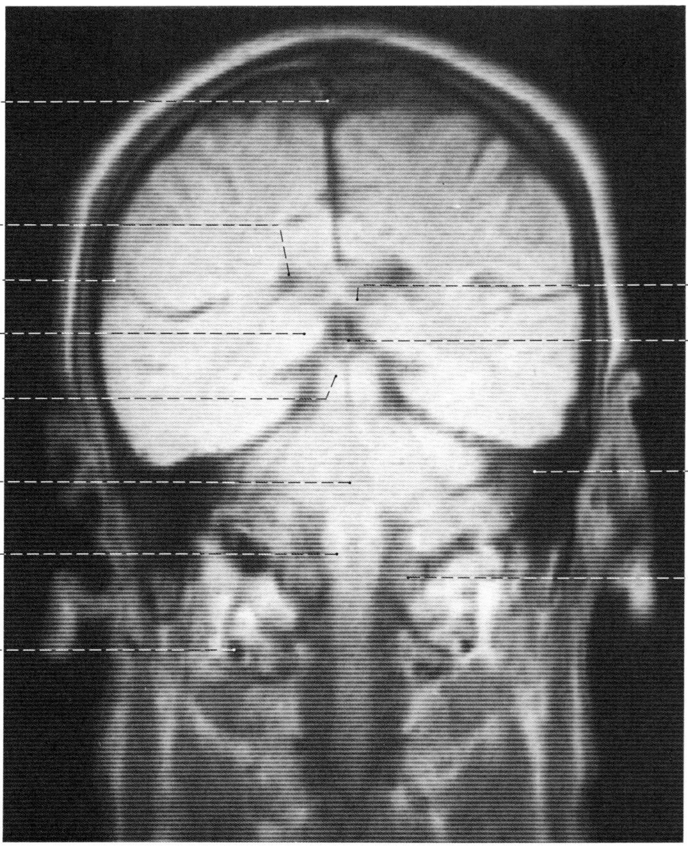

Looking into the posterior apex of the third ventricle, one can appreciate the habenular commissure, pineal recess and the antero-superior portion of the aqueduct of Sylvius. The internal cerebral veins course as paired midline structures in the velum interpositum and may be quite evident in enhanced CT studies, where they appear white, or in MRI imaging where they appear black.

The difficult-to-visualize medial and lateral geniculate nuclei are seen lateral to the cerebral peduncles and hugging the inferio-medial surface of temporo-occipital areas, forming the roof of the initial segment of the choroid fissure. The retrolenticular course of the auditory radiations from (and to) the medial geniculate nucleus to (and from) the transverse temporal (Heschl's) gyrus lie in this plane as well as the origin of the visual radiations from the lateral geniculate sweeping lateral to the temporal horn of the lateral ventricle into the temporal lobe. The posterior extension of the uncus, the parahippocampal gyrus, is noted in its close relationship to the edge of the tentorium or tentorial notch; it is simple to see how "uncal herniation" can occur with this anatomical relationship from increased supratentorial intracranial pressure. It is also anatomically evident that the major part of the medial temporal lobe is supplied by the posterior cerebral artery arching around the cerebral peduncle.

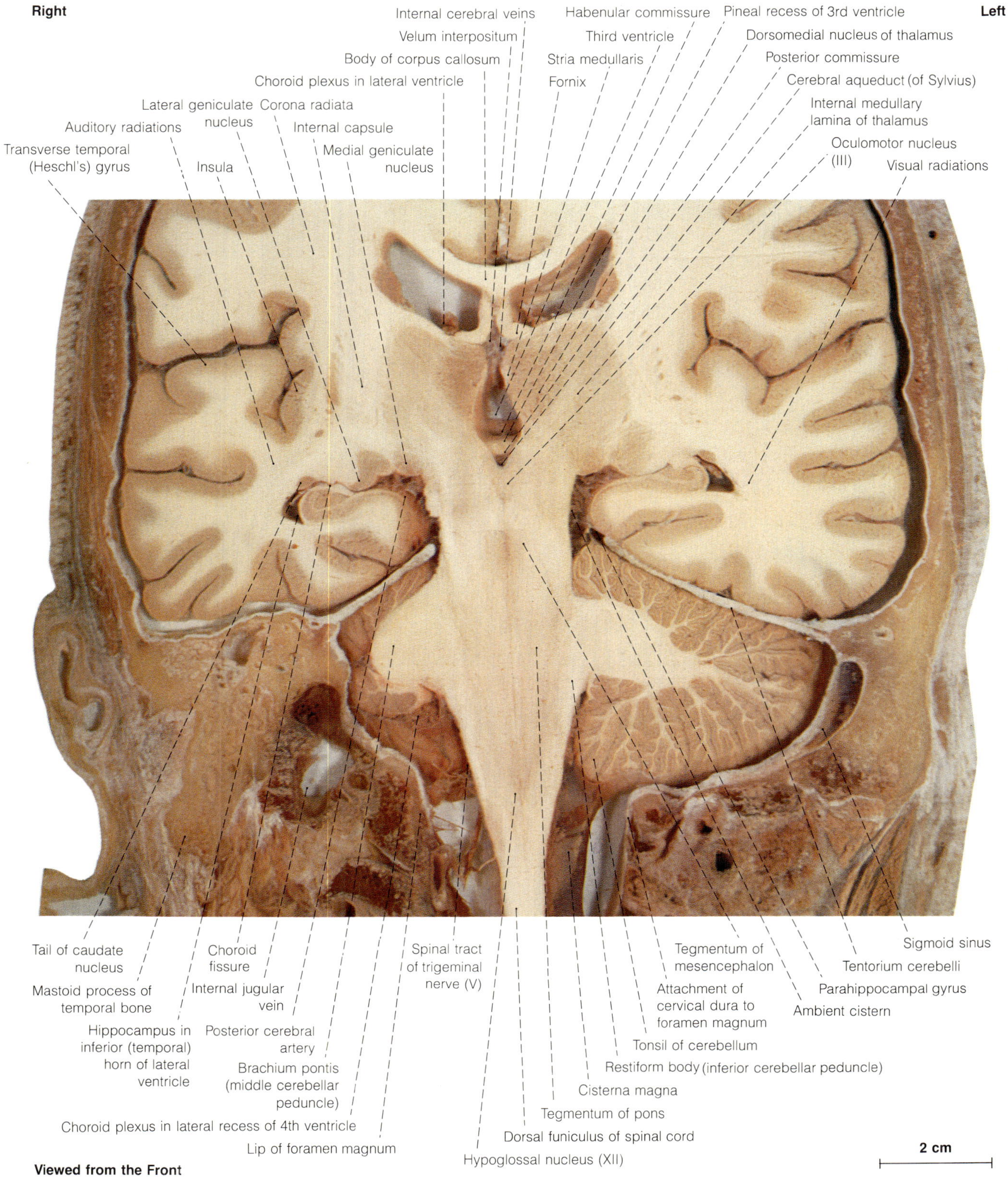

Viewed from the Front

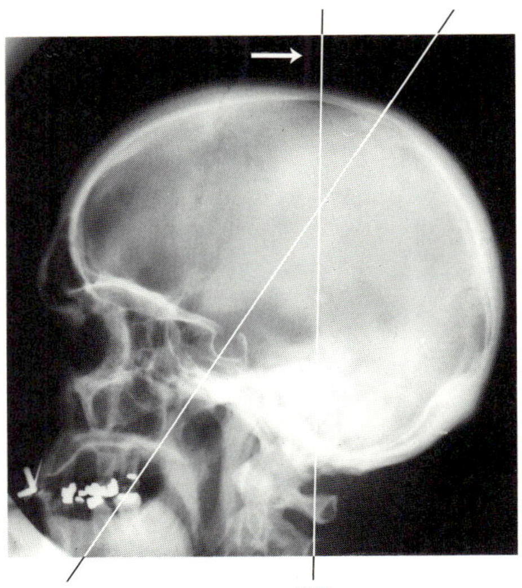

Planes of Sections

Cadaver CT Scan

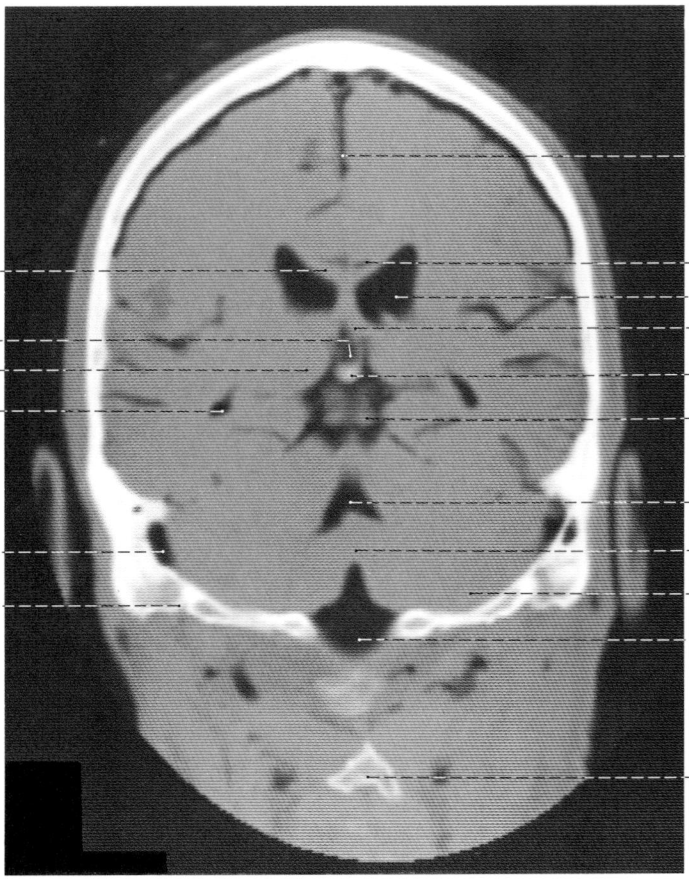

Visualized in this one slice are the lateral ventricles, posterior thalami, and fourth ventricle. The posterior columns of the fornix are completing their 180° curve from the temporal lobe into the parietal lobe at this level enroute to the medial mamillary and septal nuclei. Immediately above the pineal in this cut section, the great vein of Galen appears with clotted blood within it. Its cross-sectional area is large at this level because of the junction of veins such as the basal vein of Rosenthal and the fact that the great vein of Galen is cut on a bias in the coronal plane due to its backward curve. The posterior mesencephalon or tectum consists of two eminences, the superior and inferior colliculi. The posterior cerebral and superior cerebellar arteries and basal veins of Rosenthal are on either side of the mesencephalon in the ambient cisterns. Just lateral to the ambient cistern and forming its lateral border is the parahippocampal gyrus. The temporal horn of the lateral ventricle with the infolded hippocampus medially and visual radiations laterally is also seen in cross-section on either side.

This slice just passes through a portion of the cisterna magna and a fortuitously located branch (tonsilar) of the posterior inferior cerebellar artery (PICA) is noted running around the cerebellar tonsil on the viewer's left (right of specimen).

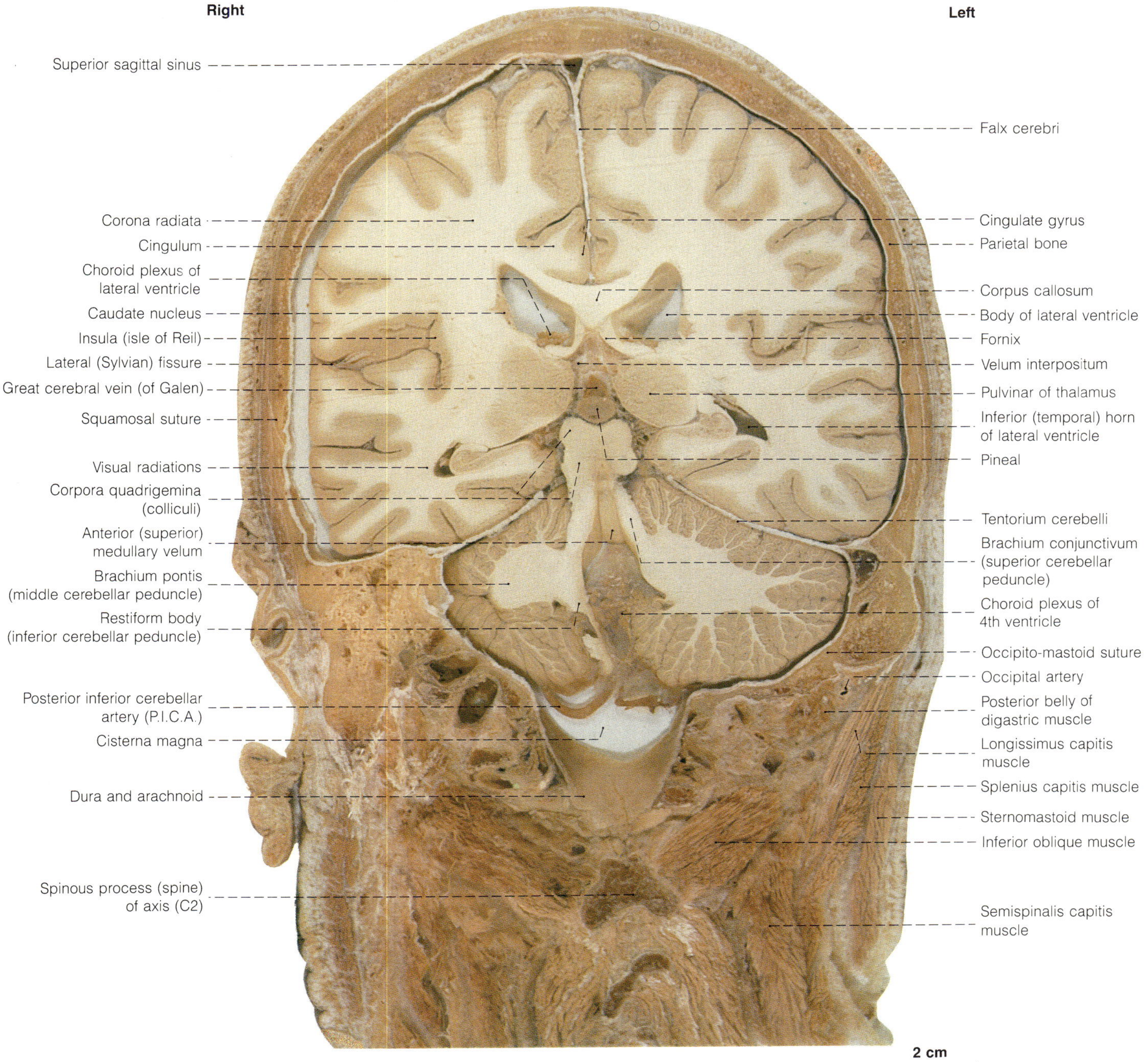

Viewed from the Front

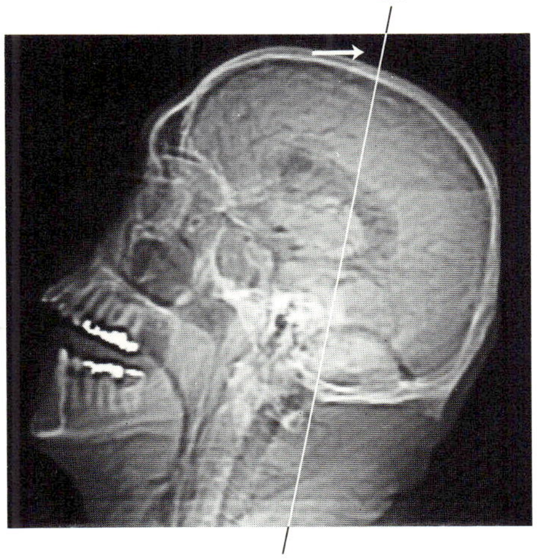

Plane of Section

Pineal and Great Cerebral Vein

Patient CT Scan

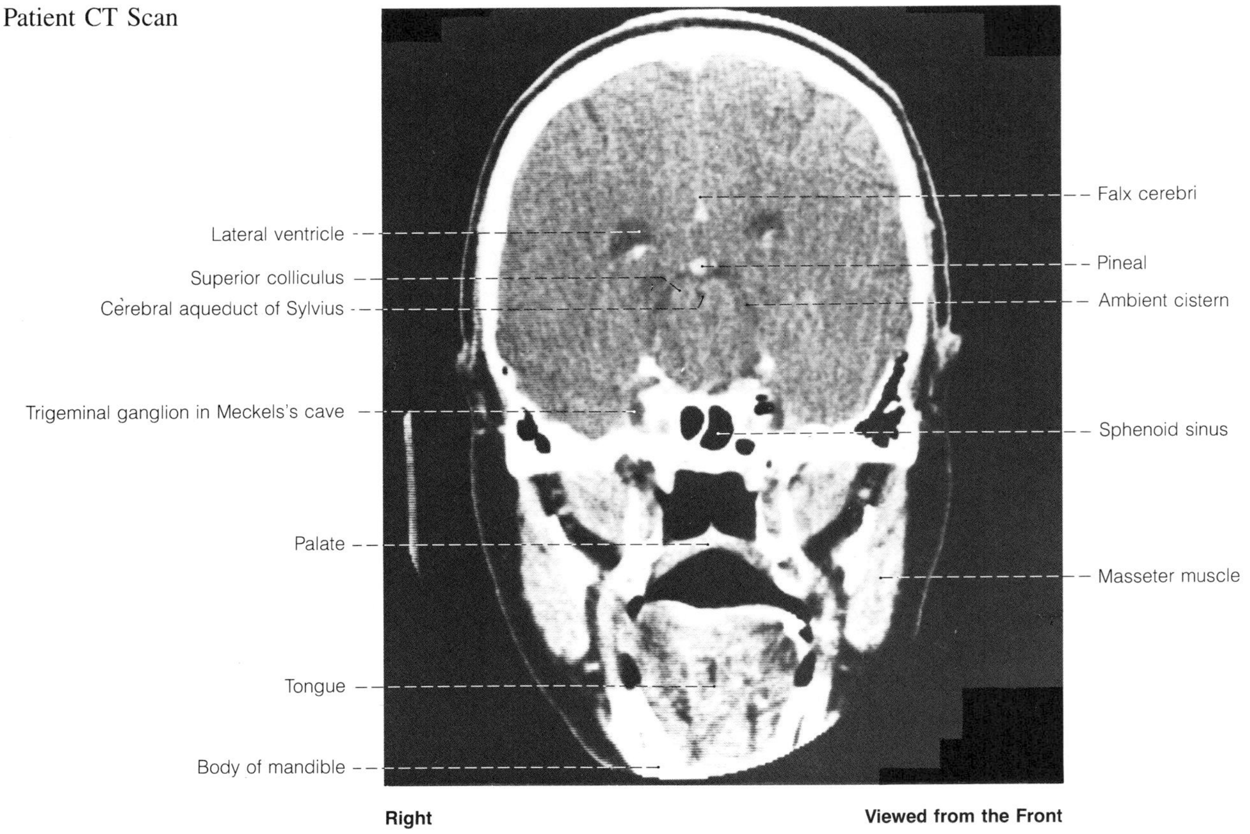

Patient MRI Scan

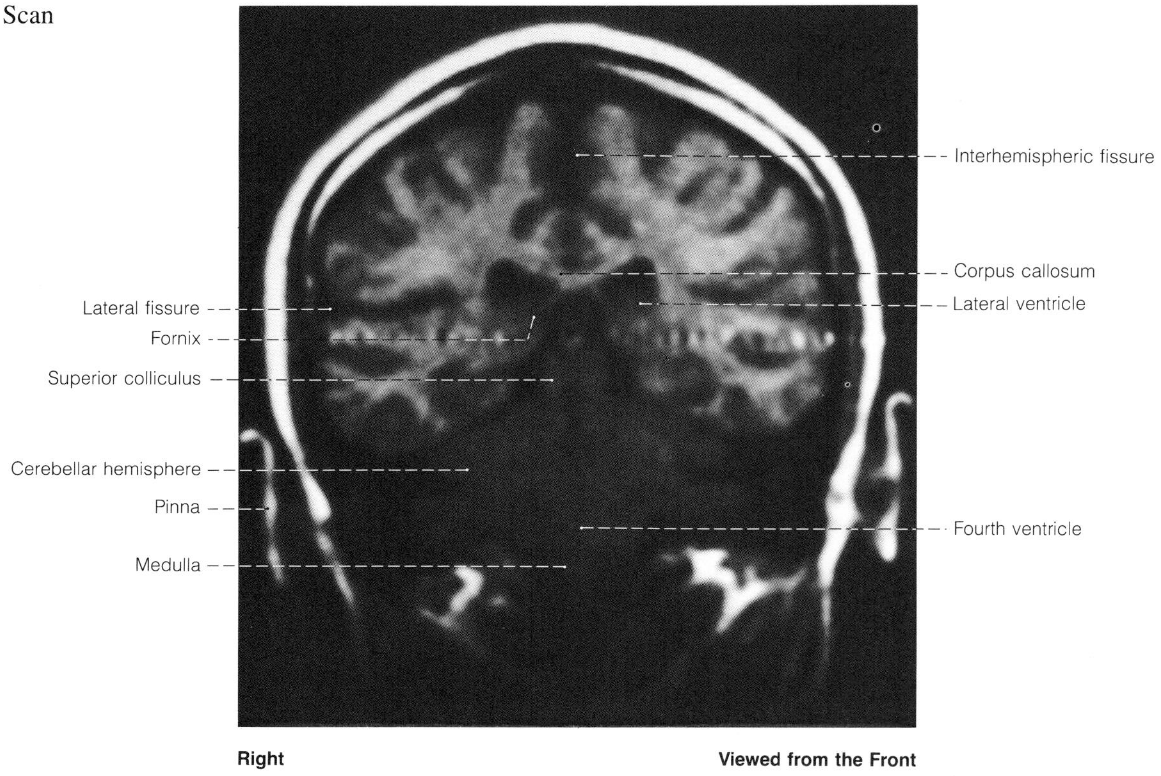

A coronal CT scan through the pineal will usually pass anterior to the cerebellum due to the angle of the patient's head. Such cuts will, however, intersect the cavernous sinus or, as shown in the CT scan, its posterior aspect with Meckel's cave and the trigeminal ganglion. In the anatomical specimen and MRI scan a true vertical coronal section is illustrated.

Passing from the infratentorial posterior fossa to supratentorial structures (note the cut edge of the tentorium) is the brachium conjunctivum or superior cerebellar peduncle, outlining the upper half of the 4th ventricle. The choroid plexus of the roof of the 4th ventricle is seen through the slice, and the inferior half of the 4th verntricle is framed by the brachia pontis or middle cerebellar peduncles and the restiform bodies (inferior cerebellar peduncles). The "arbor vitae" of the cerebellar cortex in coronal section is seen in a different projection from that usually presented sagittally through the vermis, and illustrates the homogeneity of the anatomy of the cerebellar cortex. Grey-white matter differentiation of the arbor vitae is difficult to demonstrate but appears to be readily visible with certain types of pulse sequences on MRI.

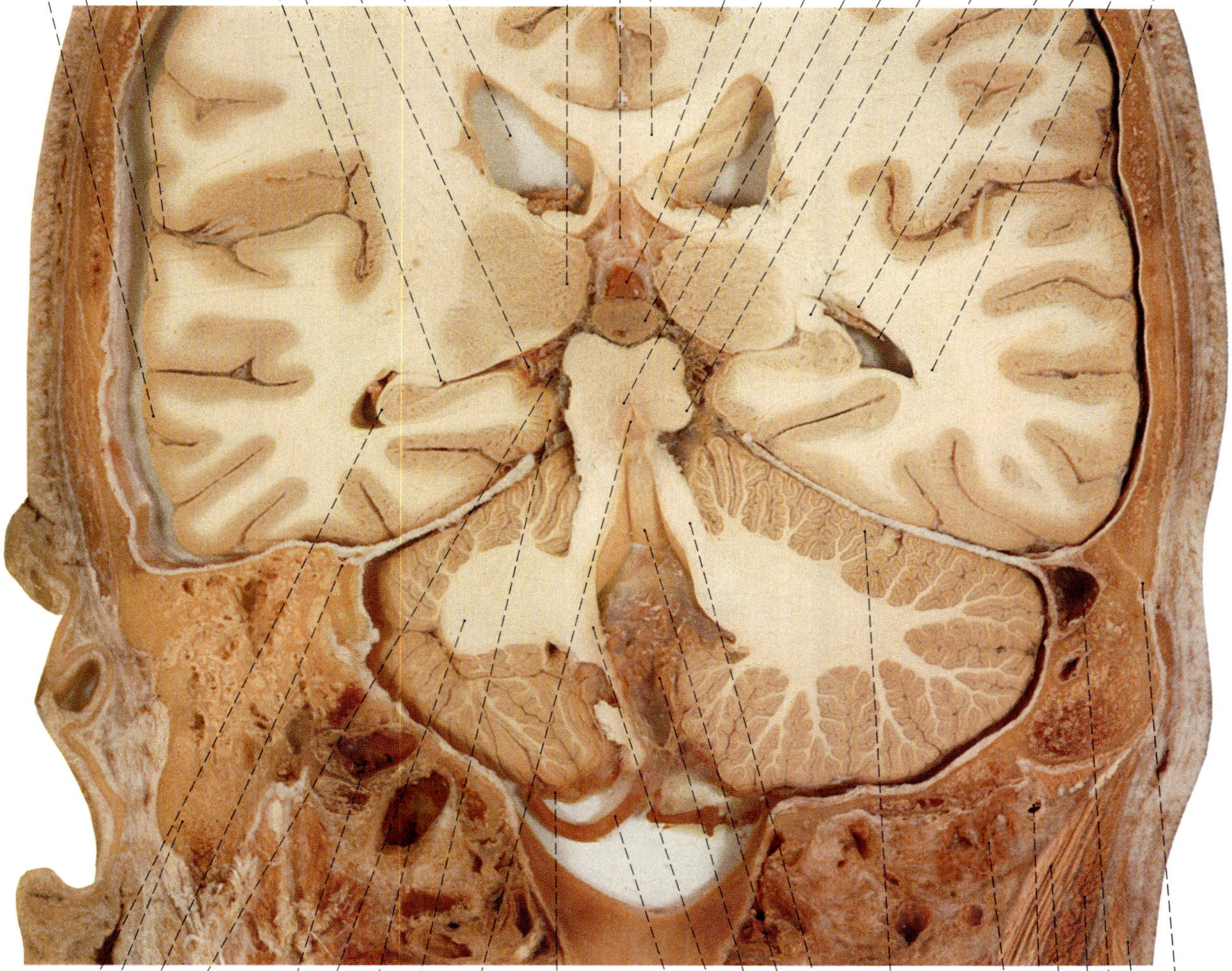

Viewed from the Front

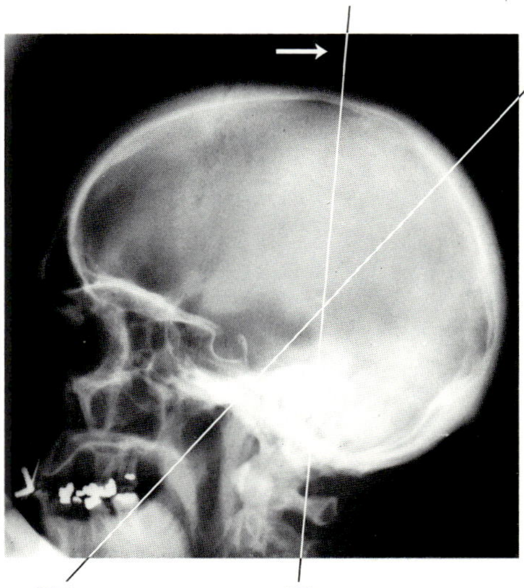

Planes of Sections

Cadaver CT Scan

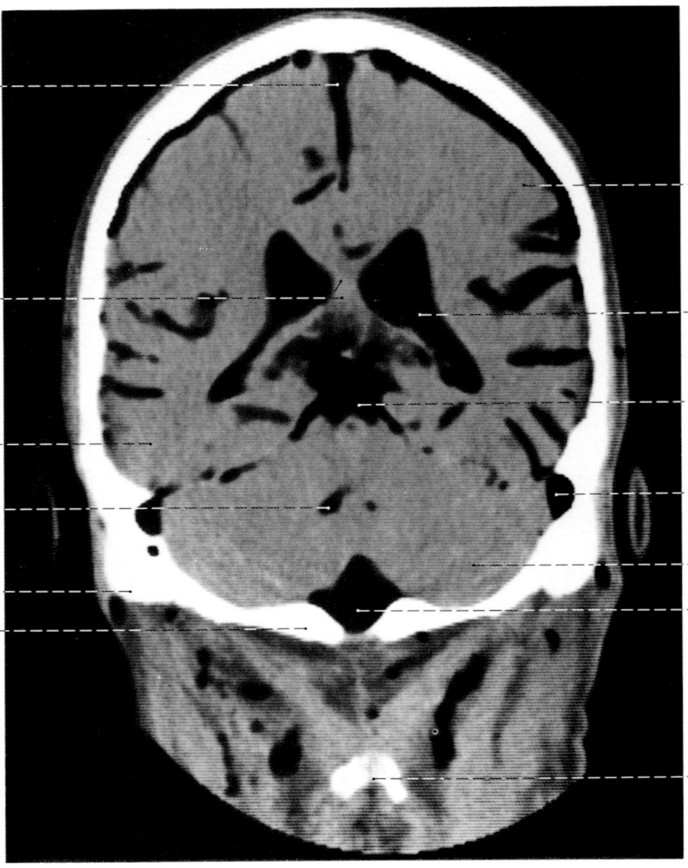

This coronal section is a cut through the trigone (atrium) of the lateral ventricle and through the curved splenium of the corpus callosum which is a dominant feature of this particular slice. Many veins, including the great vein of Galen, are embedded in the matrix of the quadrigeminal plate cistern at a point where it is contiguous with the superior cerebellar cistern, the transverse cerebral cistern and the velum interpositum. The posterior portions of the temporal lobes are present at this level and it is easy to see how temporal lobe branches arise from the posterior cerebral artery. The superior vermis of the cerebellum lies immediately within the medial infratentorial area. The vermis with the underlying cerebellar nuclei form the roof of the fourth ventricle. Because of the coronal orientation of the cut both superior and inferior vermis are seen in the same coronal cut and the indentation of the 4th ventricle by the nodulus is illustrated.

The lateral ventricles are well represented by their atria, which are clearly shown in their relation to surrounding landmarks. One relationship exceptionally well demonstrated here is of the visual radiations to the wall of the atrium (trigone of lateral ventricle).

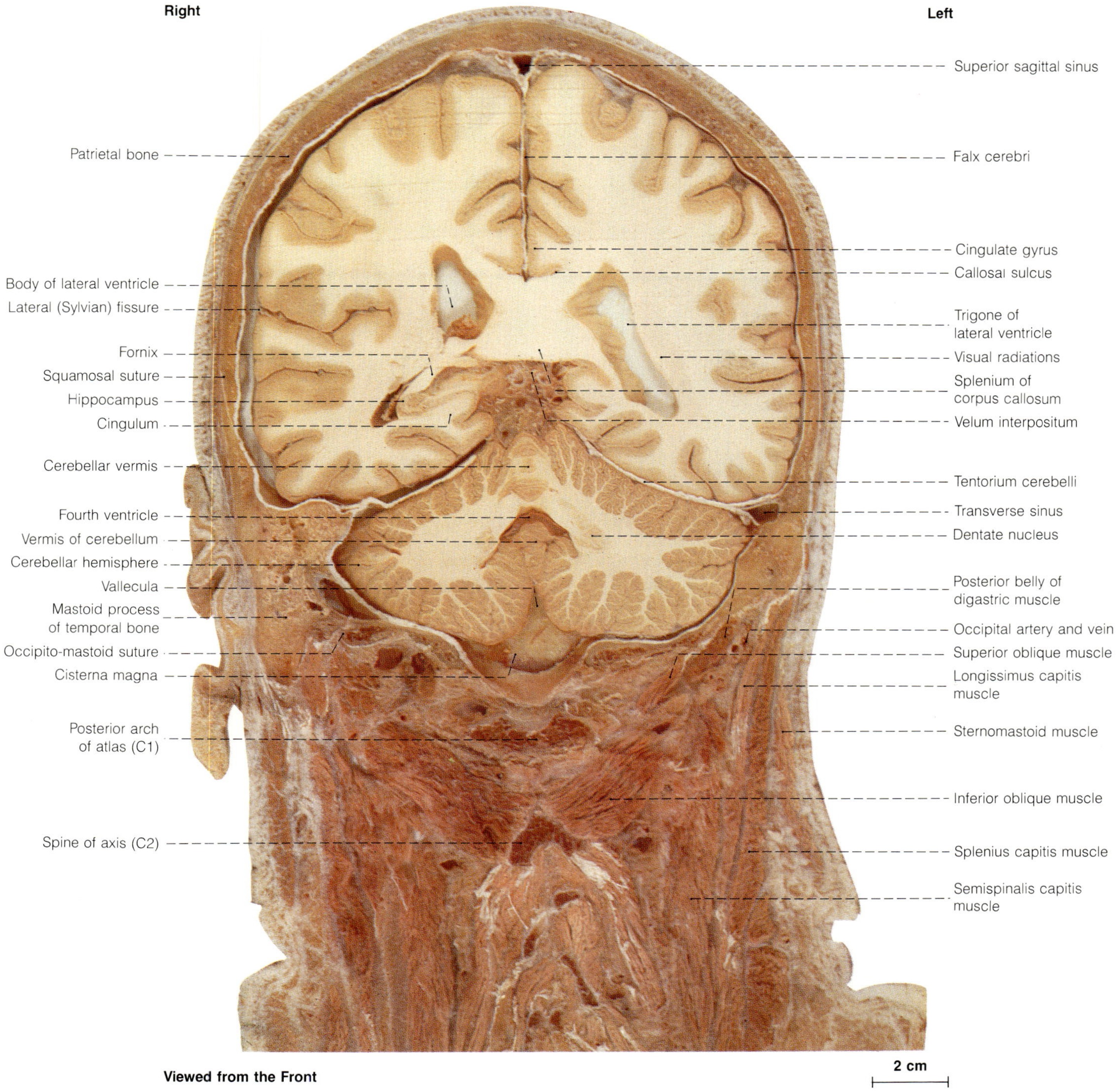

Viewed from the Front

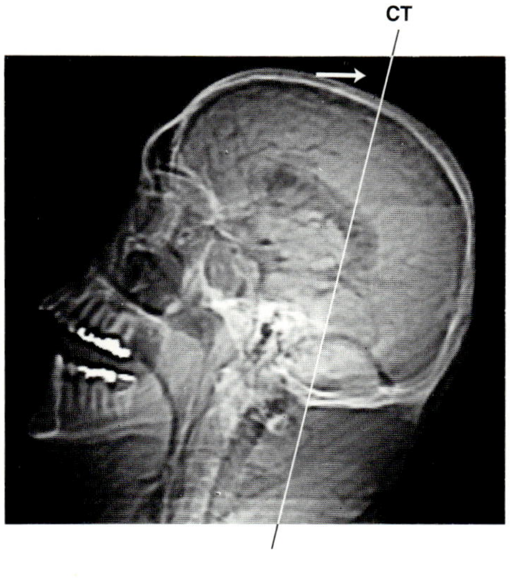

Plane of Section

Splenium of Corpus callosum

Patient CT Scan

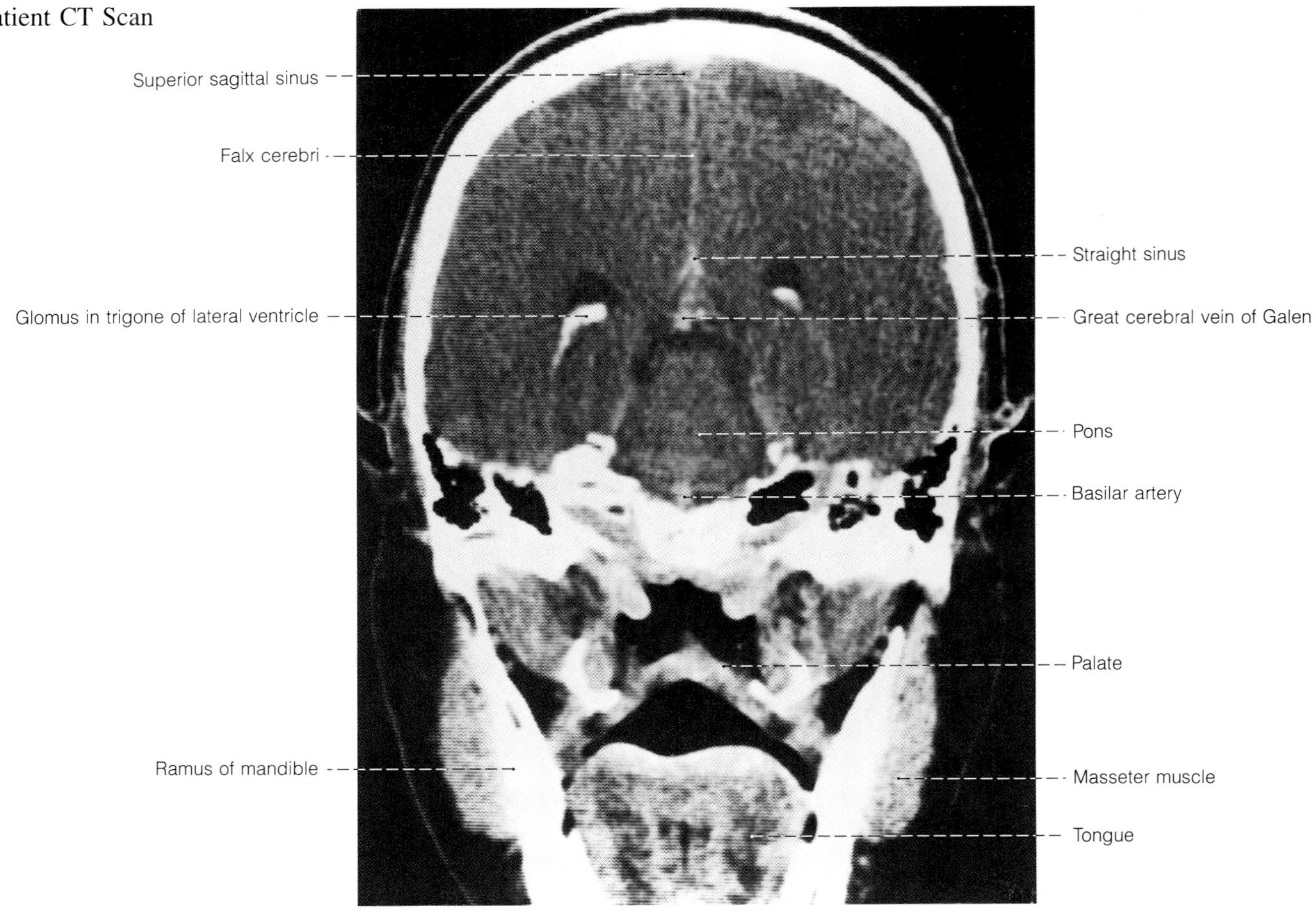

Patient MRI Scan

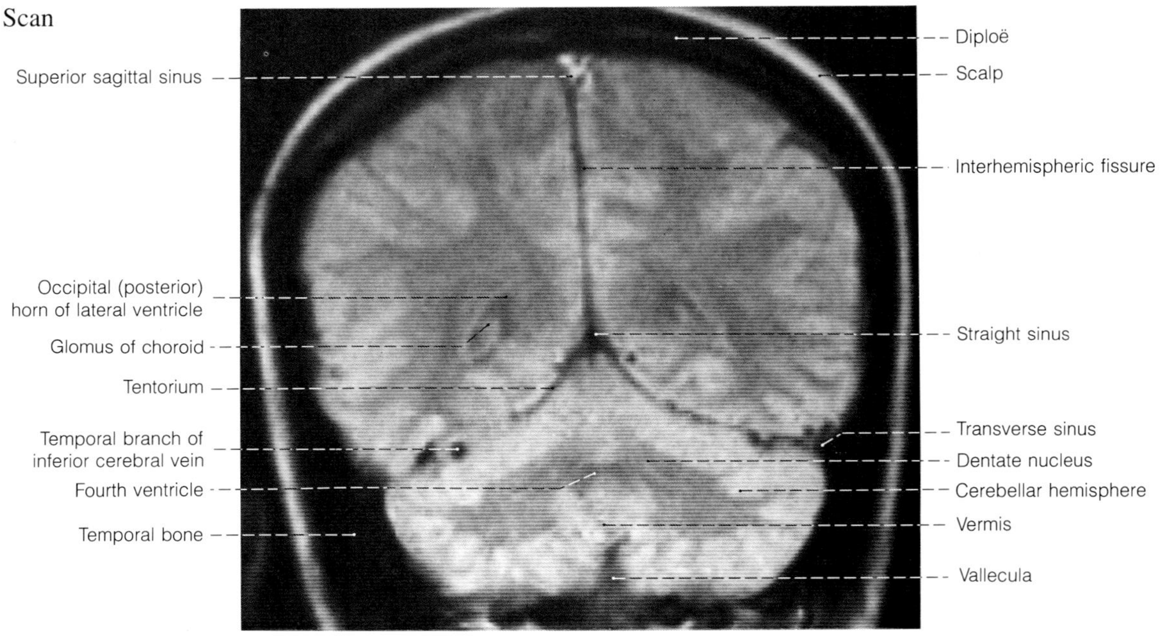

The anatomical and MRI coronal sections pass through the apex (fastigium) of the fourth ventricle and illustrate the differences in contour of the superior and inferior cerebellar surfaces. Grey white differentiation on the MRI is very good with this pulse sequence and clearly shows the "arbor vitae". The ventricular system on the MRI patient is not as enlarged as that of the specimen and the atrium of the lateral ventricle is not as well demonstrated. The dural venous sinuses at the site of entrance of cortical veins may appear gray rather than the usual black on MRI evidently because of the turbulance of flow at this junction.

Tumors arising solely in the cerebellar vermis are in the superior portion of the posterior fossa and may not displace the 4th ventricle anteriorly or posteriorly but may push it inferiorly. The cistern in which the superior vermis, pineal, and vein of Galen meet is known by several names, depending upon how close it is to adjacent structures at the naming; i.e.—ambient cistern, superior cerebellar cistern, or quadrigeminal plate cistern. Sharp boundaries of any of the cisterns are not anatomically defined and they are all parts of a continuous subarachnoid space.

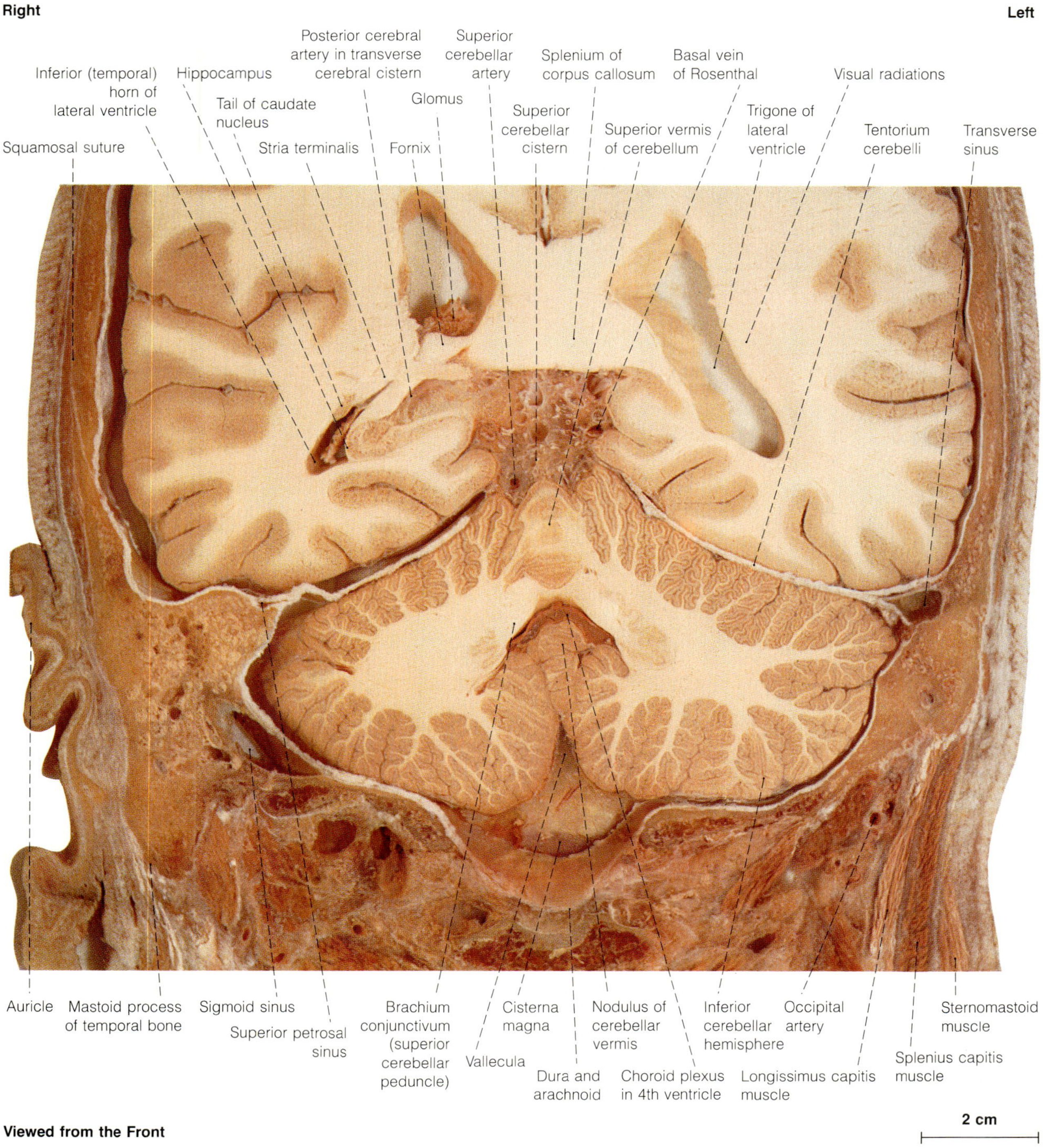

Viewed from the Front

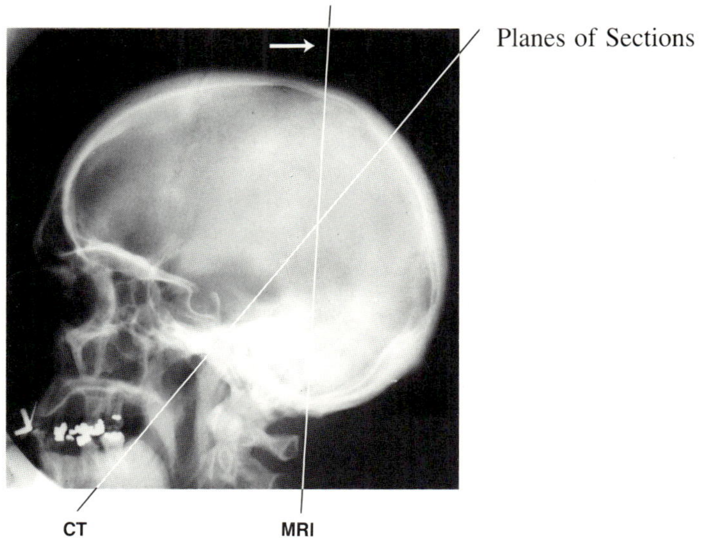

Cadaver CT Scan

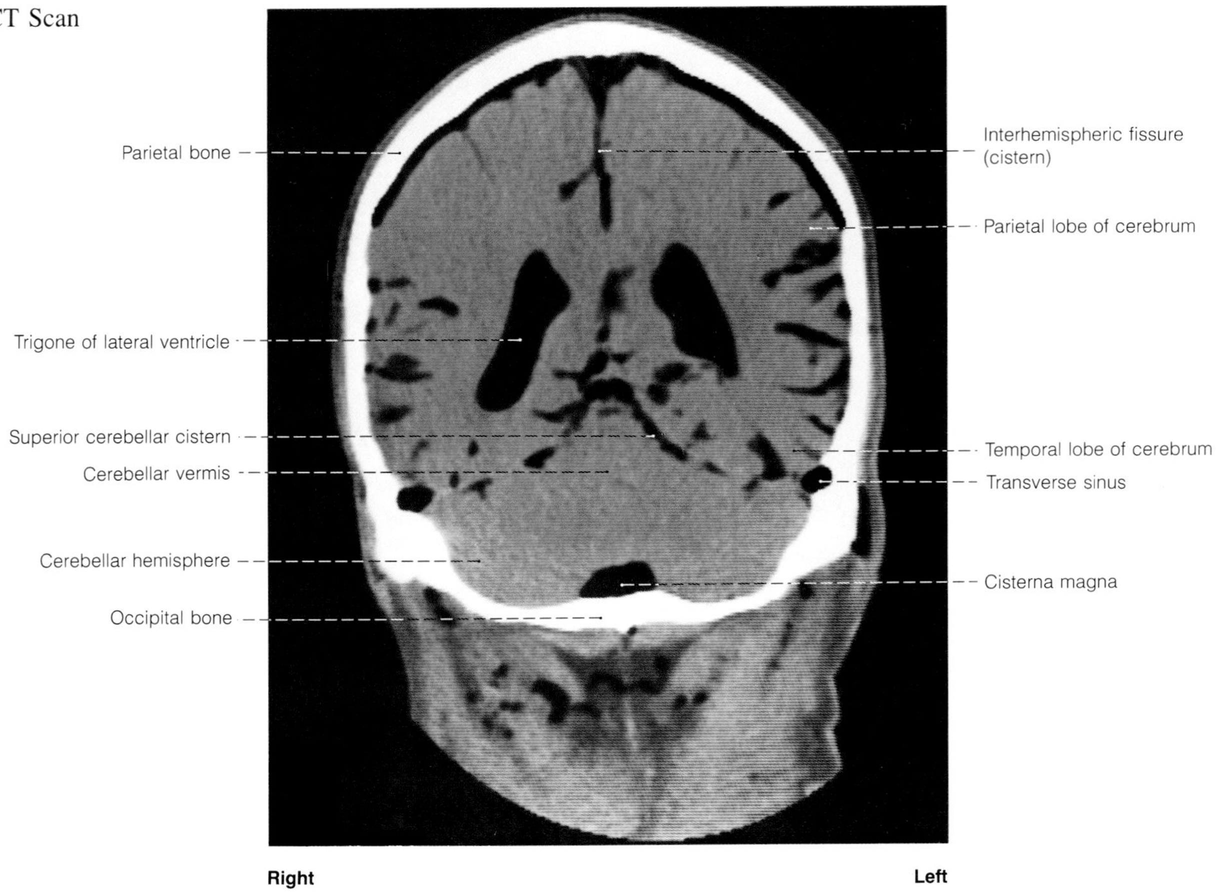

The complete form of the tentorium is evident on this cut and the reason for the name is obvious. The slope of the tent is, however, variable. The great cerebral vein of Galen is dumping into the straight sinus just caudal to this plane. The location of the transverse sinus between the leaves of tentorial dura and the location of the dentate nucleus of the cerebellum are well demonstrated in this view. Portions of the vermis are still visible in the midline. The cortex of the calcarine fissure, separating the superior and inferior visual cortices, extends nearly to the lateral ventricle where it may form a ventricular ridge known as the calcar avis.

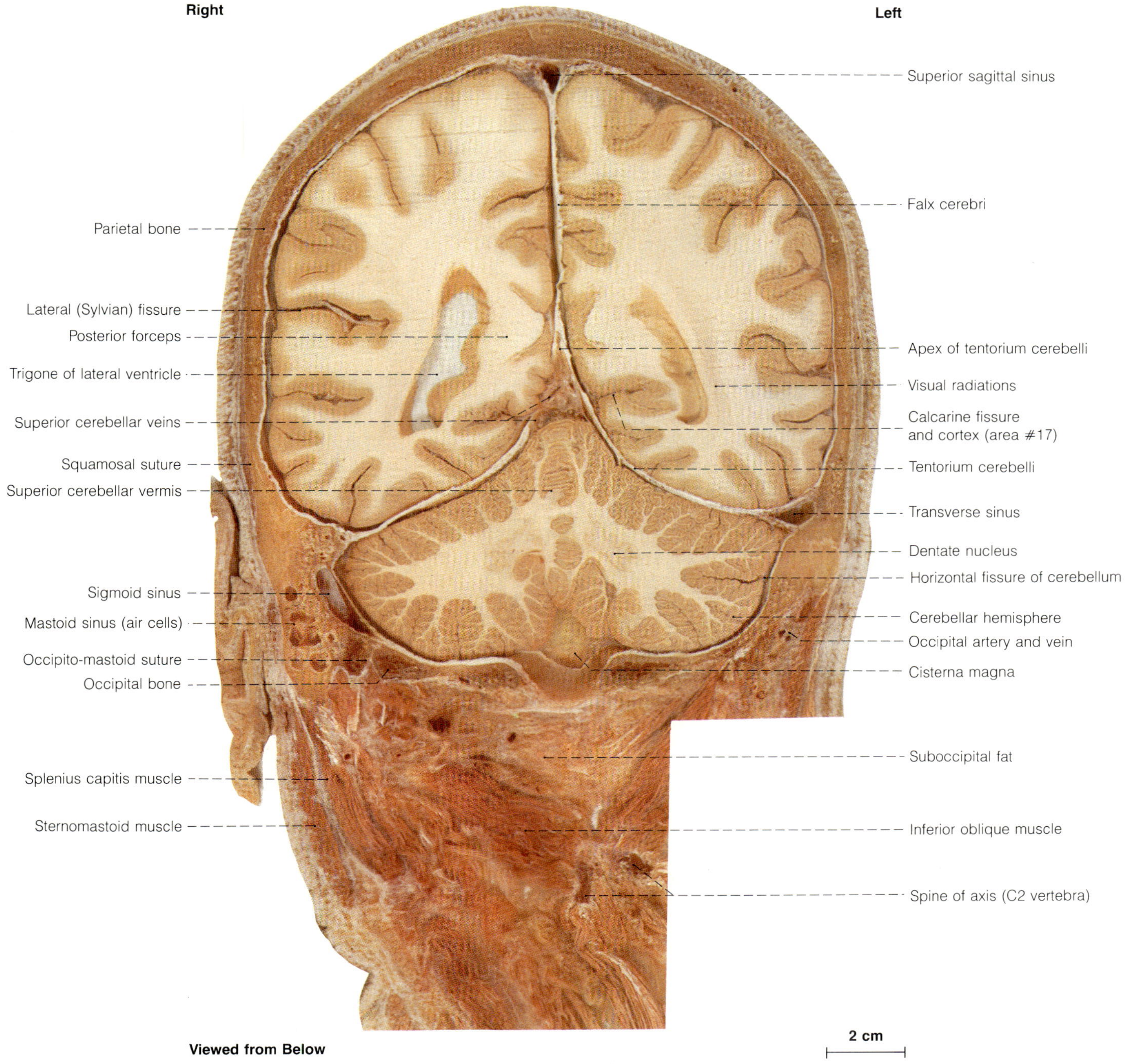

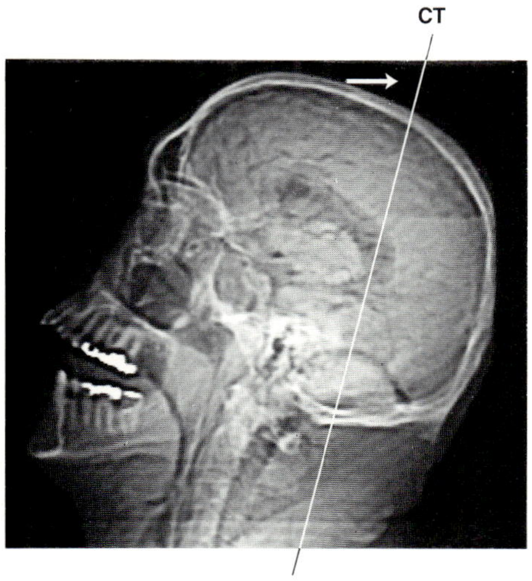

Plane of Section

Patient CT Scan

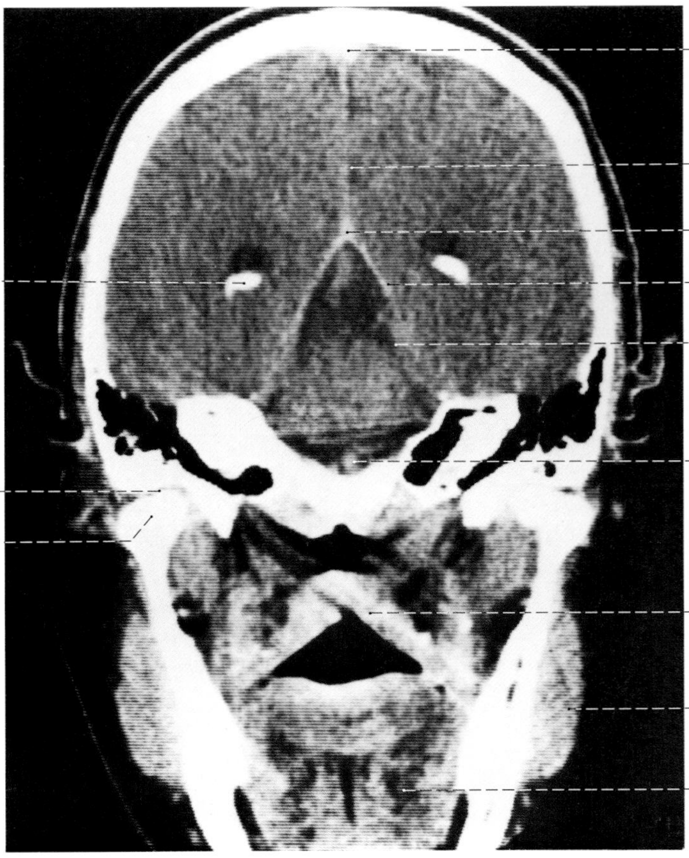

Patient MRI Scan

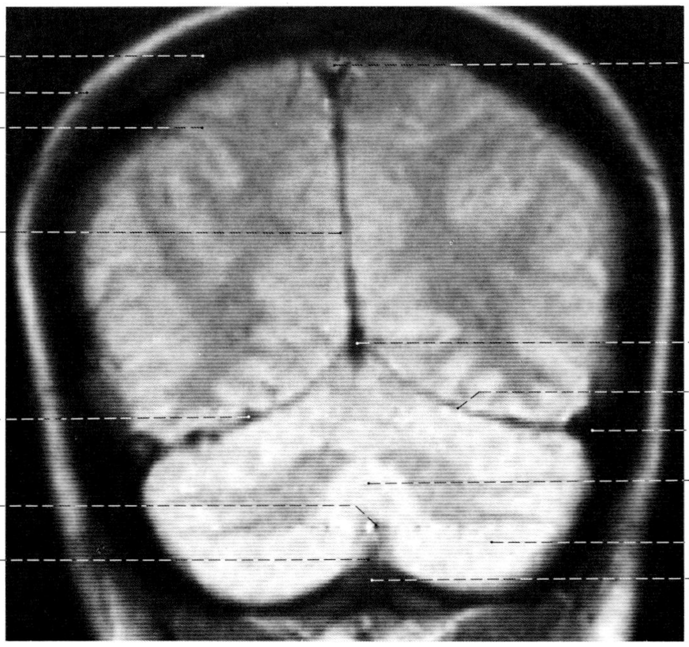

This coronal plane passes through the splenium of the corpus callosum and the parietal and temporal lobes of the cerebral hemispheres. The superior-inferior expanse of the visual radiations as they pass just lateral to the lateral ventricle into both of these lobes can be appreciated. Anatomical involvement of these visual radiations results in a reverse visual deficit (e.g. temporal radiations on the left cause a right upper homonymous quadrantanopsia).

The vessels of the brain are frequently very apparent on MRI scans and such vessels as the inferior cerebral veins in the sulci of the inferior temporal lobe are quite evident. Interesting note is made of the relatively large number of veins along the curved lateral surface of the tentorium on the viewer's left. The black (on MRI) straight sinus is centrally located.

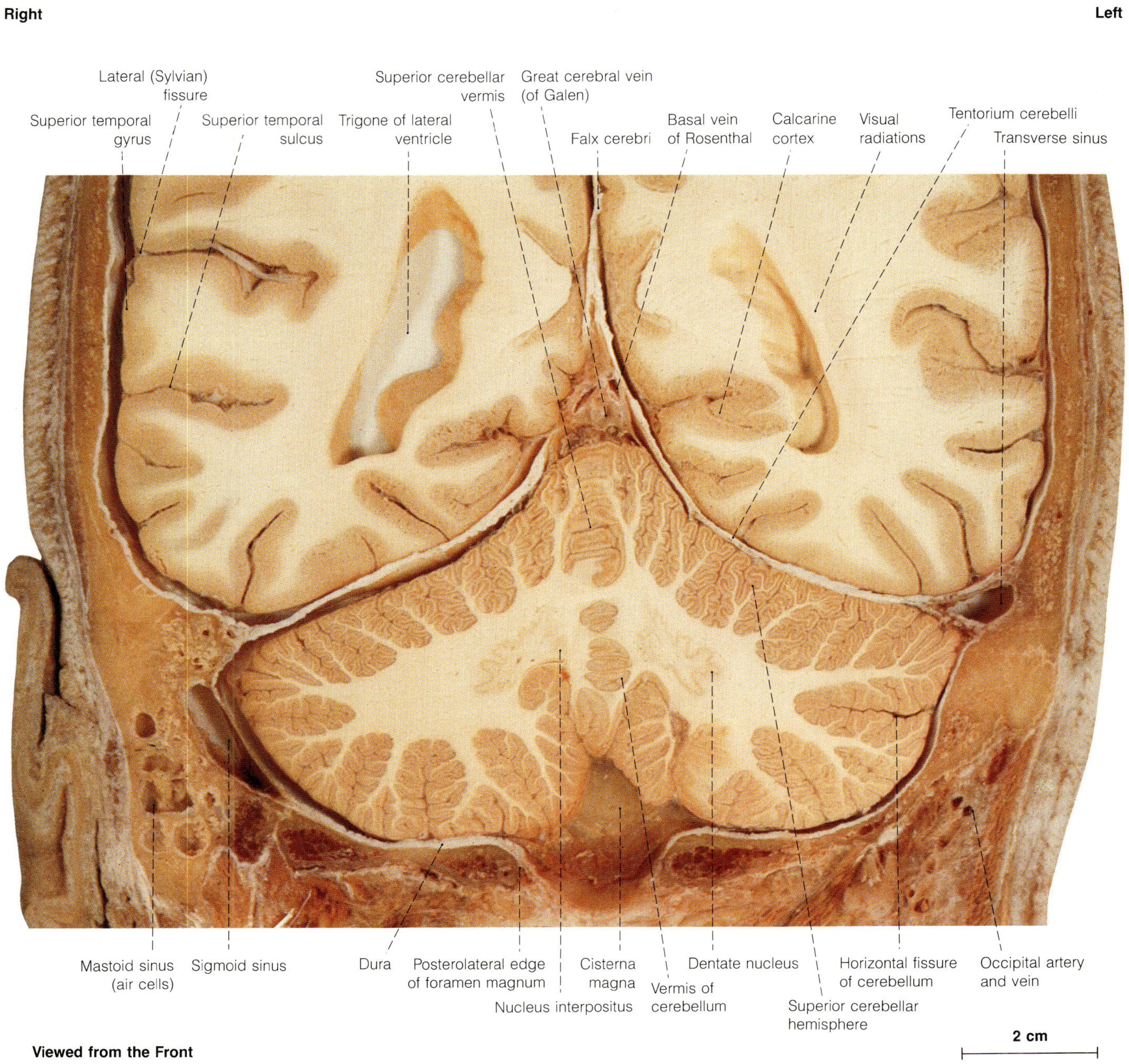

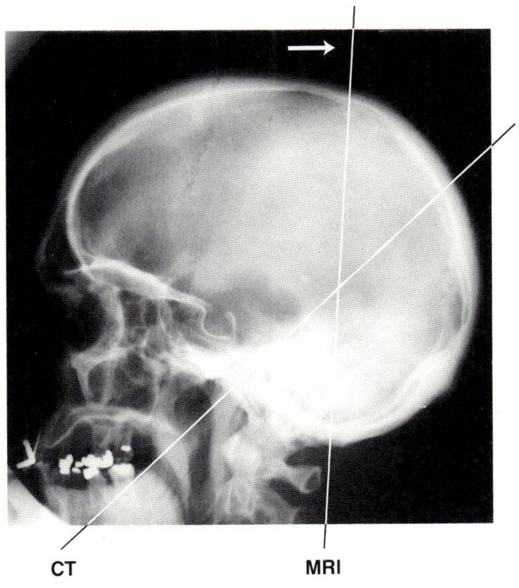

Planes of Sections

Cadaver CT Scan

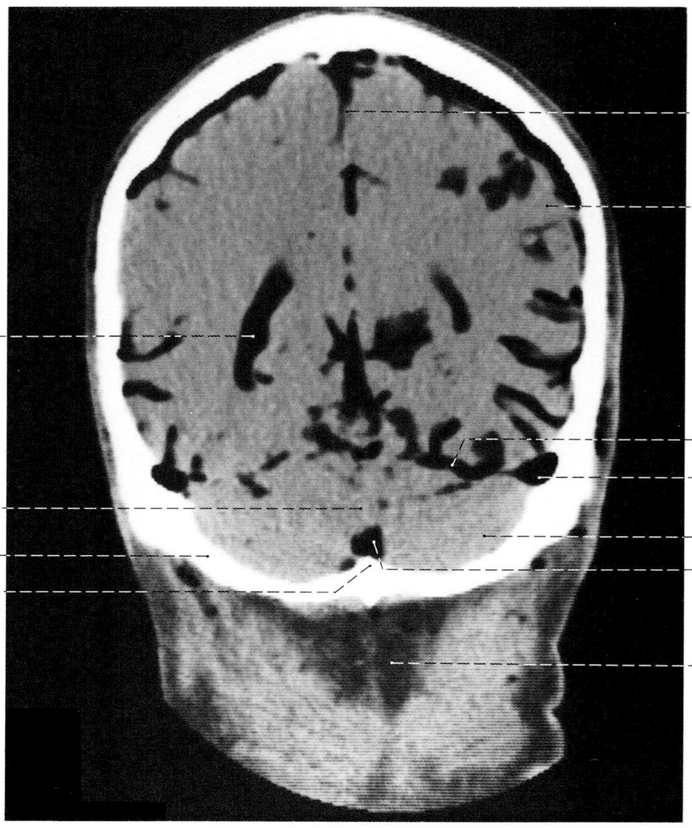

The posterior-most aspect of the occipital (posterior) horn of the lateral ventricles, lined with ependyma, is noted on the viewer's left (right side of specimen). The calcarine fissure divides upper and lower visual fields and the broad falx cerebri is fully separating right from left cerebral hemispheres. The cortex lateral to the visual radiations and the related subcortical white matter on the left are important receptive areas for language. Beneath the tentorium, the cerebellar vermis and posterior tip of the dentate nucleus are seen in this coronal section. This, the largest of the cerebellar nuclei, may also be observed in sections anterior to this plane. The dentate nuclei and lateral cerebellar hemispheres with which they are related constitute the largest anatomical mass of the cerebellum.

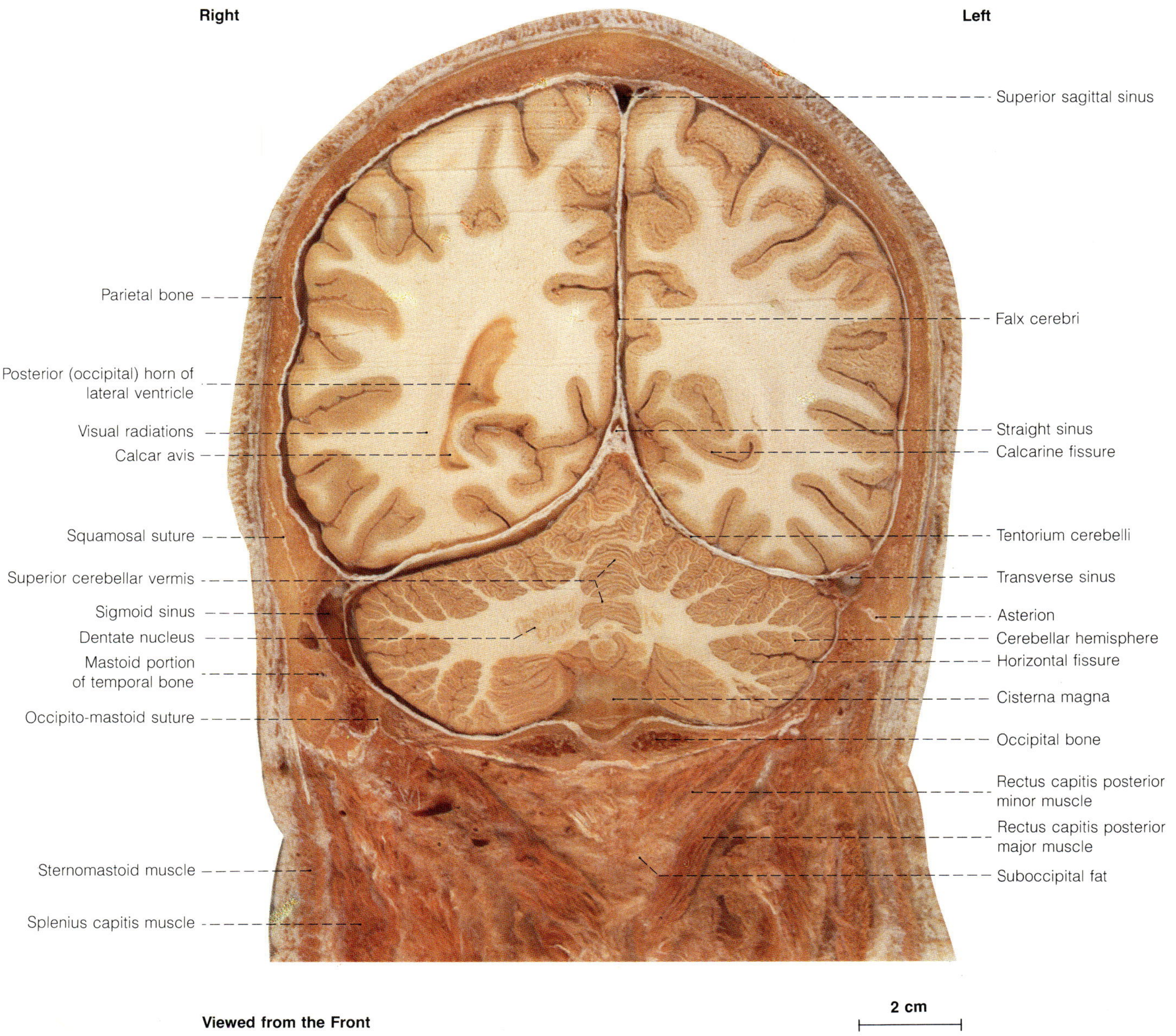

Viewed from the Front

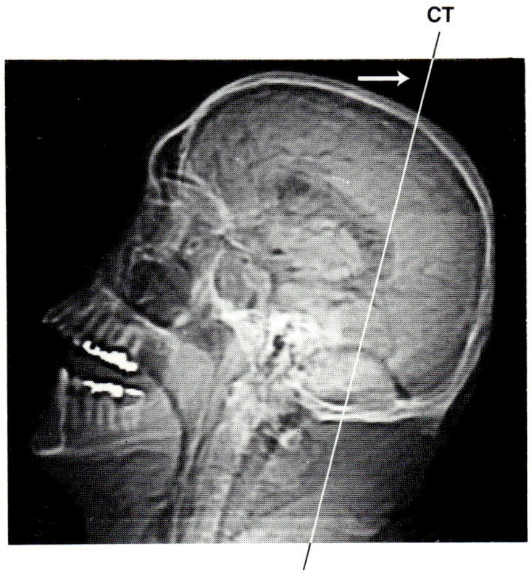

Plane of Section

Cadaver CT Scan

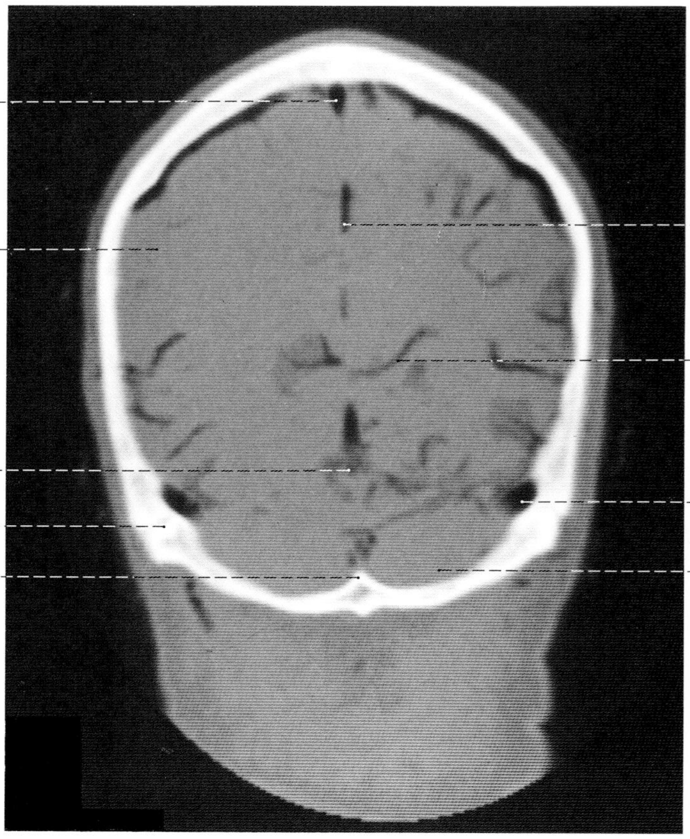

The occiptial lobes rest on the tentorium and are completely separated by the falx cerebri. In this coronal section the superior sagittal, straight, transverse, and occipital sinus may all be seen. In addition, a draining cortical vein can be seen approaching the superior sagittal sinus. It is evident that the venous drainage of this cortex may be either superiorly or inferiorly.

The stripe of Gennari (18th century Italian anatomist) characteristic of the visual cortex of the calcarine fissure may be seen in this unstained gross slice as it was undoubtedly first identified.

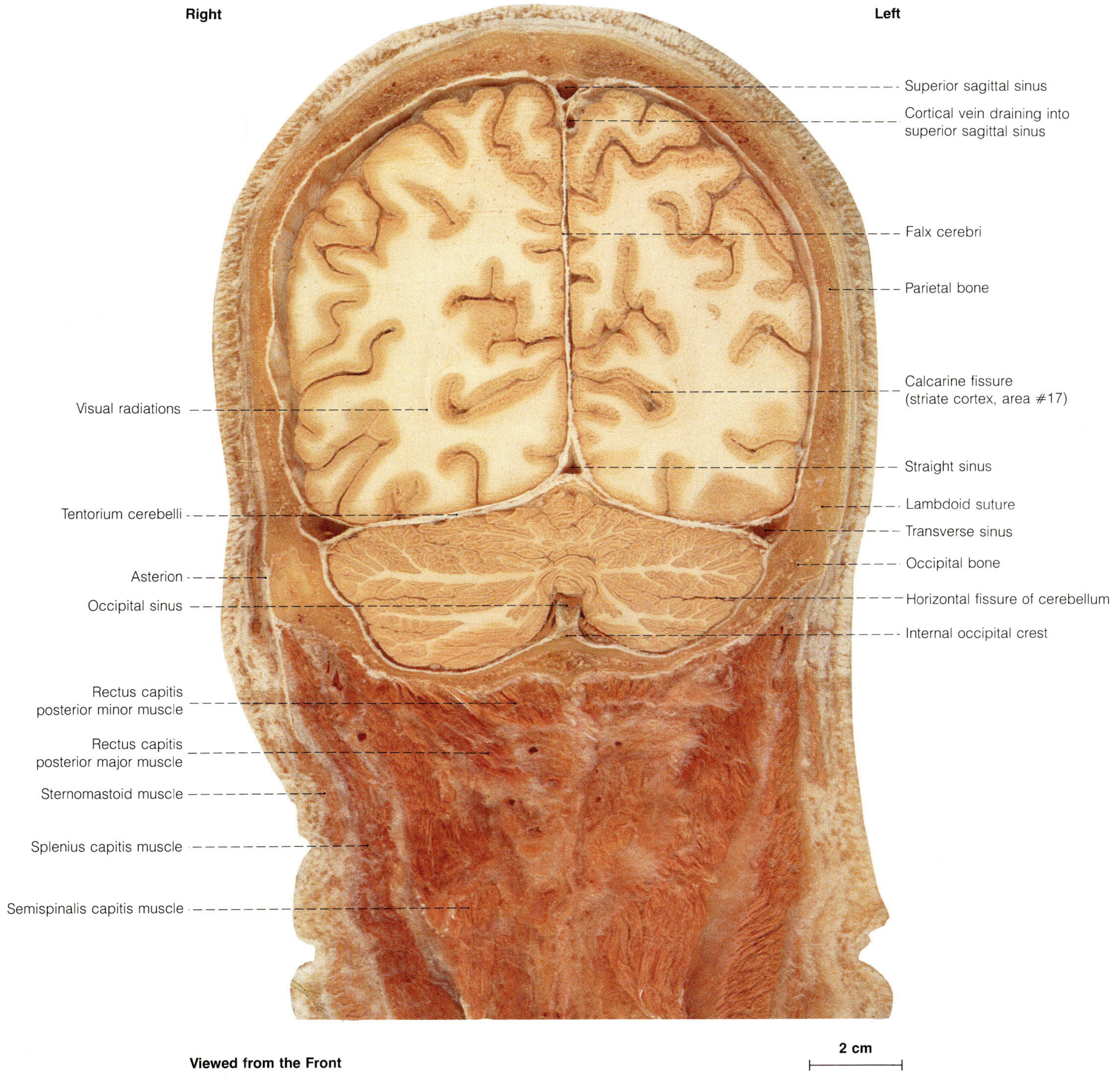

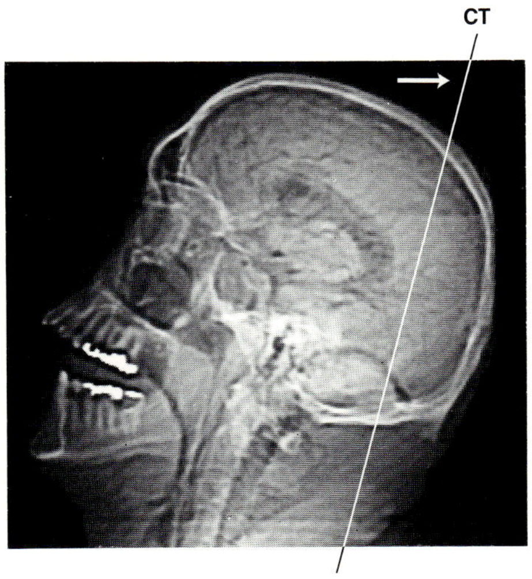

Plane of Section

Cadaver CT Scan

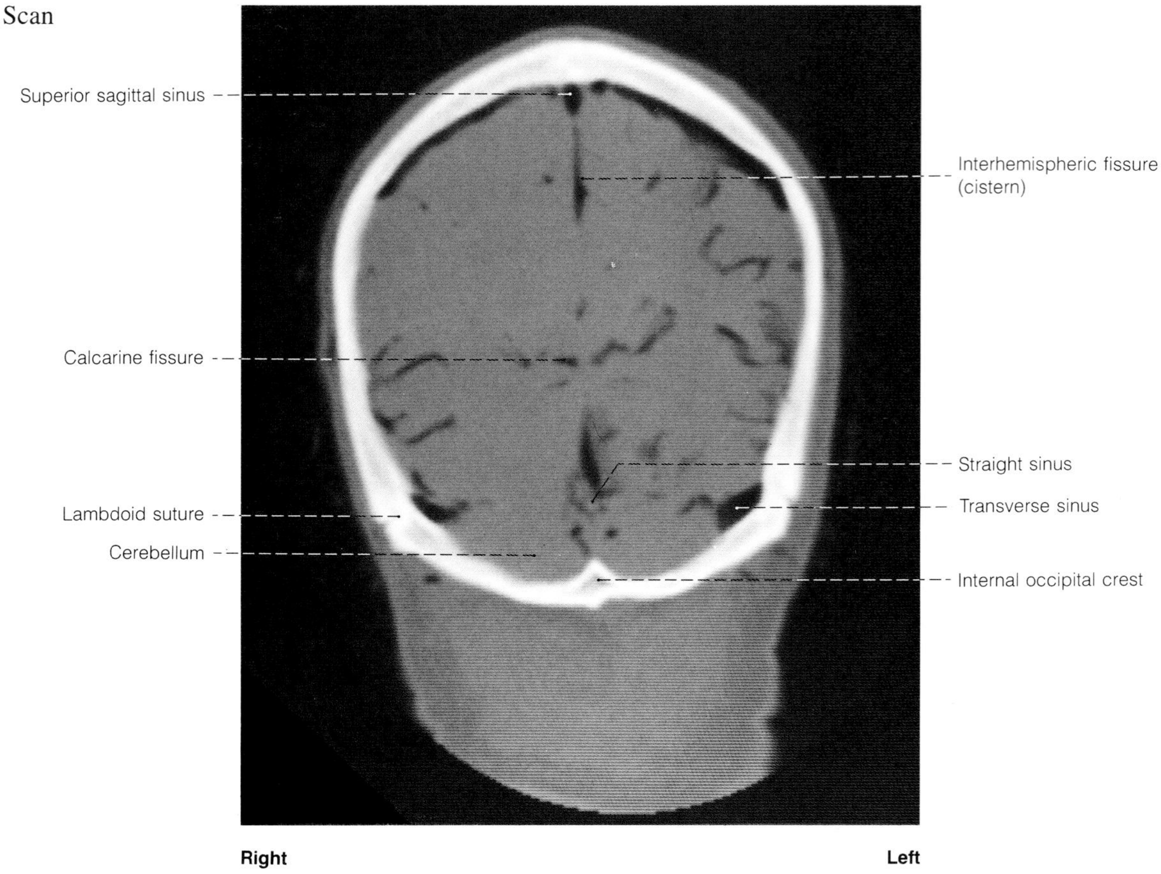

The posterior (occipital) horns of the lateral ventricles extend for quite variable distances into the occipital lobes. They are not visualized in this specimen. The subcortical white matter contains both the visual radiations and numerous associations bundles to and from the occipital lobes.

Tumors of the occipital pole are not unusual but may be prevented by the thick posterior falx and tentorium from causing significant mass effect; the effect of expansion will eventually be evident upon the choroid of the lateral ventricles, pushing them anteriorly.

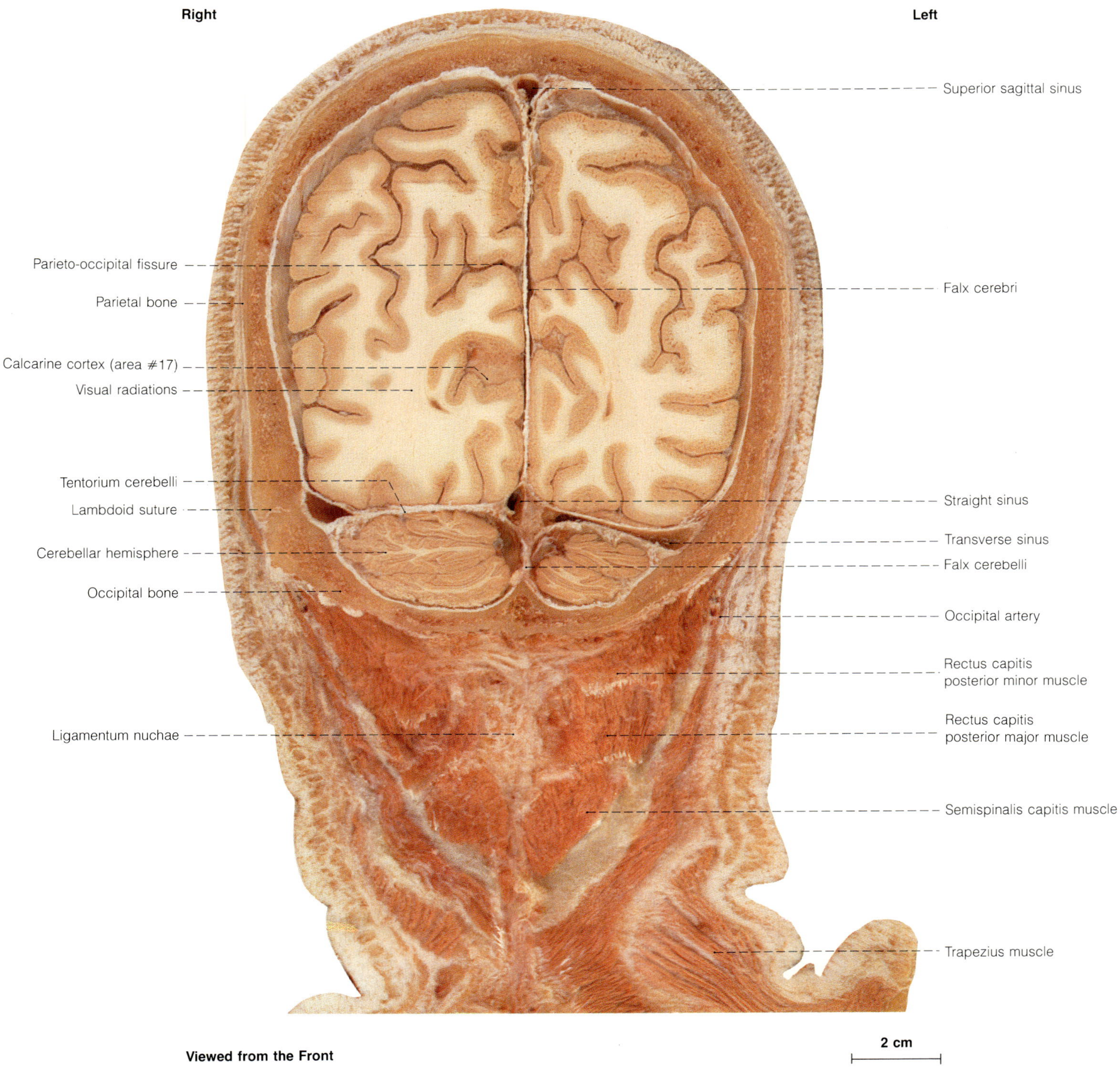

Viewed from the Front

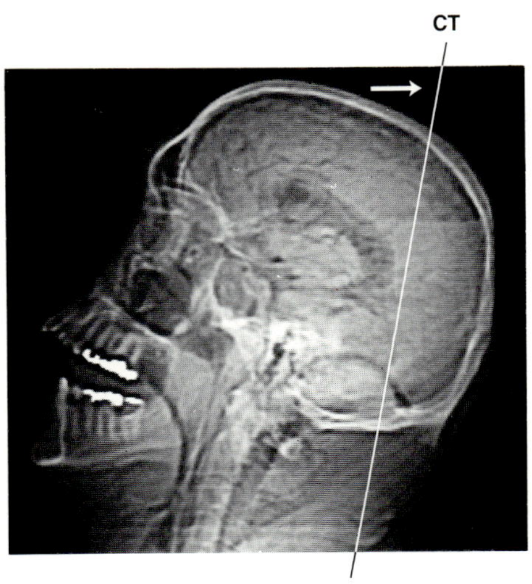

Plane of Section

Cadaver CT Scan

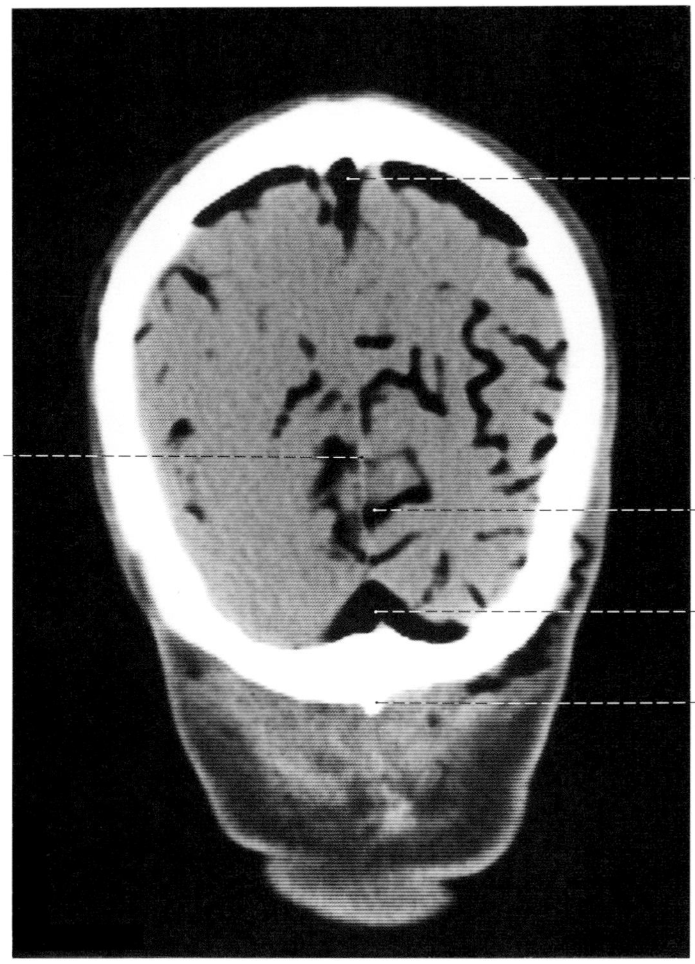

The torcular Herophili (confluence of the sinuses) is seen filled with clotted blood and the right transverse sinus is noted leading away from this level. The straight sinus usually drains into the left transverse sinus although variations are common.

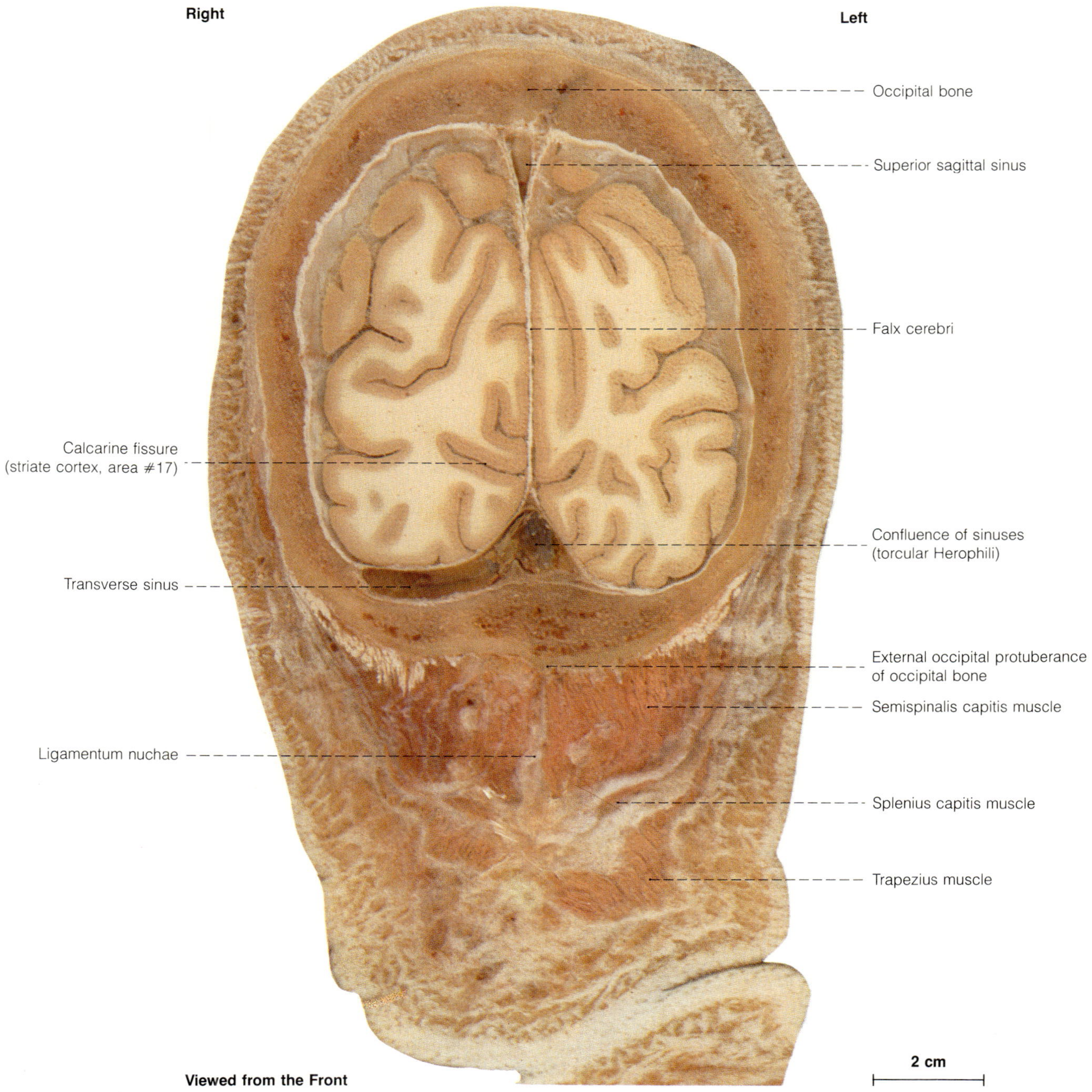

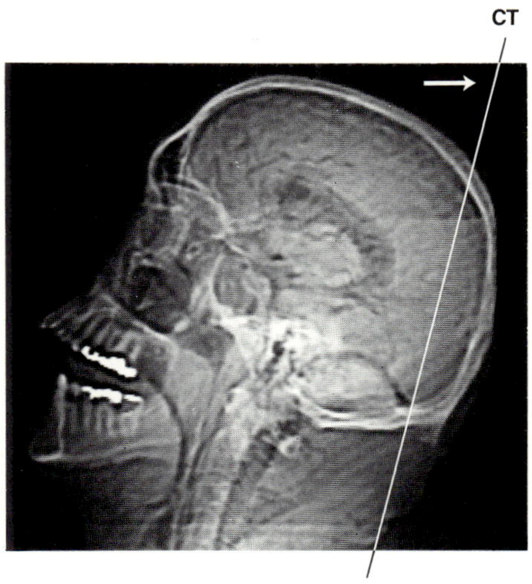

Plane of Section

Cadaver CT Scan

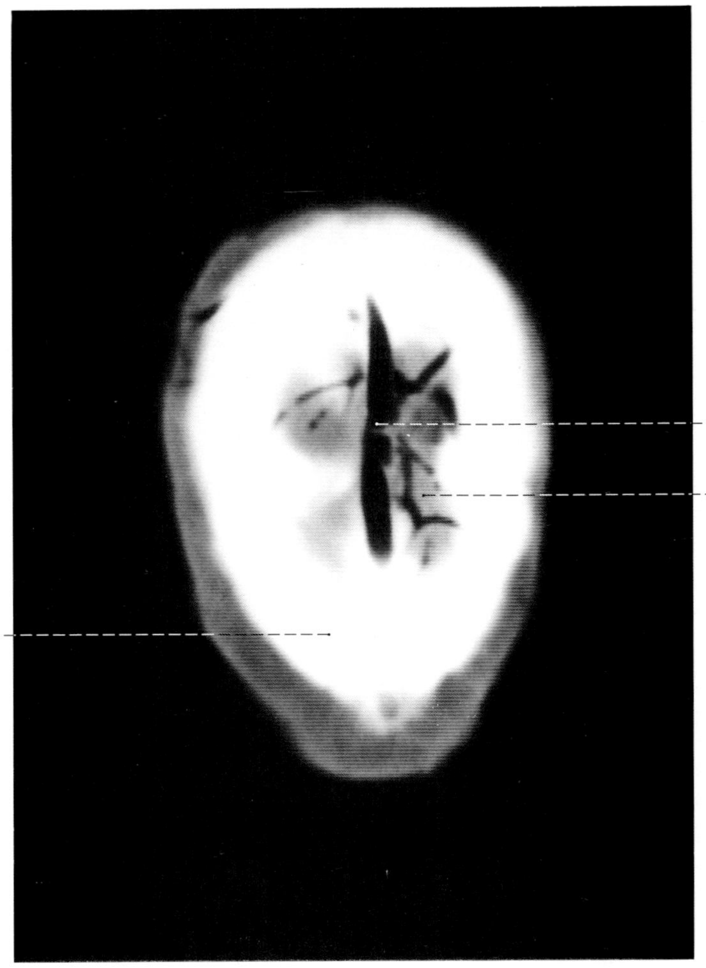

A coronal scan through the occipital pole passes through the central (macular) areas of the visual fields. Variations in the angle of the cut result in alterations of relationships which limit the usefulness of such scans. The clotted blood in the superior sagittal sinus emphasizes its size and importance in cerebral venous drainage.

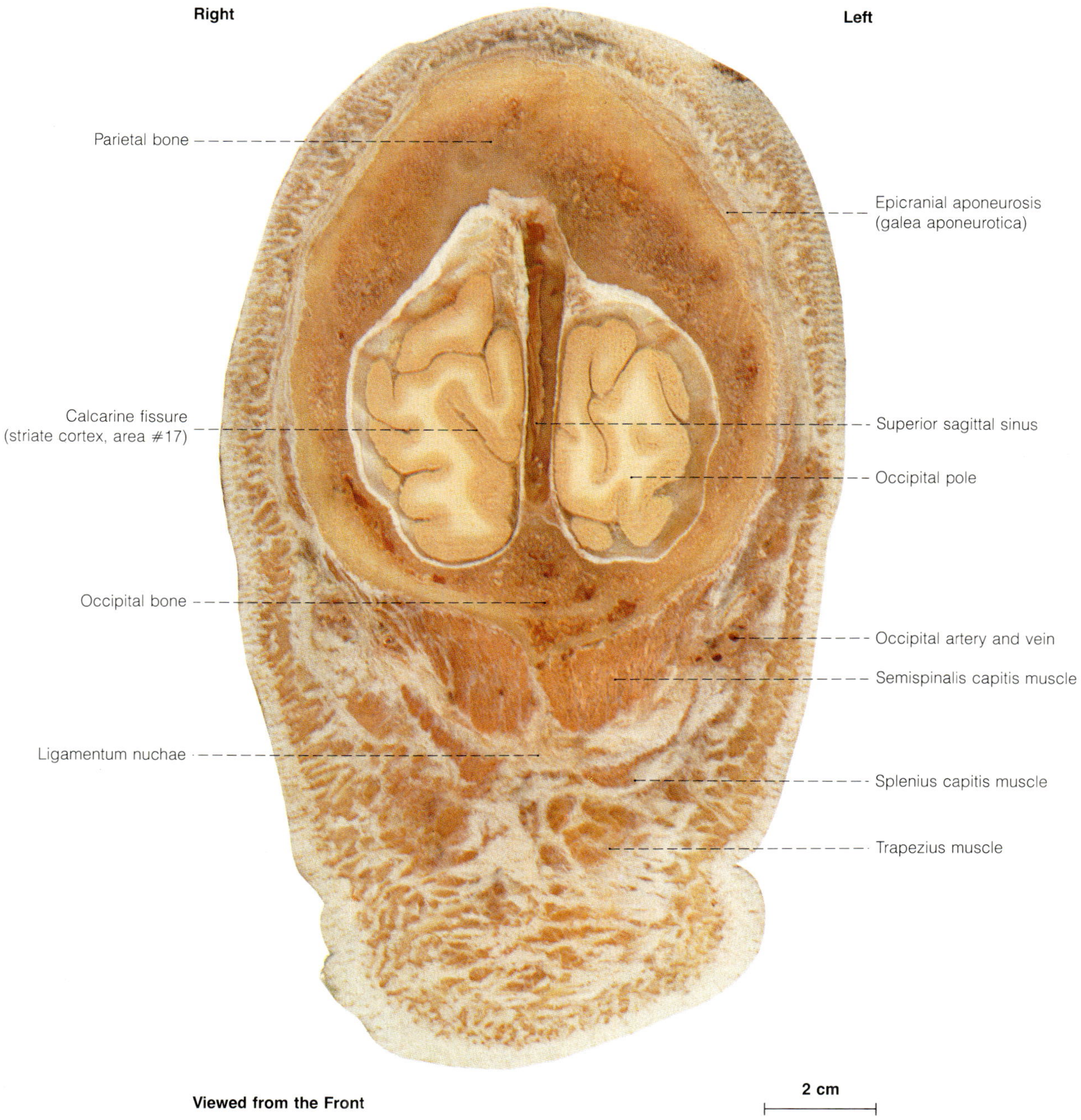

Viewed from the Front

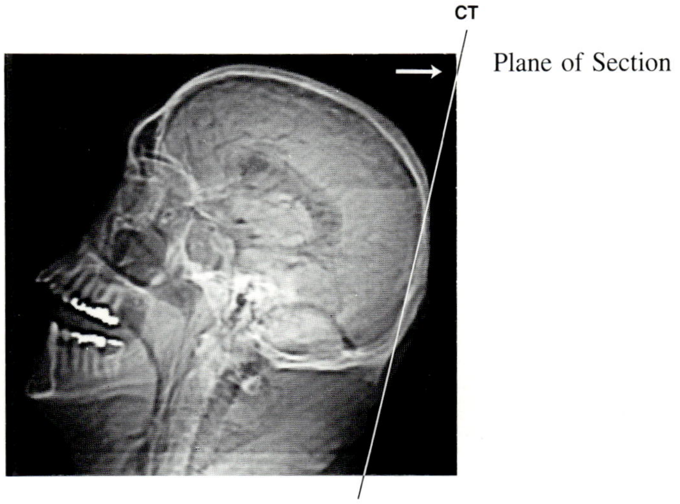

Selected Bibliography

Anderson, J. E. *Grant's Atlas of Anatomy, 8th ed*. Williams & Wilkins, Baltimore, 1983

Burrows, E. H., and N. E. Leeds. *Neuroradiology, Vol. 1*. Churchill Livingstone, N. Y., 1981.

Crosby, E. C., T. Humphrey, and E. W. Lauer. *Correlative Anatomy of the Nervous System*. The Macmillan Co., New York, 1962.

Ferner, H. *Eduard Pernkopf Atlas of Topographical and Applied Human Anatomy, 2nd ed*. Urban & Schwarzenberg, Baltimore and Munich, 1980.

Ferner, H., and J. Staubesand. *Sobotta Atlas of Human Anatomy, 10th English ed*. Translated by W. Hild. Urban & Schwarzenberg, Baltimore and Munich, 1983.

Koritké, J. G., and H. Sick. *Atlas of Sectional Human Anatomy, Vol. 1, Head, Neck, Thorax*. Urban & Schwarzenberg, Baltimore and Munich, 1983.

Lang, J. *Clinical Anatomy of the Head, Neurocranium, Orbit, Craniocervical Regions*. Trans. by R. R. Wilson and D. P. Winstanley. Springer-Verlag, Berlin, Heidelberg, N. Y., 1983

Mechan, I. *An Atlas of Anatomy Basic to Radiology*. W. B. Saunders Co., Philadelphia, 1975.

Newton, T. H., and D. G. Potts, eds. *Radiology of the Skull and Brain: Vol. 3: Anatomy and Pathology* (1975); *Vol. 4: Ventricles and Cisterns* (1978). C. V. Mosby Co., St. Louis

Newton, T. H., and D. G. Potts. *Advanced Imaging Techniques, Modern Neuroradiology, Vol. 2*. Clavadel Press, San Anselmo, Calif., 1983.

Romanes, G. J. *Cunningham's Manual of Practical Anatomy, Vol. 3: Head and Neck and Brain*. Oxford University Press, New York, 1966.

Wagner, M., and T. L. Lawson. *Segmental Anatomy, Applications to Clinical Medicine*. The Macmillan Co., New York, 1982.

Sagittal Planes

Sagittal CT images have never been practical to obtain directly on a routine basis due to positioning difficulties in the gantry, and sagittal images reconstructed from axial scans lack fine detail. It is with MRI, therefore, that we encounter for the first time detailed sagittal anatomy on a regular basis in clinical situations. The sagittal MRI images in this book match extremely well the sagittally oriented anatomical material and should be very useful in the interpretation of these scans. As in the early days of CT scanning, when we were presented with a brand-new orientation of neuroanatomy with the then-unfamiliar axial scans, we are again faced with a new and relatively unfamiliar way of viewing the brain. As the usefulness and ubiquity of MRI scanning increases, the sagittal anatomy will become second nature, but for now, the new orientation may require some study.

The cadaver used for the gross photographs was first scanned by CT (GE 8800) and a scout film obtained. This was accomplished by placing the head across the field of the scanner. The cadaver head was imbedded in gelatin, frozen and sectioned into 7 mm slices. All photographs of the gross specimen were made of the left side of each slice so that the orientation of all illustrations is with the nose to the viewer's left.

Since radiographic images have been interpreted for many years and the identification of both dense and soft tissues determined, they are useful for comparison with the newer MRI scans displaying proton density and differences in T1 & T2 times. The MRI scans were kindly provided by Fred J. Hodges III, M. D., Professor of Radiology, Edward Mallinckrodt Institute of Radiology, St. Louis, Missouri, and were performed on a Siemens Magnetom 6 K Gaus unit.

Cadaver CT Scan

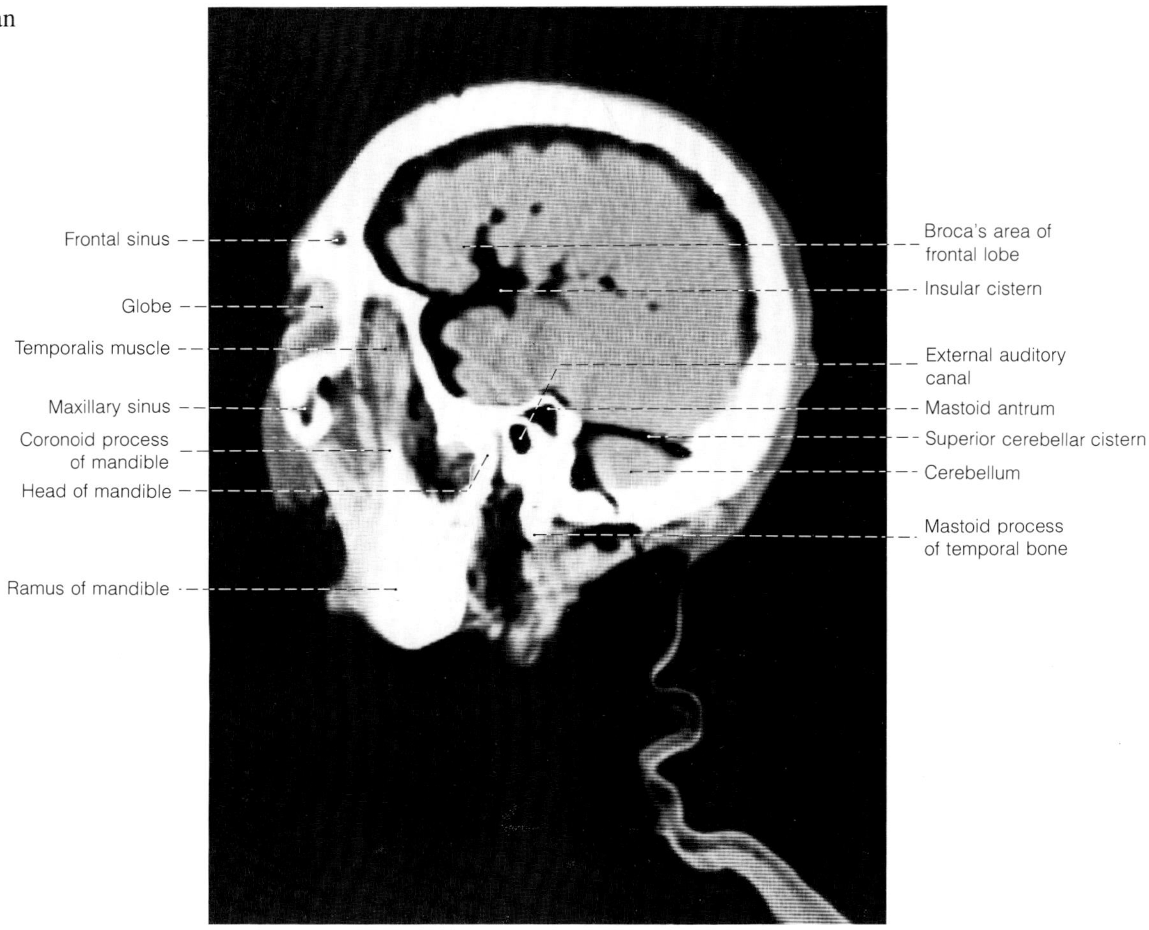

This lateral parasagittal section through the mastoid process passes through the temporomandibular (T-M) joint and infratemporal region. The AP digital radiograph of the cadaver, obtained before sectioning, provides a comparative illustration for MRI display of a patient in a comparable plane.

Lateral sagittal sections are particularly useful in demonstrating cortical surface relationships to deeper pathology and directing a neurosurgical approach with a minimum of insult to the surrounding brain. It may also be possible to visualize pathology involving the major vessels of the brain which lie largely in the cortical sulci.

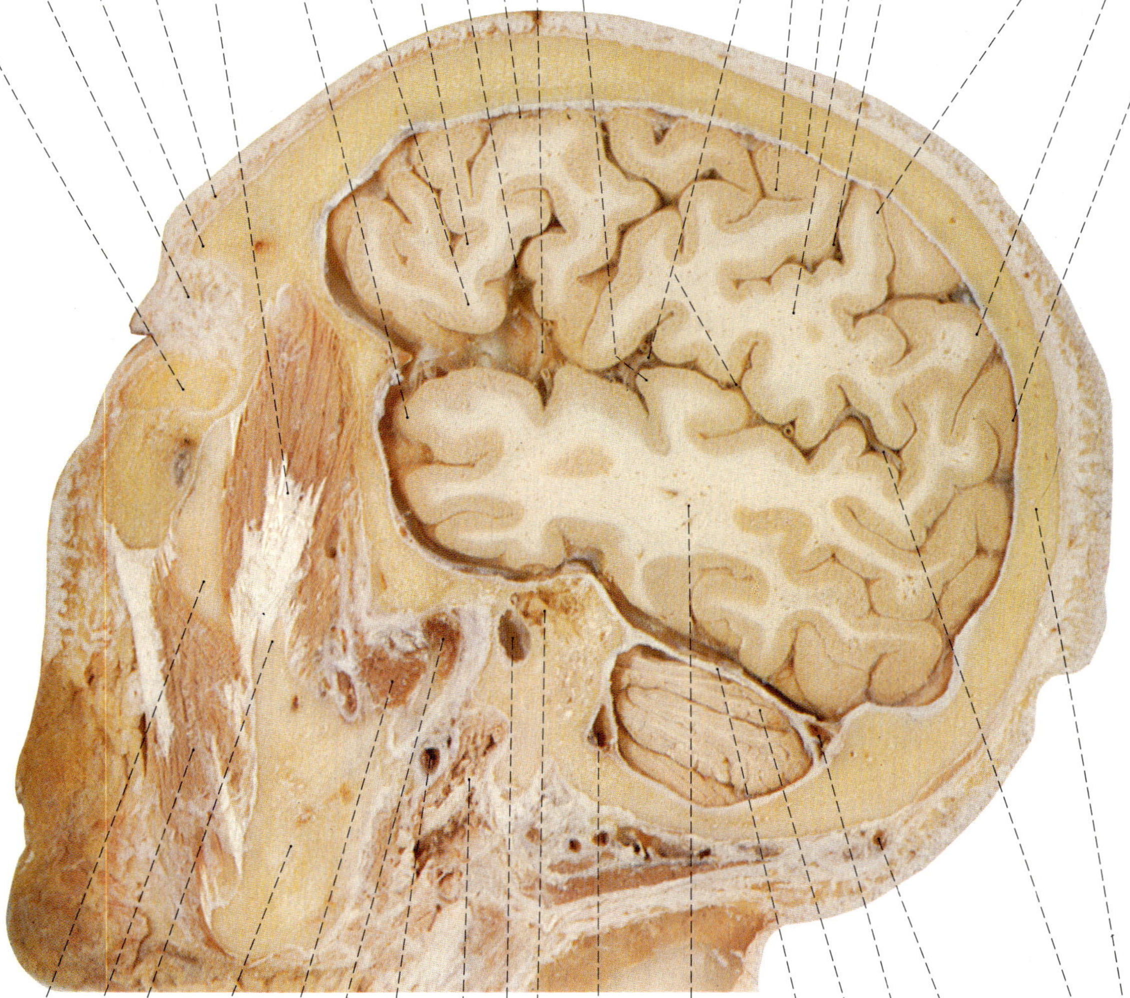

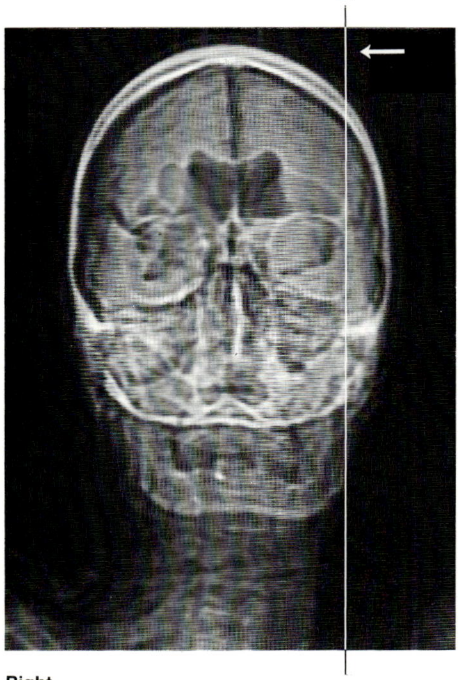

Plane of Section

Patient MRI Scan
External Auditory Canal

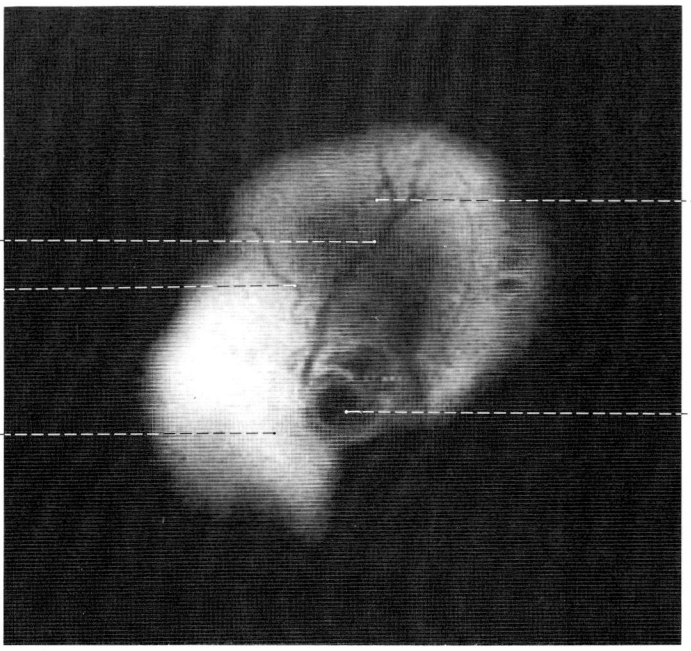

Viewed from the Left

Patient MRI Scan

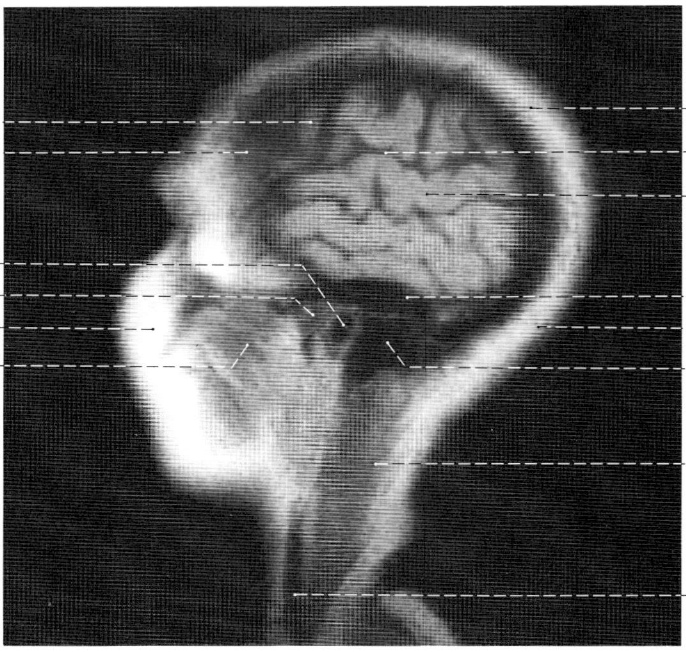

Viewed from the Left

The MRI scan at the top of the page is lateral to the MRI illustrated beneath it, the latter corresponding to the gross photograph in the plane illustrated in figures pages 159 and 161. Subcutaneous vessels are especially well visualized because of their course through fatty tissue with large portions of the superficial temporal artery and vein clearly demonstrated as black lines on the upper scan.

The cortical gyri and sulci are more easily identified in the plane shown below than in either axial or coronal planes or on deeper sagittal planes. The illustrated cut is through the temporal lobe operculum and demonstrates the Sylvian fissure along with several recognizable, clinically important fissures, sulci, and gyri. In the anatomical position with the body erect, both the lateral (Sylvian) fissure and the base of the temporal lobe are approximately horizontal to the body axis. The base of the frontal lobe conforms to the roof of the orbit and slopes downward and backward. The relationship of the temporal lobe to the temporomandibular (T-M) joint is clearly shown along with the external auditory canal. The zygomatic bone forms portions of the lateral-most aspect of the orbit on the MRI scan illustrated, the air in the mastoid air cells shows up as black, as does the surrounding bone of the mastoid portion of the temporal bone, and the air of the external auditory canal. The net result is an inability to distinguish between them on MRI. The black signal from the bone of the head of the mandible is set off from the black of the temporal bone by a rim of grey representing fibrous tissue within the temporomandibular joint.

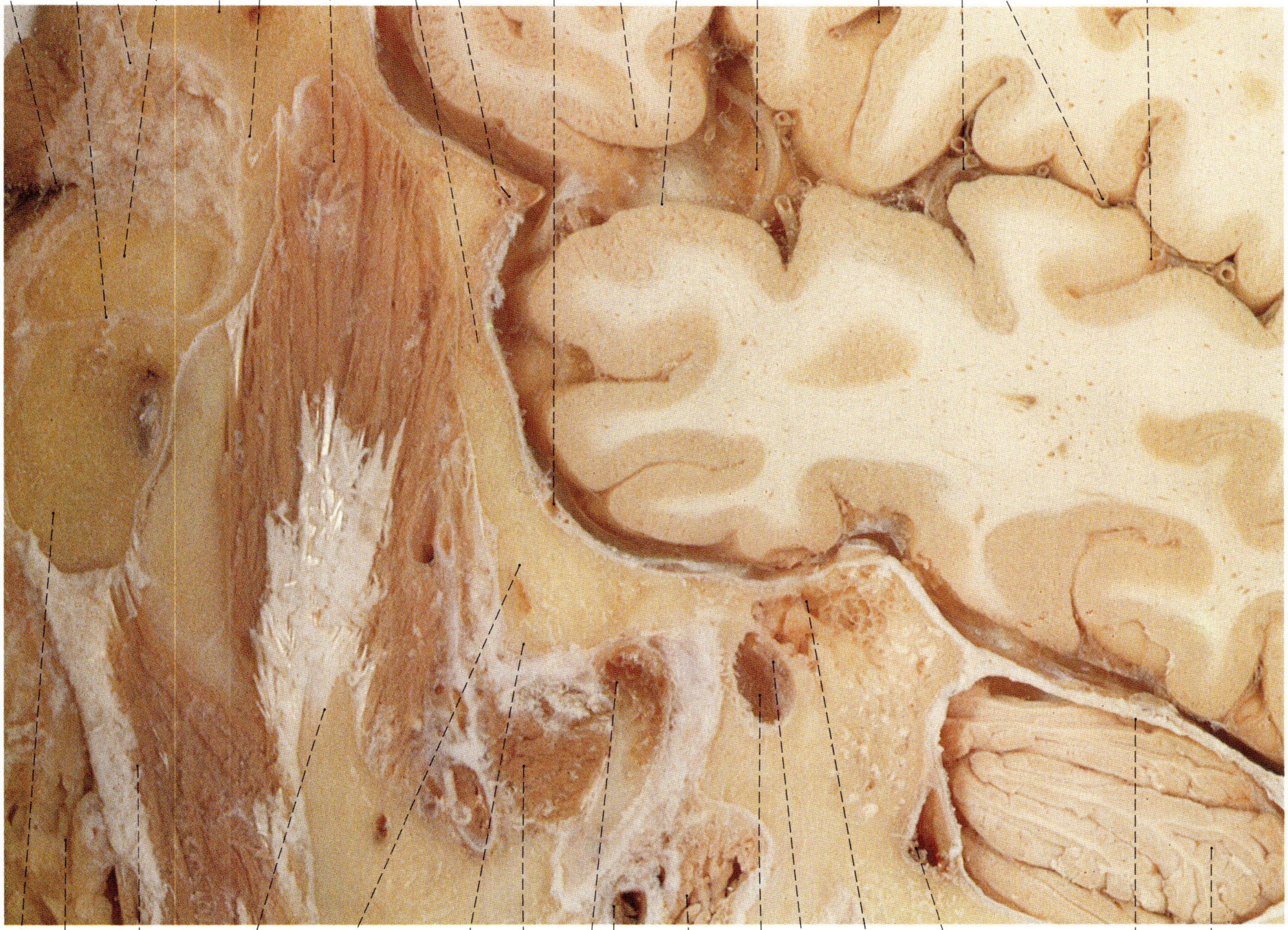
Zygomatic bone
Zygomatico-maxillary suture
Lateral canthus
Lacrimal gland
Frontal bone
Zygomatico-frontal suture
Temporalis muscle
Greater wing of sphenoid bone
Posterior branch of middle meningeal artery
Sphenoparietal sinus
Frontal operculum
Superior temporal gyrus
Insula (isle of Reil)
Precentral sulcus
Sylvian branches of middle cerebral artery
Transverse temporal (Heschl's) gyrus
Maxilla
Parotid duct
Masseter muscle
Coronoid process of mandible
Zygomatic process of temporal bone
Articular tubercle of temporal bone
Lateral pterygoid muscle
Head of mandible
External carotid artery
Parotid gland
External auditory canal
Tympanic membrane
Mastoid antrum
Sigmoid sinus
Tentorium cerebelli
Cerebellar hemisphere
2 cm

Cadaver CT Scan

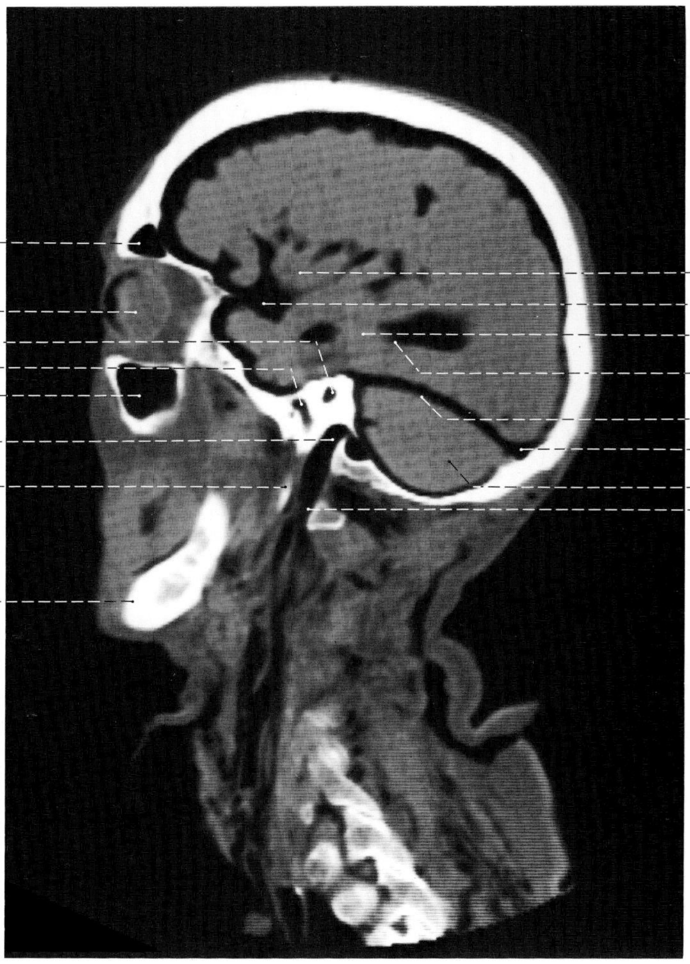

A parasagittal section through the lateral globe intersects a portion of the inferior (temporal) horn of the lateral ventricle and the insula (isle of Reil). Visual radiations flow posteriorly lateral to the atrial region of the lateral ventricle, inferior to the ventricle (Meyer's loop), and superior to the posterior horn (parietal radiations).

The cadaver CT, in the plane of the gross specimen, is to be compared with the patient MRI scan on page 164. Note especially those areas of bone and flowing blood which are both represented as black (lack of signal) with MRI. The bone is shown as black because all of the hydrogen nuclei are so tightly bound chemically in the structure of bone that relaxation after radiofrequency pulse excitation during scanning is extremely long and for all practical purposes the scanner receives no signal from those areas. Flowing blood is depicted as black (no signal) because the hydrogen nuclei that were realigned by the initial magnetization and subsequent pulse have flowed out of the plane of the cut by the time the scanner is set to receive signals to form an image. Blood which is flowing less rapidly, for example blood in the sigmoid sinus where some turbulence might be expected, would be perceived by the MRI as slightly grey because the nuclei in blood cells are not flowing out of the plane of image and so are present to give off a signal.

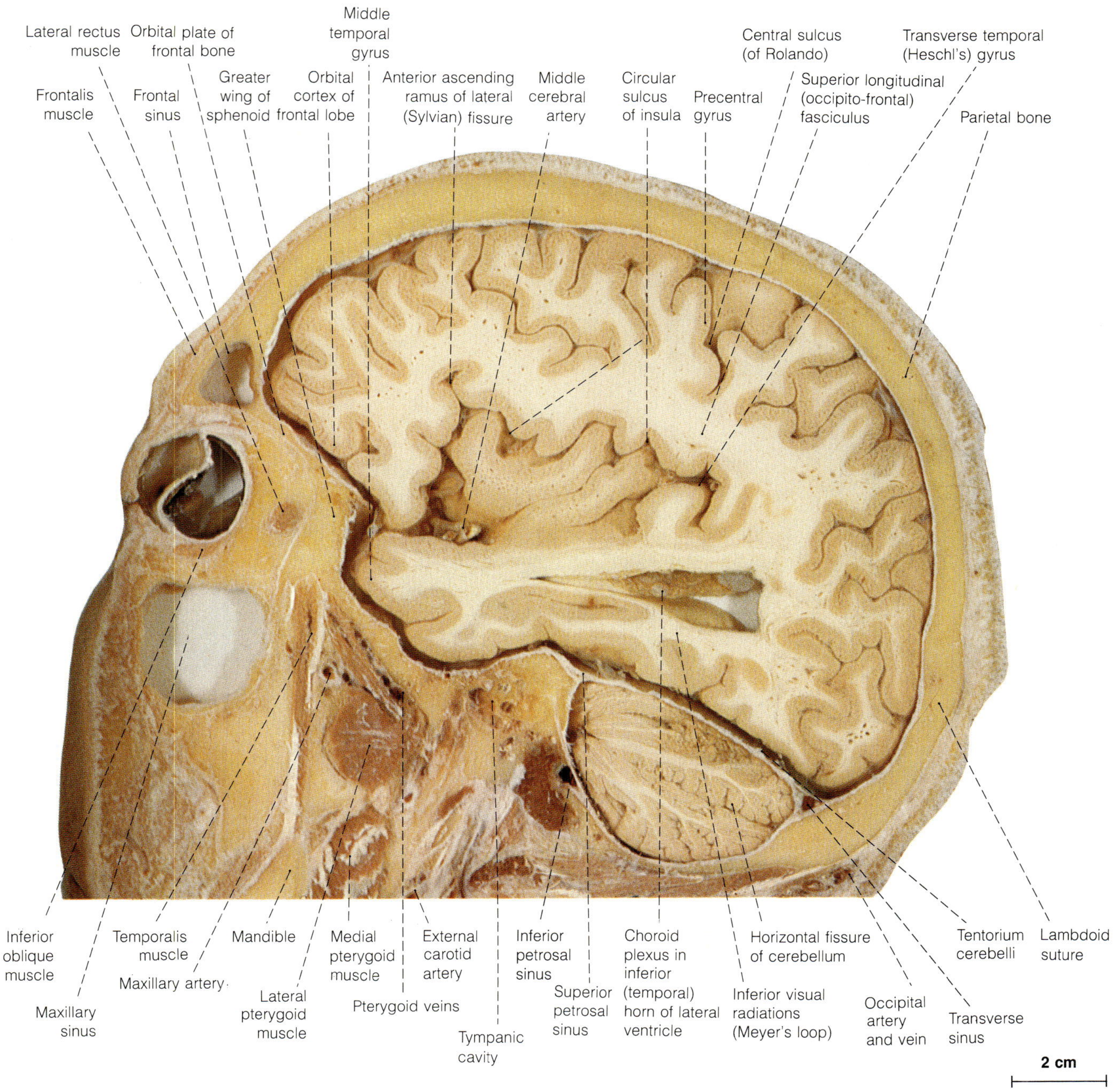

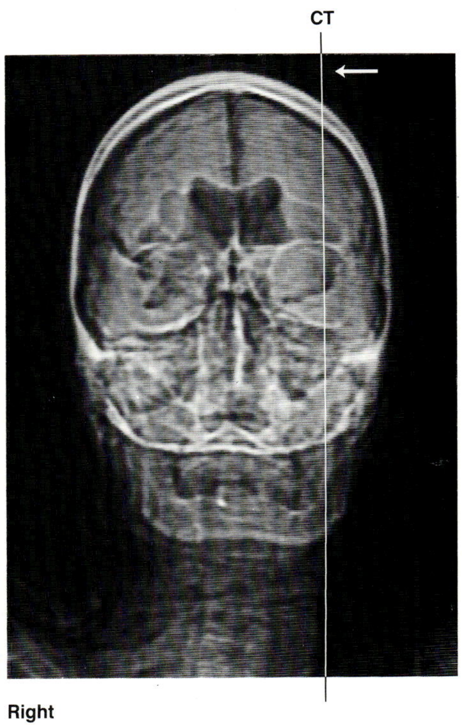

Plane of Section

Patient MRI Scan

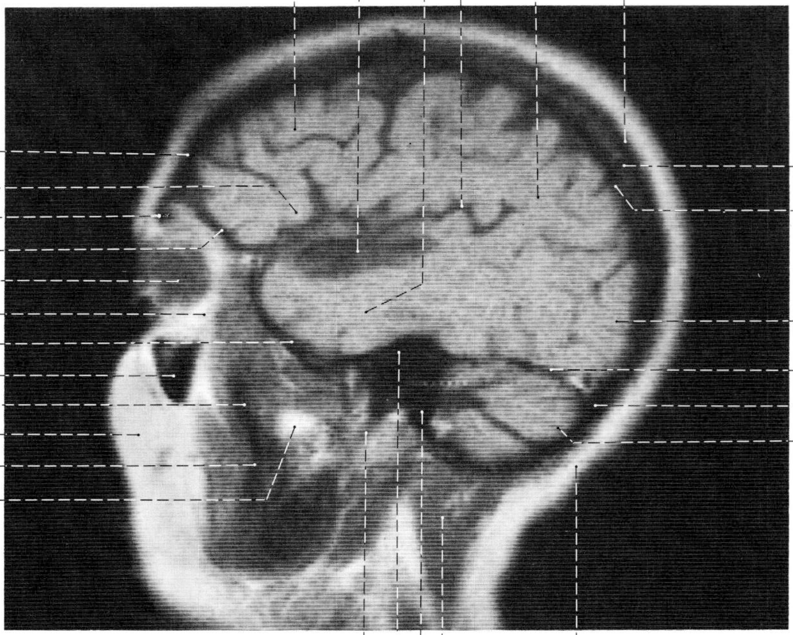

Viewed from the Left

This MRI and magnified gross photograph are in the same sagittal plane illustrated on pages 162 and 163. The limen insulae is the region of junction and continuity of the temporal, insular, and frontal lobes and the more medially located anterior perforated space. The middle cerebral artery (MCA) crosses the limen before dividing into its Sylvian branches which appear black on MRI. The cut section of the temporal (inferior) horn of the lateral ventricle in the specimen contains the hippocampus in its medial wall. Both the motor (frontal) and receptive (parieto-temporal) cortical areas for speech are within the depth of the display.

The black region beneath the temporal lobe represents the petrous bone, decreased in size in this cut compared to the one just superficial to it since the pertrous bone is tapering down to the petrous apex and will be disappearing in subsequent sections. Portions of the cerebellar hemisphere on this side with its own sulci and gyri are noted beneath the tentorium and posterior to the black petrous apex. The jugular bulb area, due to slight turbulence of blood within it, may be separated out from the total blackness of the petrous bone.

The subcutaneous fat has a white appearance on MRI and is seen to invest the entire scalp, neck, and face and also to be prominently featured within the orbit. Showing up nicely in contrast are the soft tissue densities of the globe and deep facial muscles and the black zygoma and maxillary sinus. A slight soft tissue density within the maxillary sinus could be swollen mucosal tissue associated with sinusitis.

The calvaria is also somewhat confusing, with an increased signal noted as a separate layer between the totally black outer and inner tables of calveria. The black transverse sinus is indistinguishable from the inner table of the occipital bone. One might assume that, with the patient supine for MRI imaging, venous pressure would be slightly elevated and flow may be sluggish, therefore giving off a slight signal and depictable on MRI as a small grey area if resolution is good and one looks very closely.

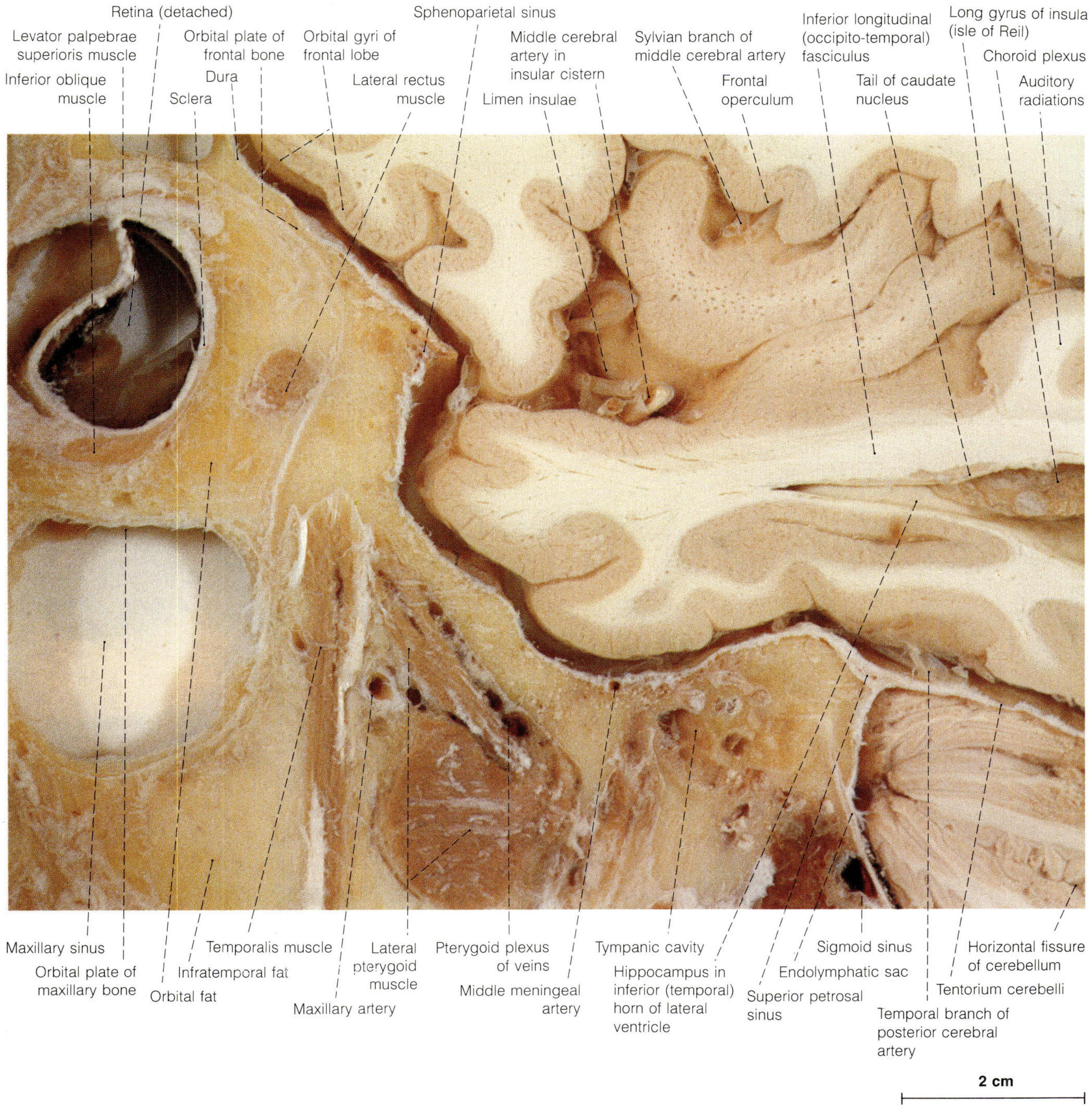
Retina (detached)
Levator palpebrae superioris muscle
Orbital plate of frontal bone
Orbital gyri of frontal lobe
Sphenoparietal sinus
Middle cerebral artery in insular cistern
Sylvian branch of middle cerebral artery
Inferior longitudinal (occipito-temporal) fasciculus
Long gyrus of insula (isle of Reil)
Choroid plexus
Inferior oblique muscle
Dura
Sclera
Lateral rectus muscle
Limen insulae
Frontal operculum
Tail of caudate nucleus
Auditory radiations
Maxillary sinus
Orbital plate of maxillary bone
Orbital fat
Temporalis muscle
Infratemporal fat
Lateral pterygoid muscle
Maxillary artery
Pterygoid plexus of veins
Middle meningeal artery
Tympanic cavity
Hippocampus in inferior (temporal) horn of lateral ventricle
Superior petrosal sinus
Sigmoid sinus
Endolymphatic sac
Temporal branch of posterior cerebral artery
Horizontal fissure of cerebellum
Tentorium cerebelli
2 cm

Cadaver CT Scan

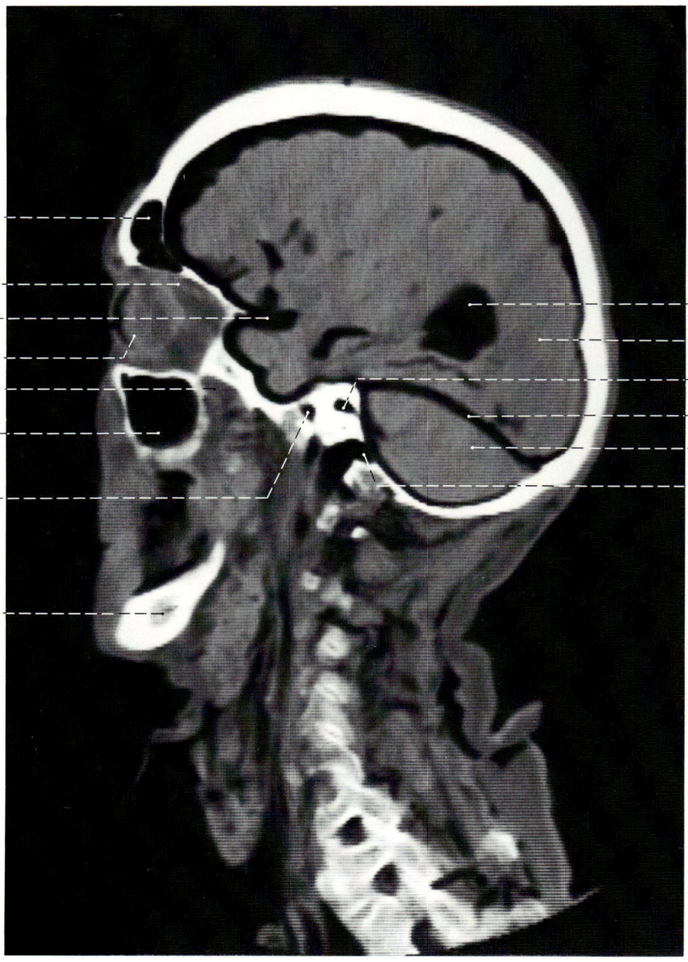

This lateral parasagittal section through the middle of the globe intersects the inferior horn and trigone (atrium) of the lateral ventricle. The hippocampus, along the medial wall of the temporal horn, is seen as it abuts the amygdala anteriorly. The internal auditory meatus (porus acusticus interna) with its facial (VII) and auditory (VIII) cranial nerves is less than 1 cm posterior to the internal carotid artery. Also nicely demonstrated on the gross specimen is the manner in which grey matter of the calcarine cortex indents the atrium of the occipital horn of the lateral ventricle to help form the calcar avis.

Supratentorially, the corona radiata streams centrally to pass medial to the lenticular nucleus and form the internal capsule. These fibers of the corticospinal tract are uncrossed at this level and a portion of the posterior limb of the internal capsule is already visualized. In more medial cuts more of the internal capsule will become visible.

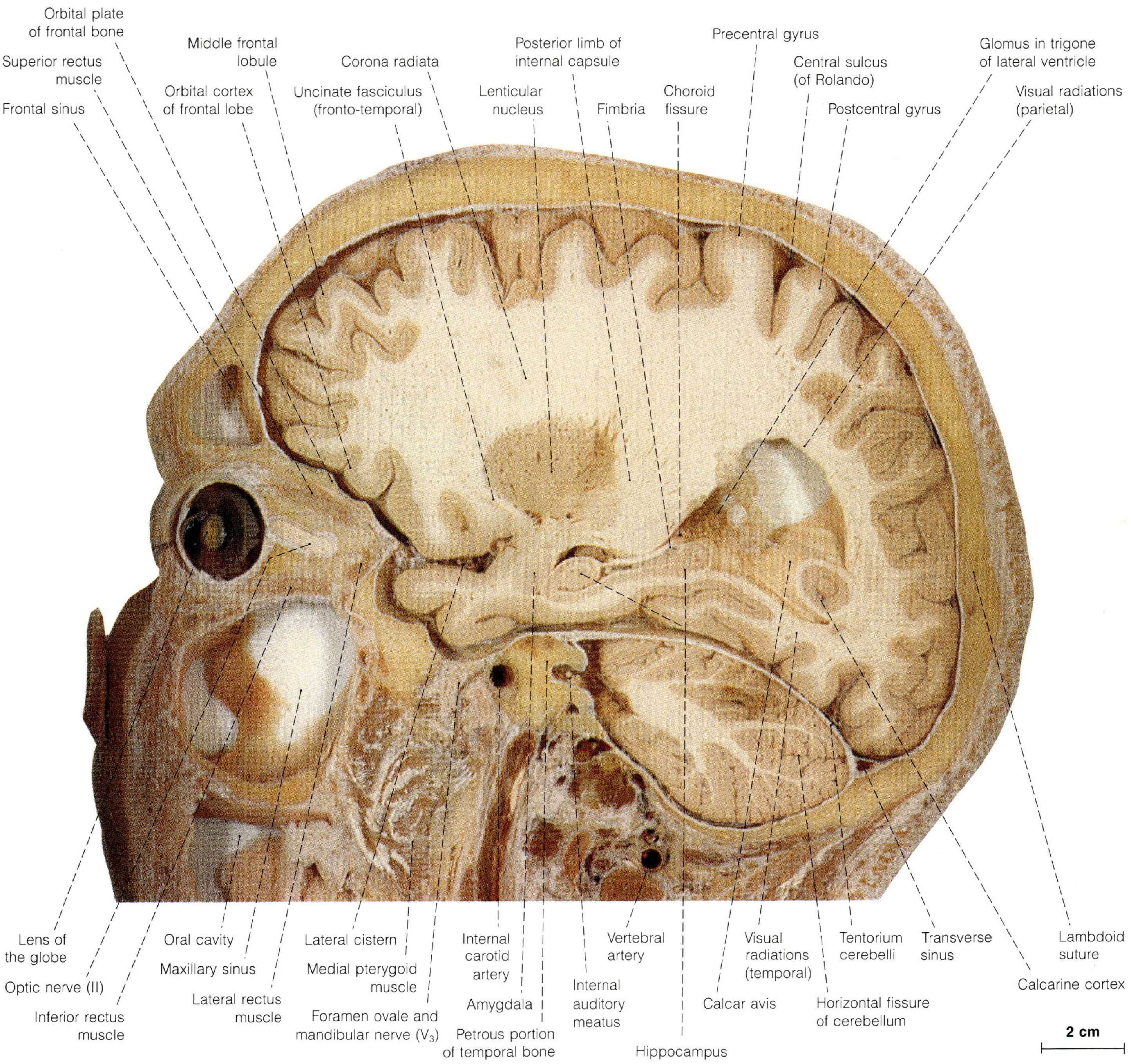

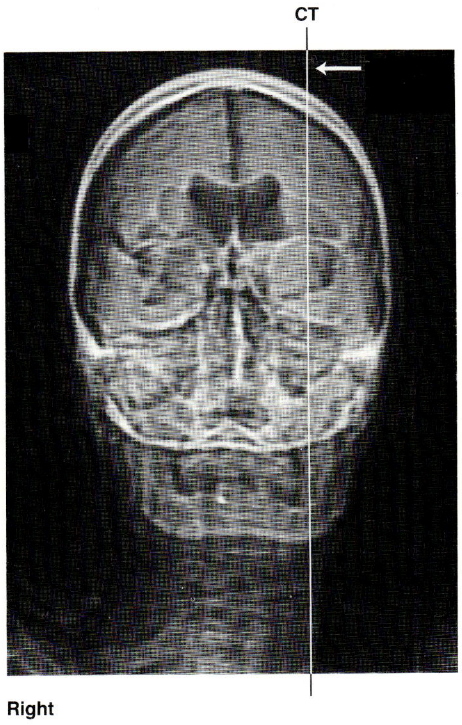

Plane of Section

Patient MRI Scan

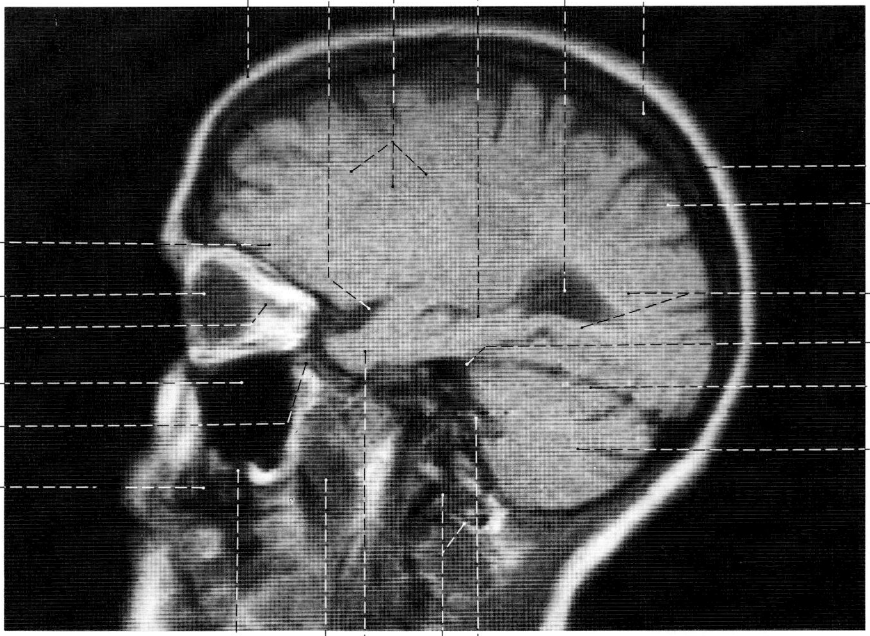

Viewed from the Left

This MRI scan of a patient is in a parasagittal plane comparable to the gross slice illustrated. The relationships of temporal lobe pathology to such limbic structures as the amygdala and hippocampus can be most easily appreciated in this plane. The gross specimen is a fortuitous cut through the foramen ovale and its mandibular division (V_3) of the trigeminal nerve. Their relationships posteriorly with the petrous part of the internal carotid artery, the Eustachian tube, and the internal auditory meatus are more evident in these parasagittal sections than in other planes.

The trigone of the lateral ventricle, containing CSF with a relatively long relaxation characteristic, is clearly delineated from the surrounding brain. With this sequence, grey-white matter differentiation is not high, but parenchymal CSF differences are enhanced. In particular, the fissure of the lateral horn leading to the hippocampal area is well seen containing CSF and matches with the gross section.

The arbor vitae is well seen on the gross section in the posterior fossa and might be better appreciated with a different pulse sequence on MRI. The petrous apex has almost vanished in this slice but an interesting representation of a totally black, tortuous vertebral artery containing rapidly flowing blood is seen in the cervical region outside the cranial contents.

In the orbit, a white signal from the abundant orbital fat sets the globe and extraocular muscles in high relief.

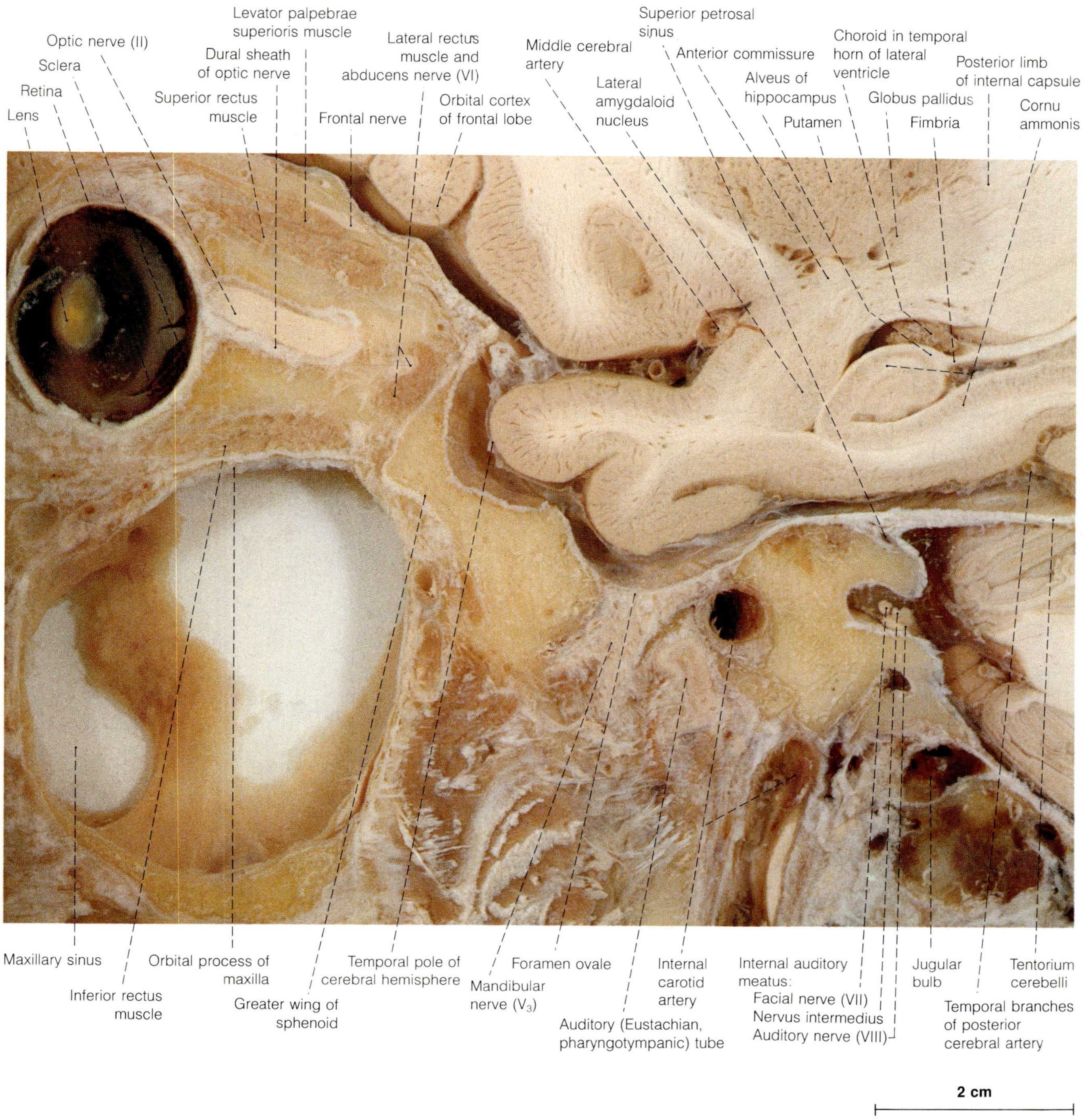
Levator palpebrae superioris muscle
Superior petrosal sinus
Optic nerve (II)
Lateral rectus muscle and abducens nerve (VI)
Middle cerebral artery
Choroid in temporal horn of lateral ventricle
Sclera
Dural sheath of optic nerve
Anterior commissure
Posterior limb of internal capsule
Retina
Alveus of hippocampus
Lateral amygdaloid nucleus
Superior rectus muscle
Orbital cortex of frontal lobe
Globus pallidus
Cornu ammonis
Lens
Frontal nerve
Putamen
Fimbria
Maxillary sinus
Orbital process of maxilla
Temporal pole of cerebral hemisphere
Foramen ovale
Internal carotid artery
Internal auditory meatus:
Jugular bulb
Tentorium cerebelli
Inferior rectus muscle
Greater wing of sphenoid
Mandibular nerve (V_3)
Facial nerve (VII)
Nervus intermedius
Auditory nerve (VIII)
Temporal branches of posterior cerebral artery
Auditory (Eustachian, pharyngotympanic) tube
2 cm

Cadaver CT Scan

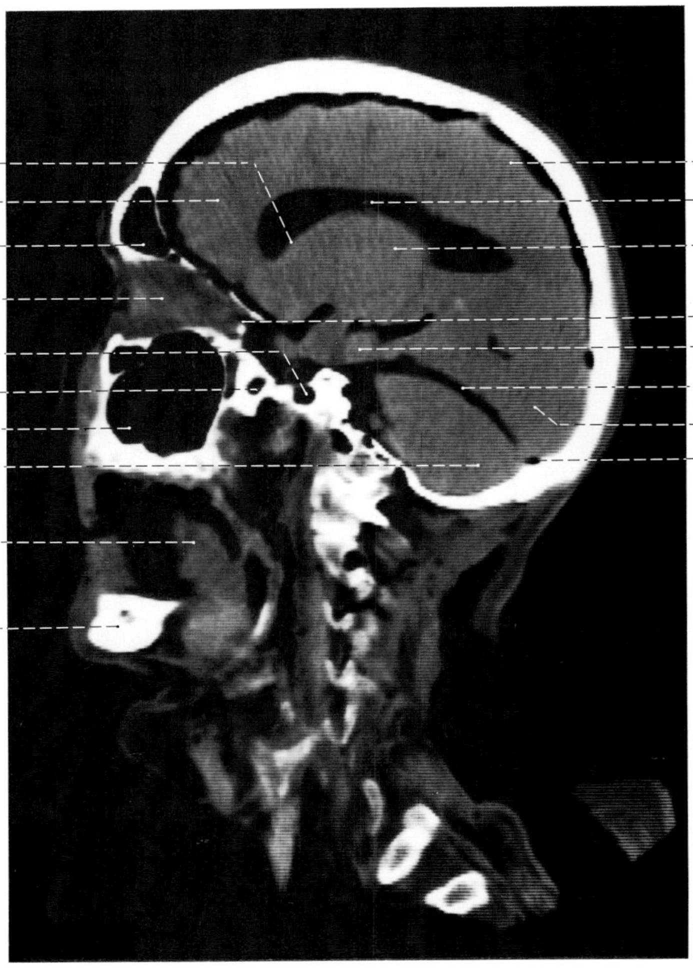

This parasagittal section through the medial globe and lateral ventricle exposes the lateral aspect of the caudate nucleus and, beneath and behind it, the internal capsule. Although the cadaver CT does not differentiate the caudate and lenticular nuclei from the internal capsule and thalamus, their location can be inferred from the ventricular and cisternal configuration displayed.

Infratentorially, the trigeminal nerve is seen on the gross specimen and the MRI image on page 172 as it emerges from the pons, passes over the medial border of the apex of the petrous part of the temporal bone, and enters the trigeminal (semilunar or Gasserian) ganglion in Meckel's cave. This depiction of Meckel's cave may be the most graphic possible since it is not well visualized in cuts in any other plane.

White matter fibers forming the trunks of the arbor vitae of the cut surface of the cerebellum are noted to be coursing laterally and posteriorly from the middle cerebellar peduncle (brachium pontis).

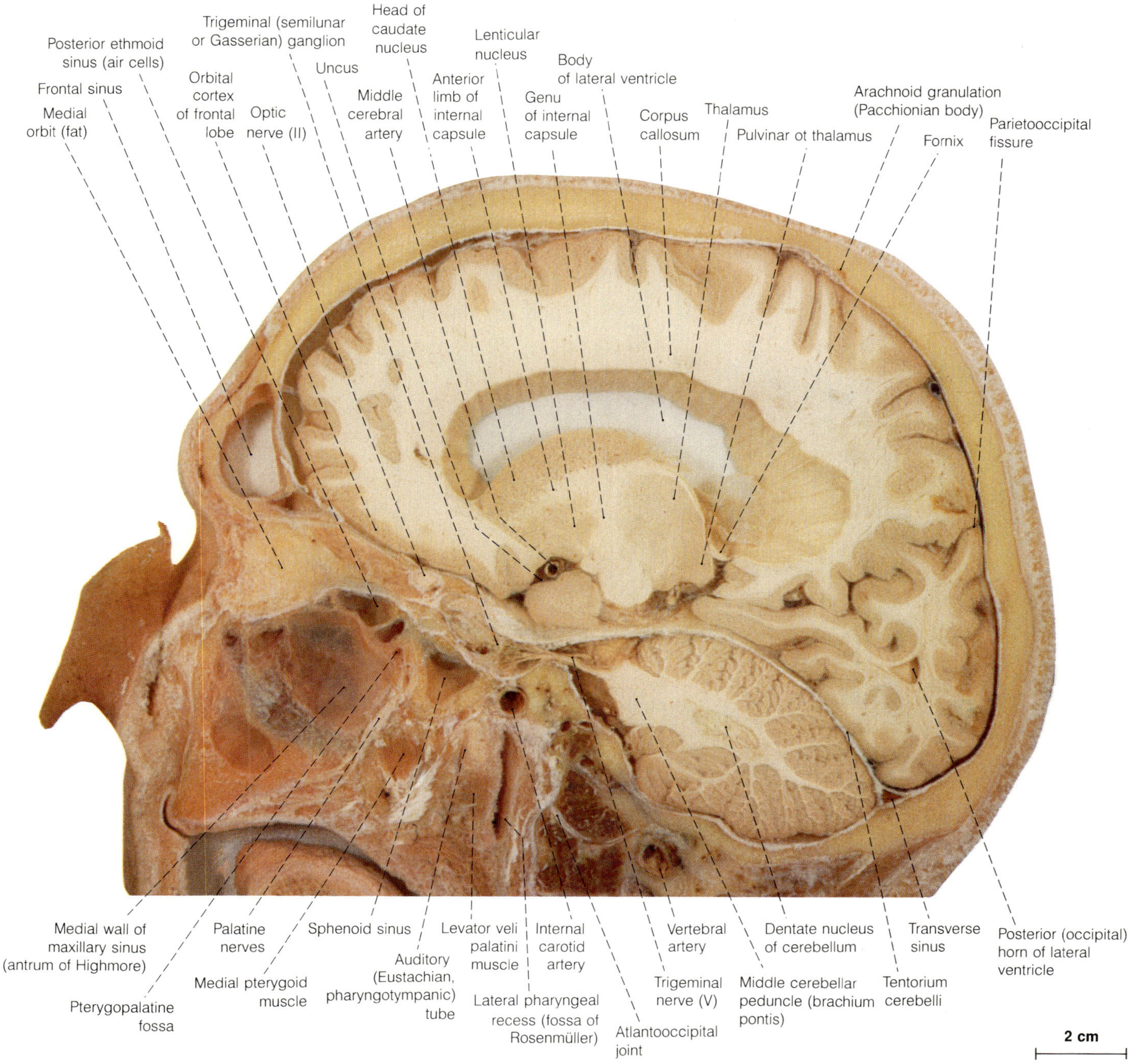

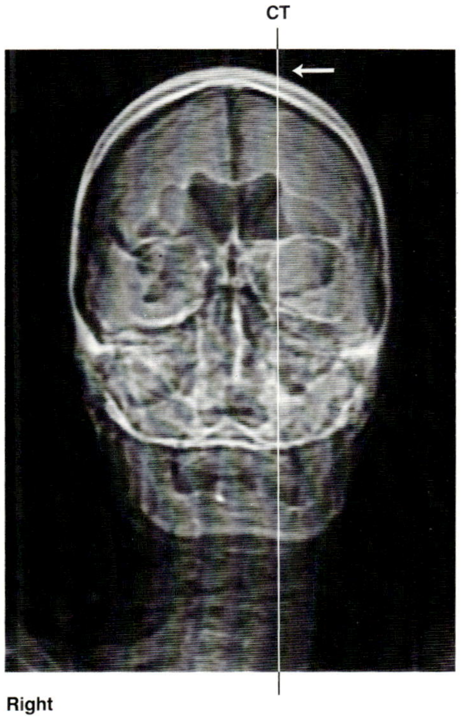

Plane of Section

Patient MRI Scan

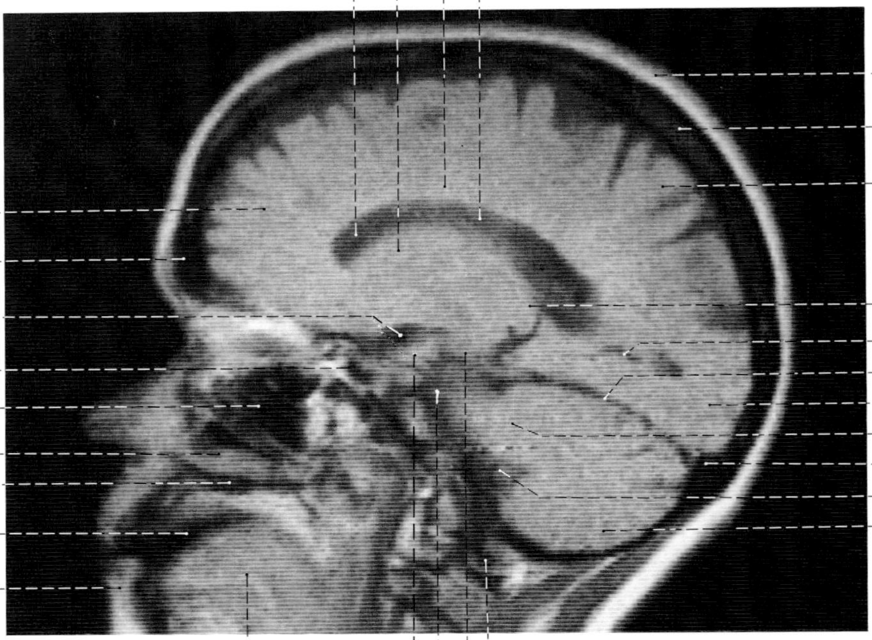

Viewed from the Left

The close anatomical relationships of the internal carotid artery in the canal, the Eustachian tube, and the trigeminal ganglion in Meckel's cave, all just rostral to the mass of the petrous portion of the temporal bone, can be easily appreciated in the gross specimen. Although their identification is more difficult with the recovery technic used for the MRI, their positions may be inferred from the visualized cerebral peduncle and cavernous carotid.

The middle cerebral artery as it enters the Sylvian fissure gives rise to the lenticulostriate vessels which are not well seen here due to their small size but which supply the striatal and internal capsular areas above. The posterior cerebral artery, curving around the peduncle, supplies the thalamus and posterior limb of the internal capsule as well as the medial temporal and occipital lobes including the calcarine (visual) cortex.

An interesting finding on both the gross specimen and MRI is the appearance of just the tip of the uncus in this sagittal plane, illustrating the characteristics of this portion of the temporal lobe which makes it the most medial portion of that lobe and the first to herniate with increases of supratentorial pressure. Just infero-posterior to the uncus, the trigeminal nerve (CN V) can be seen on both MRI and gross to be leaving the pons. Black regions on MRI representing ethmoid sinus air cells have no differentiation possible between their bony walls and the air they surround.

The black curvilinear shape defining the posterior portion of the thalamus (pulvinar) is a vascular structure possibly a composite lack of signal from the basal vein of Rosenthal and the posterio-lateral choroidal artery which lie in close relationship to each other in this location.

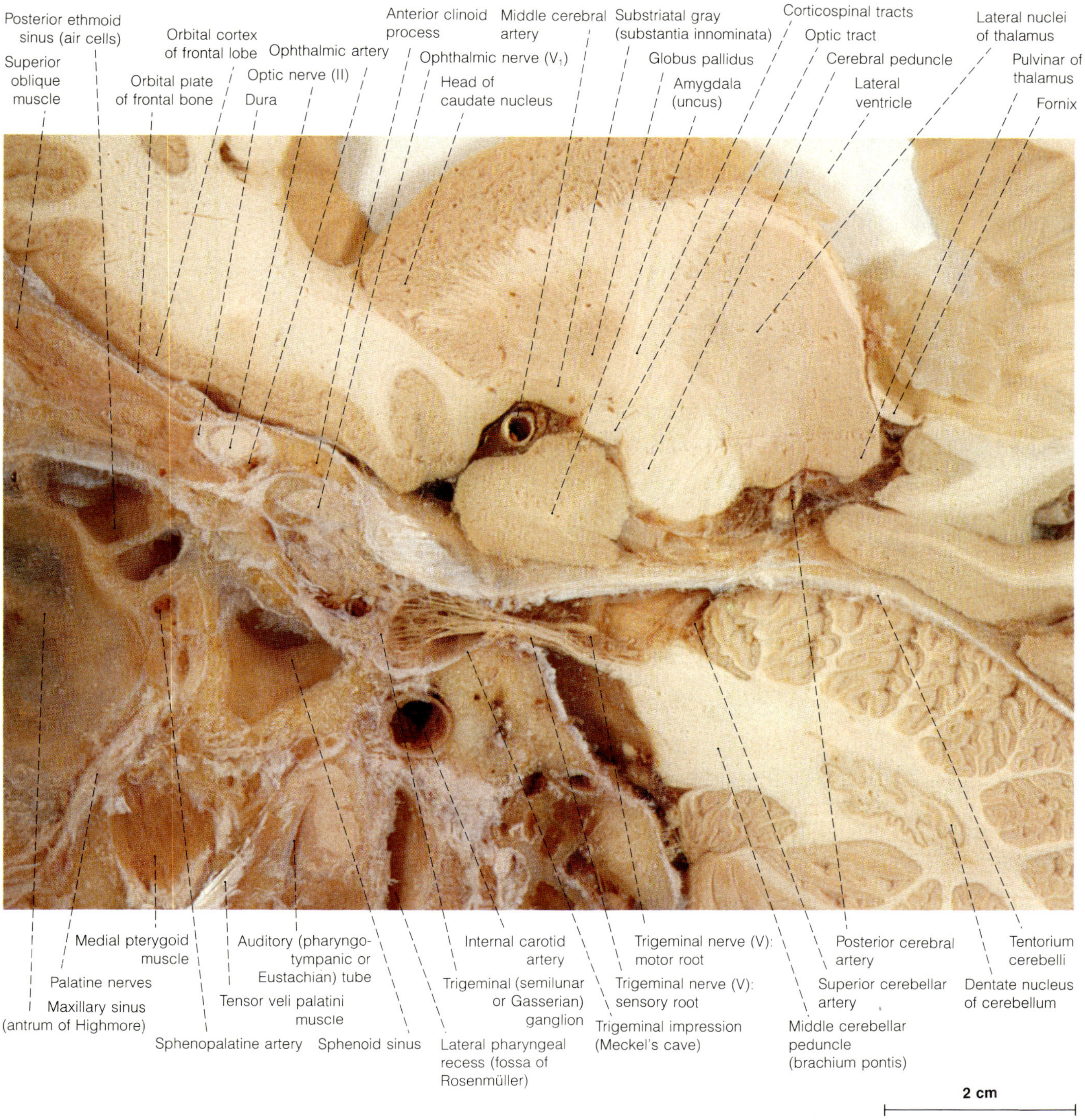

Posterior ethmoid sinus (air cells)
Superior oblique muscle
Orbital cortex of frontal lobe
Orbital plate of frontal bone
Ophthalmic artery
Optic nerve (II)
Dura
Anterior clinoid process
Ophthalmic nerve (V_1)
Head of caudate nucleus
Middle cerebral artery
Substriatal gray (substantia innominata)
Globus pallidus
Amygdala (uncus)
Corticospinal tracts
Optic tract
Cerebral peduncle
Lateral ventricle
Lateral nuclei of thalamus
Pulvinar of thalamus
Fornix
Maxillary sinus (antrum of Highmore)
Palatine nerves
Medial pterygoid muscle
Sphenopalatine artery
Tensor veli palatini muscle
Auditory (pharyngotympanic or Eustachian) tube
Sphenoid sinus
Internal carotid artery
Trigeminal (semilunar or Gasserian) ganglion
Lateral pharyngeal recess (fossa of Rosenmüller)
Trigeminal nerve (V): motor root
Trigeminal nerve (V): sensory root
Trigeminal impression (Meckel's cave)
Posterior cerebral artery
Superior cerebellar artery
Middle cerebellar peduncle (brachium pontis)
Tentorium cerebelli
Dentate nucleus of cerebellum
2 cm

Cadaver CT Scan

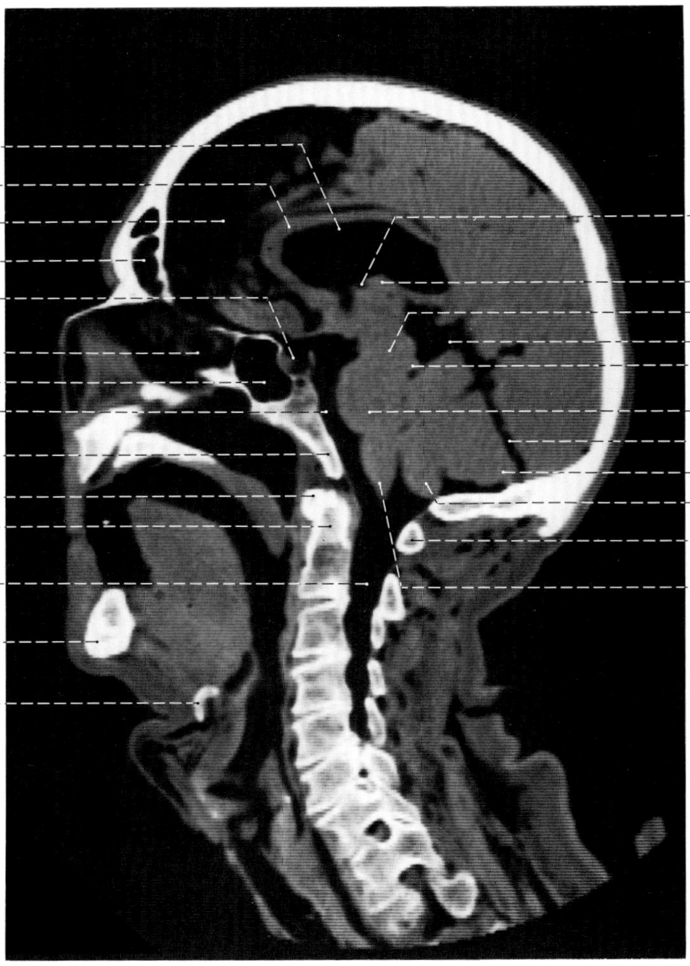

This parasagittal section is just to the left of the midline and illustrates the brainstem and the thalamic relationships lateral to the third ventricle. The surface of the gross slice is through the cavernous sinus; however, the CT scan also includes the adjacent sella turcica in its display.

The relatively posterior position in the head of the interventricular foramen of Monro and its relationship to the sella and the optic chiasm may be appreciated in such a sagittal cut.

The contiguity of the frontal, ethmoidal and sphenoidal sinuses is evident as are their relations to the adjacent brain. The relatively large size of the quadrigeminal cistern may permit pathological processes in the region, such as tumors arising in the region of the pineal, to attain some size before presenting as neurological symptoms. Important adjacent colliculi, thalamus, corpus callosum, and cerebellum are most evident in this plane.

The brainstem, particularly the pons, now has the familiar appearance on cut section that one associates with these central structures. The 4th ventricle is visible and easily recognized as a posterior fossa landmark, with the brachium conjunctivum (superior cerebellar peduncle) forming the antero-lateral wall of the ventricle.

Other recognizable, parasagittal features are now visible including the transverse fibers of the corpus callosum, seen here in cut cross-section.

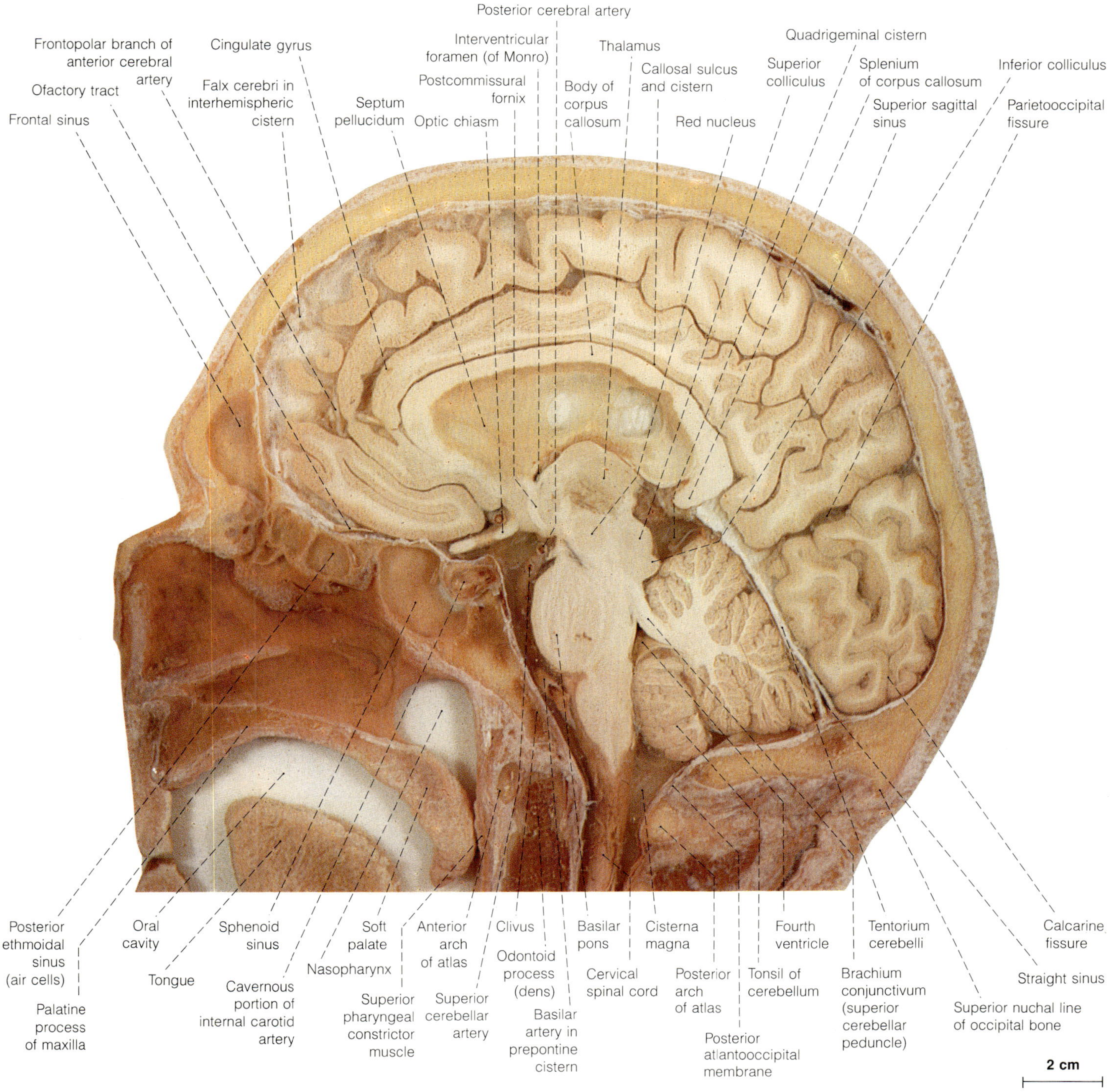

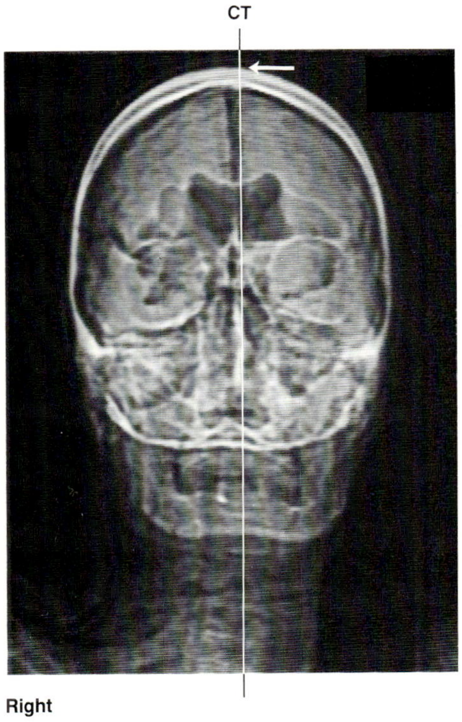

Plane of Section

Patient MRI Scan

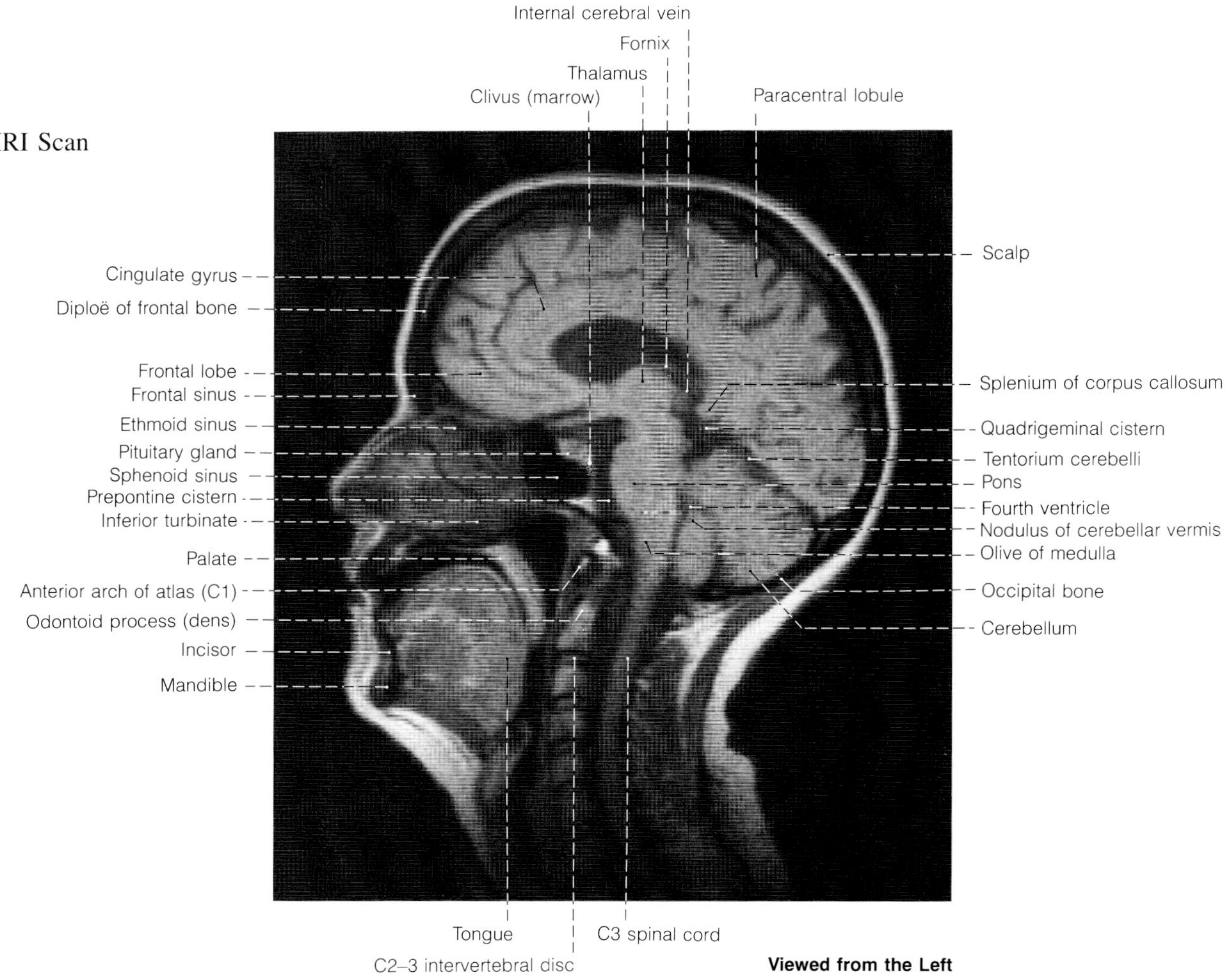

Viewed from the Left

The parasagittal scan is just barely off the midline and shows the thalamus, brainstem, and their nuclei and tracts. This particular scan was performed with a slightly different recovery sequence which allows some grey-white differentiation. It is to be expected that future developments in sequencing techniques and resolution (i.e., larger matrix) might afford an even more detailed look at brainstem nuclei *in vivo*. The pituitary gland appears as a proton dense area above the posterior part of the sphenoid sinus. This slice passes through the fornix as it arches in front of the interventricular foramen of Monro and then posteriorly into the mamillary nuclei. Of particular interest is the excellent visualization of the pituitary, outlined on three sides by thin, black plates of sella turcica bone.

Curvilinear black structures deep in the brain represent the course of an internal cerebral vein and possibly a splenial branch of the posterior cerebral artery. The extreme black of the basilar artery is set off by the less-than black appearance of the CSF in the anterior prepontine cistern, just dorsal to the very white appearance (short T2) of the fat in the marrow of the clivus.

The cervical discs have characteristic alignment and show MRI to be an excellent modality for evaluating the cervical spine as well as the cervical spinal cord.

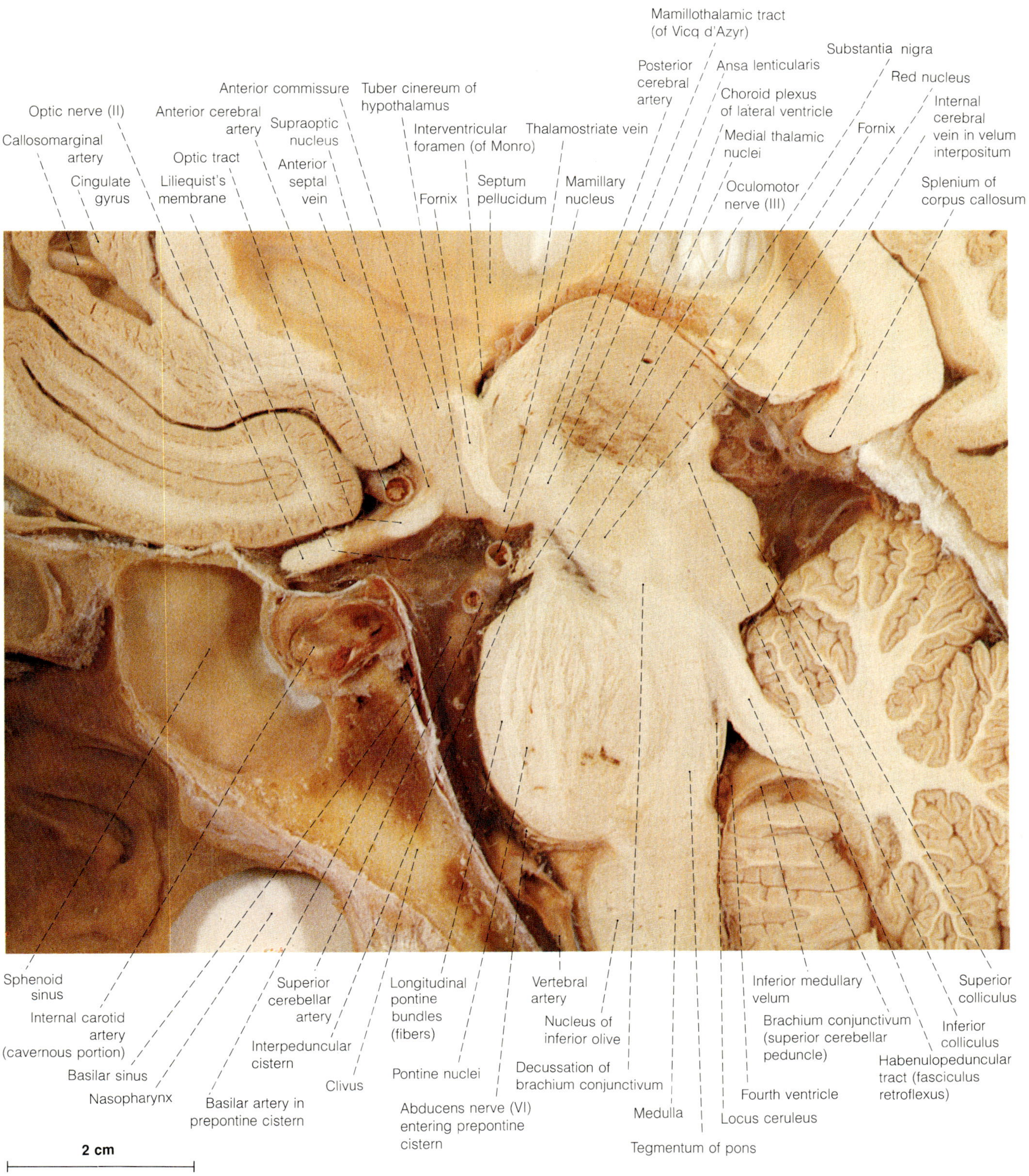
Mamillothalamic tract (of Vicq d'Azyr)
Substantia nigra
Posterior cerebral artery
Ansa lenticularis
Red nucleus
Anterior commissure
Tuber cinereum of hypothalamus
Choroid plexus of lateral ventricle
Internal cerebral vein in velum interpositum
Optic nerve (II)
Anterior cerebral artery
Supraoptic nucleus
Interventricular foramen (of Monro)
Thalamostriate vein
Fornix
Callosomarginal artery
Medial thalamic nuclei
Optic tract
Anterior septal vein
Cingulate gyrus
Liliequist's membrane
Fornix
Septum pellucidum
Mamillary nucleus
Oculomotor nerve (III)
Splenium of corpus callosum
Sphenoid sinus
Internal carotid artery (cavernous portion)
Basilar sinus
Nasopharynx
Superior cerebellar artery
Interpeduncular cistern
Basilar artery in prepontine cistern
Clivus
Longitudinal pontine bundles (fibers)
Pontine nuclei
Abducens nerve (VI) entering prepontine cistern
Vertebral artery
Nucleus of inferior olive
Decussation of brachium conjunctivum
Medulla
Tegmentum of pons
Inferior medullary velum
Brachium conjunctivum (superior cerebellar peduncle)
Fourth ventricle
Locus ceruleus
Superior colliculus
Inferior colliculus
Habenulopeduncular tract (fasciculus retroflexus)
2 cm

Cadaver CT Scan

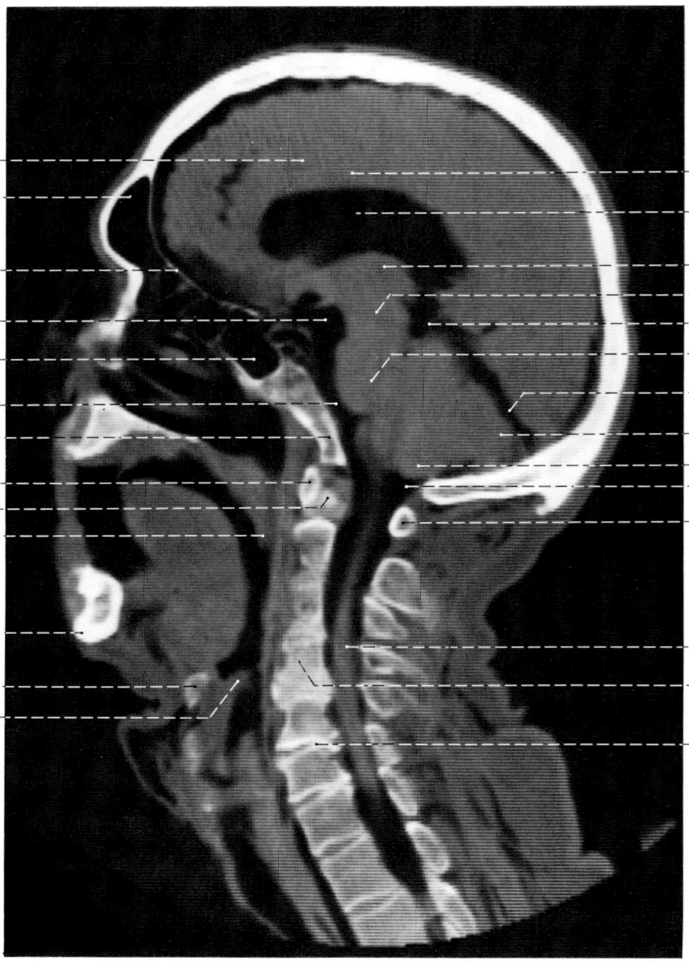

The parasagittal section viewed from the left is approximately 3 mm to the left of the midline cranially but, because of the cervical scoliosis, approaches a midsagittal plane in the neck.

The head of the caudate is viewed from its medial surface as it bulges into the anterior horn of the lateral ventricle. The vertical alignment of the thalamus, mesencephalon, pons, medulla and spinal cord with the telencephalon above and cerebellum behind are nicely displayed in this section.

An almost midline appearance of the cervical cord and medulla is seen on the gross specimen. It is to be expected that pathological processes such as brainstem or cord tumors or syringomyelia would be diagnosed by this modality. The gross specimen shows severe cervical degenerative disease and spondylosis.

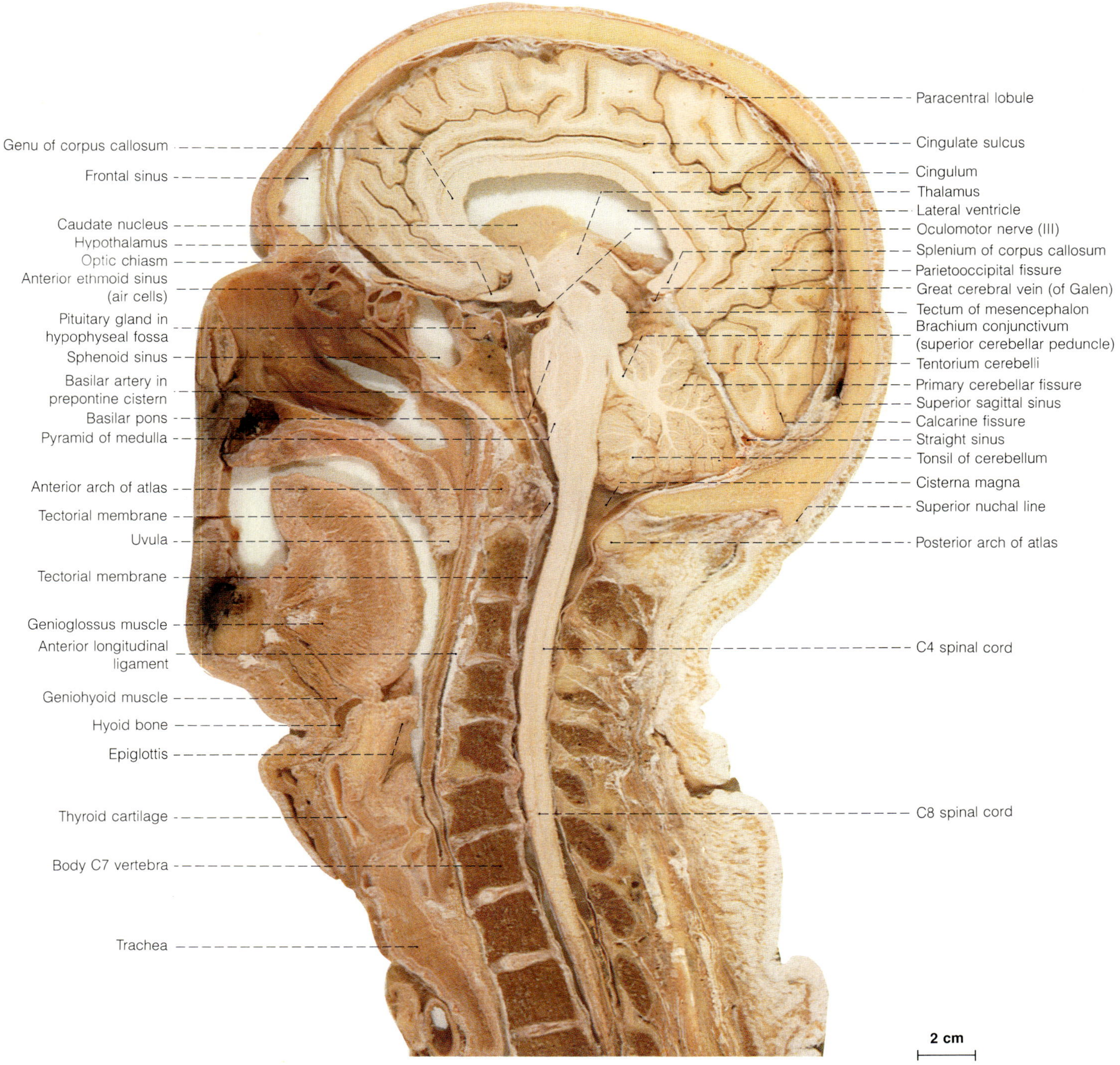

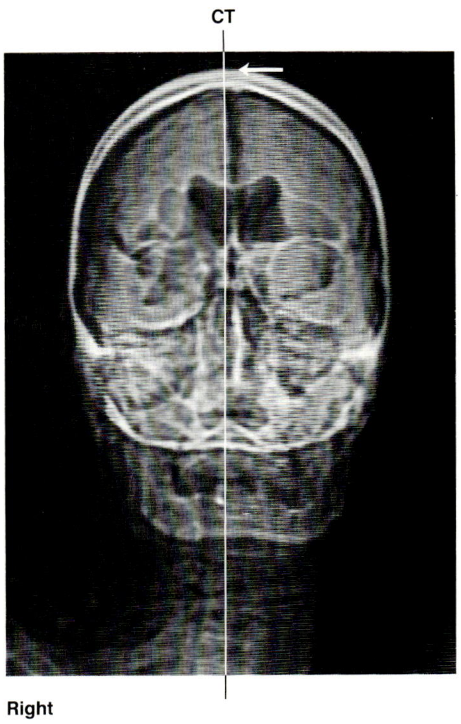

Plane of Section

Patient MRI Scan

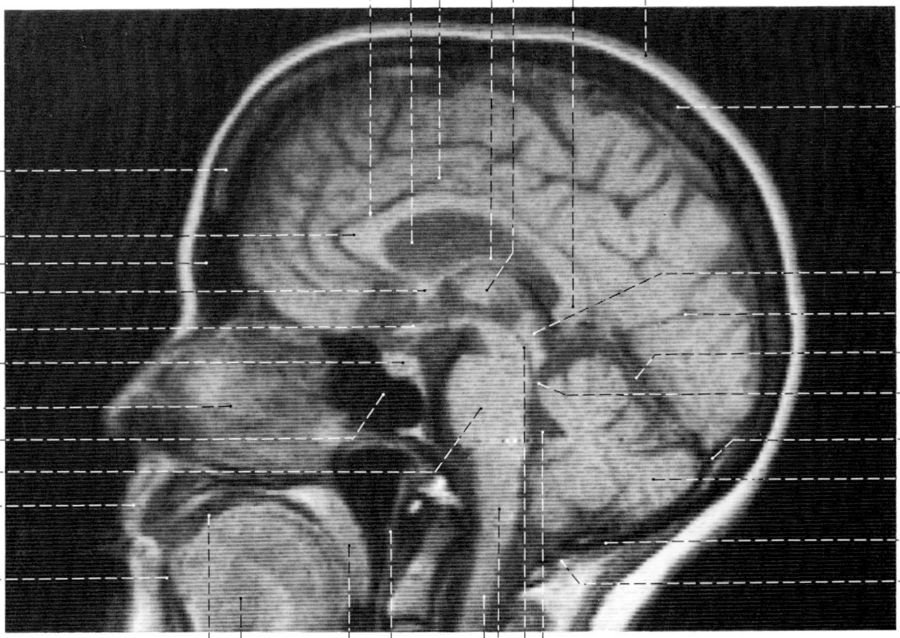

Viewed from the Left

The MRI scan and the photograph of the anatomical specimen are near the midline. Medial cortical gyri and the corpus callosum interconnecting the cerebral hemispheres are advantageously displayed in such planes as are the more ventral pituitary and perisellar regions. The resolution of the MRI scan, especially with this technique which enhances CSF brain differences rather than grey-white matter delineation, is so good that most of the structures visualized on the specimen can be identified on the MRI. Of particular interest is the intensely dark curved course of the internal cerebral vein and the black basilar artery barely set off against the slightly less black CSF of the prepontine cistern.

The bulk of the pituitary is noted and with certain pulse sequences even the anterior and posterior lobes of the pituitary may be differentiated.

The aqueduct of Sylvius has a slightly curved course through the tectum of the midbrain, leading into the characteristically shaped 4th ventricle. Midline cerebellar vermian structures are evident as are the sulci and gyri of the medial surface of the cerebral hemisphere.

The decussation of the pyramids within the foramen magnum marking the transition from the brain to the spinal cord may be depicted as outside the skull if a horizontal line is passed posteriorly from the anterior margin of the foramen magnum. This relationship may be an important consideration in evaluating fractures of the anterior arch of the atlas and the related odontoid process (dens).

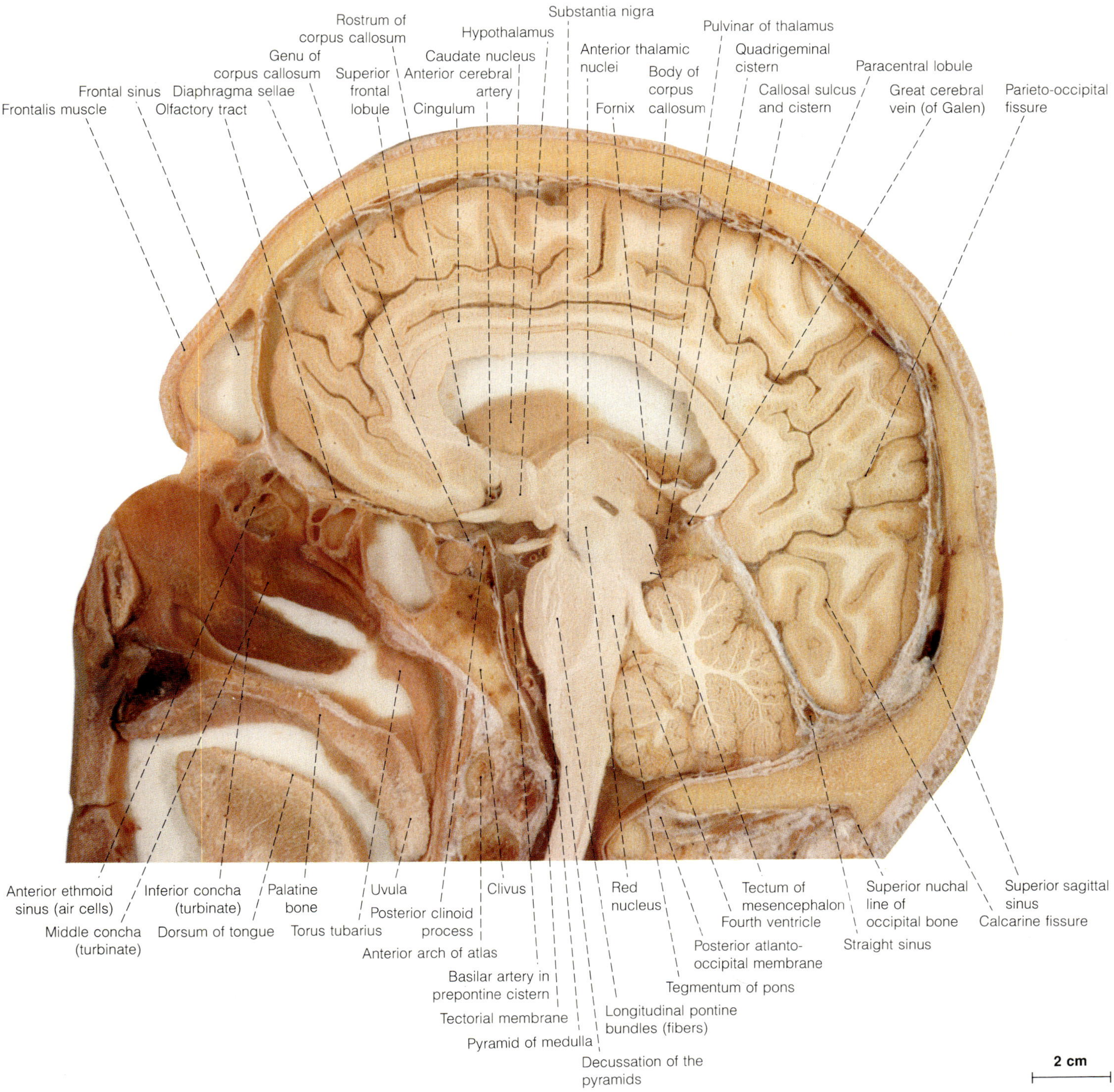
Rostrum of corpus callosum
Substantia nigra
Hypothalamus
Pulvinar of thalamus
Caudate nucleus
Anterior thalamic nuclei
Quadrigeminal cistern
Genu of corpus callosum
Superior frontal lobule
Anterior cerebral artery
Body of corpus callosum
Paracentral lobule
Frontal sinus
Diaphragma sellae
Callosal sulcus and cistern
Great cerebral vein (of Galen)
Parieto-occipital fissure
Frontalis muscle
Olfactory tract
Cingulum
Fornix
Anterior ethmoid sinus (air cells)
Inferior concha (turbinate)
Palatine bone
Uvula
Clivus
Red nucleus
Tectum of mesencephalon
Superior nuchal line of occipital bone
Superior sagittal sinus
Posterior clinoid process
Fourth ventricle
Calcarine fissure
Middle concha (turbinate)
Dorsum of tongue
Torus tubarius
Anterior arch of atlas
Posterior atlanto-occipital membrane
Straight sinus
Basilar artery in prepontine cistern
Tegmentum of pons
Tectorial membrane
Longitudinal pontine bundles (fibers)
Pyramid of medulla
Decussation of the pyramids
2 cm

Patient MRI Scan

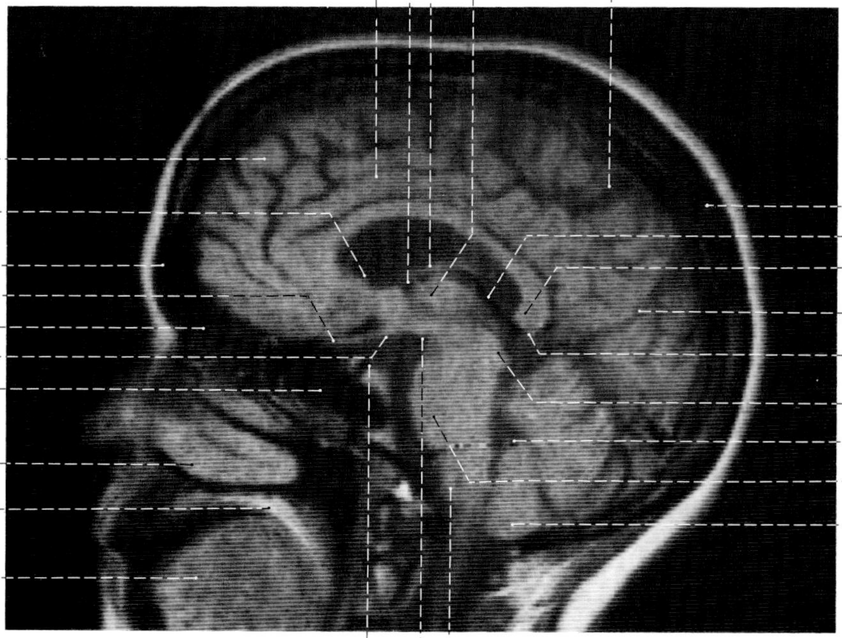

Viewed from the Left

In MRI scans the vascular channels are especially prominent when surrounded by proton dense soft tissues. The internal cerebral veins draining into the great cerebral vein are nicely depicted in the MRI illustrated and can be seen draining into a portion of the vein of Galen. Cortical vessels may likewise enhance the contrast of the sulci. Because the superior sagittal sinus and the adjacent inner table of the calvaria are perceived as black, the two cannot be differentiated easily.

The course of the oculomotor nerve (III) from the interpeduncular fossa to the wall of the cavernous sinus is well visualized in the gross specimen. Both anterior and posterior lobes of the pituitary are also distinguishable below the diaphragma sellae. The optic chiasm is frequently 1 cm above the diaphragma although in the specimen illustrated it is somewhat less. The course of the optic nerve can be traced into the chiasm and around the hypothalamus in the MRI scan.

Since this slice is just off midline the aqueduct is no longer visible but the quadrigeminal plate remains a prominent feature. The cerebellar tonsil on this side is also well differentiated and its relationships to the dorsal aspect of the medulla and the lip of the foramen magnum can be appreciated.

Another structure which has protons so tightly bound that they will not resonate so that a signal can be perceived under current pulse sequences is the densely fibrous dura. Hence, the tentorium is visualized as a dark band separating supra and infratentorial structures. Within it, in a random fashion, are even blacker regions which represent cortical veins of the interior surface of the posterior temporal and occipital lobes.

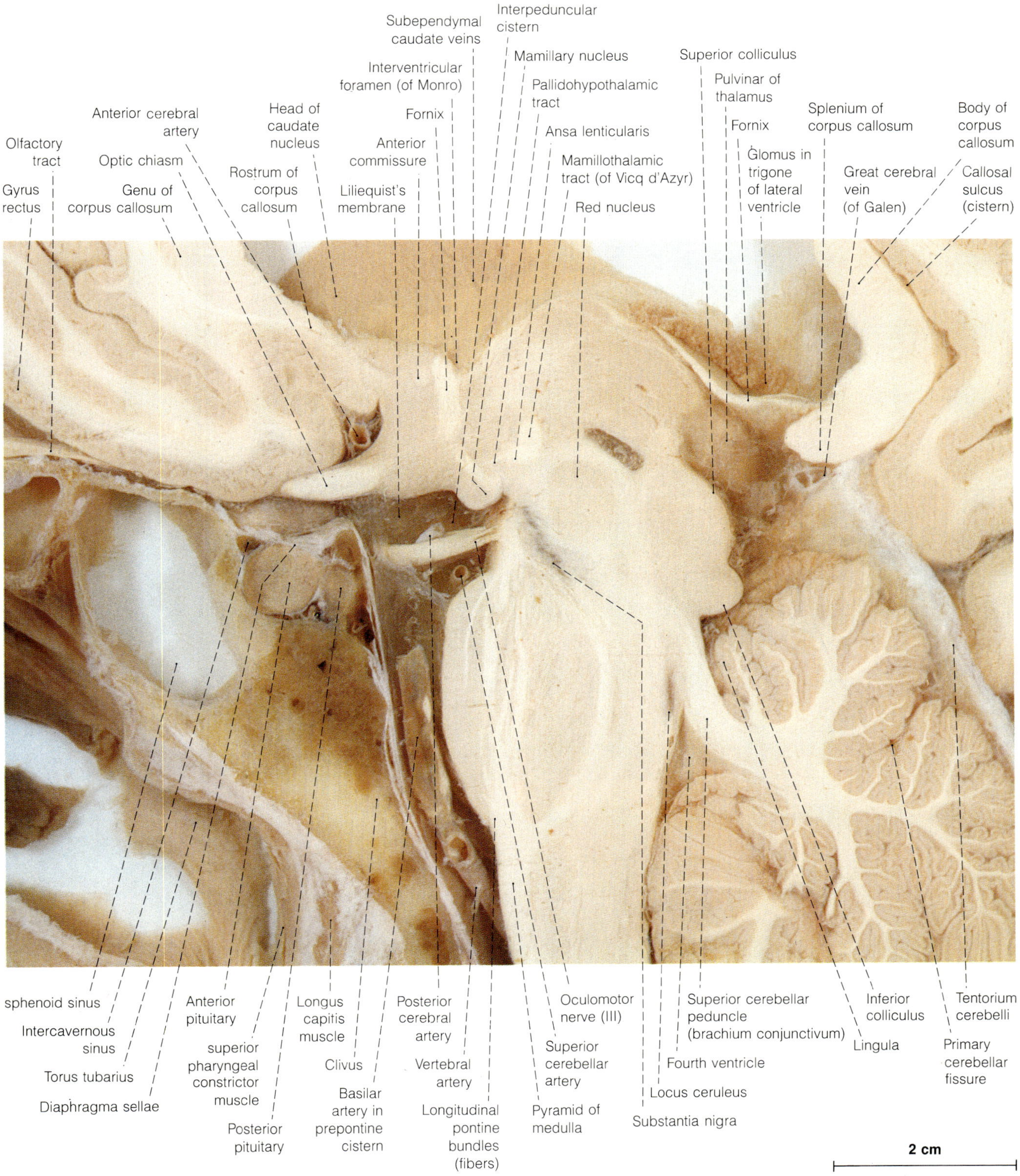
Subependymal caudate veins
Interpeduncular cistern
Interventricular foramen (of Monro)
Mamillary nucleus
Superior colliculus
Pallidohypothalamic tract
Pulvinar of thalamus
Anterior cerebral artery
Head of caudate nucleus
Fornix
Splenium of corpus callosum
Body of corpus callosum
Ansa lenticularis
Fornix
Olfactory tract
Anterior commissure
Optic chiasm
Mamillothalamic tract (of Vicq d'Azyr)
Glomus in trigone of lateral ventricle
Rostrum of corpus callosum
Great cerebral vein (of Galen)
Callosal sulcus (cistern)
Gyrus rectus
Genu of corpus callosum
Liliequist's membrane
Red nucleus
sphenoid sinus
Anterior pituitary
Longus capitis muscle
Posterior cerebral artery
Oculomotor nerve (III)
Superior cerebellar peduncle (brachium conjunctivum)
Inferior colliculus
Tentorium cerebelli
Intercavernous sinus
superior pharyngeal constrictor muscle
Clivus
Vertebral artery
Superior cerebellar artery
Lingula
Primary cerebellar fissure
Torus tubarius
Fourth ventricle
Basilar artery in prepontine cistern
Diaphragma sellae
Locus ceruleus
Longitudinal pontine bundles (fibers)
Pyramid of medulla
Posterior pituitary
Substantia nigra
2 cm

Cadaver CT Scan

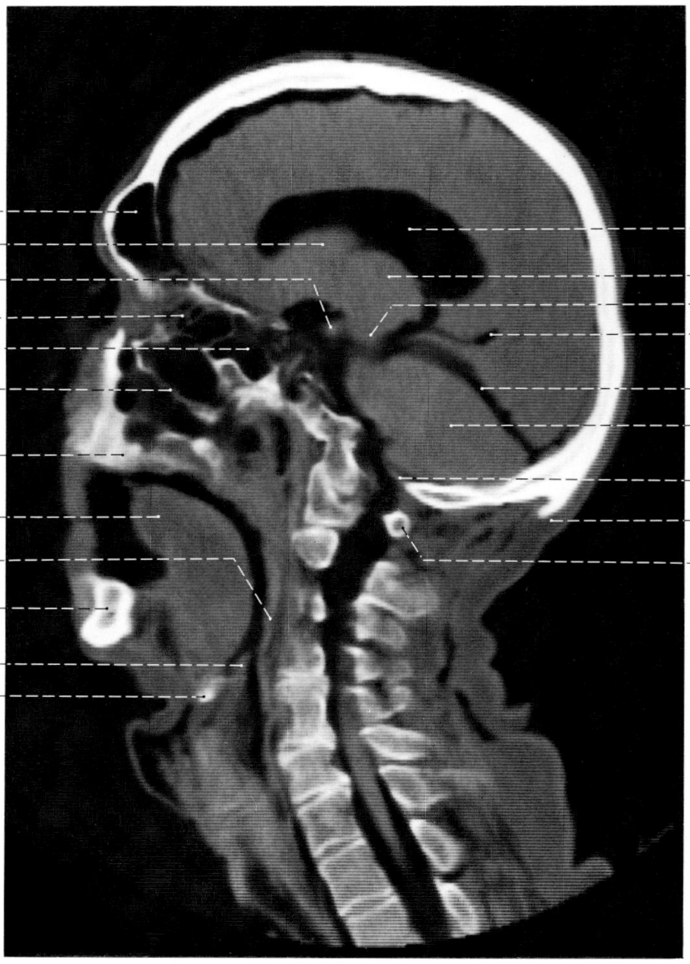

The parasagittal section is through the right cavernous sinus viewed from the medial side. Such a slice exposes the lateral free margin of the tentorium (tentorial notch) as it arches around the mesencephalon and illustrates the relation of the uncus and optic tract to the tentorial notch. The genu of the internal capsule containing the pyramidal bundles is shown here in its continuity with the cerebral peduncle.

The relatively medial position of the cerebellar dentate nucleus which gives rise to most of the superior cerebellar peduncle (brachium conjunctivum) illustrates why lesions of the medial cerebellum might produce more profound symptoms than those more lateral involving only the cerebellar hemispheres.

This view looking laterally from a more medial perspective is useful as an adjunct to the previous slices which were viewed as if one were moving from lateral to medial.

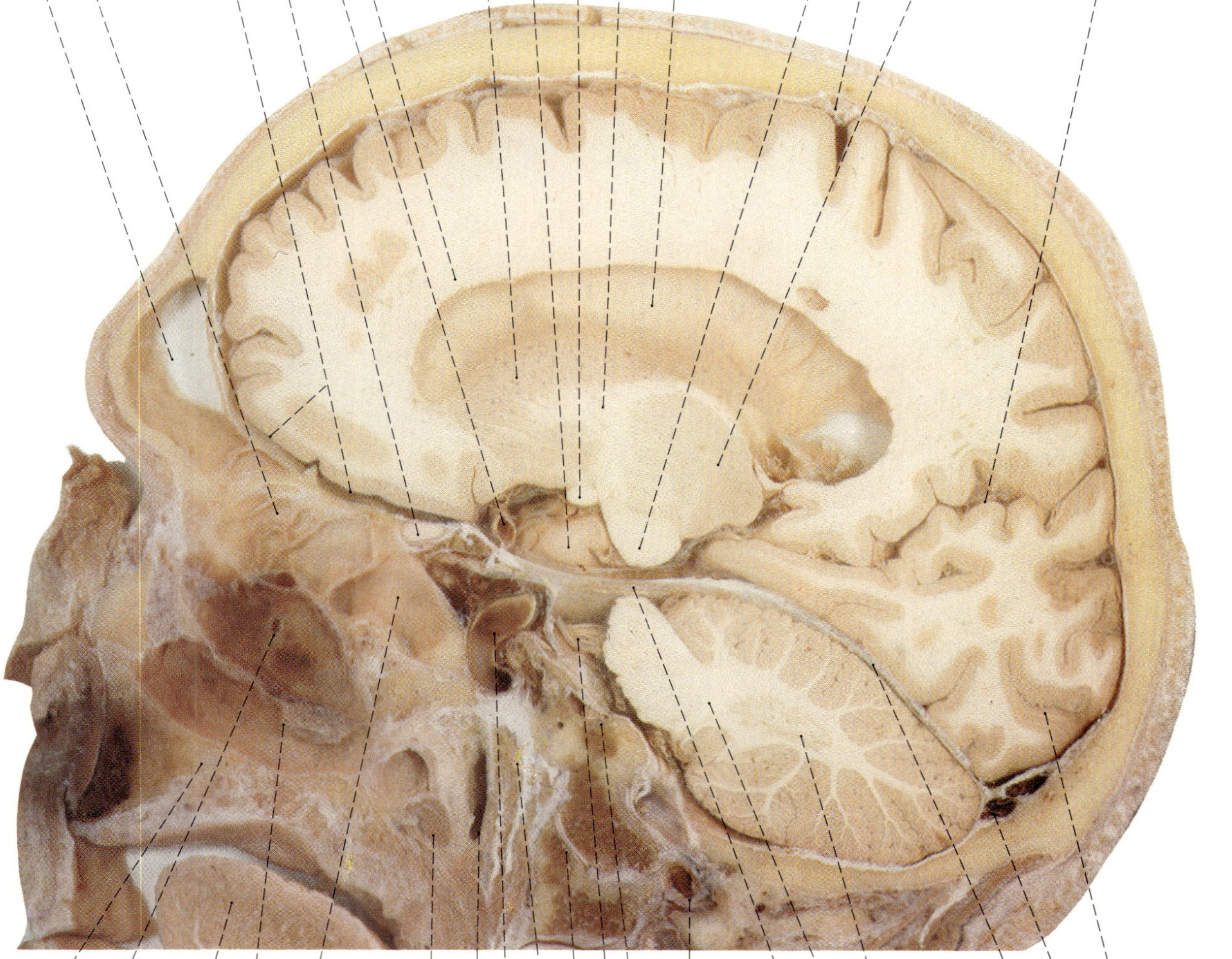

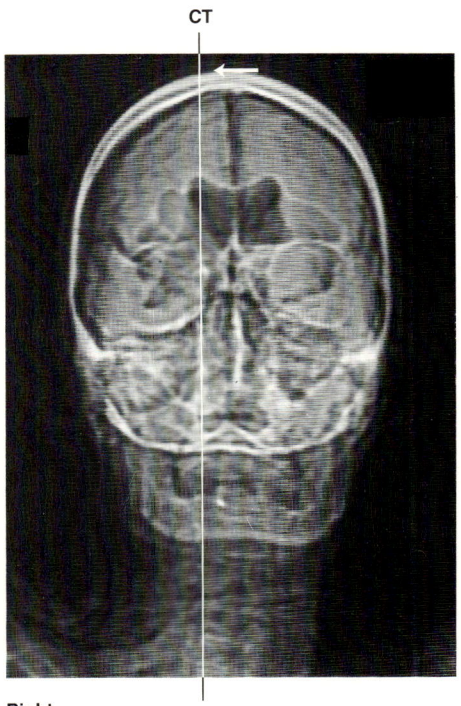

Plane of Section

Patient MRI Scan

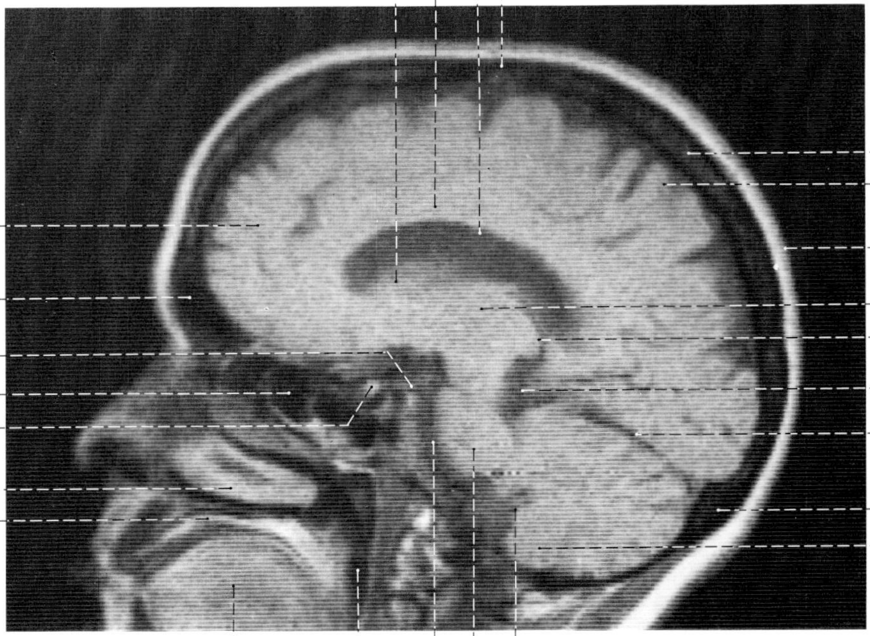

Viewed from the Left

Eleven of the cranial nerves appear in this slice: The optic (II) as it enters the optic foramen; the oculomotor (III) in the wall of the cavernous sinus; the trochlear (IV) along the free margin of the tentorium; the abducens (VI) in Dorello's canal; the facial (VII) and auditory (VIII) nerves entering the internal auditory meatus; the glossopharyngeal (IX), vagus (X), and spinal accessory (XI) as they enter the jugular foramen; and the hypoglossal (XII) in the anterior condylar foramen. Since this section is slightly lateral to the midline, the region of the olfactory bulbs and cribriform plate is not seen.

Sagittal anatomy is particularly useful for envisioning the relationship of cortical hemispheres to brainstem nuclei and basal ganglia; we have found that a presentation of anatomy in this plane often adds significantly to one's mastery of anatomy in the axial and coronal planes.

Although the pulse sequence used for the MRI display does not differentiate grey and white matter, some nuclei and fiber bundles can be easily identified because the cisterns and ventricles are quite evident and certain anatomical relationships are constant.

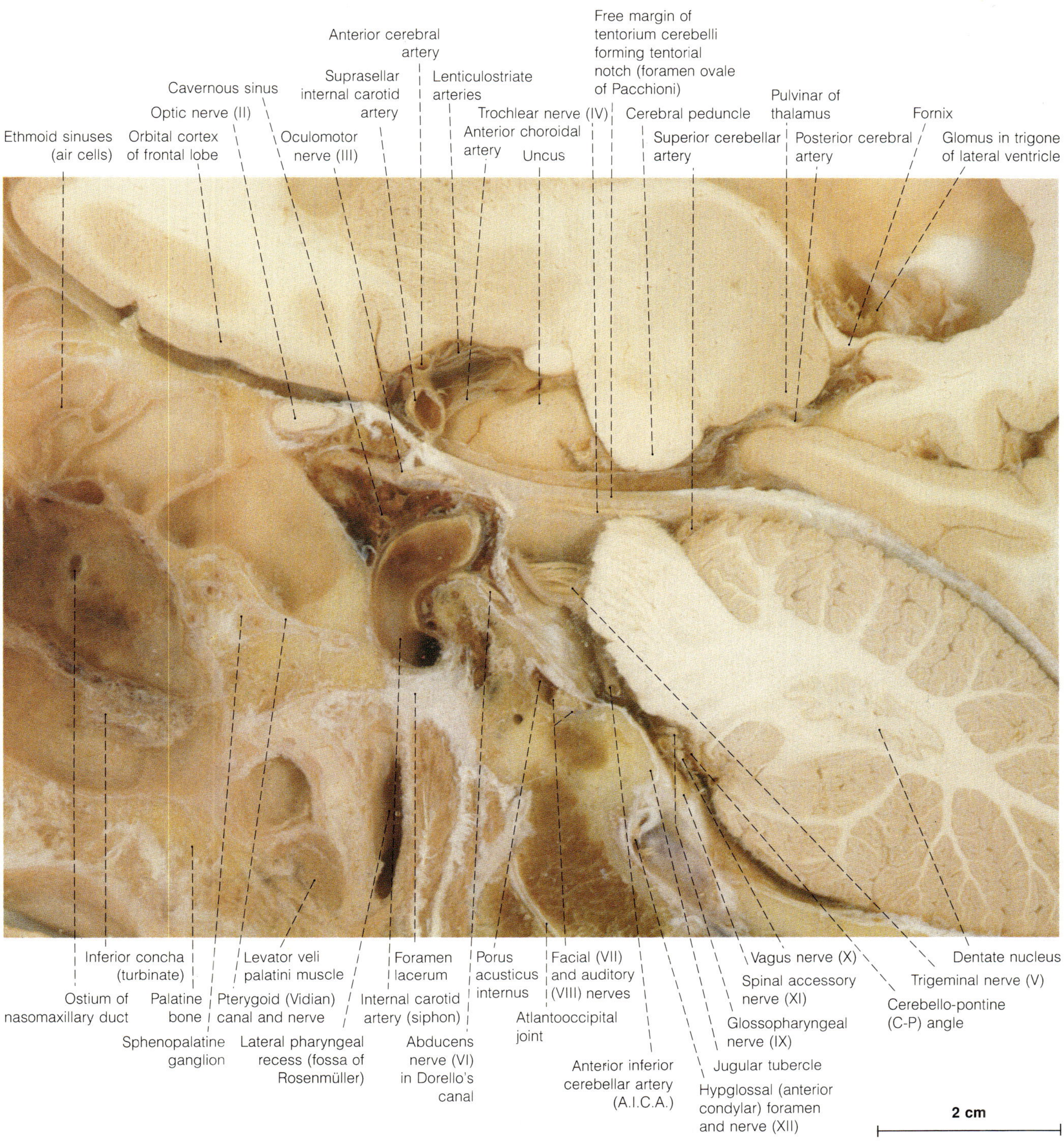
Anterior cerebral artery
Free margin of tentorium cerebelli forming tentorial notch (foramen ovale of Pacchioni)
Cavernous sinus
Suprasellar internal carotid artery
Lenticulostriate arteries
Pulvinar of thalamus
Optic nerve (II)
Trochlear nerve (IV)
Cerebral peduncle
Fornix
Ethmoid sinuses (air cells)
Orbital cortex of frontal lobe
Oculomotor nerve (III)
Anterior choroidal artery
Uncus
Superior cerebellar artery
Posterior cerebral artery
Glomus in trigone of lateral ventricle
Inferior concha (turbinate)
Levator veli palatini muscle
Foramen lacerum
Porus acusticus internus
Facial (VII) and auditory (VIII) nerves
Vagus nerve (X)
Dentate nucleus
Ostium of nasomaxillary duct
Palatine bone
Pterygoid (Vidian) canal and nerve
Internal carotid artery (siphon)
Spinal accessory nerve (XI)
Trigeminal nerve (V)
Cerebello-pontine (C-P) angle
Atlantooccipital joint
Glossopharyngeal nerve (IX)
Sphenopalatine ganglion
Lateral pharyngeal recess (fossa of Rosenmüller)
Abducens nerve (VI) in Dorello's canal
Jugular tubercle
Anterior inferior cerebellar artery (A.I.C.A.)
Hypglossal (anterior condylar) foramen and nerve (XII)
2 cm

Cadaver CT Scan

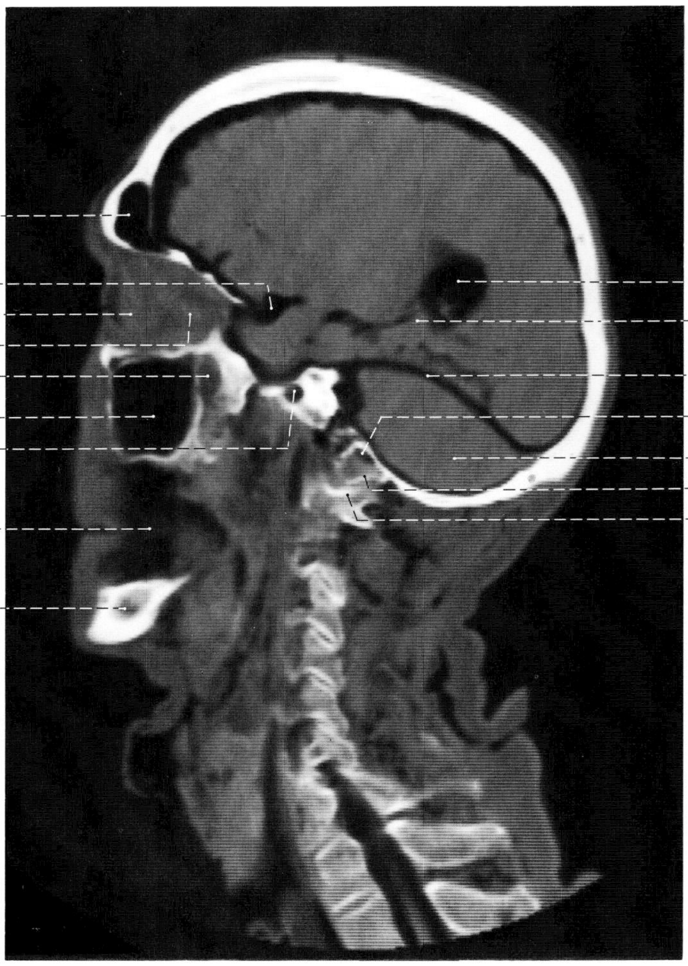

This parasagittal section of the right side is viewed from the medial aspect. The inferior (temporal) horn of the lateral ventricle is transected exposing the hippocampus indenting the anterior tip of the ventricle. The amygdala is also in contiguity with the lenticular nucleus above.

The section also passes through the pterygopalatine fossa with communications inferiorly into the oral cavity, medially with the nasal cavity, superiorly and anteriorly with the orbit, posteriorly with middle cranial fossa and laterally with the infratemporal fossa.

Of interest, as on the left side, are the relative relationships of the putamen, globus pallidus, and internal capsule. Students commonly see these presented in coronal and axial planes but their relationships in a sagittal plane can be surprising. Here, for example, the central, more medial, globus pallidus merges supero-anteriorly with the more lateral putamen and postero-inferiorly with the posterior limb of the internal capsule. Because of artifactual separation in the gross specimen, some of the long fiber tracts of the internal capsule are separated from each other illustrating their linear nature.

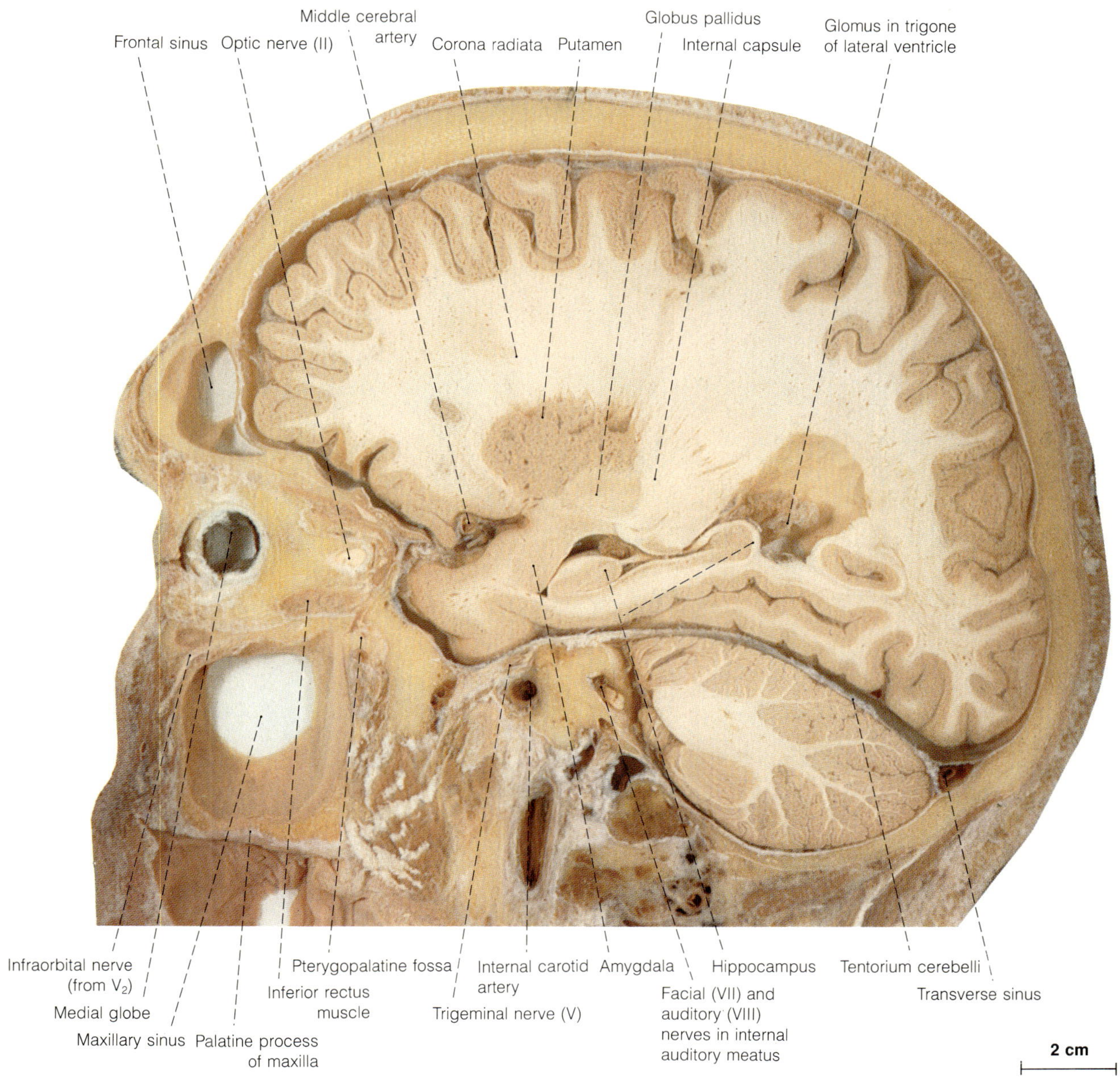

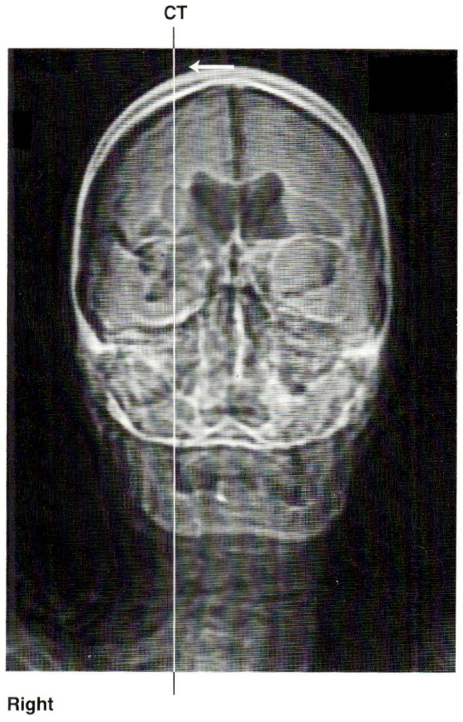

Plane of Section

Patient MRI Scan

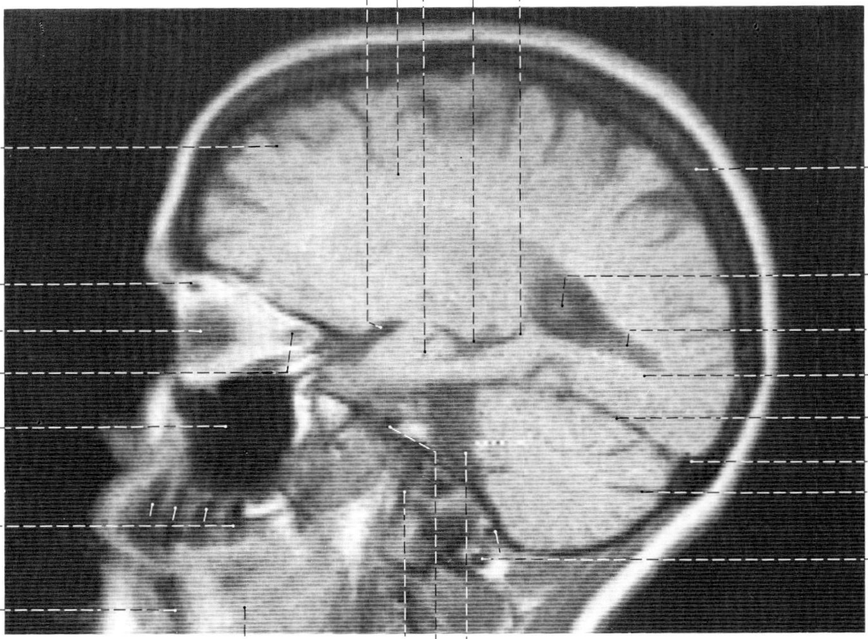

Viewed from the Left

MRI, unhampered by metal fillings in the teeth or dense bone, permits visualization of the roots of teeth adjacent to the floor of the maxillary sinus and the vertebral artery as it loops over the atlas to penetrate the posterior atlantooccipital membrane and enter the posterior fossa.

Particularly well shown in the MRI slice is the transverse sinus with its envelope of dura. The latter has about the same signal characteristic (black) as the moving blood in the sinus but the overall complex is easily visualized because of its characteristic shape and contrast with brain parenchyma.

The dark grey area anterior to the cerebellum probably represents CSF in the cerebello-pontine angle cistern; air or metrizamide contrast CT scans will probably no longer be necessary to diagnose CP angle masses with the availability of MRI.

As on the left side, facial structures here have their characteristic appearance. The CSF-containing atrium of the lateral ventricle and occipital horn are nicely shown with a glomus of choroid within the ventricle. A fissure leads antero-inferiorly to the temporal lobe and a vascular structure identified within it as a black curve might represent the posterolateral choroidal artery.

The lentriculostriate (anterior-lateral perforating) arteries arise from the middle cerebral artery as it passes superior to the amygdala. These vessels supply the overlying basal nuclei and adjacent internal capsule.

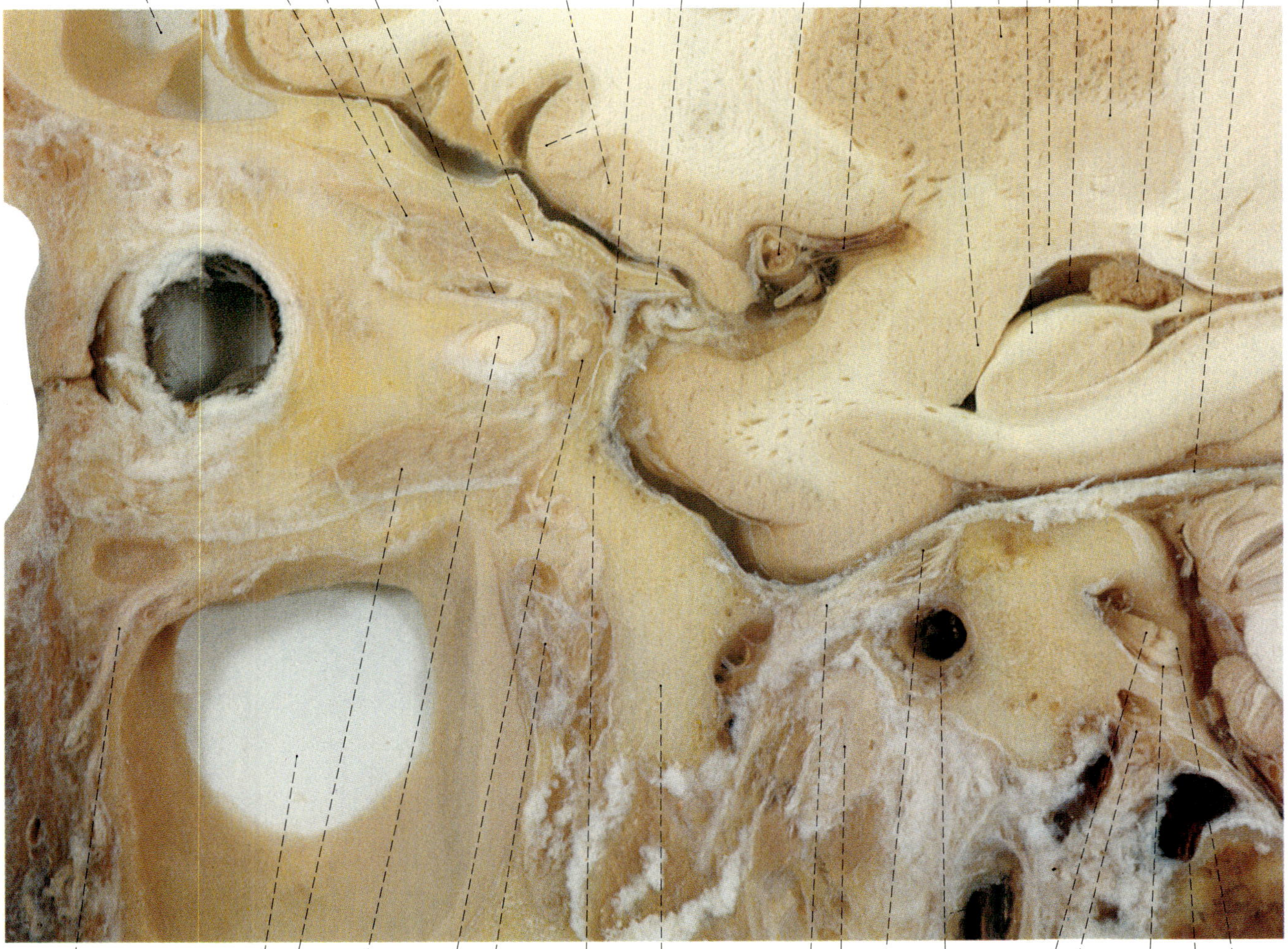
Substriatal gray
Inferior (temporal) horn of lateral ventricle
Hippocampus
Globus pallidus
Orbital plate of frontal bone
Amygdala
Tentorium cerebelli
Middle cerebral artery
Levator palpebrae superioris muscle
Superior ophthalmic vein
Lateral aspect of anterior clinoid process
Fimbria
Sphenoparietal sinus
Lenticulostriate arteries
Frontal sinus
Frontal nerve
Orbital gyri
Putamen
Choroid
Infraorbital nerve in infraorbital canal
Optic nerve (II)
Greater wing of sphenoid
Lateral pterygoid plate
Internal carotid artery
Jugular bulb
Inferior rectus muscle
Maxillary sinus
Pterygopalatine fossa
Mandibular nerve (V_3) in foramen ovale
Trigeminal nerve (V)
Acoustic part of auditory nerve (VIII)
Lateral rectus muscle and abducens nerve (VI)
Pharyngotympanic (auditory or Eustachian) tube
Vestibular part of auditory nerve (VIII)
Facial nerve (VII)
Glossopharyngeal nerve (IX)
2 cm

Cadaver CT Scan

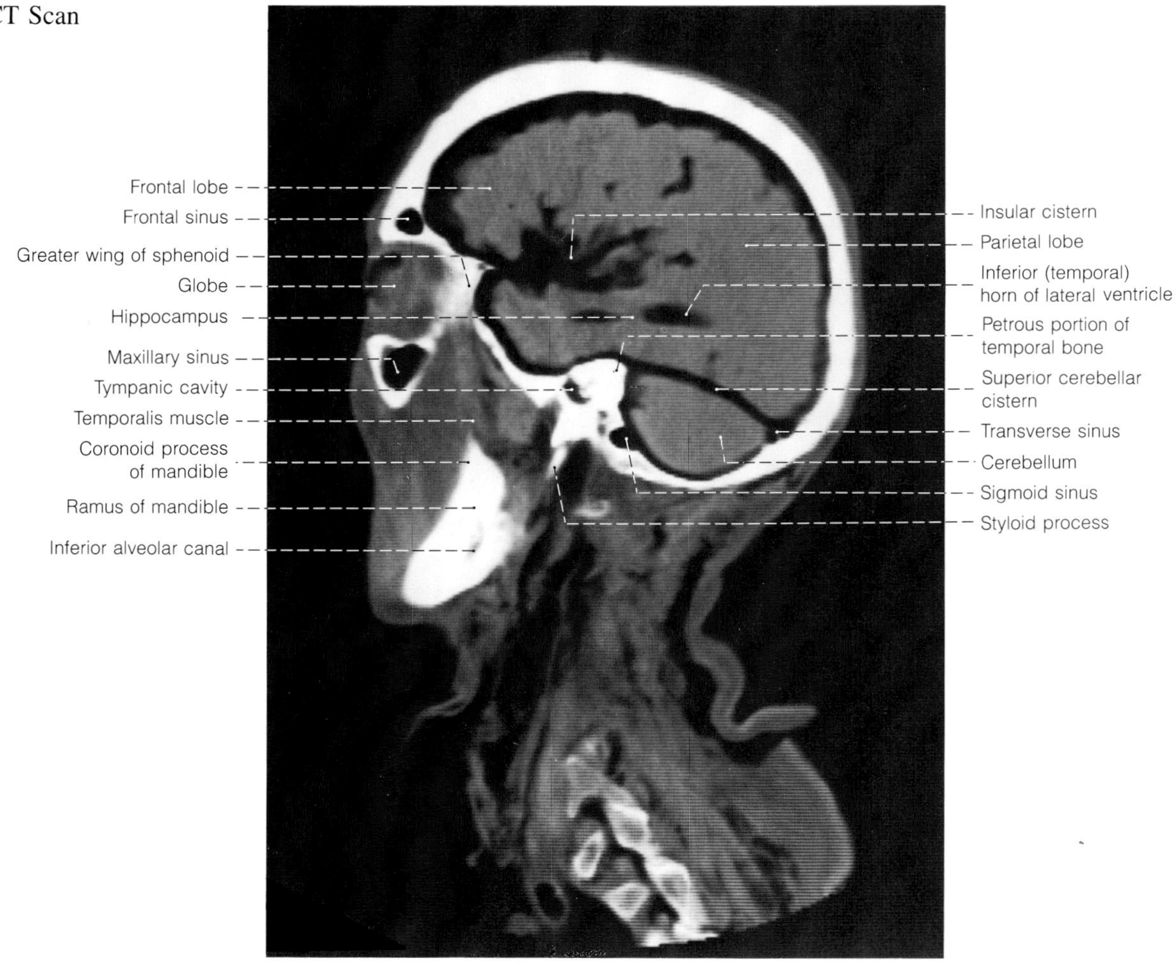

The parasagittal sections (CT and anatomical specimen) are medial views of slices through the right hemisphere exposing the temporal (inferior) horn of the lateral ventricle and the insula. A portion of the hippocampus is seen within the temporal horn and the cochlea is transected within the petrous part of the temporal bone. Basically the anatomy is similar to that noted on the left side but here the medial viewpoint offers a different perspective.

Also of particular interest are the fiber tracts of the visual radiations which have separated slightly in the fixing and freezing process.

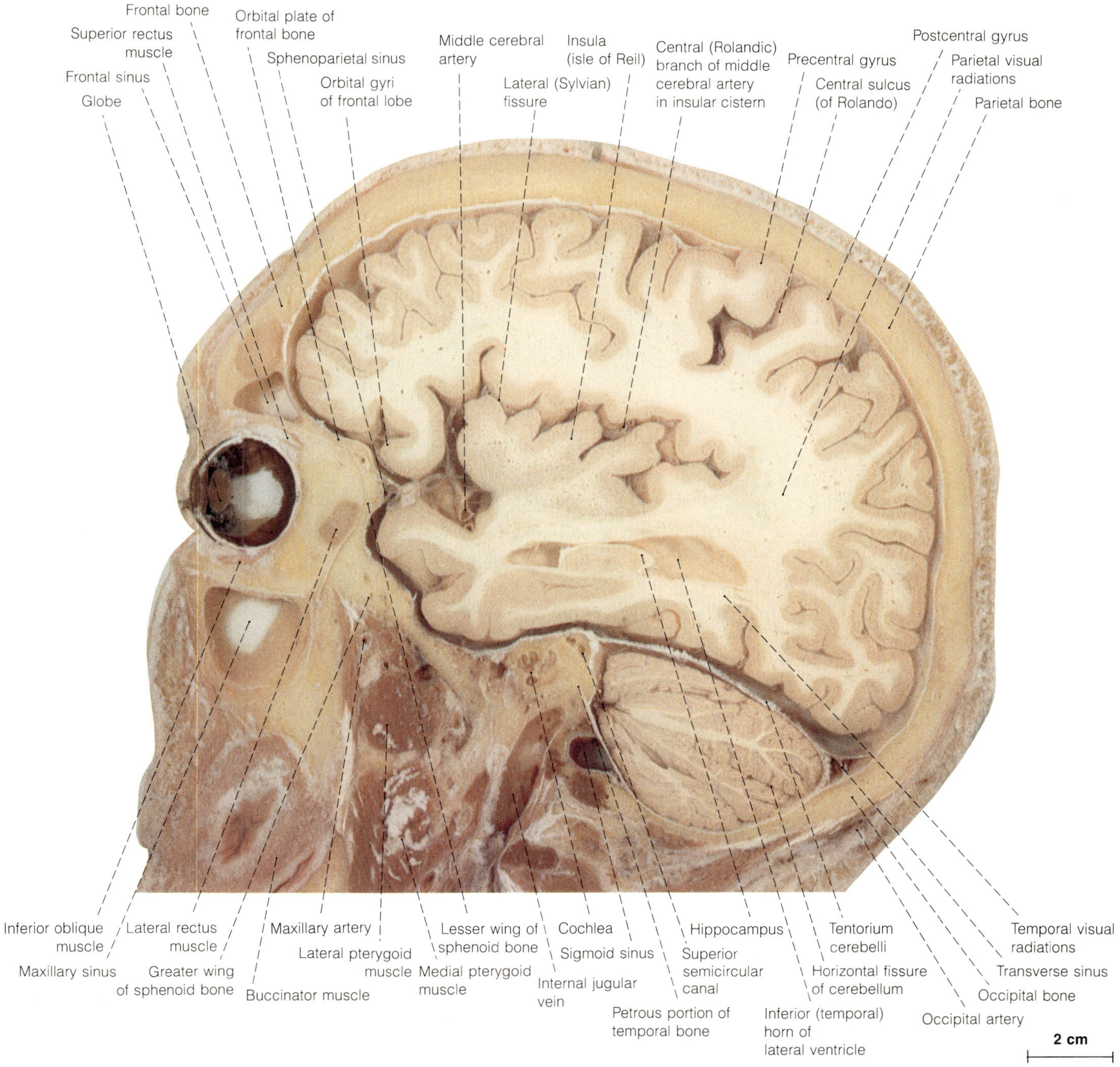

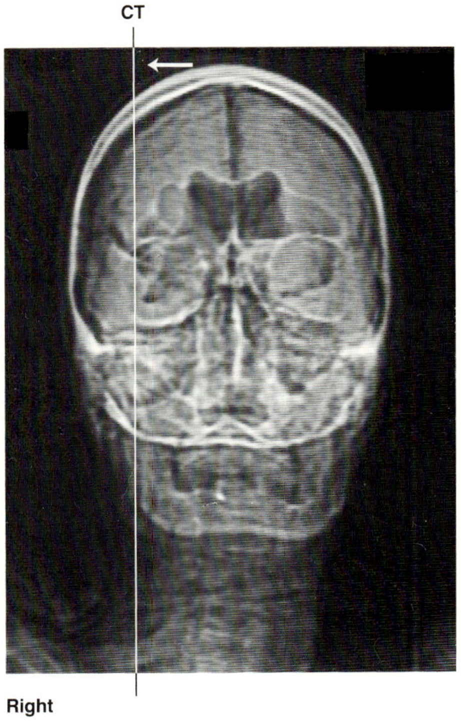

Plane of Section

Patient MRI Scan

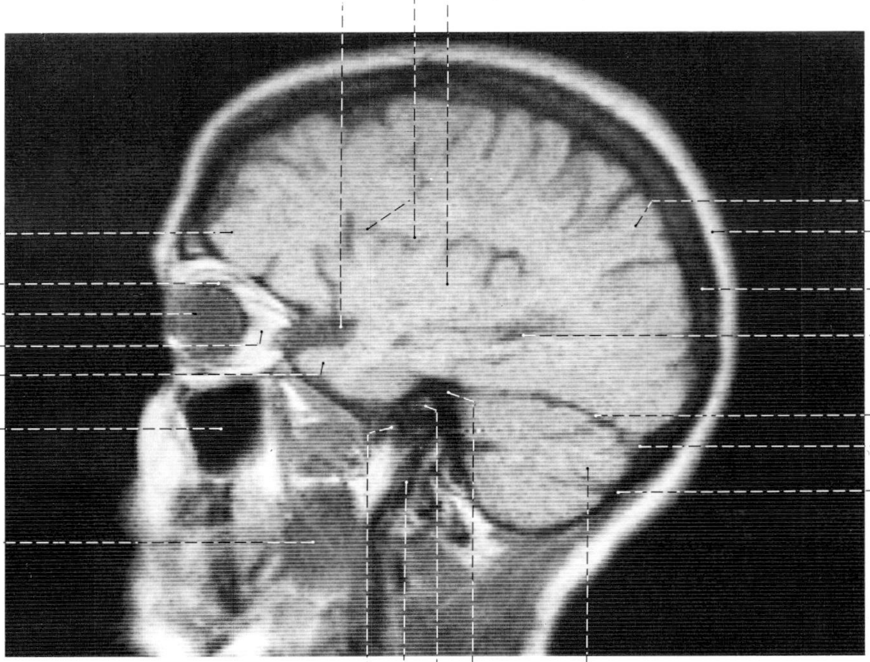

Viewed from the Left

This parasagittal MRI correlates nicely with the anatomical specimen. Particularly well seen in both (although completely different individuals) are the dark convolutions of the insular lobe and the CSF-containing spaces of the narrow trigone of the lateral ventricle.

An interesting phenomenon is present in the cerebellopontine angle cistern area where blackness due to the bone of the petrous apex completely surrounds a rounded soft tissue mass which is interpreted to represent the facial (VII) and auditory (VIII) nerve complex on cut section traveling into the plane of the MRI scan.

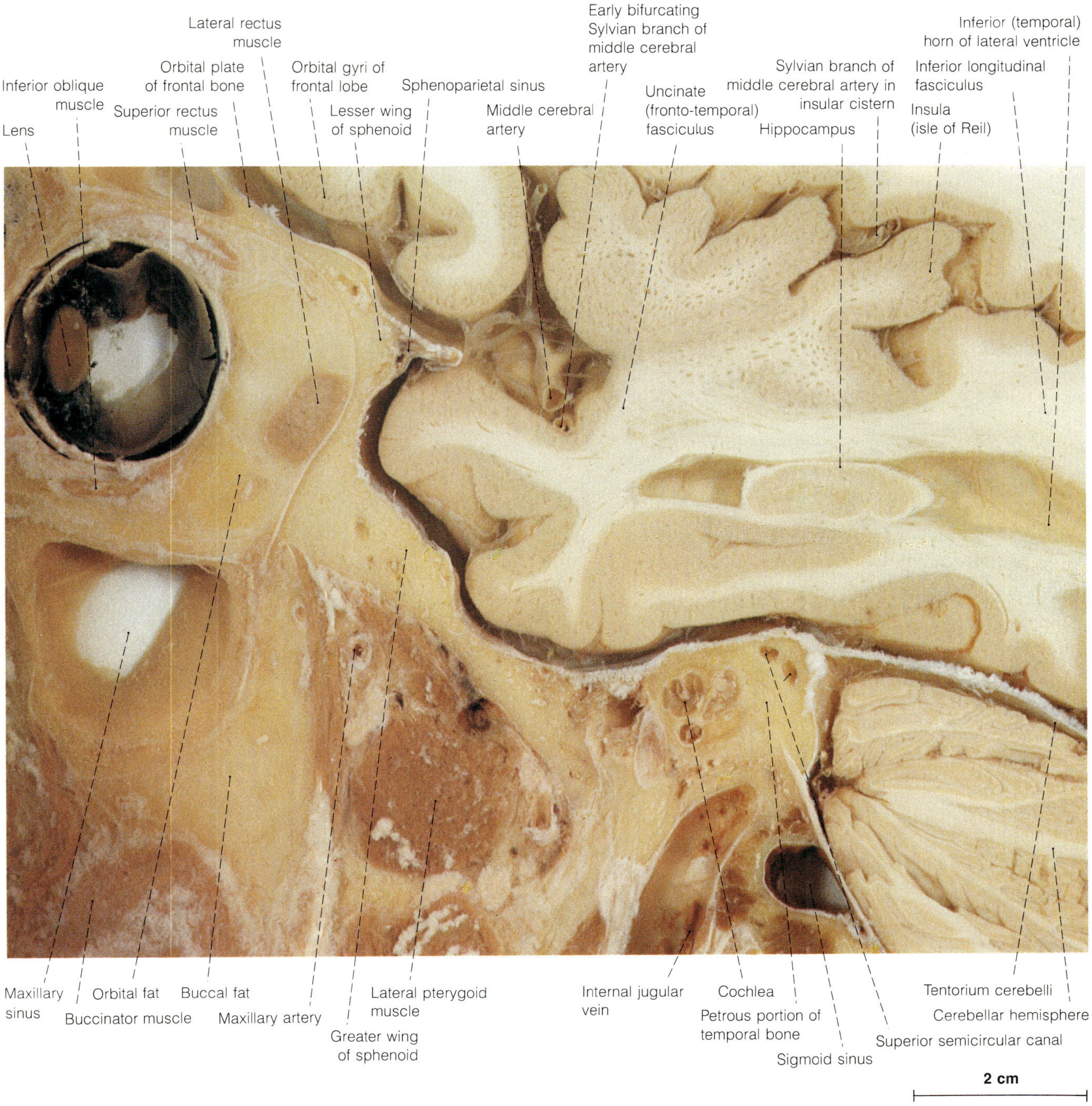
Lateral rectus muscle
Orbital plate of frontal bone
Inferior oblique muscle
Lens
Superior rectus muscle
Orbital gyri of frontal lobe
Lesser wing of sphenoid
Sphenoparietal sinus
Early bifurcating Sylvian branch of middle cerebral artery
Middle cerebral artery
Uncinate (fronto-temporal) fasciculus
Sylvian branch of middle cerebral artery in insular cistern
Hippocampus
Inferior (temporal) horn of lateral ventricle
Inferior longitudinal fasciculus
Insula (isle of Reil)
Maxillary sinus
Buccinator muscle
Orbital fat
Buccal fat
Maxillary artery
Greater wing of sphenoid
Lateral pterygoid muscle
Internal jugular vein
Cochlea
Petrous portion of temporal bone
Sigmoid sinus
Superior semicircular canal
Tentorium cerebelli
Cerebellar hemisphere
2 cm

Cadaver CT Scan

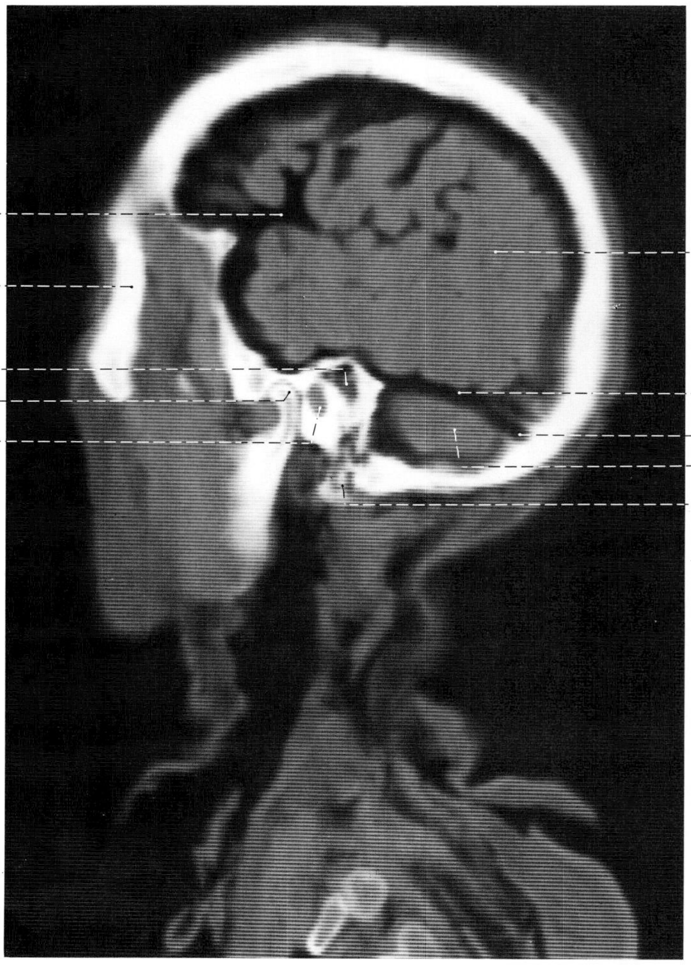

This anatomical slice is dominated by the lateral or Sylvian fissure and the bulk of the temporal lobe. Looking into the Sylvian fissure from its medial aspect, the medial surface of the opercular cortex is visible.

The external auditory canal and head of the mandible in the temporomandibular joint are seen in their characteristic close approximation. The ridge of the lesser and greater wings of the sphenoid are also appreciated in this section which passes through the lateral wall of the orbit and globe.

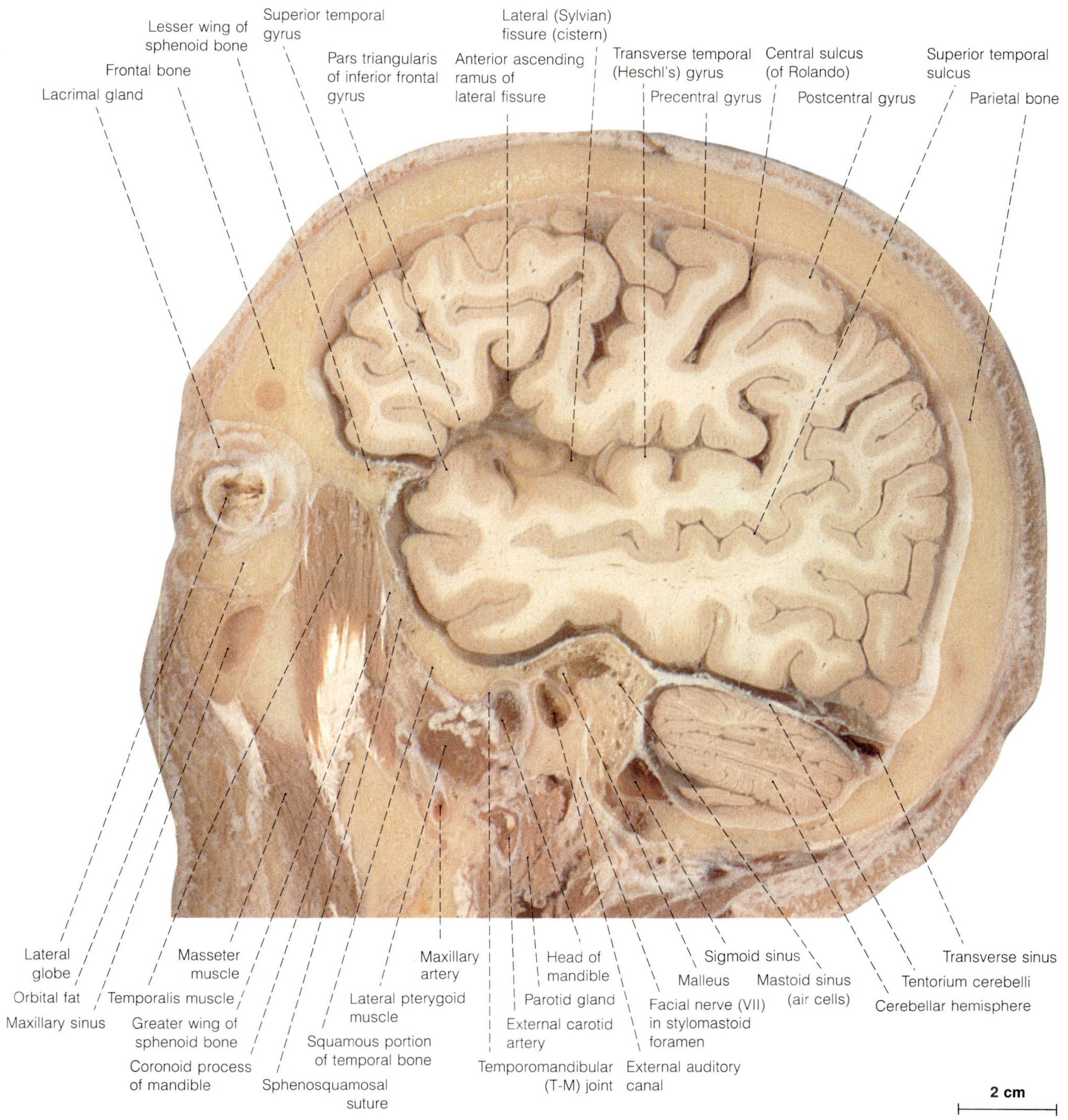

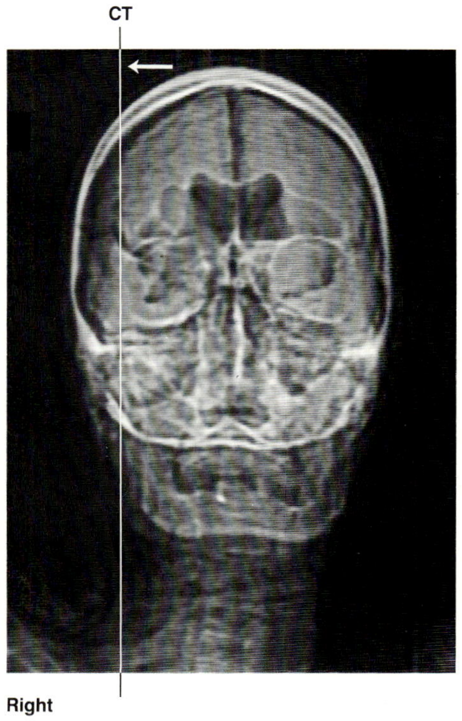

Plane of Section

Patient MRI Scan

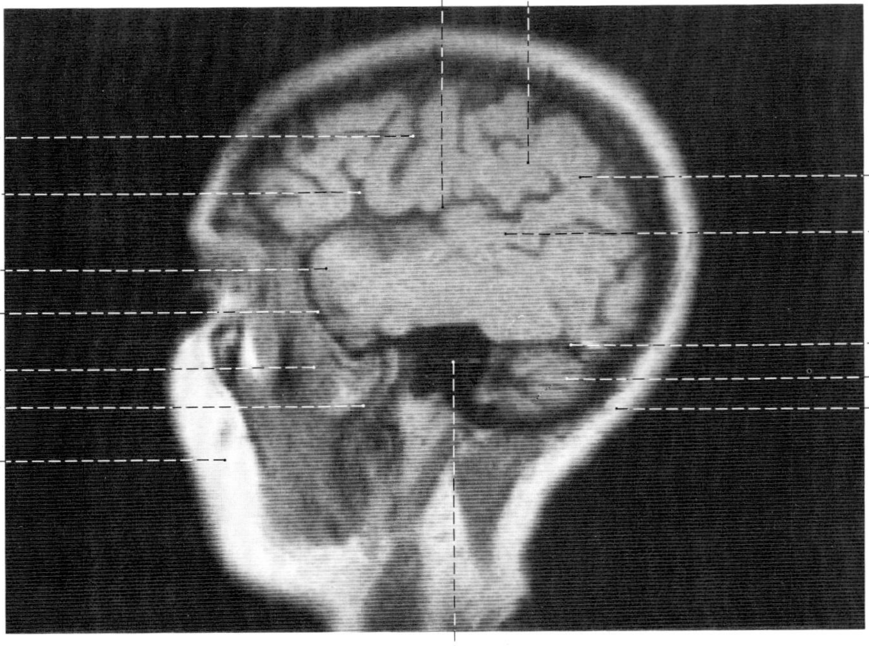

Viewed from the Left

The plane of the patient MRI scan approximates the anatomical section with a large black area representing the temporal bone and venous sinuses closely apposed to or running through the temporal bone.

The ridge of the sphenoid has a black line representing its cortex. Most of the grey echo below this is probably due to the contents of the infratemporal fossa and the marrow (diploë) within the sphenoid bone.

The bulk of the temporal lobe dominates the anatomy of the slice, and although this particular pulse sequence does not allow differentiation of grey and white matter, the gyri and sulci and Sylvian fissure are particularly well displayed.

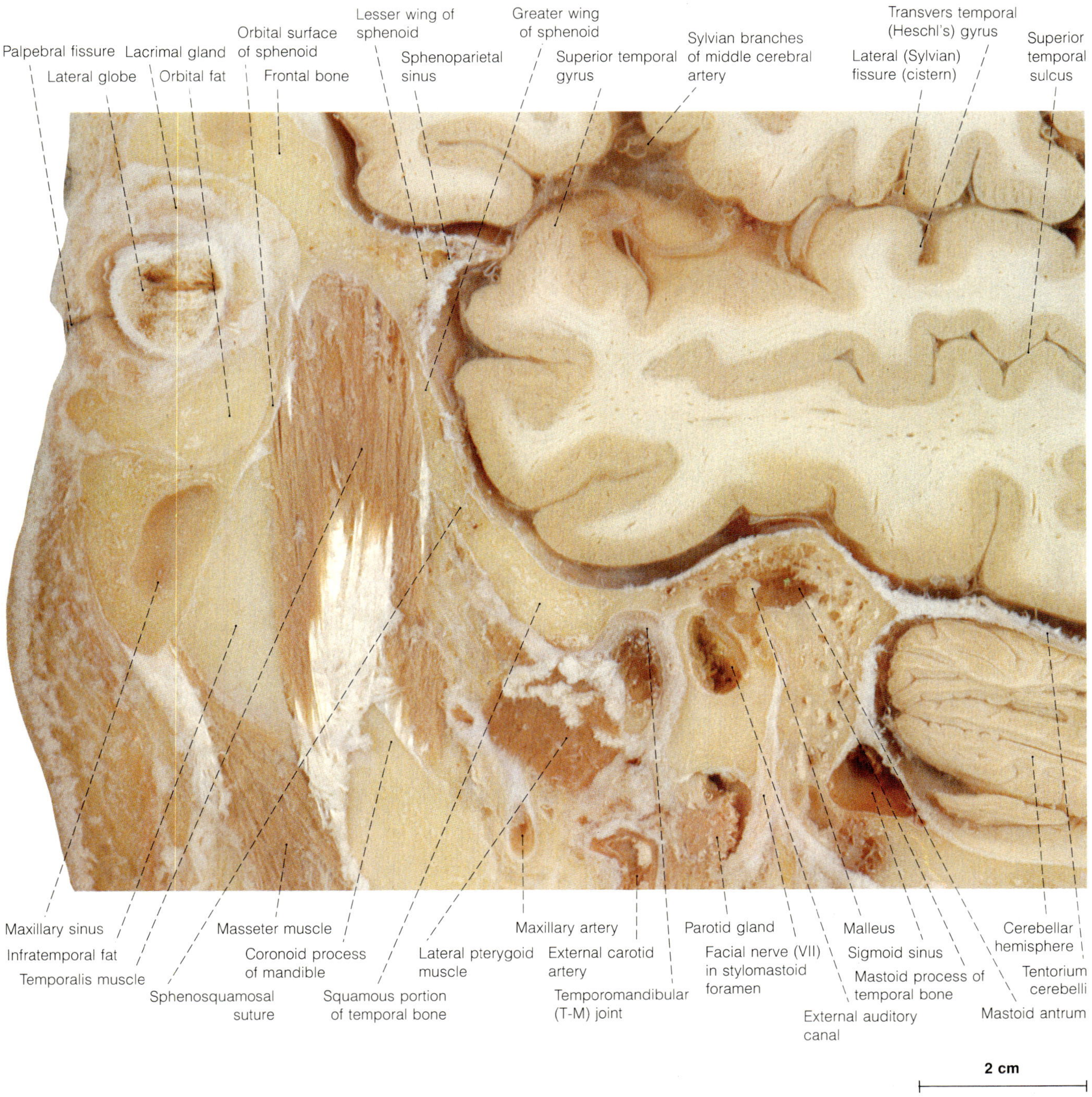
Palpebral fissure
Lateral globe
Lacrimal gland
Orbital fat
Orbital surface of sphenoid
Frontal bone
Lesser wing of sphenoid
Sphenoparietal sinus
Greater wing of sphenoid
Superior temporal gyrus
Sylvian branches of middle cerebral artery
Transvers temporal (Heschl's) gyrus
Lateral (Sylvian) fissure (cistern)
Superior temporal sulcus
Maxillary sinus
Infratemporal fat
Temporalis muscle
Sphenosquamosal suture
Masseter muscle
Coronoid process of mandible
Squamous portion of temporal bone
Lateral pterygoid muscle
Maxillary artery
External carotid artery
Temporomandibular (T-M) joint
Parotid gland
Facial nerve (VII) in stylomastoid foramen
Malleus
Sigmoid sinus
Mastoid process of temporal bone
External auditory canal
Cerebellar hemisphere
Tentorium cerebelli
Mastoid antrum
2 cm

Selected Bibliography

Anderson, J. E. *Grant's Atlas of Anatomy, 8th ed.* Williams & Wilkins, Baltimore, 1983.

Burrows, E. H., and N. E. Leeds. *Neuroradiology, Vol. 1.* Churchill Livingstone, N. Y., 1981.

Ferner, H. *Eduard Pernkopf Atlas of Topographical and Applied Human Anatomy, 2nd ed.* Urban & Schwarzenberg, Baltimore and Munich, 1980.

Ferner, H., and J. Staubesand. *Sobotta Atlas of Human Anatomy, 10th English ed.,* Translated by W. Hild. Urban & Schwarzenberg, Baltimore and Munich, 1983.

Koritké, J. G., and H. Sick. *Atlas of Sectional Human Anatomy, Vol. 1, Head, Neck, Thorax.* Urban & Schwarzenberg, Baltimore and Munich, 1983.

Lang, J. *Clinical Anatomy of the Head, Neurocranium, Orbit, Craniocervical Regions.* Trans. by R. R. Wilson and D. P. Winstanley. Springer-Verlag, Berlin, Heidelberg, N. Y., 1983.

Mechan. I. *An Atlas of Anatomy Basic to Radiology.* W. B. Saunders Co., Philadelphia, 1975.

Newton, T. H., and D. G. Potts. *Advanced Imaging Techniques, Modern Neuroradiology, Vol. 2.* Clavadel Press, San Anselmo, Calif., 1983.

Wagner, M., and T. L. Lawson, *Segmental Anatomy, Applications to Clinical Medicine.* the Macmillan Co., New York, 1982.

Woodburne, R. T. *Essentials of Human Anatomy.* Oxford University Press, New York, 1973.

Orbits

T. L. Reid, M.D.

The bony orbit has the shape of a four-sided pyramid, with the medial wall of each orbital cavity parallelling the sagittal plane. The orbit lies immediately below the anterior cranial fossa, lateral to the nasal cavity and ethmoidal air sinuses, and just above the maxillary sinus with the axis directed forward and laterally. The apex of the pyramid is usually described as either the optic foramen or the medial end of the superior orbital fissure (fig. 13).

The roof or vault of the orbit, sloping downward and backward, is formed mostly by the thin orbital plate of the frontal bone (fig. 1). Posteriorly, the lesser wing of the sphenoid contributes to the orbital roof medial to the superior orbital fissure. The fossa for the lacrimal gland (fig. 2) lies at the antero-lateral angle, bounded inferiorly by the zygomaticofrontal suture at the junction of the lateral wall and roof. The capsule of the gland is attached to the periosteum of the orbital plate. Antero-medially, the concavity of the lacrimal fossa is between the anterior and posterior lacrimal crests and ends in the nasolacrimal canal containing the nasolacrimal duct (fig. 2).

The fovea for the trochlea (fig. 15) of the superior oblique muscle forms a tiny depression on the frontal bone at the junction of the roof and medial wall and is frequently characterized by a small trochlear spine. The foveal spine represents the attachment of the trochlea through which the tendon of the superior oblique muscle passes.

The floor of the orbit is also the roof of the maxillary sinus (fig. 13). The inferior orbital fissure separates the floor from the lateral wall of the orbit. Extending anteriorly from the inferior orbital fissure is the infraorbital sulcus (fig. 11) which is continuous with the infraorbital canal. The canal opens at the infraorbital foramen, through which the maxillary nerve and infraorbital artery pass.

The medial wall of the orbit, or lamina papyracea (figs. 5, 11), is formed primarily by the very thin orbital lamina of the ethmoid bone, with lesser contributions of lacrimal bone, frontal process of the maxilla, and body of the sphenoid. The lateral orbital wall is formed by the orbital surfaces of the greater wing of the sphenoid posteriorly and the zygomatic bone anteriorly (fig. 7).

Numerous openings connect the orbit with adjacent regions. The superior orbital fissure serves as a communication between the middle cranial fossa and the orbit. The wide part of the superior orbital fissure lies below and lateral to the optic foramen and transmits the oculomotor (III), trochlear (IV), and abducens (VI) nerves, the superior ophthalmic vein (figs. 1, 16), and the ophthalmic division (V_1) of the trigeminal nerve. The spine for an attachment of the lateral rectus is located at the junction of the two limbs of the fissure. The inferior orbital fissure (fig. 9) lies between the greater wing of the sphenoid and the orbital portion of the maxilla and opens posteriorly into the pterygopalatine fossa. The infraorbital nerve, the zygomatic nerve, and the inferior ophthalmic vein traverse the inferior orbital fissure. Ethmoidal branches of the ophthalmic artery pierce the lamina papyracea and enter the anterior cranial fossa through the anterior ethmoidal foramen. The posterior ethmoidal canal (foramen) contains the posterior ethmoidal nerve and artery. The optic canal (fig. 14) is bordered laterally by the lesser wing of the sphenoid, and is separated from the medial end of the superior orbital fissure by a bar of bone serving as a point of attachment for the common tendinous ring (anulus tendineus communis). The optic canal transmits both the optic nerve and, inferolaterally, the ophthalmic artery.

The globe located anteriorly in the orbit has an average vertical diameter of 23 mm and a horizontal diameter of 23.5 mm. Orbital fat fills the retrobulbar space and has a characteristic absorption coefficient on CT scans. The optic nerve has a delicate, concave medial curve from the optic canal to the globe. The two ophthalmic nerve branches, the lacrimal and frontal, enter the orbital cavity via the superior orbital fissure, above the muscle cone. The frontal nerve divides into a lateral supraorbital and medial supratrochlear nerve, both of which emerge at the upper rim of the orbit to supply the forehead. The trochlear nerve also enters the superior orbital fissure and turns medially to reach the superior oblique muscle.

The four rectus muscles are attached posteriorly at the orbital apex to the common tendinous ring of Zinn. The levator palpebrae superioris (figs. 2, 16) arises in conjunction with the superior rectus muscle and is difficult to separate from it even on the best CT. The superior rectus (fig. 3) passes forward and somewhat laterally to pierce Tenon's capsule, and inserts into the sclera above and behind the sclerocorneal junction. The inferior rectus (fig. 4) runs forward and laterally and, after penetrating the bulbar sheath, passes above the inferior oblique to insert anteriorly on the globe. The inferior rectus is below its nerve supply, the inferior division of the oculomotor nerve.The lateral rectus (fig. 12), lateral to its abducens nerve (VI) and the ciliary ganglion and ophthalmic artery, inserts into the sclera on the lateral side of the eyeball. The medial rectus passes forward along the medial wall of the orbit, just below the superior oblique muscle to attach to the medial side of the sclera. In the rostral orbit the superior oblique passes forward, adjacent to the lamina papyracea, to the trochlea (fig. 15) where it bends posterolaterally, at an angle of 55° and pierces Tenon's capsule, passing deep to the superior rectus and inserting behind the equator in the lateral globe. The inferior oblique (fig. 2) arises from the floor of the orbit, lateral to the nasolacrimal duct, and progresses laterally backwards, to curve around the lower lateral quadrant of the posterior sclera.

The ophthalmic artery (fig. 15), in addition to supplying the orbital contents, has several anastomotic relations with branches of the external carotid artery. These may be important sources of collateral flow in cerebral vascular diseases. The lacrimal branch of the ophthalmic artery can anastomose with a branch of the middle meningeal and the deep anterior temporal arteries. The supraorbital branch has anastomoses with the supratrochlear and superficial temporal arteries. The anterior ethmoidal artery gives off the anterior artery of the falx. The nasal branch of the ophthalmic artery has anastomoses with the angular branch of the facial artery. The venous interconnections may provide potential conduits for bacterial agents in infection. The inferior ophthalmic vein receives communications from the veins in the orbital floor, angular vein, superior ophthalmic vein, lower bulbar muscle veins, pterygoid plexus of veins, and the infraorbital vein. The superior ophthalmic vein (fig. 16) originates with the union of the nasofrontal vein and a branch of the supraorbital vein. The ethmoidal veins are branches from the superior orbital vein. The superior and inferior ophthalmic veins usually unite and leave the orbit through the superior orbital fissure and may be major egress points for arterial blood in carotid cavernous fistulae.

Planes of Sections

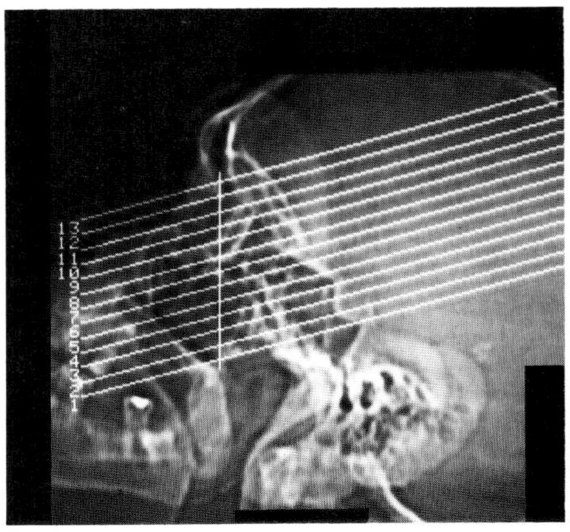

Patient CT Scans

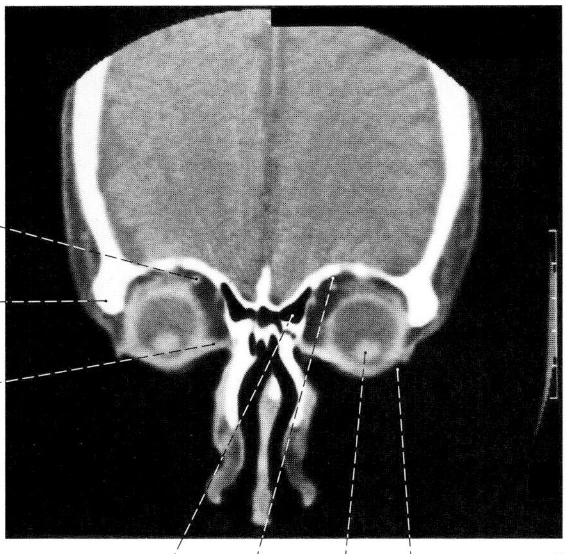

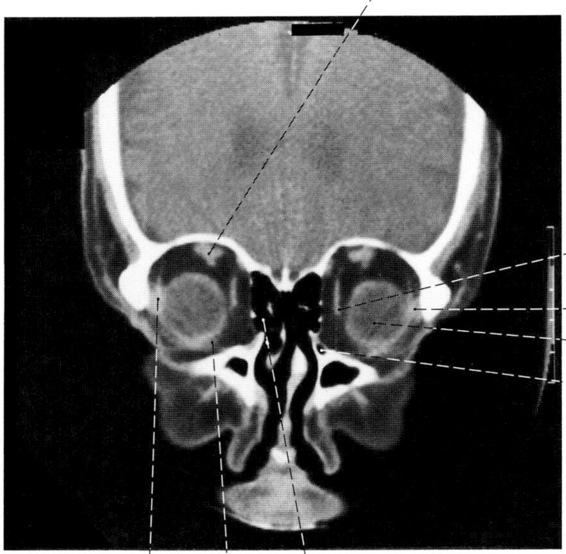

These coronal sections are 5 mm thick with 2 mm overlap. They do not represent true coronal cuts, as there is a limitation on the degree of comfortable extension of the neck within the gantry, and allowances are made for fillings in teeth.

Sinuses are well visualized. The frontal sinuses appear as wing-shaped structures anteriorly (fig. 1). The ethmoidal sinuses are located medial to the orbit below the thin orbital plate of the frontal bone, posterior and inferior to the frontal sinus. Ethmoidal sinusitis may predispose a patient to the development of orbital cellulitus, and sinus masses may impinge on orbital structures. The lamina papyracea is poorly identified in mid-orbital sections with the window settings used (fig. 5). The sphenoidal sinuses lie behind the ethmoidal air cells and anterior to the pituitary fossa. The maxillary sinus is located ventromedially to the orbit above the dental roots. The mid-orbital cut illustrated (fig. 3) passes through the lamina cribosa, the zygomatic and maxillary contributions to the orbital limits, and the infraorbital foramen.

Intraorbital contents visualized include the biconvex lens and cornea, within the globe, and the nasolacrimal duct and lacrimal gland. The optic nerve, noted in the caudal orbit, is best visualized when the patient directs his gaze upward during CT scanning. Optic nerve tumors may appear as enlargement of its diameter or a mass within the muscle cone. The superior ophthalmic vein is superiomedial to the anterior globe on enhanced slices, and the ophthalmic artery is superiolateral to the optic nerve.

The temporalis muscle (fig. 6) and the zygomatic arch buttress the lateral orbital wall. The maxillary artery which may anastomose with the ophthalmic artery courses through the infratemporal fossa. The horizontally inclined vidian canal is medial and inferior to the foramen rotundum. The foramen rotundum, containing the maxillary nerve, passes into the pterygopalatine fossa from the middle cranial fossa.

On coronal slices, the optic chiasm is usually 1 cm above and behind the curvilinear chiasmatic groove, lateral to which are the anterior clinoid processes (fig. 7). The most posterior cut (fig. 8) illustrated passes through the cavernous sinus, anterior hypophyseal fossa, and the cavernous portion of the internal carotid artery.

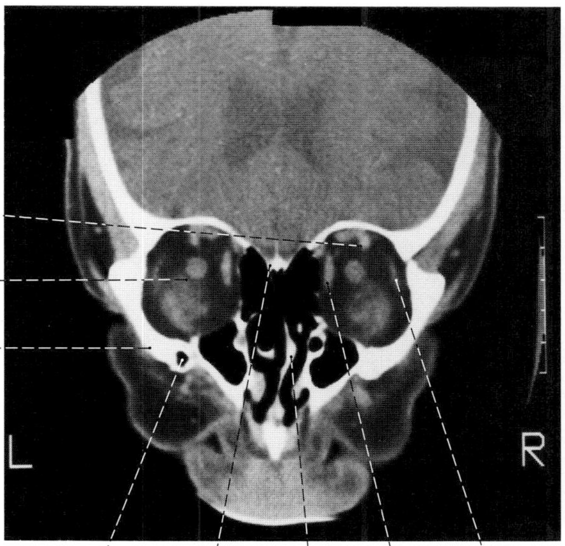
Superior rectus muscle and levator palpebrae superioris
Optic Nerve (II)
Maxillary bone
Infraorbital foramen
Cribriform plate
Nasal septum
Superior oblique muscle
Lateral rectus muscle
L
R

3

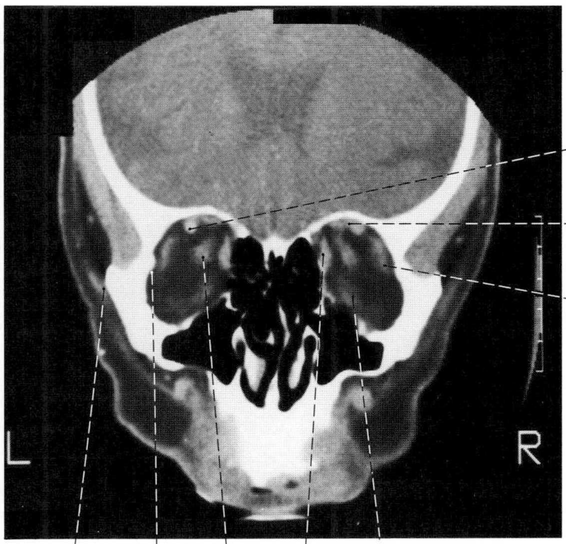
Superior ophthalmic vein
Superior rectus muscle
Lateral rectus muscle
Zygomatic tubercle
Inferior orbital tubercle
Optic nerve
Superior oblique muscle
Inferior rectus muscle
L
R

4

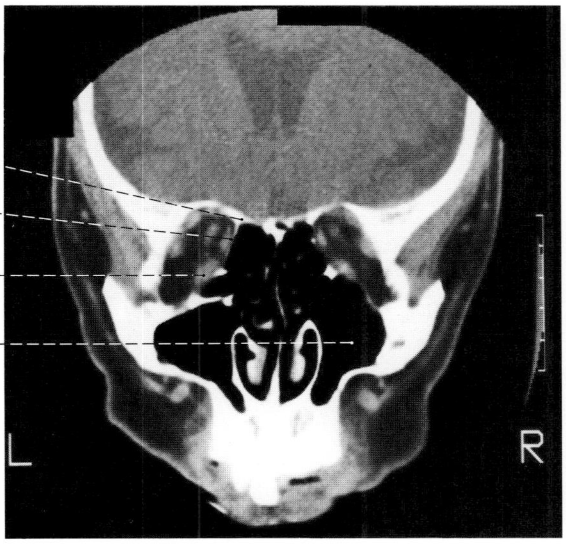
Planum sphenoidale
Lamina papyracea
Inferior rectus muscle
Maxillary sinus
L
R

5

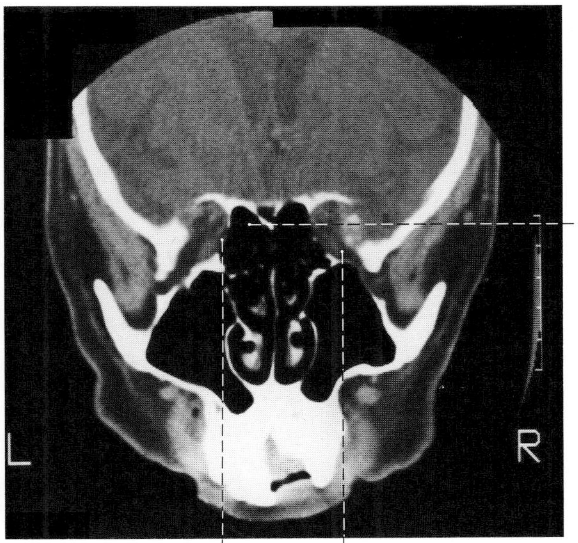
Sphenoid sinus
Medial orbital wall
Inferior orbital fissure
L
R

6

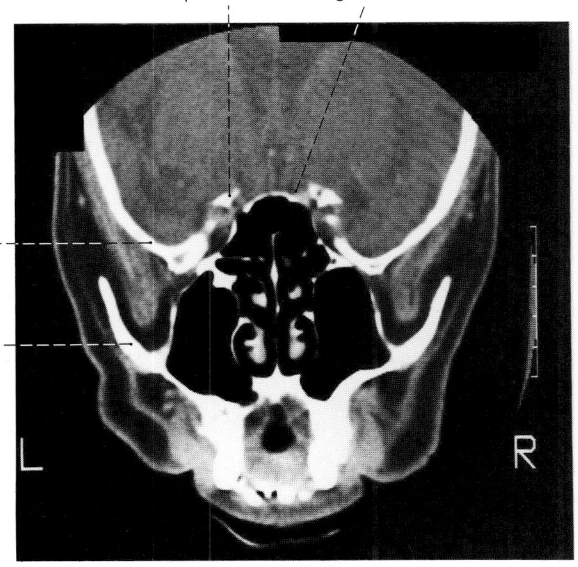
Anterior clinoid process
Chiasmatic groove
Greater wing of sphenoid bone
Zygoma
L
R

7

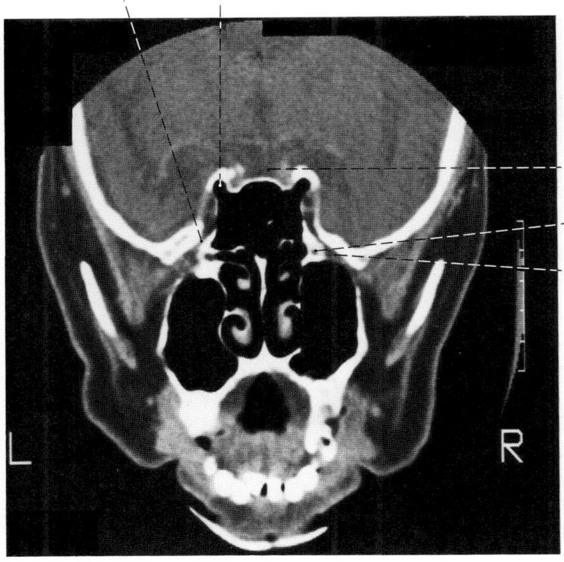
Superior orbital fissure
Sphenoid sinus in anterior clinoid process
Hypophyseal fossa
Vidian canal
Pterygopalatine fossa
L
R

8

Axial CT of the Orbit

Planes of Sections

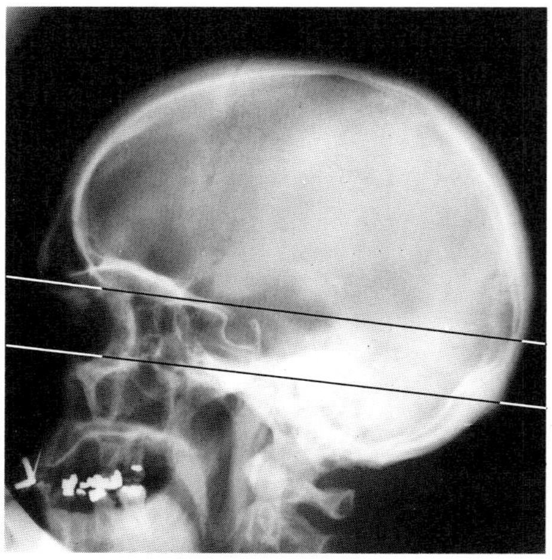

Patient CT Scans

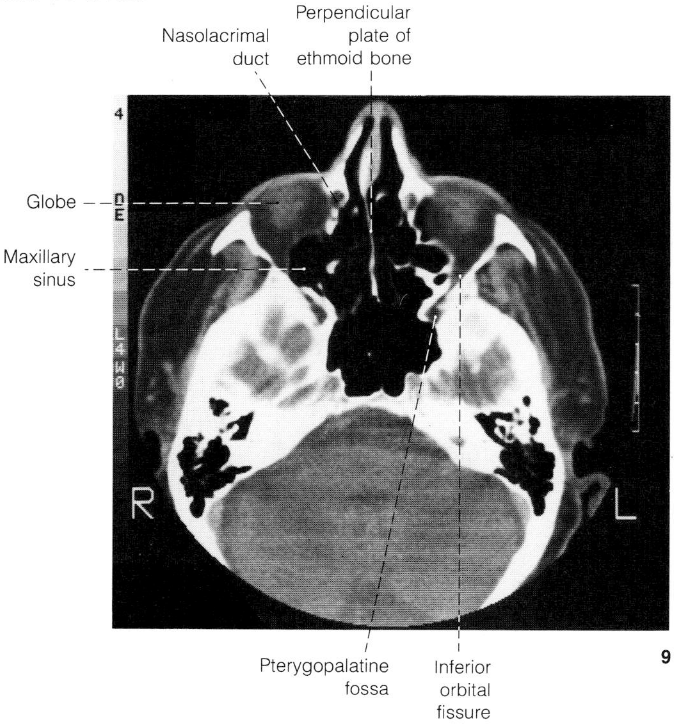

9

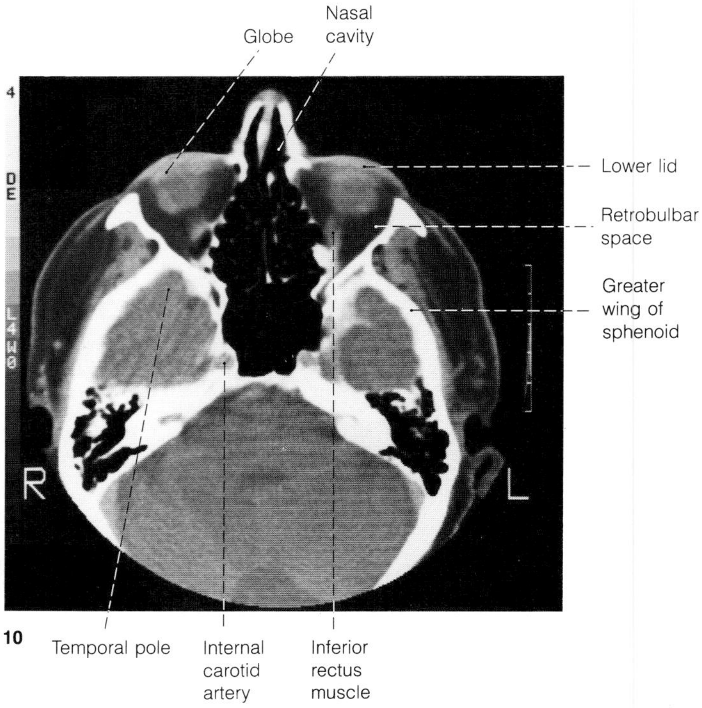

10

The axial sections are 5 mm thick with 2 mm overlap. These produce good spatial resolution and are expeditious, although thinner slices yield less volume averaging. Intraorbital vessels, optic nerve, and muscles are particularly well delineated. The optic nerve is highlighted in the retrobulbar fat. Increased retrobulbar fat, soft tissue deposits, and enlargement of the rectus muscles (usually unilateral) can be a consequence of an inflammatory or infectious process. The globe and lens are well defined within the orbit. The ophthalmic artery (fig. 15), after entering the orbit, usually ascends lateral to the optic nerve and gives off the lacrimal artery. The superior ophthalmic vein crosses the optic nerve, and lies above the ophthalmic artery. The posterior clinoid, supraclinoid internal carotid artery, and pentagonal cistern are evident (fig. 16) behind the orbit. The superior oblique, trochlea, and insertional tendon are seen in the slice below (fig. 15), at the level of the dorsum sella. The anterior clinoid processes are penetrated by sphenoid air cells. The sieve-like lamina cribosa, the lowest part of the floor of the anterior cranial fossa, is bisected by the crista galli (fig. 15). Suprasellar and parasellar masses, such as tumor or aneurysm, may extend to compromise the optic nerve or chiasm. The optic canal, a rounded aperture in the middle cranial fossa, is separated from the sphenoid sinus by only a thin plate of bone (fig. 14). The inferior orbital fissure (fig. 9) is seen at the level of its conduit to the pterygopalatine fossa (fig. 9). The rounded, widened portion of the superior orbital fissure is inferolateral to the optic canal (fig. 13).

The cavernous sinuses are between and below the medial and lateral petroclinoid ligaments. Pathology within the sinus may lead to sixth nerve palsy, as cranial nerve VI courses through the sinus just lateral to the internal carotid artery. Compression of the sinus wall may lead to compromise of the trochlear (IV), oculomotor (III), and ophthalmic (V_1) and maxillary (V_2) divisions of the trigeminal nerve.

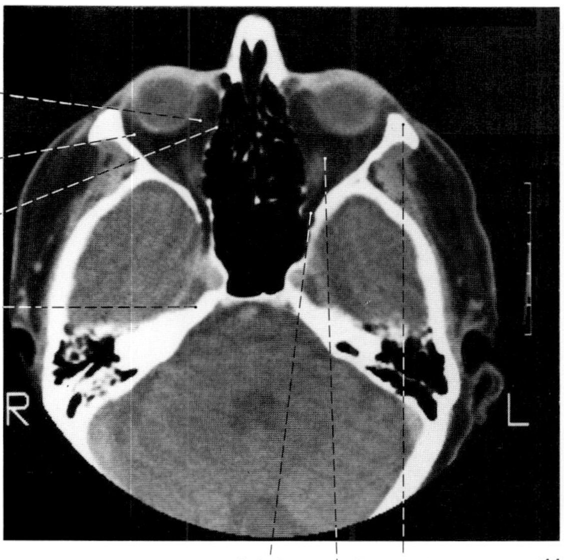

11

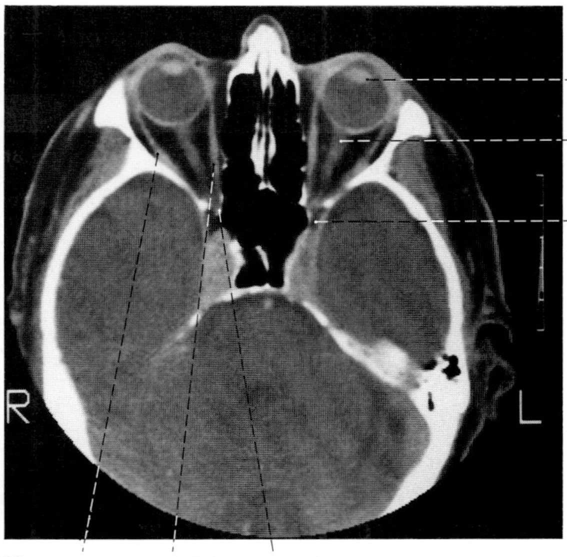

12

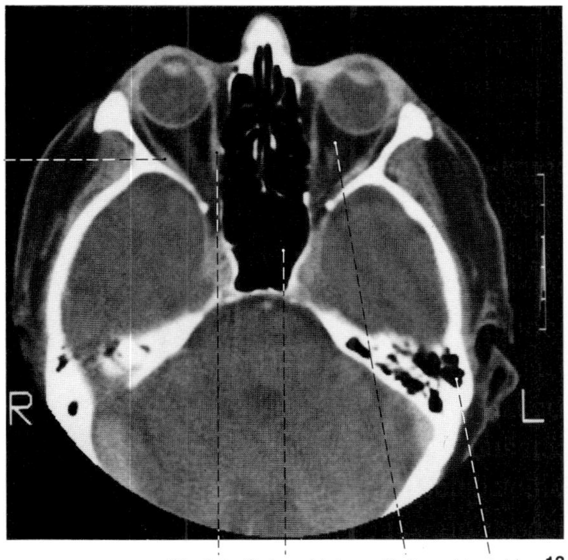

13

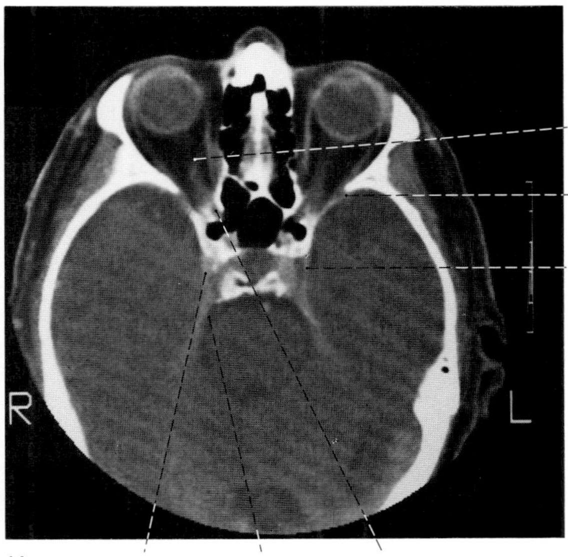

14

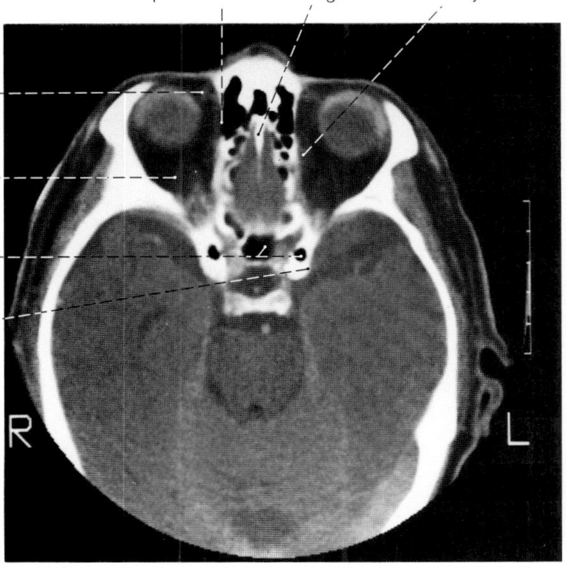

15

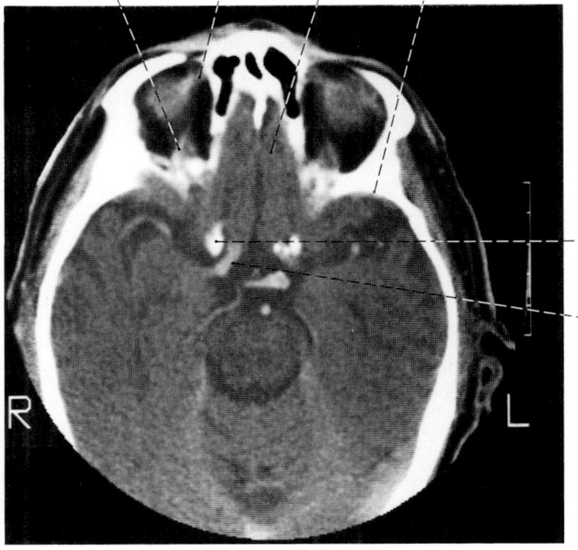

16

Selected Bibliography

Bossi, R. and Pisan, C. Collateral cerebral circulation through the ophthalmic artery. *British Journal of Radiology* 28: 462–469, 1955.

Forbes, G. Computed tomography of the orbit. *Radiological Clinics of North America* 20: 37–42, March 1982.

Grant, J. C. B. *An Atlas of Anatomy,* 6th ed. The Williams and Wilkins Co., Baltimore, 1972.

Hollinshead, W. H. *Textbook of Anatomy*. Harper and Row, Hagerstown, Maryland, 1967.

Jacobs, L. and Weisberg. *Computerized Tomography of the Orbit and Sella Turcica*. Raven Press, New York, 1980.

Meschan, Isadore. *An Atlas of Anatomy Basic to Radiology*. W. B. Saunders Co., Philadelphia, 1975.

Schnitzlein, H. N., Hartley, E. W., Murtagh, R. *Computerized Tomography of the Head and Spine*. Urban and Schwarzenberg, Baltimore, 1983.

Wolff, E. *Anatomy of the Eye and Orbit,* 7th ed. W. B. Saunders Co., Philadelphia, 1978.

Temporal Bone

C. P. Shah, M.D.

With the development of high resolution computed tomography capable of visualizing delicate bony structures previously inaccessible without surgery in patients, the detailed anatomy of the temporal bone has assumed a broader clinical importance. Computed tomography is able to routinely demonstrate such structures as the tympanic membrane, epitympanic recess, ossicles, aditus ad antrum, mastoid air cells, cochlea, vestibule, semicircular canals, round and oval windows, and internal auditory canal. Scans also demonstrate the course of the facial nerve and relationships of the carotid artery and jugular vein within the temporal bone.

The complex structural relations are usually better displayed and understood with images obtained in the axial and coronal planes which are widely used clinically. Oblique variations of these planes, however, may be on occasion advantageous to demonstrate certain anatomical structures or pathological processes.

The superficial gross anatomical features of the temporal bone are illustrated on pages 210 and 211. Selected axial planes are compared with color photographs of comparable anatomical slices on pages 212–221. A complete series of axial CT images of the right temporal bone of an adult patient are arranged on pages 222–223. Coronal CT scans are compared with gross anatomical specimens on pages 224–227 and a series of coronal CT scans of an adult patient are found on pages 228–229.

Lateral View

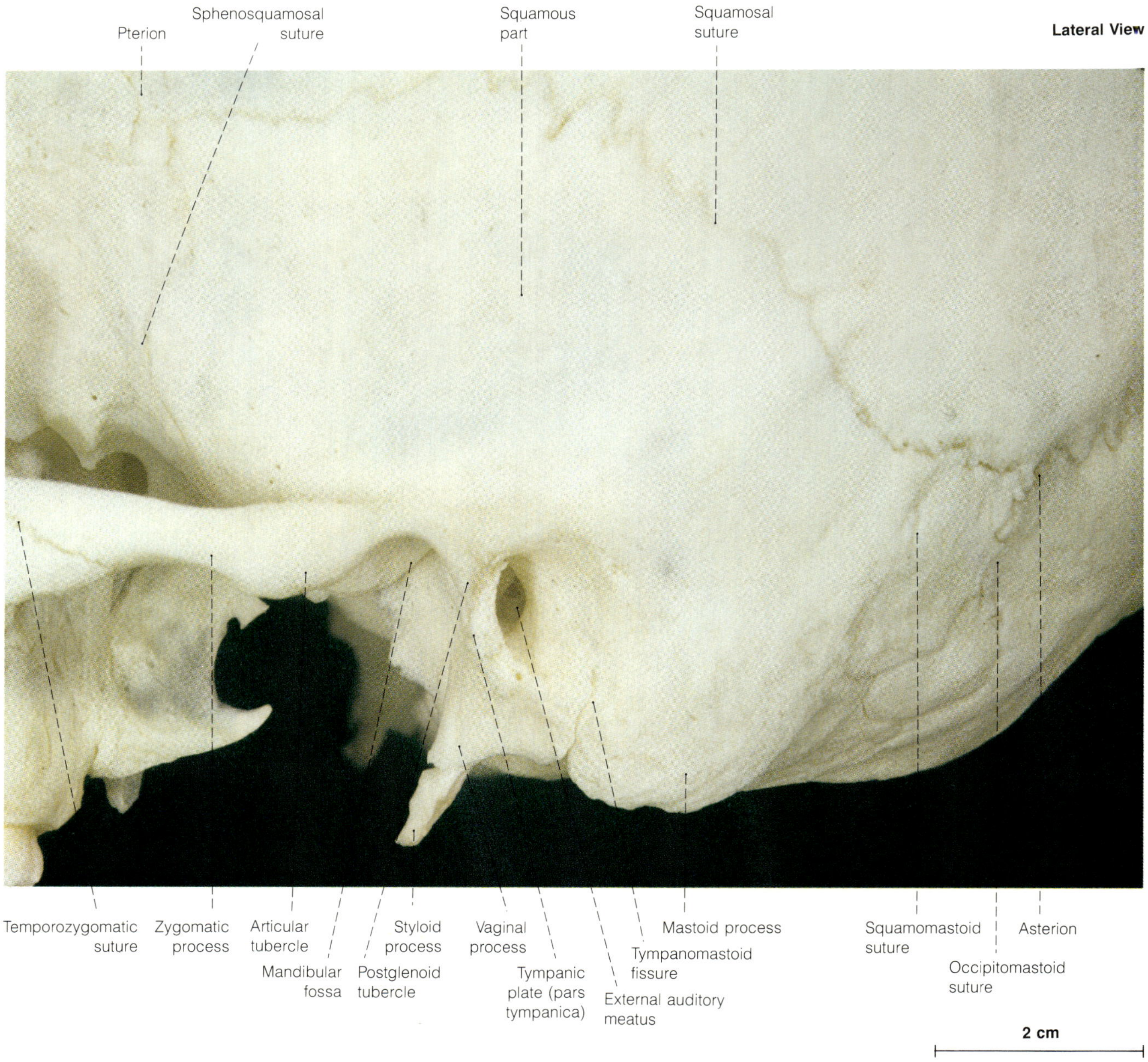

The temporal bone is usually described as consisting of *squamous, mastoid,* and *petrosal* portions. These lateral, superior and inferior views of a skull illustrate its external markings and bony articulations.

Superior View

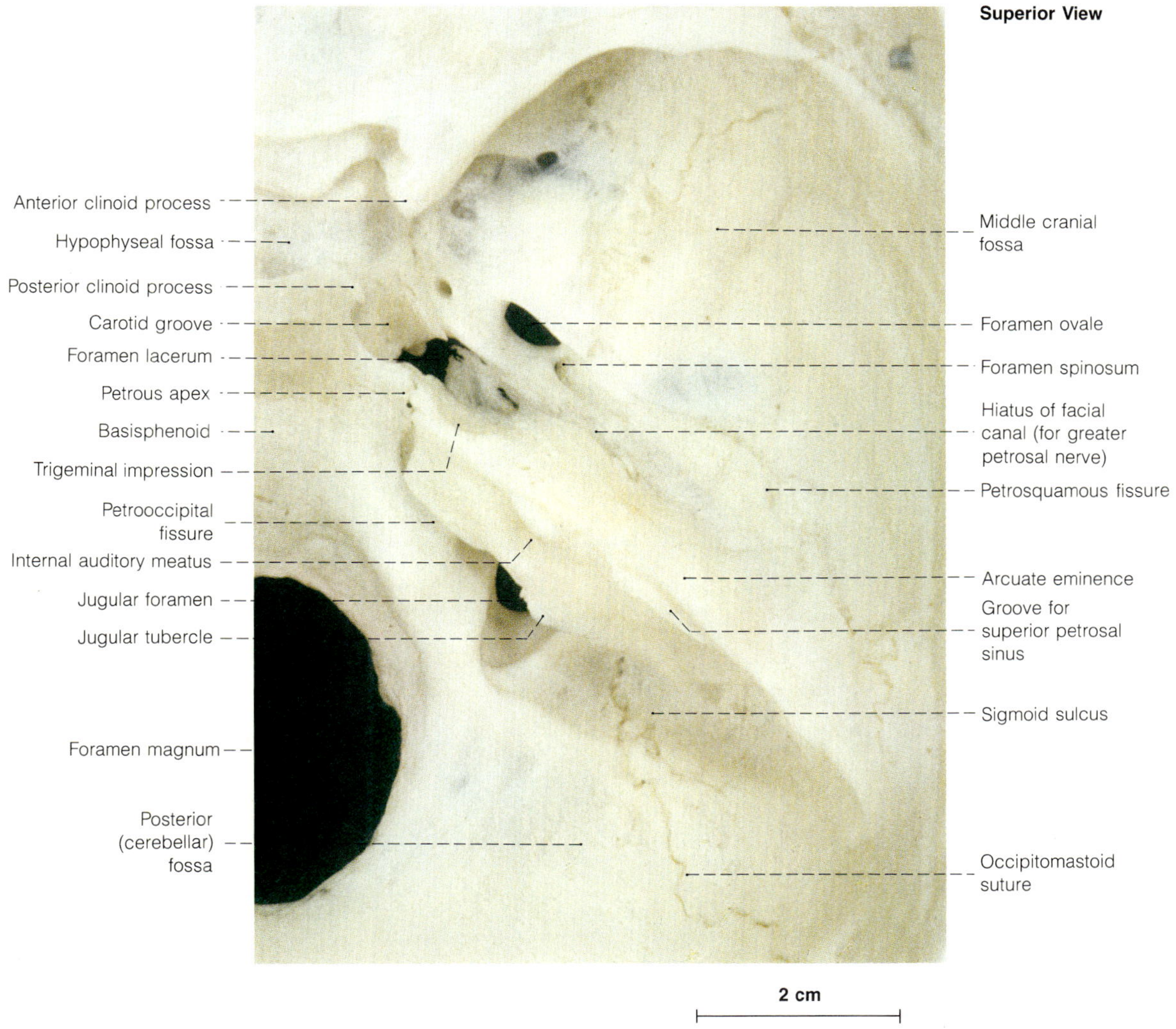

Inferior View

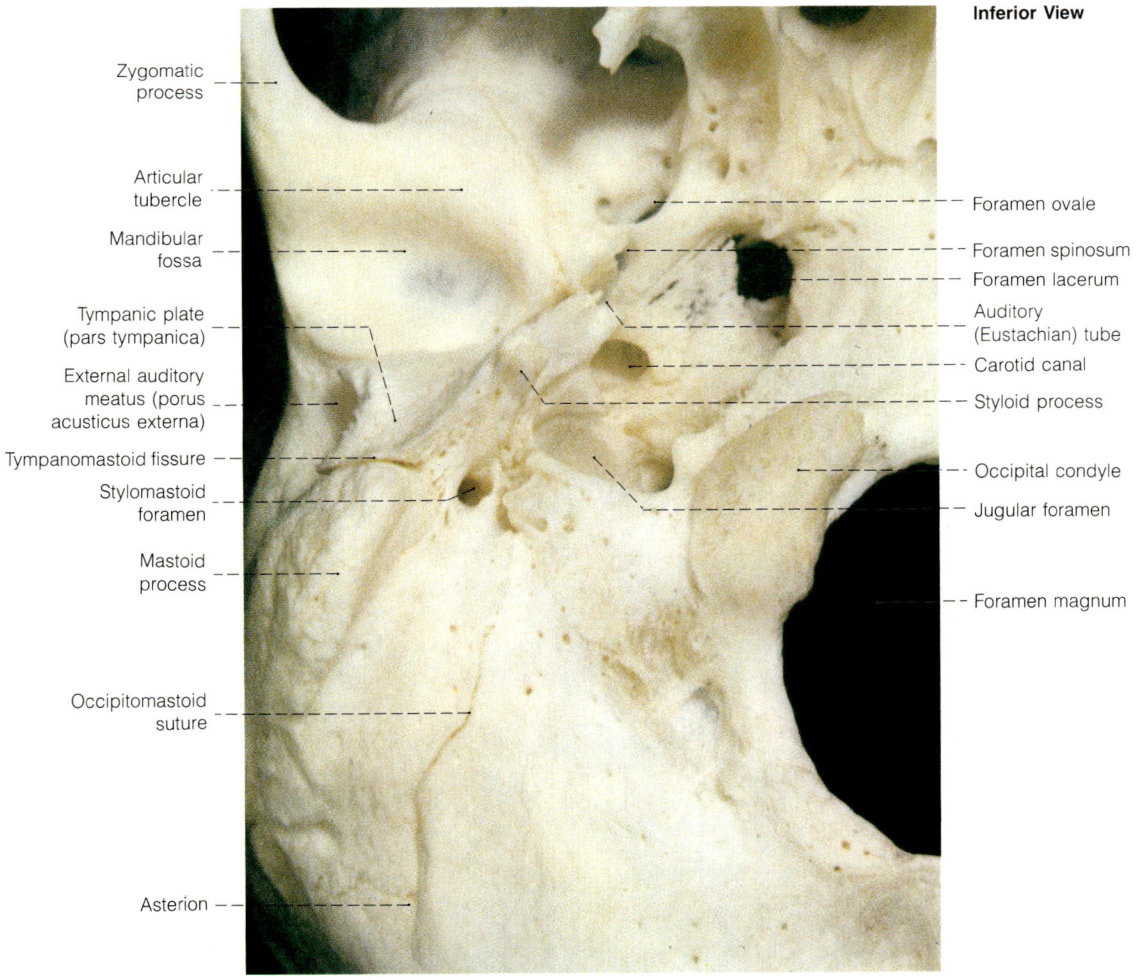

Patient CT Scan

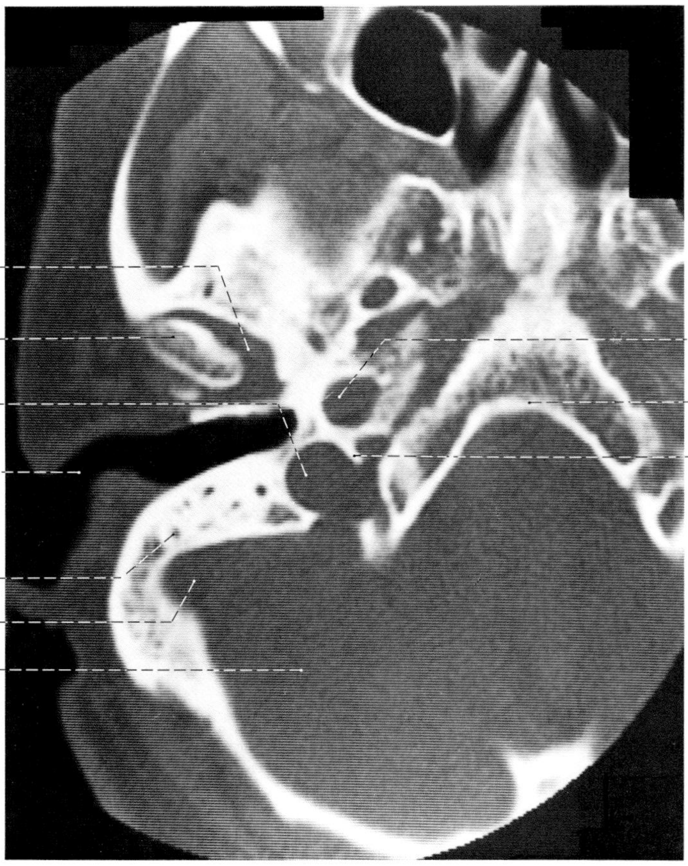

This 1.5 mm thick axial CT section of an adult right temporal bone passes through its inferior portion at the level of the external auditory canal as indicated on the "scout" view. The gross anatomical photograph is in a comparable plane and is also viewed from below.

The external auditory canal directed medially and slightly antero-superiorly is approximately 2.5 cm in length in an adult. This cylindrical canal is completely surrounded by tympanic bone except superiorly where it is covered by squamous temporal bone. The temporo-mandibular articulation (T-M joint) constitutes its anterior relationship and the mastoid process and air cells (sinus) are adjacent posteriorly. Medially the tympanic membrane separates the external canal from the tympanic (middle ear) cavity.

The jugular bulb (fossa) lies medial to the mastoid portion of the temporal bone. The complete bony margin of the fossa may be visualized with CT with only a thin bony plate separating it from the middle ear cavity. Antero-medial to the jugular fossa lies the carotid canal. They are separated by the carotico-jugular spine. This plane also demonstrates the close proximity of the mastoid air cells (sinus) with the sigmoid sinus and other posterior fossa structures, especially the cerebellar hemisphere. Erosion of the mastoid by a pathological process resulting in a cerebellar abscess is easily visualized in these normal anatomical illustrations.

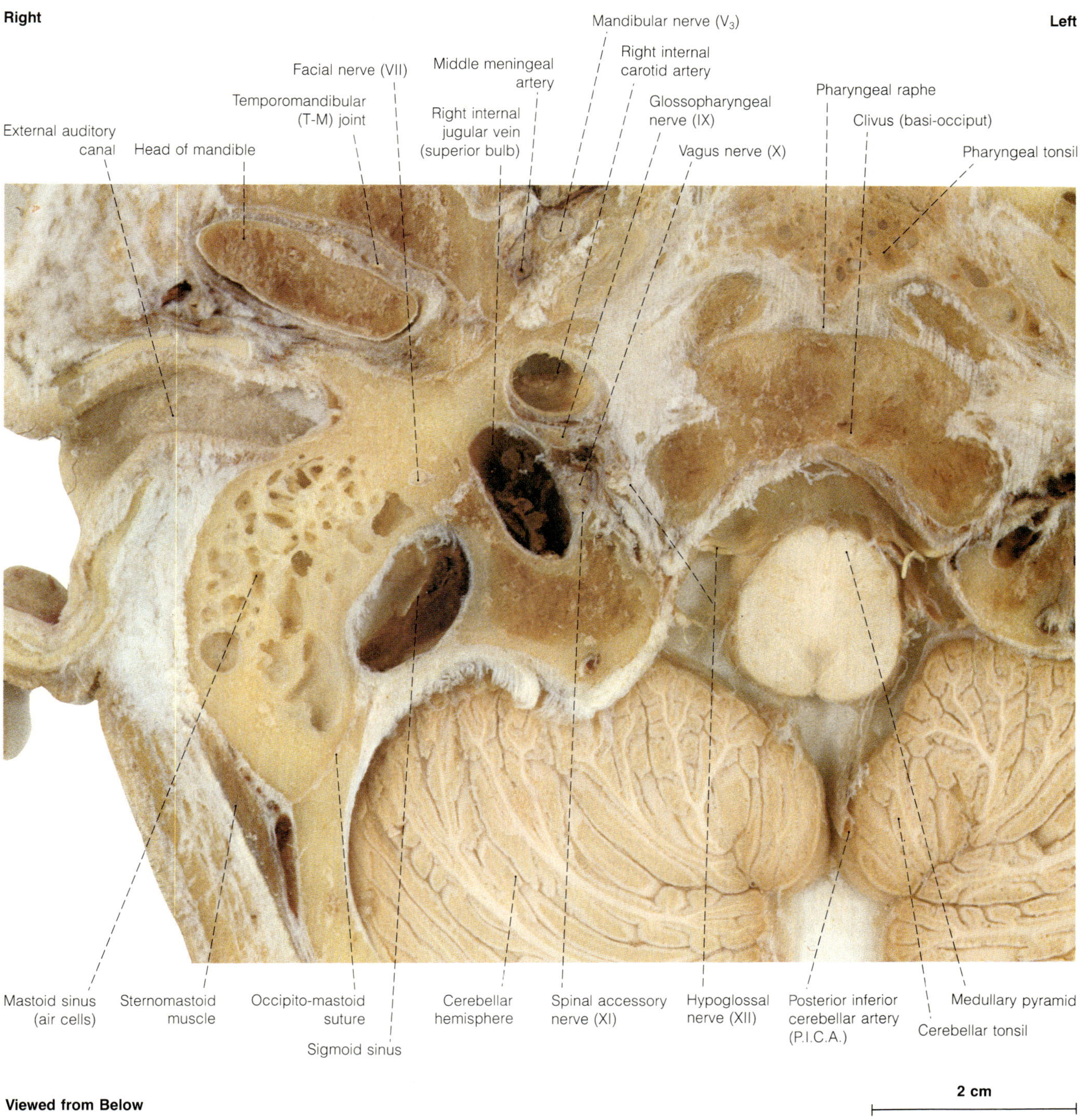

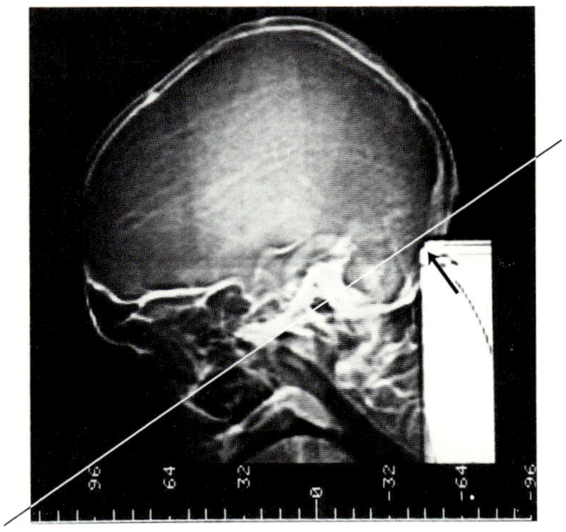

Plane of Section

Cadaver CT Scan

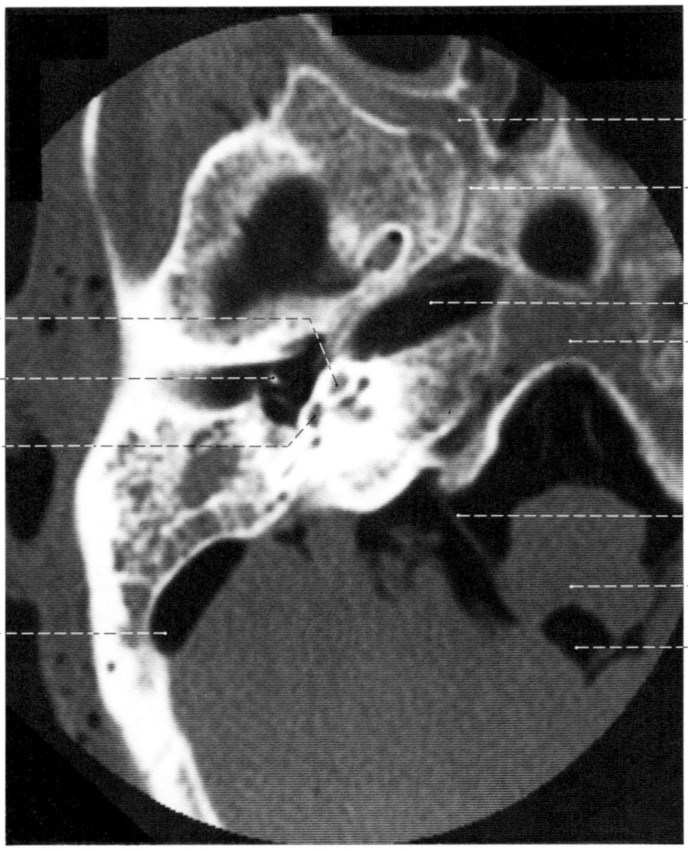

Right

Patient CT Scan

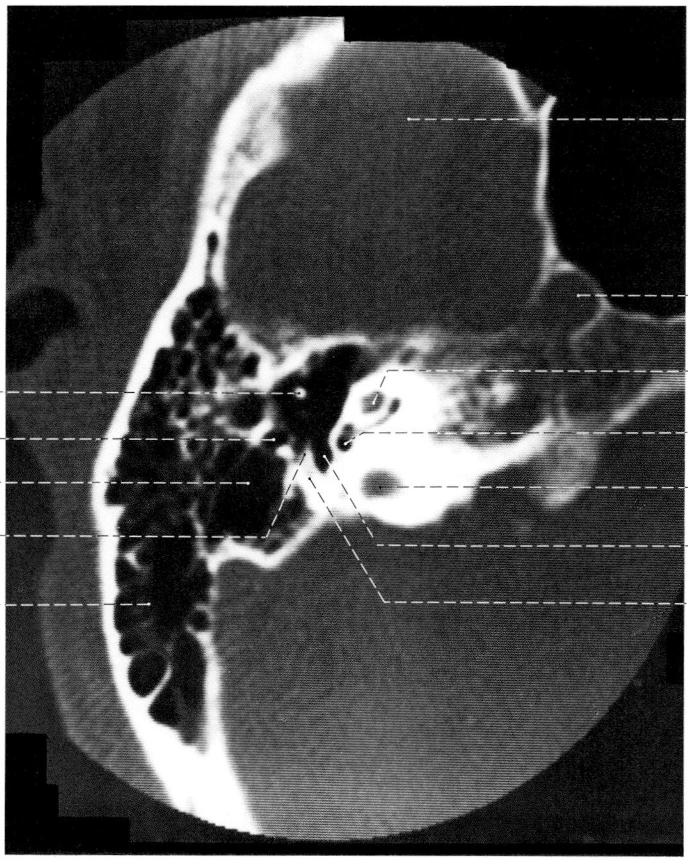

Right

These figures are approximately 5 mm superior to those illustrated on pages 212 and 213. The patient axial CT scan is 1.5 mm thick.

The middle ear is divided into the mesotympanum, the epitympanum (the epitympanic recess), and the hypotympanum. The mesotympanum is the region of the middle ear cavity directly contiguous with the tympanic membrane. The ossicles for the most part lie in the epitympanic recess. The handle of the malleus and long process of the incus, however, extend downward into the mesotympanum. The epitympanic recess communicates with the mastoid antrum and air cells via the aditus ad antrum.

Anteriorly the middle ear cavity has two openings, the Eustachian (auditory or pharyngotympanic) tube and the semicanal for the tensor tympani muscle (see also page 222). These structures are parallel and adjacent to the carotid canal which lies more medially. The semicanal is immediately lateral and superior to the Eustachian tube and is separated from it by a bony septum.

The promontory, the labyrinthine capsule covering the basal (or 1st) turn of cochlea, forms the medial wall of the middle ear. The round window's niche (fenestra rotunda) is slightly dorsal to the basal turn of the cochlea. Immediately posterior and lateral to the

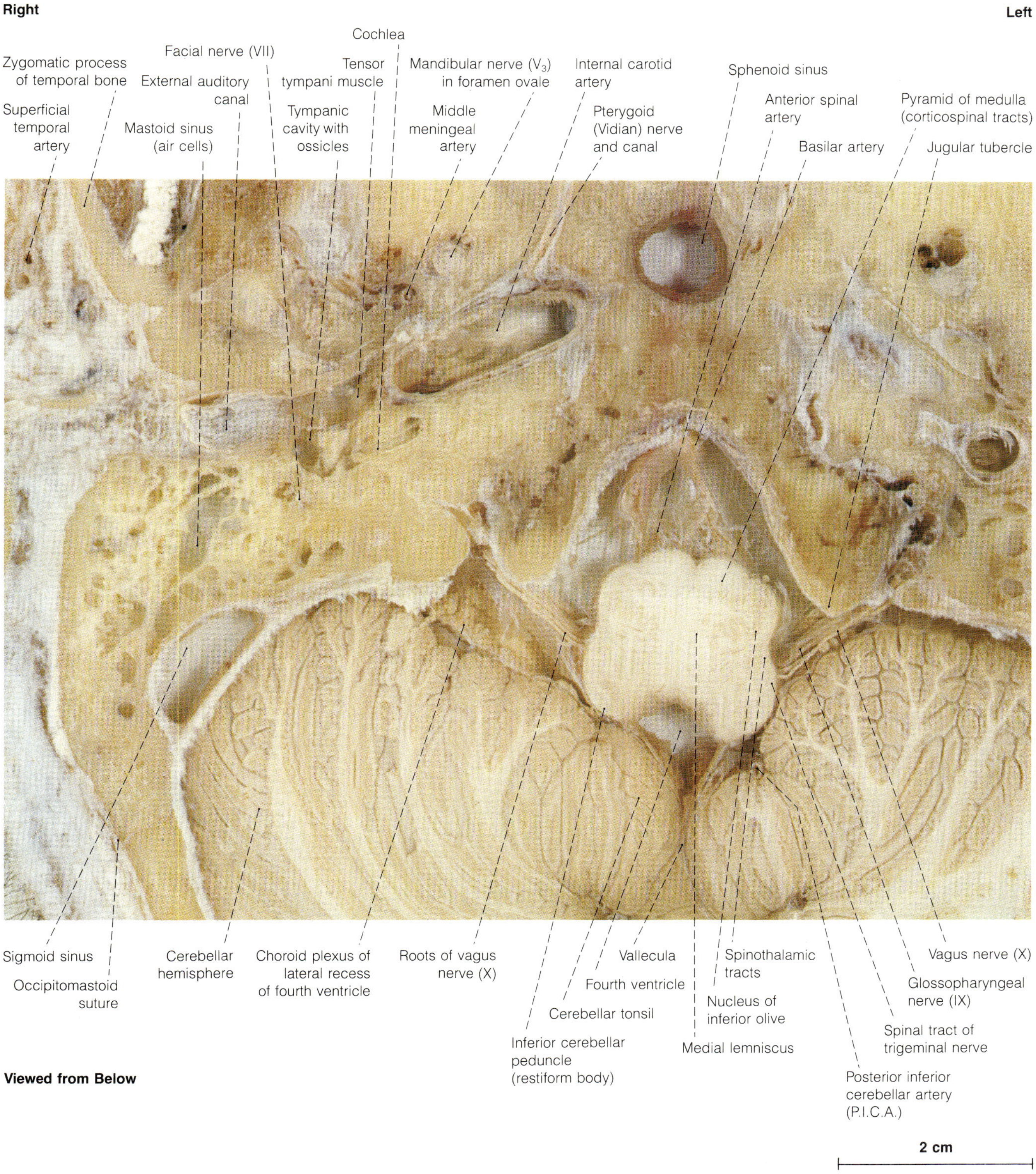

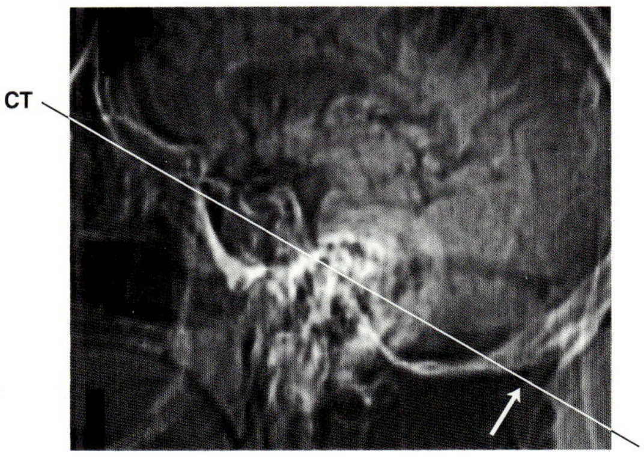

Plane of Section

basal turn of the cochlea is the sinus tympani. Lateral to the sinus tympani is the pyramidal eminence. Behind the pyramidal eminence lies the vertical segment of the facial nerve in the facial canal.

The dome of the jugular fossa is postero-inferior to the cochlea. Just medial to the jugular fossa lies the cochlear aqueduct. Additional important relationships can be visualized on adjacent 1.5 mm CT scans illustrated on page 222.

Cadaver CT Scan

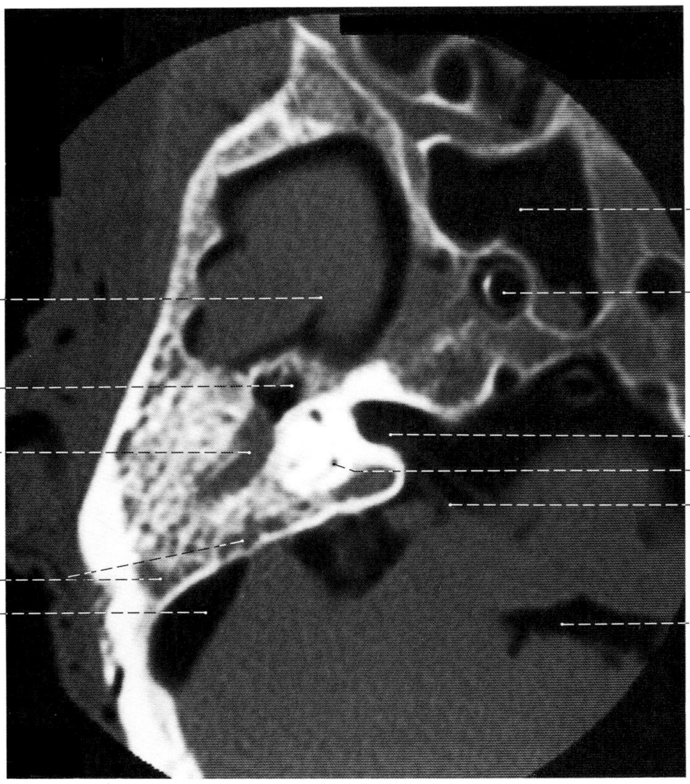

Patient CT Scan

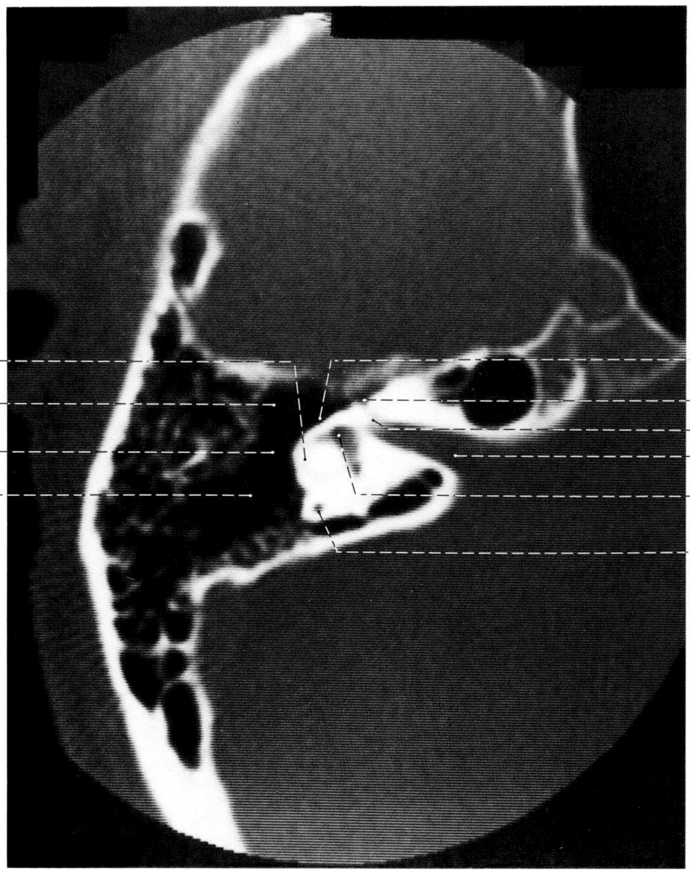

These figures are approximately 5 mm superior to those illustrated on pages 214 and 215. The patient CT scan is a 1.5 mm thick axial section of an adult right temporal bone. Mastoid air cells surround the mastoid antrum and extend lateral to the epitympanic recess. The posterior semicircular canal extends postero-laterally from the crus commune. The entire lateral semicircular canal is visualized in this axial plane. It opens into the vestible and forms the medial wall of the aditus ad antrum.

The cochlea lies anterior to the fundus of the internal auditory canal (or meatus). The facial and superior vestibular nerves occupy the anterior and posterior compartments respectively of the superior portion of internal auditory canal. The cochlear and inferior vestibular nerves lie in the anterior and posterior compartments respectively of the inferior portion of the internal auditory canal.

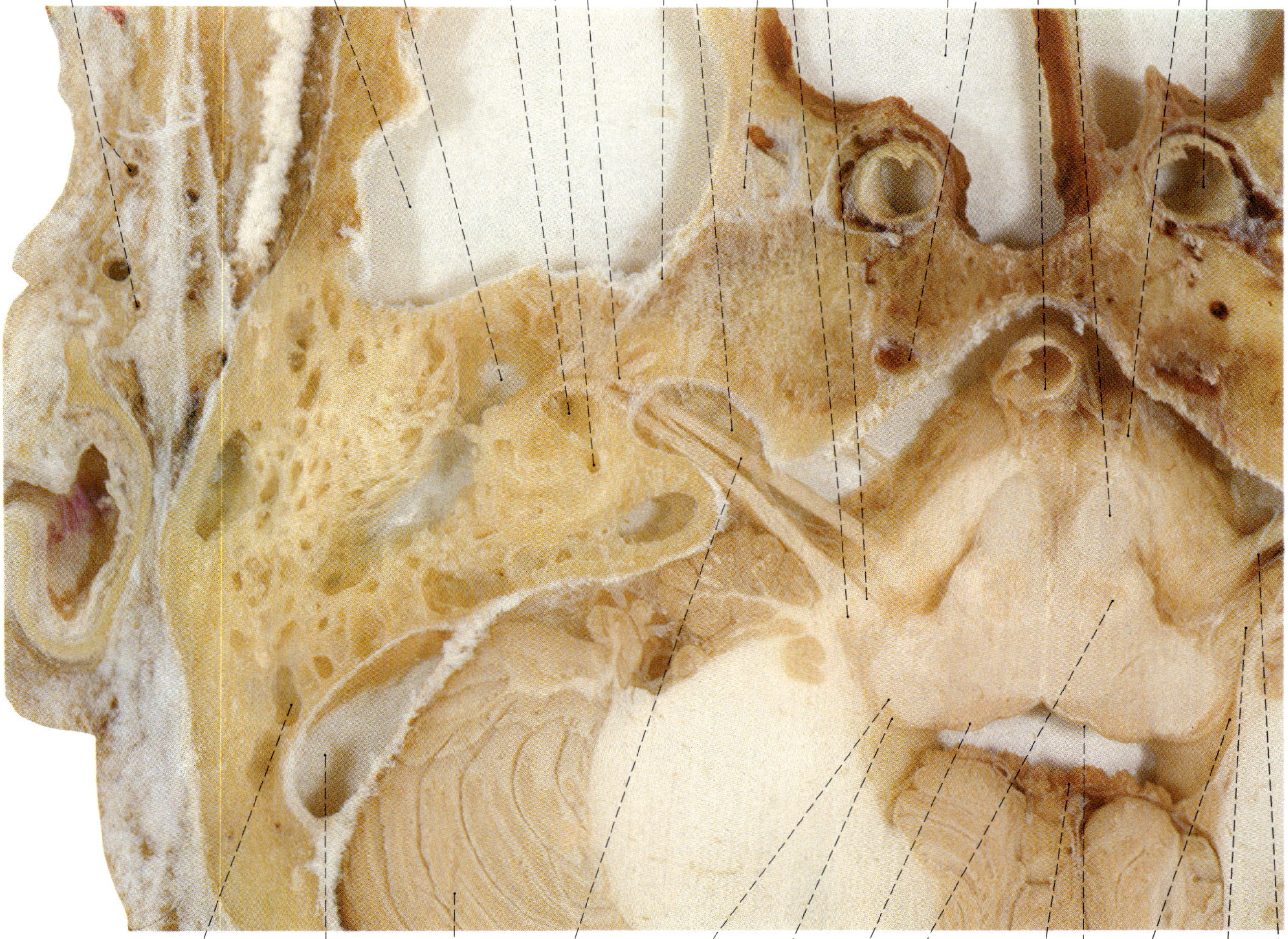

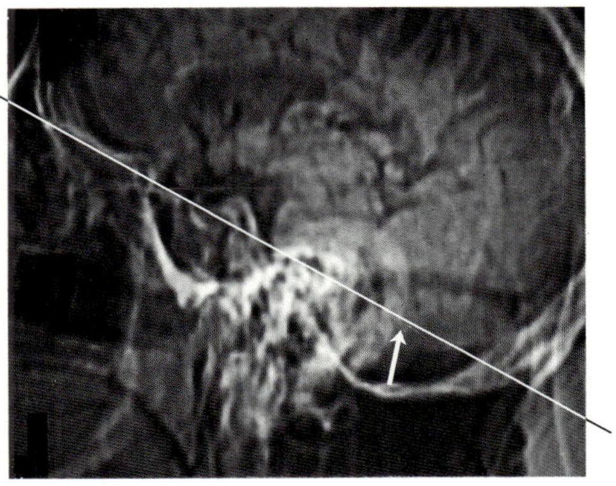

Plane of Section

The first part of the facial nerve begins at the fundus of the internal auditory canal (in its antero-superior compartment). It courses antero-laterally superior to the cochlea and ends at the geniculate ganglion where the facial nerve makes a hairpin turn and courses postero-laterally along the medial wall of middle ear cavity to the pyramidal eminence. This constitutes the second part of the facial nerve. Posterior to the pyramidal eminence the facial canal turns sharply downward (vertical segment) to exit via the stylomastoid foramen. The vertical segment of the facial canal may be difficult to identify in the axial plane due to surrounding mastoid air cells but is well visualized in coronal or sagittal planes (figure 3, page 228).

Cadaver CT Scan

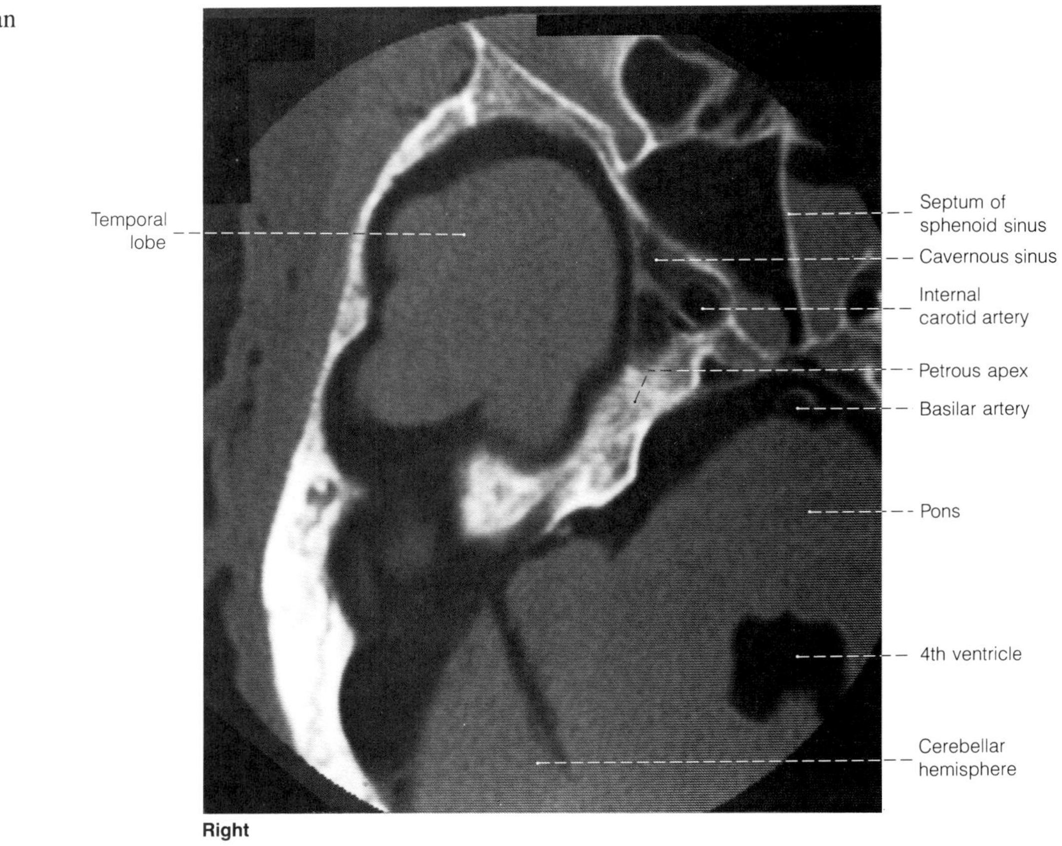

Patient CT Scan

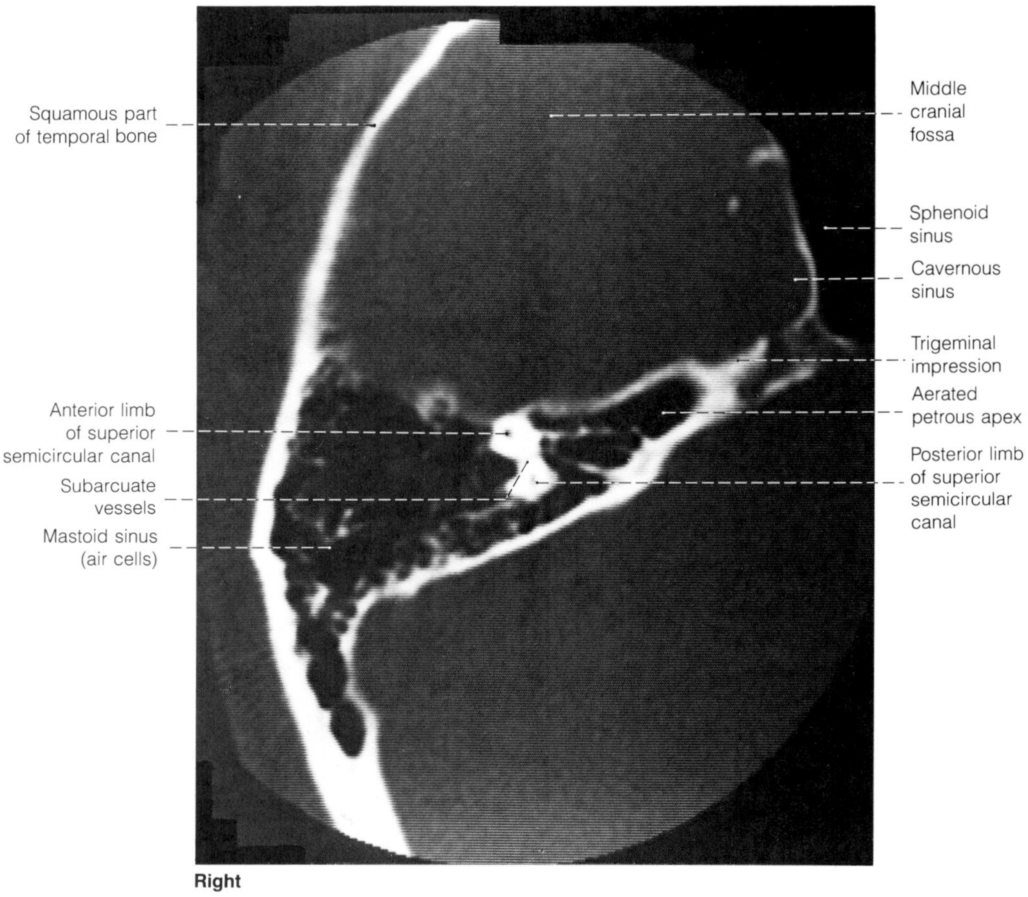

These figures in the axial plane are approximately 5 mm above those illustrated on pages 216–217. The scan of the patient is a 1.5 mm thick axial section of an adult right temporal bone passing above the level of the epitympanic recess and mastoid antrum.

The mastoid air cells (sinus) occupy the major portion of the section. Note that the aeration extends medially in this individual to involve the petrous apex but may not be so extensive in other patients. The close relationship of these air cells to the middle and posterior cranial fossa and the potential for mastoid pathology to extend into temporal lobe and cerebellum is clearly illustrated.

The anterior and posterior limbs of the superior semicircular canal are near the center of the petrous part of the temporal bone. The subarcuate vessels pass between these limbs of the superior semicircular canal.

The sigmoid sinus lies postero-lateral to the mastoid air cells and the trigeminal impression for the semilunar (Gasserian or trigeminal) ganglion is located anteriomedial to the aerated petrous apex in the patient illustrated.

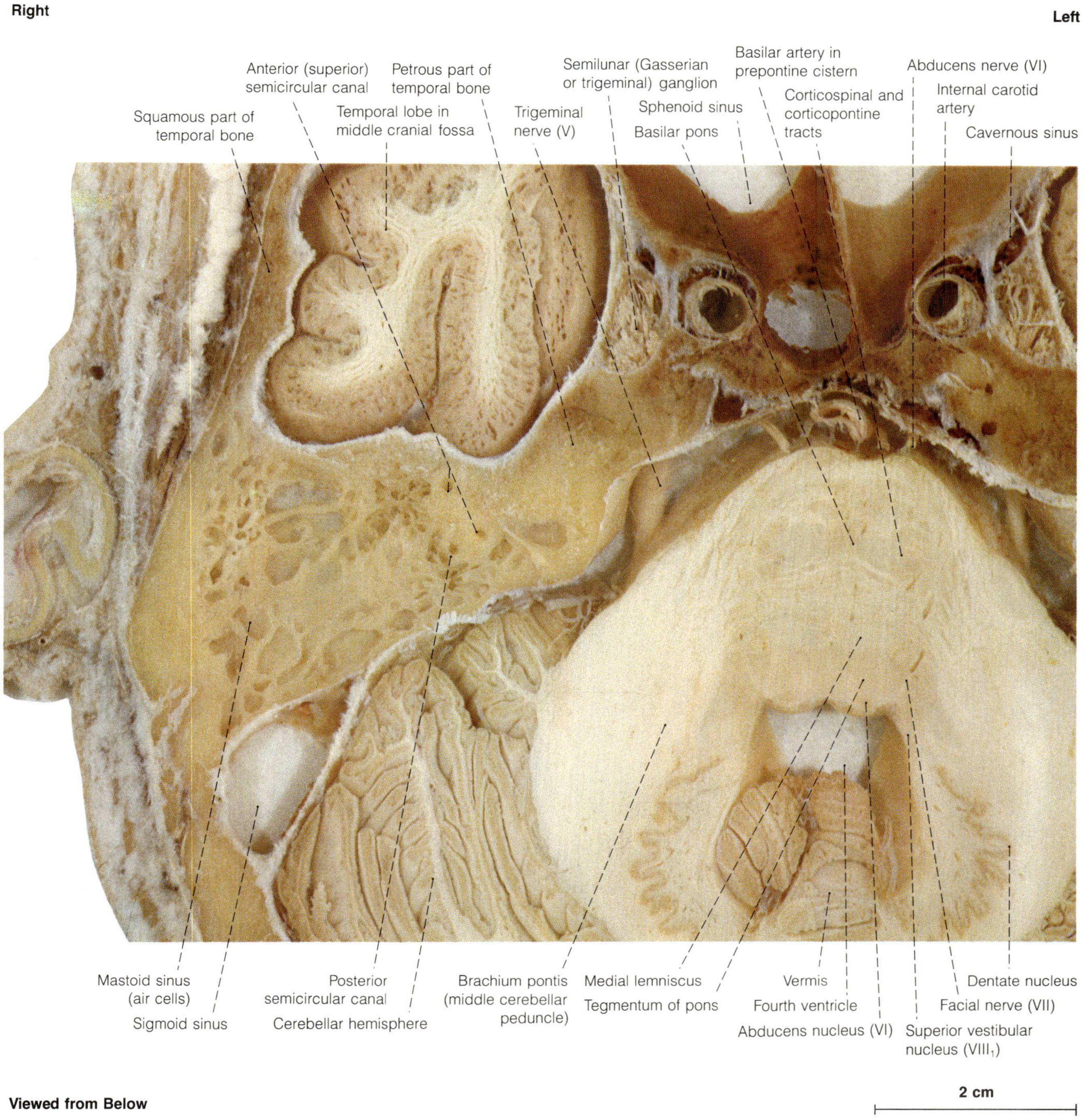

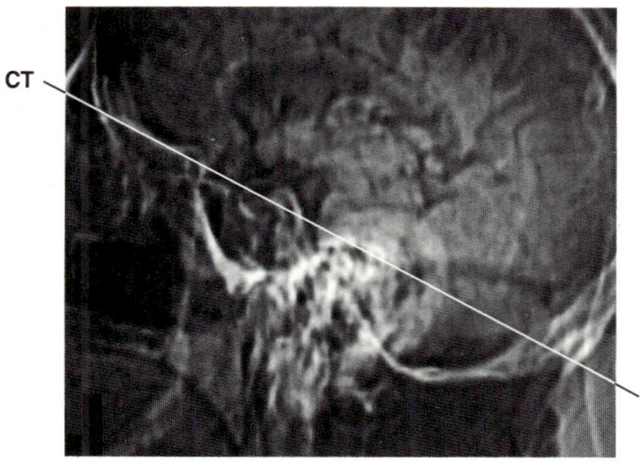

Plane of Section

Patient CT Scan

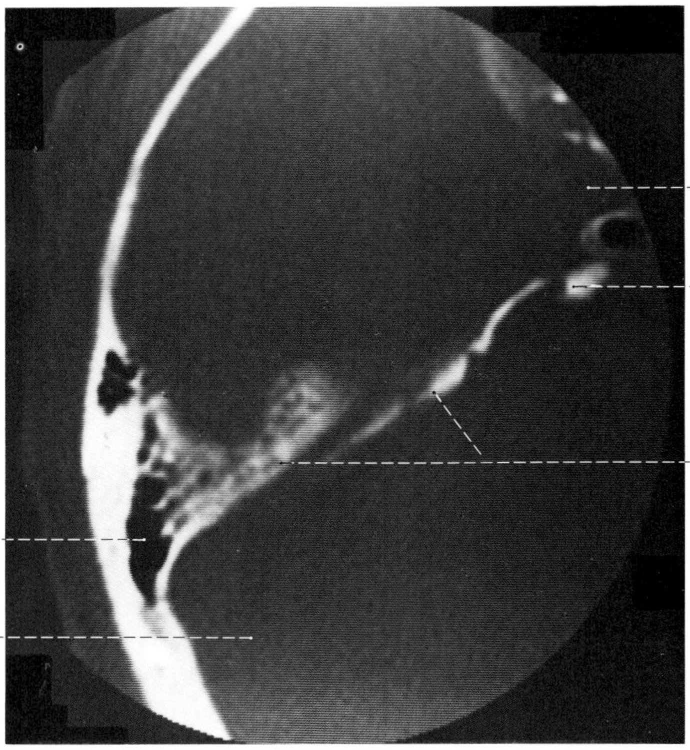

Right

These figures are approximately 5 mm above those illustrated on pages 218–219. The CT section is 1.5 mm thick of an adult temporal bone passing through the apex of the petrous bone and attachment of the tentorium cerebelli; the superior petrosal venous sinus parallels this apex as it passes from the cavernous sinus to the sigmoid sinus. In planes superior to those illustrated, the temporal lobe is separated from the cerebellum by the tentorium.

Right **Left**

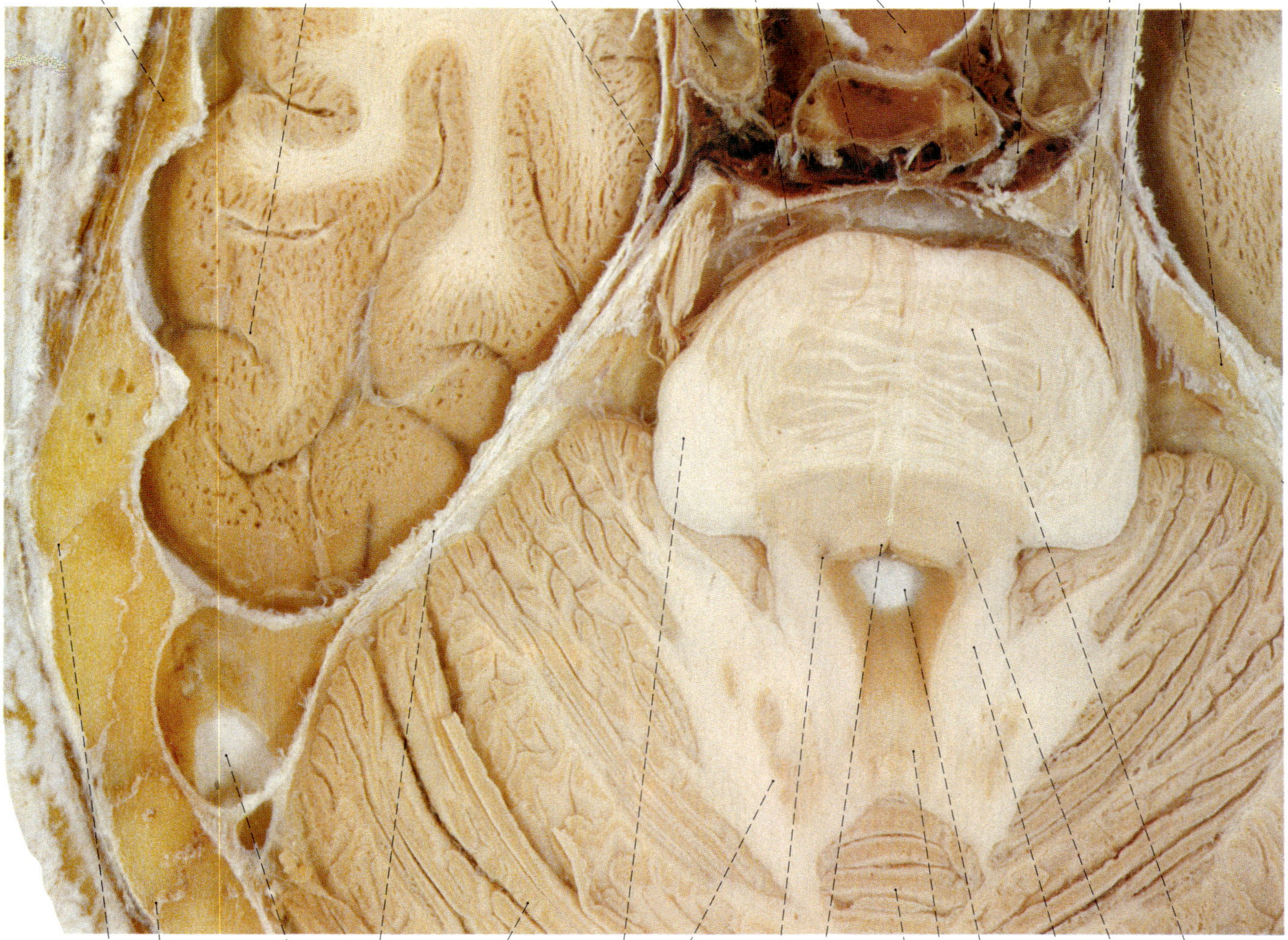

Viewed from Below

2 cm

Plane of Section

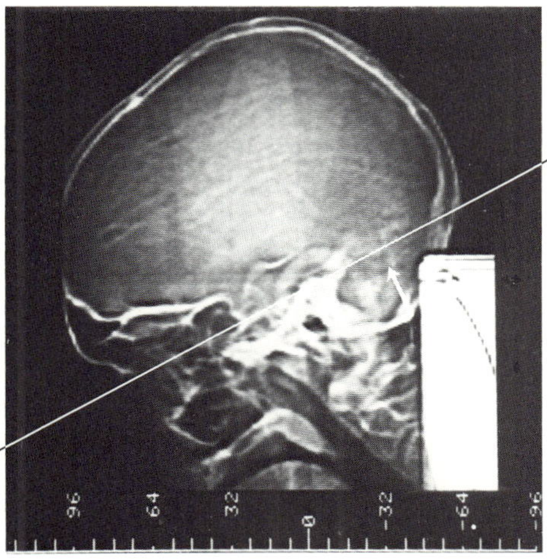

Planes of Sections

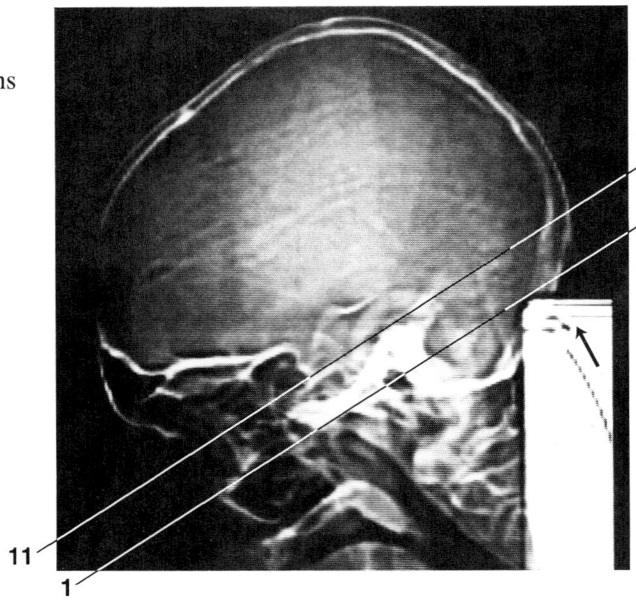

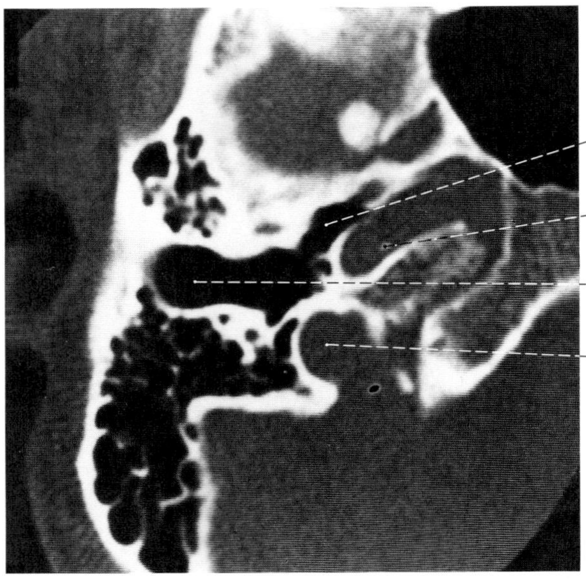

1

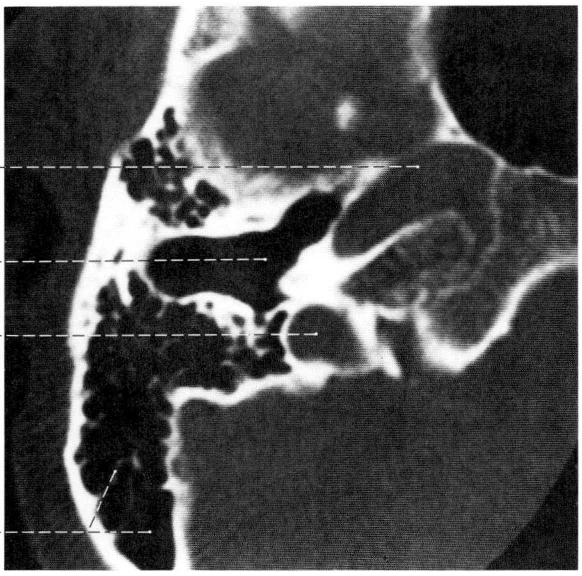

2

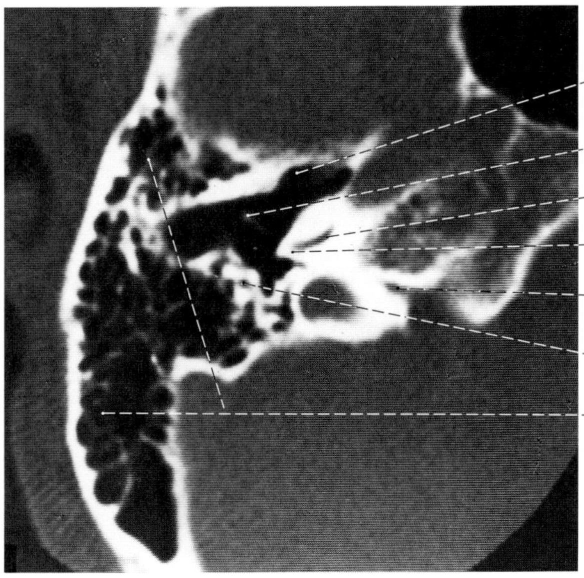

3

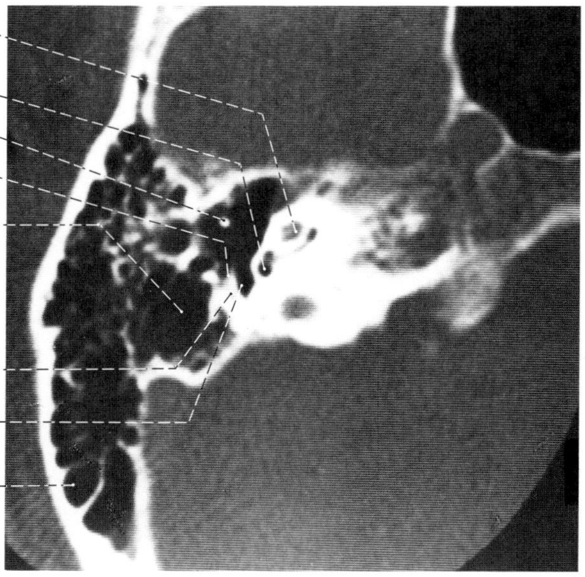

4

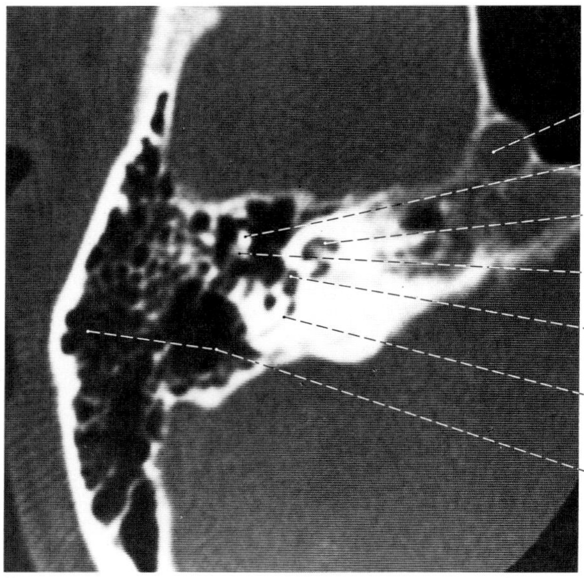

5

The figures on pages 222–223 are a series of axial CT scans of the right adult temporal bone. The planes are within the double lines superimposed on "scout" film. The first image is the most inferior. Each subsequent image is 1.5 mm superior to the preceding image.

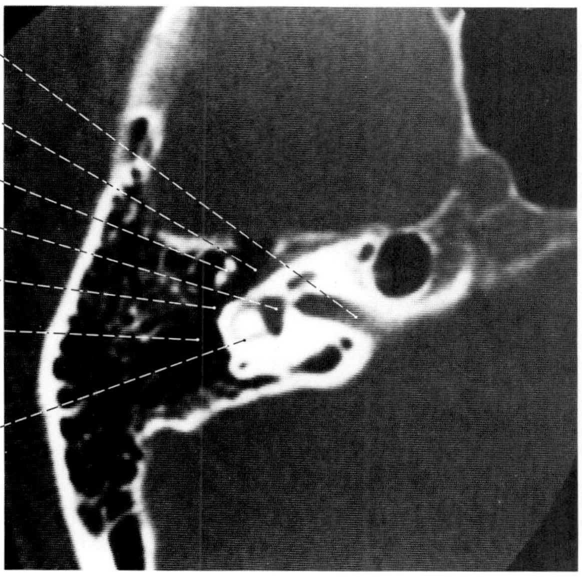
Internal auditory canal
Epitympanic recess
Incudo-malleolar joint
Vestibule
Aditus ad antrum
Antrum
Lateral semicircular canal

6

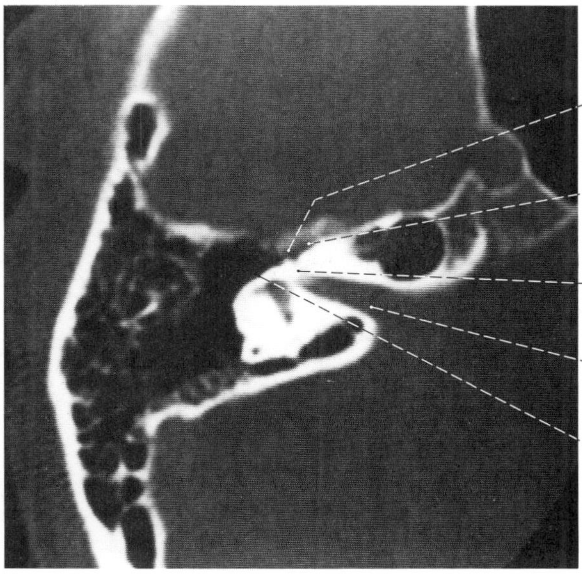
Geniculate ganglion
Canal for greater petrosal nerve
Facial nerve (1st part)
Internal auditory canal
Facial nerve (2nd part)

7

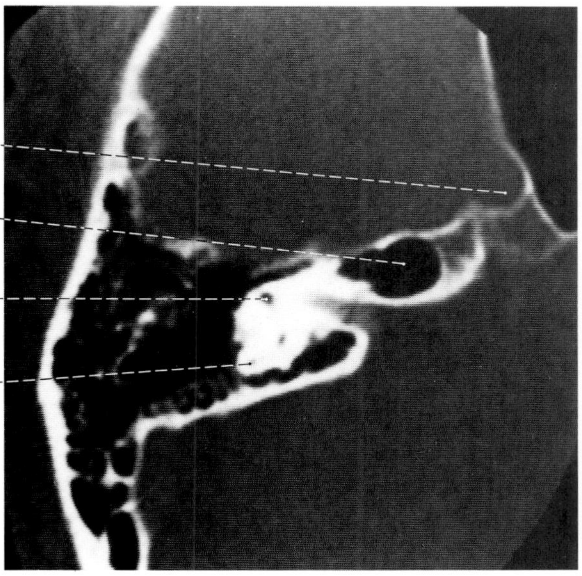
Carotid canal
Aerated petrous apex
Superior semicircular canal
Posterior semicircular canal

8

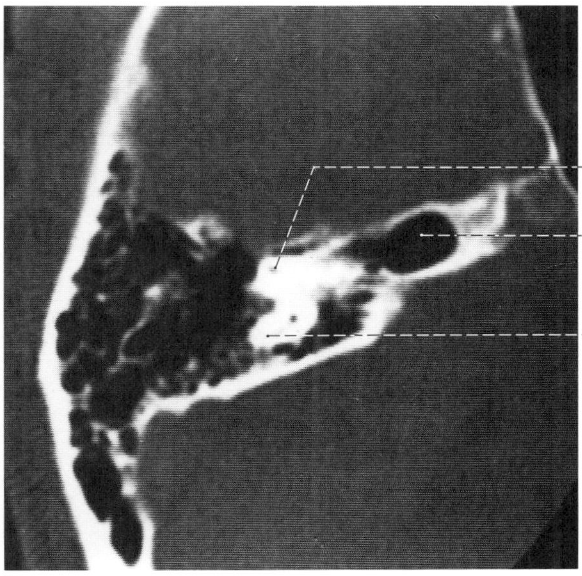
Superior semicircular canal
Air cell
Posterior semicircular canal

9

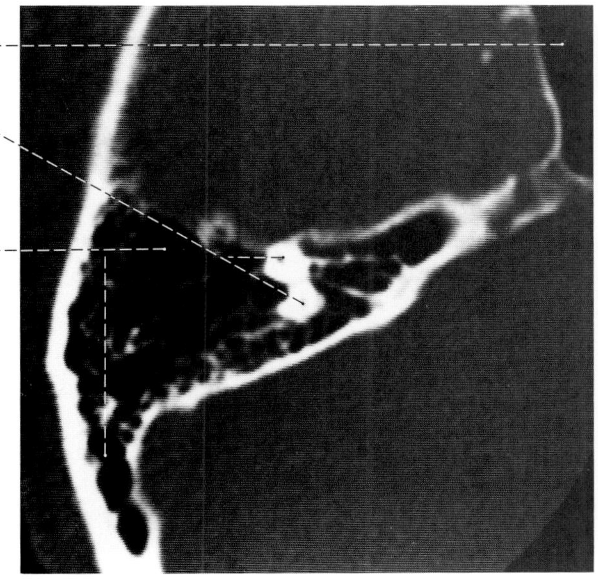
Sphenoid sinus
Superior semicircular canal
Mastoid sinus (air cells)

10

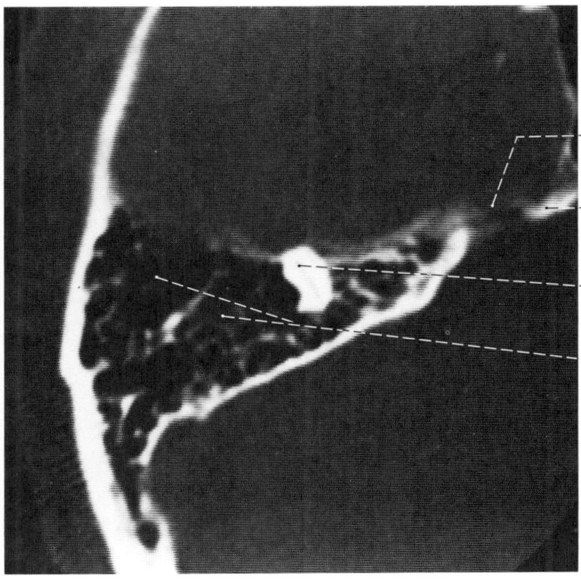
Meckel's cave
Posterior clinoid process
Superior semicircular canal
Mastoid sinus (air cells)

11

Patient CT Scan

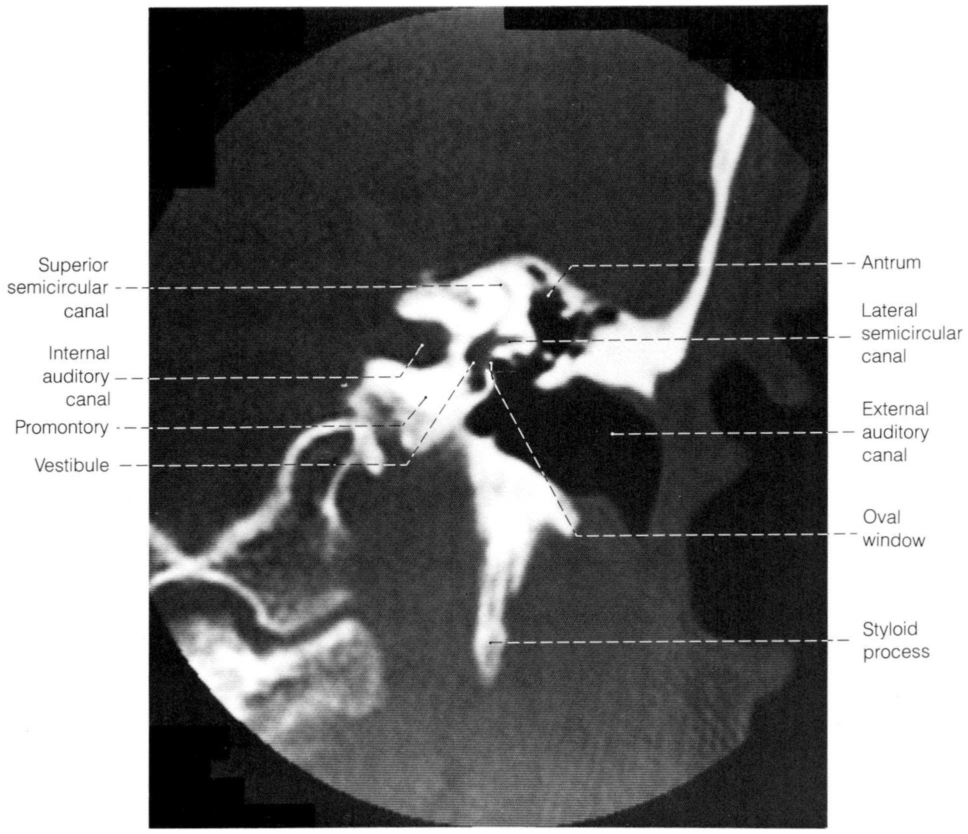

Patient CT Scan

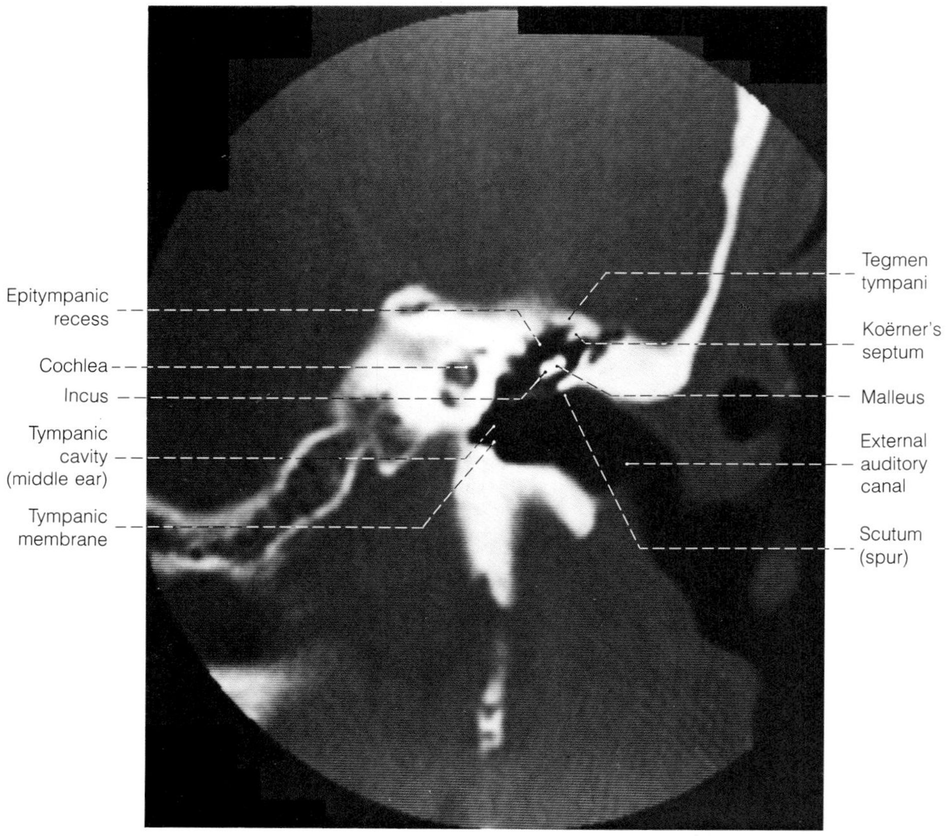

The top figure is a 1.5 mm thick coronal section of a left adult temporal bone at the level of the internal auditory canal 3 mm posterior to the bottom figure. The color photograph of the gross anatomical section is a fortuitous cut viewed from posterior through the middle ear cavity containing the malleus.

The CT sections show the posterior wall of the external auditory canal. The supero-lateral portion of the tympanic membrane attaches to the scutum, (tympanic spur or tympanic spine) of the external canal. A horizontal line extending medial from the scutum separates the mesotympanum from the epitympanic recess of the middle ear. The ossicles, for the most part, are located within the epitympanic recess with the handle of the malleus and long process of incus extending into the mesotympanum. The epitympanic recess and mastoid antrum are separated from the temporal lobe by a thin bony plate called the tegmen tympani. The Koërner's septum, representing the remnant of the petrosquamosal suture, projects from the tegmen tympani into the mastoid antrum.

All the inner ear structures are very well visualized in these sections and the series of coronal CT scans illustrated on pages 228–229. The inner ear contains the cochlea, vestibule, semicircular canals and internal auditory canal. The promontory of the basal turn of the cochlea forms the medial wall of middle ear. Postero-superiorly lies the vestibule. The bony vestibule has an opening called the oval window (vestibular window or fenestra ovalis) on

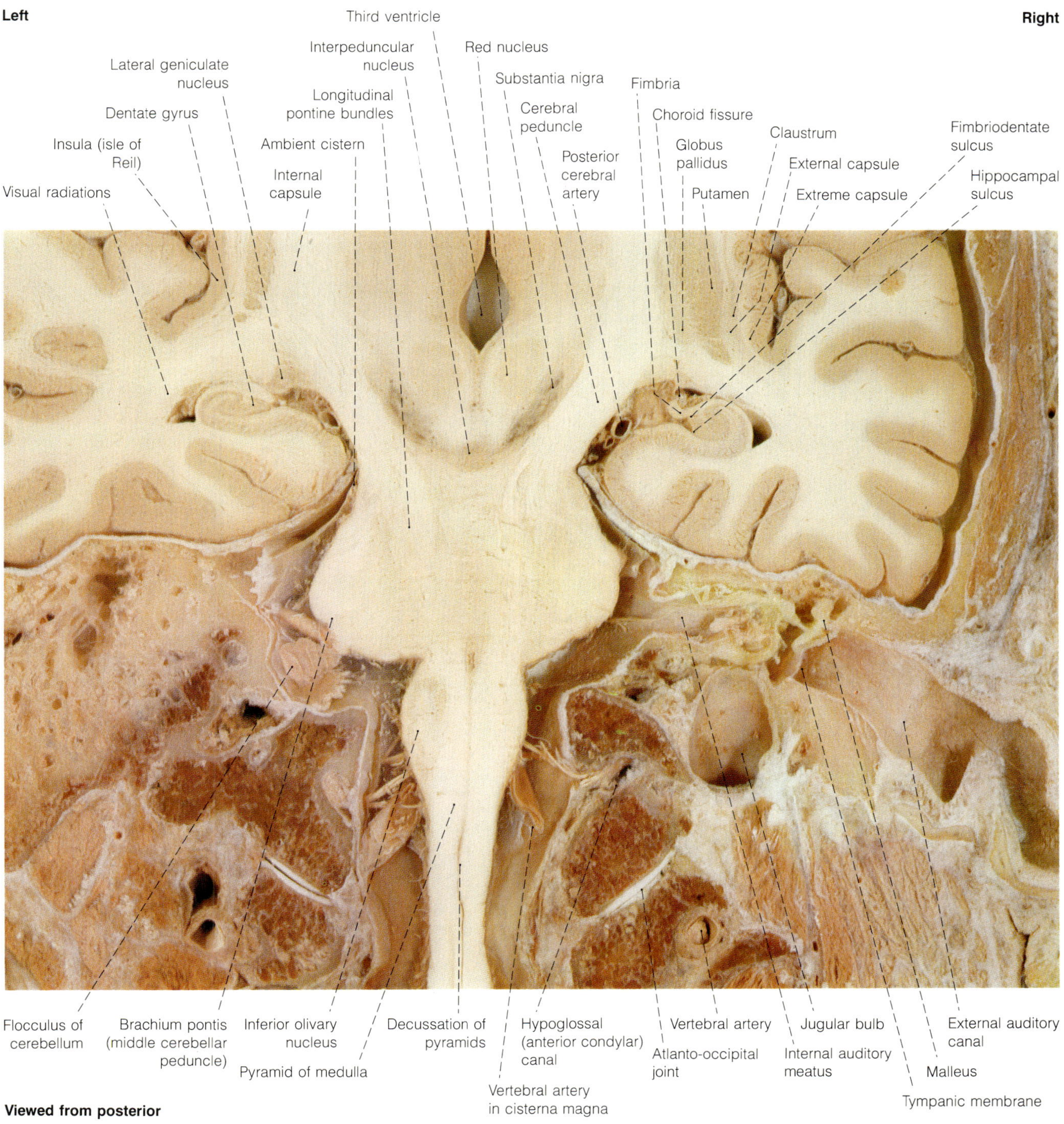

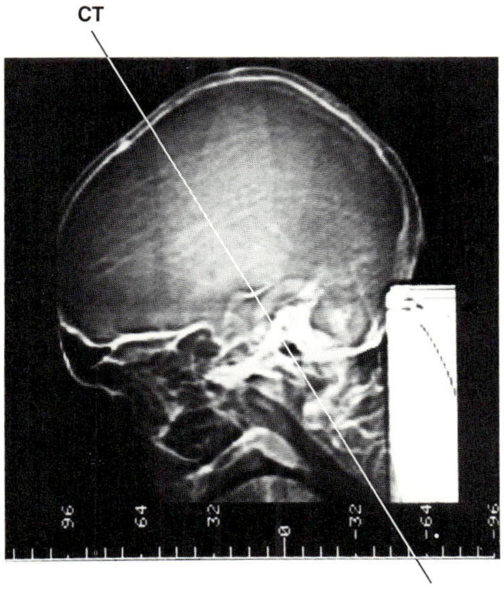

Plane of Section

its lateral aspect. The shape of the window conforms to the shape of the foot plate of the stapes. The superior and lateral semicircular canals are connected with the vestibule. The tympanic portion of the facial nerve lies inferior to the lateral semicircular canal. The internal auditory canal, medial to the cochlea and vestibule, is divided into superior and inferior compartments by the crista falciformis (falciform crest).

Patient CT Scan

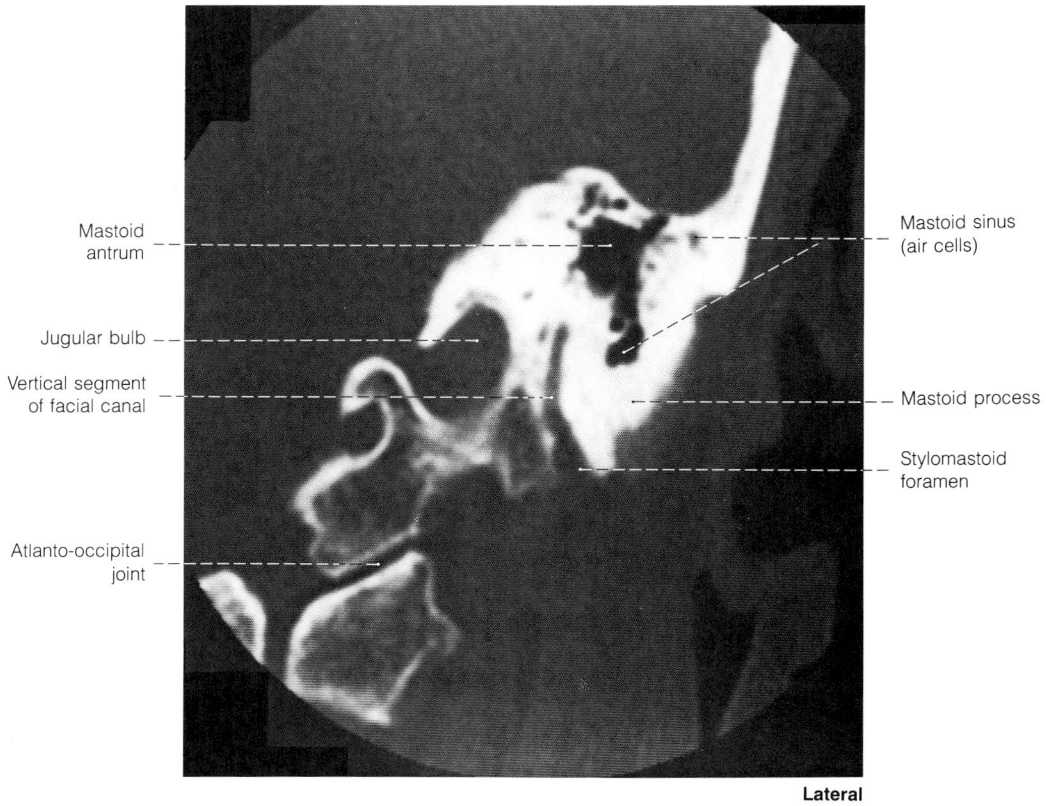

Patient CT Scan

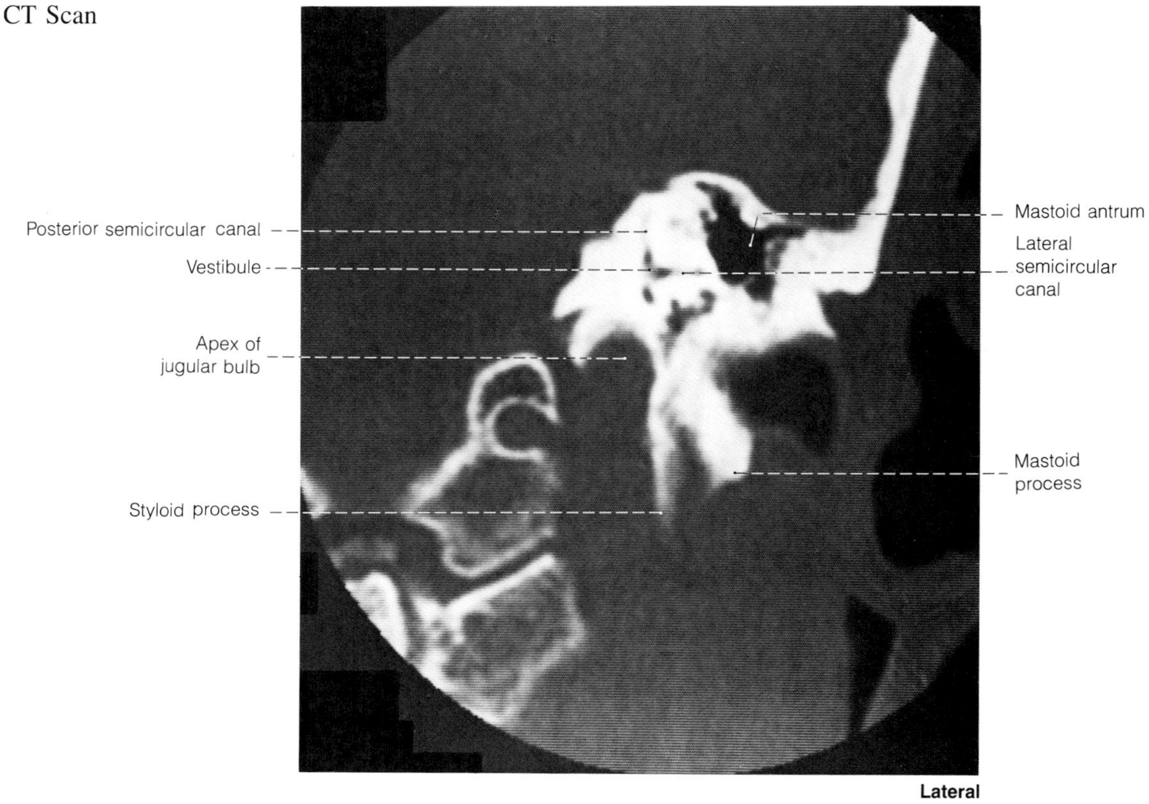

The top figure is a 1.5 mm coronal CT section of a left adult temporal bone at the level of the vertical segment of the facial canal and nerve. The facial nerve (VII) descends inferior to the lateral semicircular canal towards the stylomastoid foramen between the styloid process and the mastoid sinus through which it exits. The jugular fossa lies medial to the facial canal and infero-medial to the posterior semicircular canal. The posterior portion of the mastoid antrum is also visualized. The mastoid air cells extend for varying distances superiorly and laterally from the mastoid antrum.

The bottom figure is a 1.5 mm coronal CT section of the left adult temporal bone approximately 2 mm anterior to the first figure. The section passes through postero-medial portion of external auditory canal and posterior portion of the middle ear.

The mastoid antrum and surrounding air cells are well delineated. Medial to the antrum, the loop of the posterior semicircular canal is identified in the petrous portion of the temporal bone. The lateral (horizontal) semicircular canal protrudes into the mastoid antrum and its medial end is displayed as it opens into the vestibule. The posterior semicircular canal joins the crus commune above the vestibule.

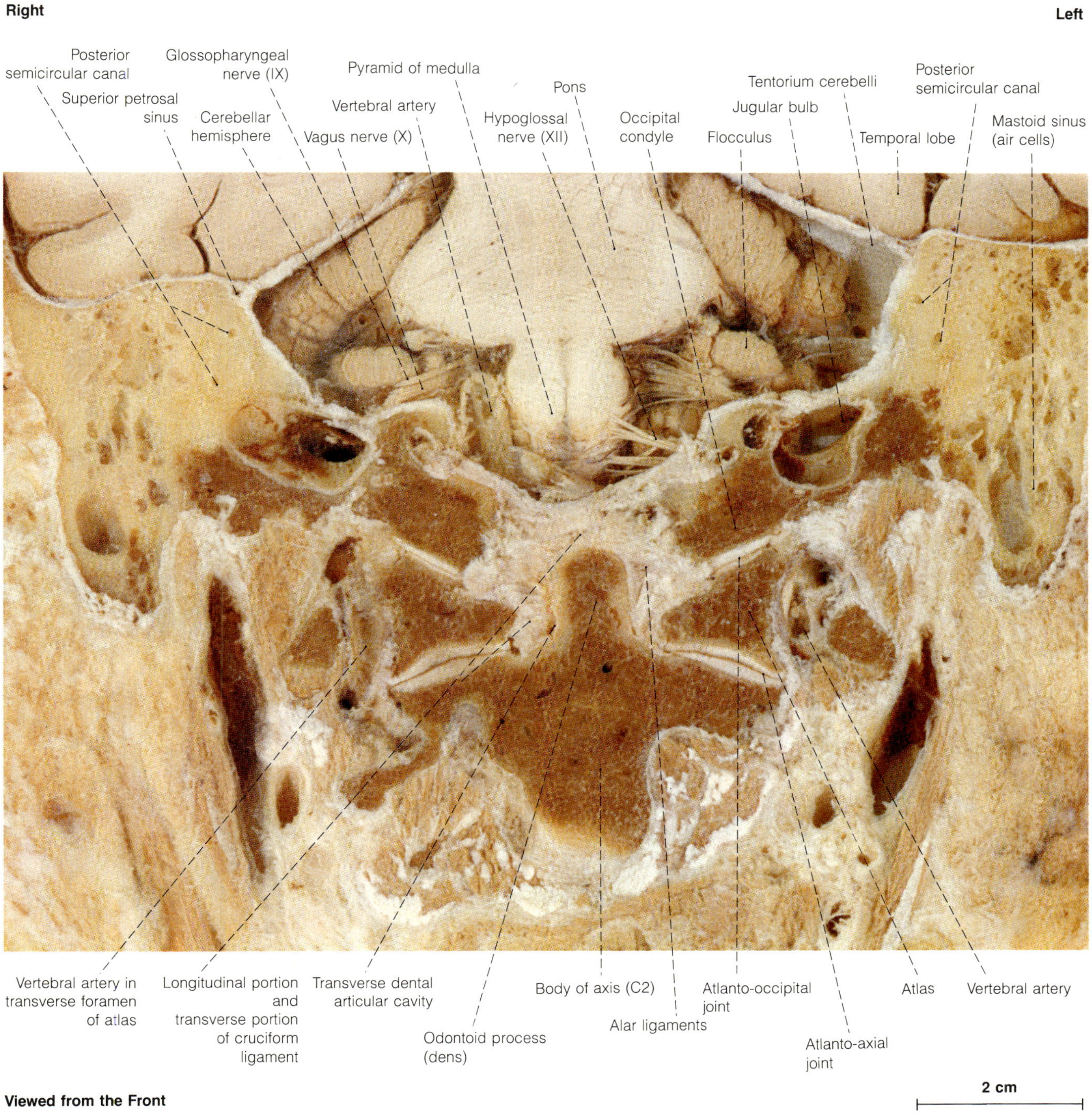

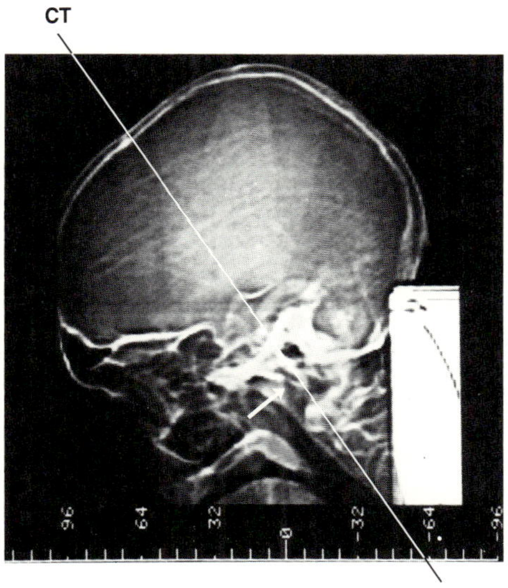

Plane of Section

Planes of Sections

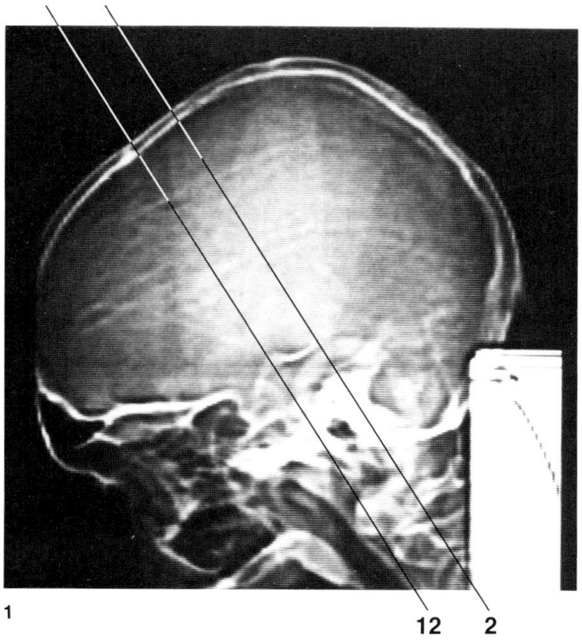

1

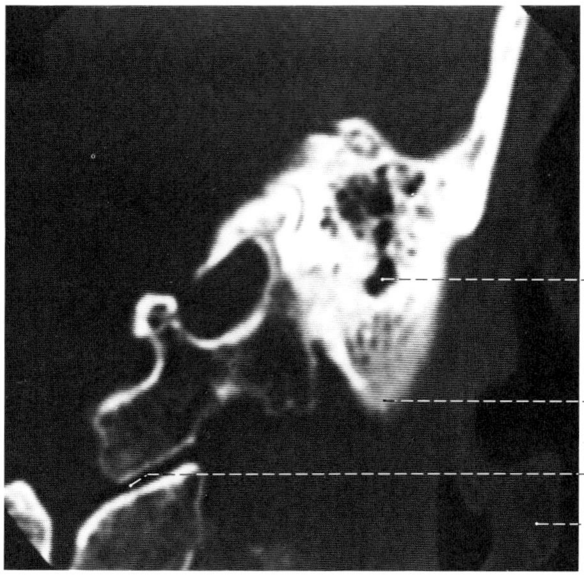

2 Lateral

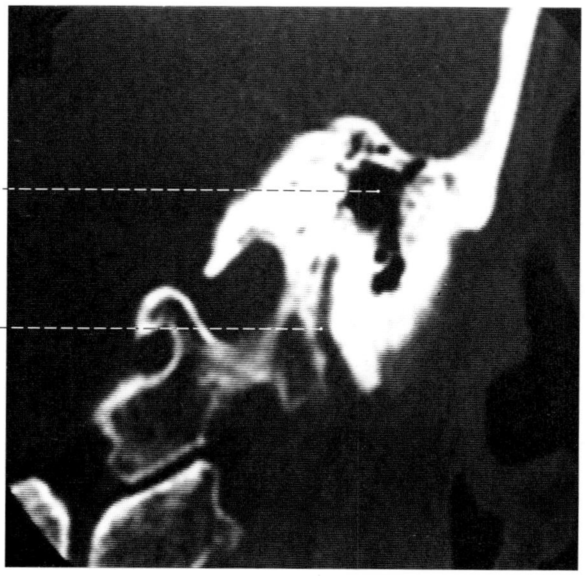

3 Lateral

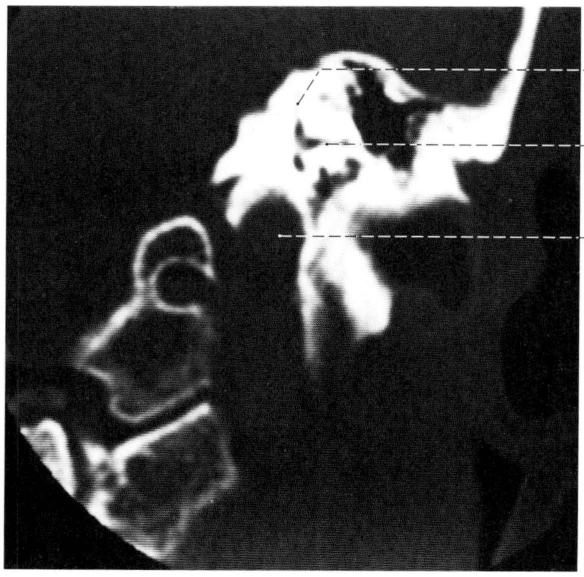

4 Lateral

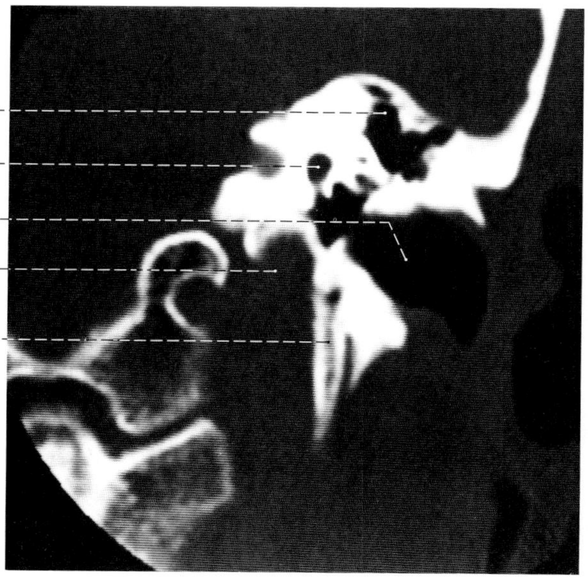

5 Lateral

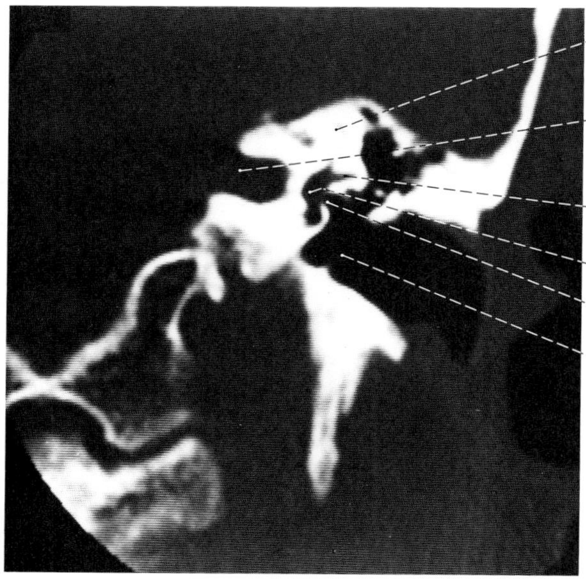

6 Lateral

The figures illustrated on pages 228–229 are a series of coronal CT scans through the temporal bone arranged from posterior to anterior. Such planes are especially advantageous in showing some relationships of the middle ear.

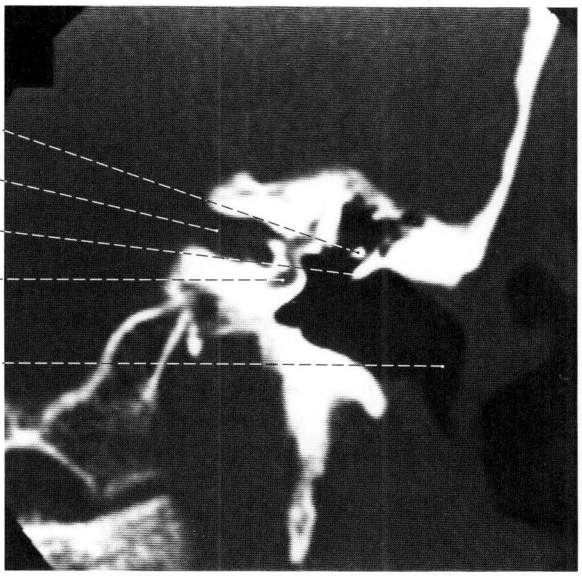

7 Lateral

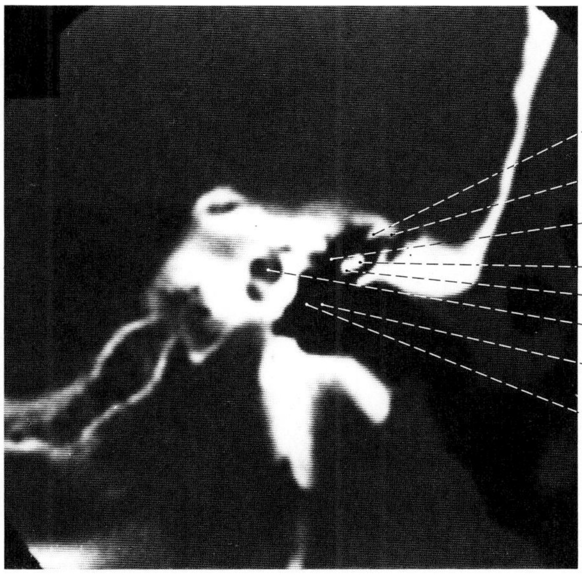

8 Lateral

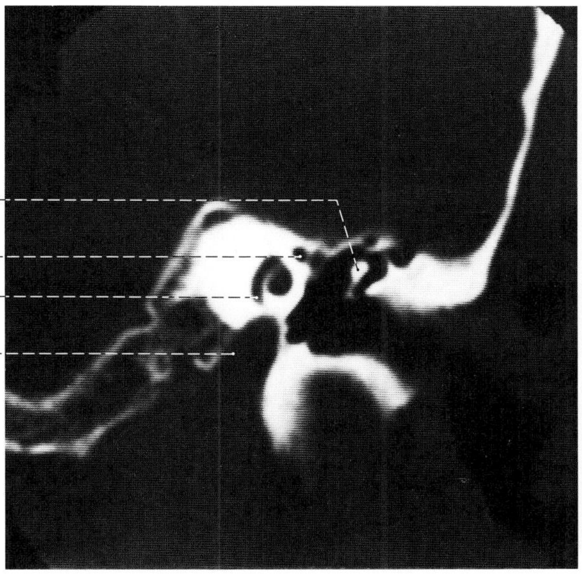

9 Lateral

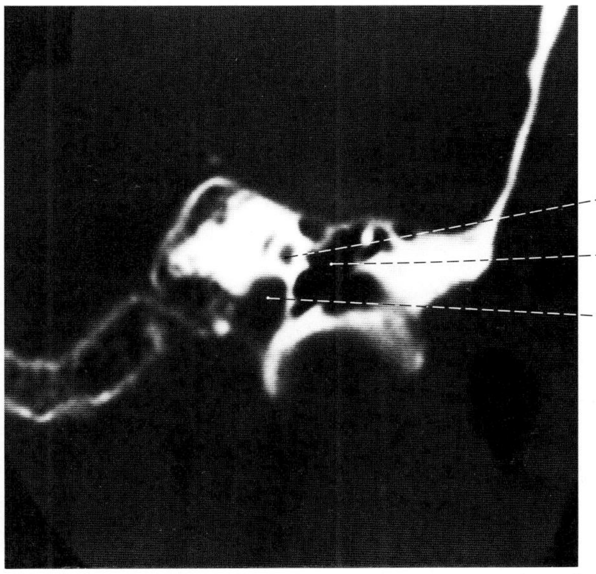

10 Lateral

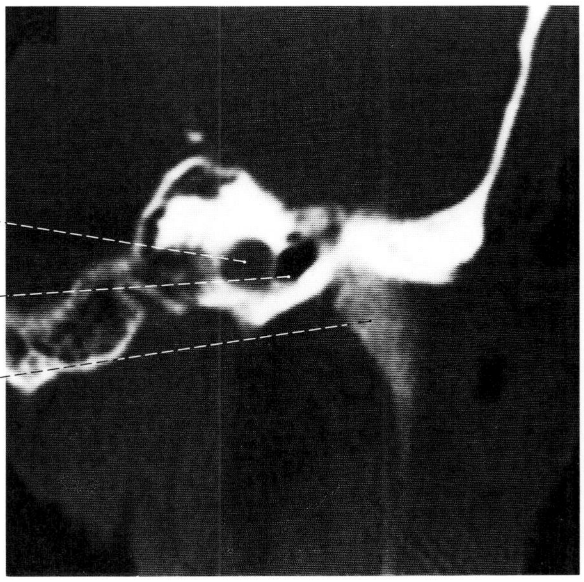

11 Lateral

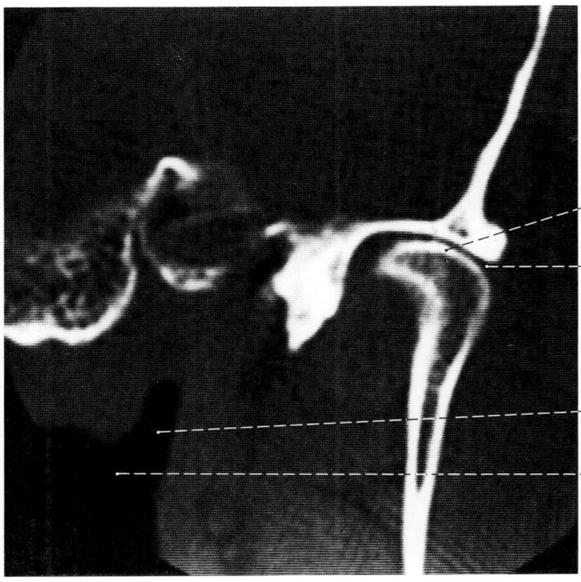

12 Lateral

Selected Bibliography

Anderson, J. E. *Grant's Atlas of Anatomy,* 8th ed., Williams & Wilkins, Baltimore, 1983.

Anson, B. J. and J. A. Donaldson. *Surgical Anatomy of the Temporal Bone,* 3rd ed., W. B. Saunders Co., Philadelphia, 1981.

Galdino, E. V. and R. A. Buckingham. *Tomography and Cross Sections of the Ear.* W. B. Saunders Co., Philadelphia, 1975.

Pernkopf, E. *Atlas of Topographic and Applied Human Anatomy,* 2nd ed., H. Ferner, ed. Urban & Schwarzenberg, Baltimore, 1980.

Schaeffer, J. P. *Morris' Human Anatomy.* The Blakiston Co., New York and Toronto, 1953.

Taylor, S. *The Petrous Temporal Bone (Including the Cerebellopontine* Angle). Rad. Clin. N. Am. 20: 67–86, 1982.

Virapongse, C. et al. *Computed Anatomy of the Temporal Bone.* Am. J. Roent. 139: 739–749, 1982.

Zonneveld, F. W., et al. *Direct Multiplanar C. T. of the Petrous Bone.* Radiographics, Vol. 3, No, 3, 1983.

Ventricles and Cisterns

John A. Arrington, M.D.

Cerebrospinal fluid (CSF) bathes the entire pial surface of the brain and spinal cord and fills the ventricular spaces of the brain. It is elaborated partially by the choroid plexuses of the lateral, third and fourth ventricles and partially by brain supportive tissues, then is resorbed through the arachnoid granulations into the venous sinuses. CSF performs primarily a supportive function for the CNS but may also act as a lymphatic analogue in waste removal. An outline of the ventricles is presented in tabular form on pages 232–233 and of the cisterns on page 237.

The ventricles of the brain and basal subarachnoid cisterns were well explored during the period of pneumoencephalography, a procedure no longer generally performed, and fascinated medieval anatomists, as well as the earliest neuroradiologists. The CSF-containing spaces are readily apparent on both routine CT and MRI scans and, since they can now be routinely well visualized, the relationships and contents of the cisterns and ventricles have become very useful landmarks. The ventricles are superimposed on a sagittal MRI illustration in the figure on page 233 and displayed in the figures on pages 234–235 in CT images in the axial plane. The cisterns are illustrated in the figures on pages 238–241 in both axial and coronal planes. Contrast media such as Metrizamide ® or air in the subarachnoid space enhances their visualization.

For overall orientation an outline of the ventricular system has been superimposed on a mid-sagittal MRI display in the figure on page 233. The position of the choroid plexuses is indicated in red.

The choroid plexus is formed by close apposition and infolding of vascular pia (tela choroidea) and ependyma of the ventricles. Lateral ventricle choroid extends posteriorly from the interventricular foramen of Monro to the trigone of each lateral ventricle where it then curves around the pulvinar of the thalamus along the choroid fissure into the inferior horn of the lateral ventricle. The choroid plexus of the third ventricle is attached to the stria medullaris thalami along the medial surface of the thalamus on each side and projects into the roof of the third ventricle. The choroid plexus in the inferior medullary velum of the fourth ventricle extends from the tip of the foramen of Magendie superiorly toward the cerebellum and projects laterally into each lateral recess emerging through the foramina of Luschka.

According to Milorhat and others, cerebrospinal fluid (CSF) is produced by the choroid plexus of the lateral, third and fourth ventricles and by brain parenchyma producing a net flow of fluid into the ventricular system. CSF travels from the lateral ventricles through the interventricular foramen of Monro into the third ventricle. From there it passes through the cerebral aqueduct into the fourth ventricle where it then flows into the subarachnoid cisterns surrounding the brain and spinal canal via the median and lateral apertures of the fourth ventricle, the foramina of Magendie and Luschka respectively.

Each lateral ventricle consists of a body in the fronto-parietal region, and anterior (or frontal), posterior (or occipital), and inferior (or temporal) horns in the frontal, occipital, and temporal lobes respectively. The trigone is where the occipital and temporal horns diverge from the body of the lateral ventricle and within which is usually found a large aggregation of choroid known as the glomus.

The body of each lateral ventricle (figures 1, 2) extends from the interventricular foramen of Monro to the splenium of the corpus callosum. The body of the corpus callosum forms the roof; the body of the caudate nucleus lies in the ventrolateral wall; and the septum pellucidum, (figures 2–5) extending from the fornix to the corpus callosum, constitutes the medial wall of the lateral ventricle. Where the septum pellucidum ends approximately 1.5 cm posterior to the interventricular foramen and the fornix is attached to the body of the corpus callosum, the medial walls of both ventricles diverge laterally and inferiorly.

The anterior or frontal horns (figures 2–5) extend anteriorly, laterally, and slightly inferiorly from the interventicular foramen into the frontal lobes. The head of the caudate nucleus forms a prominent bulge into the lateral wall of each anterior horn. The septum pellucidum and the parolfactory or septal cortex area in front of the lamina terminalis delimit the anterior horn medially.

The posterior or occipital horn (figure 3) projects posteriorly and medially from the trigone into the occipital lobe. Its size is somewhat variable and frequently asymmetrical. Fibers of the corpus callosum (tapetum and forceps major) form the roof and the optic radiations are adjacent to the lateral wall. There are sometimes two longitudinal ridges visualized on the medial surface of the occipital horn, the upper ridge due to the forceps major while the lower ridge represents the depth of the calcarine (visual) cortex (area #17) and is called the calcar avis.

Ventricular System

Cavity	Anatomical relations
Lateral ventricles	In telencephalon (cerebral hemispheres)
Anterior (frontal) horn	Lateral wall – Caudate nucleus forms a bulge Anterior and superior – Corpus callosum (genu) Medial – Septum pellucidum or medial frontal lobes, septal nuclei Inferior – Nucleus accumbens
Body	Roof – Corpus callosum Ventral part of the lateral wall – Caudate nucleus (body) Ventral part of medial wall – Fornix and attached choroid Medial, separating the ventricles – Septum pellucidum
Trigone	Contains glomus Medial – Hippocampus Lateral – Visual radiations
Posterior (occipital) horn	Superior, lateral and inferior – Visual radiations Medial – Calcar avis and calcarine cortex
Inferior (temporal) horn	Medial – Hippocampus, fimbria and choroid fissure Roof – Tail of caudate nucleus Anterior – Amygdala (basolateral nucleus) indents tip anteriorly from medial side Lateral – Temporal parenchyma including association tracts anteriorly and visual radiations (Meyer's loop) posteriorly
Interventricular foramen (of Monro)	Connects third and lateral ventricles Contains choroid plexus and associated thalamostriate and internal cerebral veins passing from lateral to third ventricle Anteriosuperior – Fornix as it arches behind anterior commissure Anteriolateral – Head of caudate nucleus Lateral – Genu of internal capsule and globus pallidus Posterior – Diencephalon (thalamus including massa intermedia)
Third ventricle	In diencephalon, between hypothalami and thalami Anterior limit – lamina terminalis Floor (inferior), from anterior to posterior – supraoptic recess and optic chiasm, infundibular recess and region, tuber cinereum, and mamillary nuclei Roof (superior) – Stria medullaris on sides with interconnecting choroid, paired internal cerebral veins course in medullary velum Posterior and superior – Pineal recess between the habenular and posterior commissures Posterior and inferior – Tegmentum of mesencephalon including red nucleus Medially – may be interrupted by massa intermedia (interthalamic adhesion)

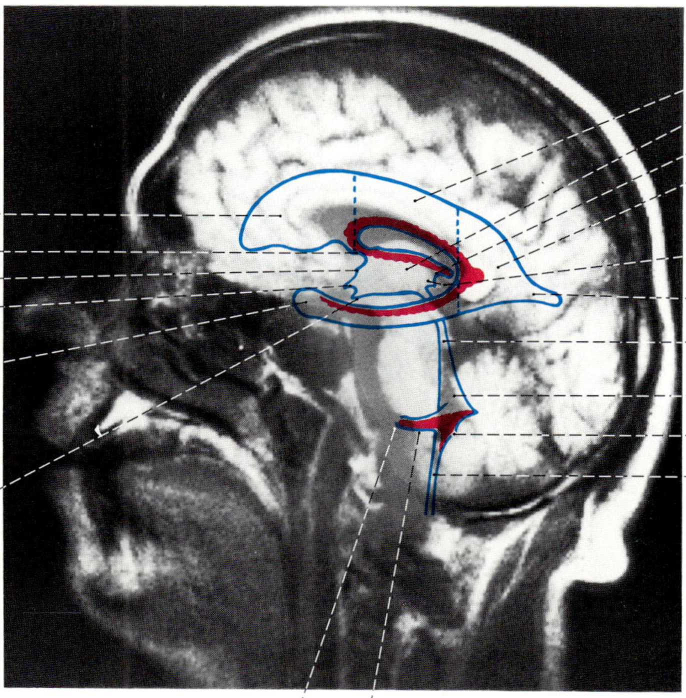

Cavity	Anatomical relations
Cerebral aqueduct (of Sylvius) (Iter)	In mesencephalon, between third and fourth ventricles Roof – Posterior commissure and colliculae (corpora quadrigemina or tectum) Floor – Oculomotor (III) and trochlear (IV) nuclei and medial longitudinal fasciculus (MLF) Anterior – Tegmentum of mesencephalon including red nucleus and brachium conjunctivum
Fourth ventricle	Related to pons, cerebellum and medulla
Superior part	Roof – Superior (anterior) medullary velum with superior vermis just above it Lateral – Brachium conjunctivum (superior cerebellar peduncle) Floor – Locus ceruleus and MLF of upper pons
Middle part	Lateral wall – Brachium pontis (middle cerebellar peduncle) and restiform body (inferior cerebellar peduncle) Roof – Cerebellar vermis and central cerebellar nuclei Floor – Facial colliculus (and abducens [VI] nucleus) MLF, and vestibular nuclei
Lateral recess	Extends below inferior cerebellar peduncle (restiform body) into C-P angle cistern with flocculus of cerebellum, auditory (VIII) and facial (VII) nerves Contains lateral foramen of Luschka Vestibular and cochlear nuclei are at medial junction with fourth ventricle
Apex of roof	Fastigium
Inferior part	Roof – Formed by inferior medullary velum (choroid) with median foramen of Magendie opening into vallecula. Indented by nodulus of vermis. As retromedullary posterior inferior cerebellar artery (PICA) becomes retrotonsilar, small choroidal arteries arise at the "choroid point". Floor – Hypoglossal nuclei (XII), vagal nuclei (X), and MLF
Obex	Caudal point of fourth ventricle Lateral walls – area postrema and gracile nuclei Floor – Hypoglossal nuclei (XII) and MLF
Central canal	In lower medulla and spinal cord Most sensory nuclei are dorsal Most motor nuclei are ventral Most tracts (e.g. pyramidal and spinothalamic) decussate ventral to canal Sacral tip may be duplicate canal

Related cavities of the brain

Cavum septi pellucidi	Sometimes found between leaves of septum pellucidum
Cavum vergae	Posterior part of enlarged cavum septi pellucidi above fornix and posterior to interventricular foramen. Communicates with cavum septi pellucidi. Occasionally present.
Cavum of velum interpositum	Rostral extension of quadrigeminal cistern below fornix and above pulvinar of thalamus and choroid of third ventricle. Does not communicate with cavum septi pellucidi or cavum vergae. Occasionally present.

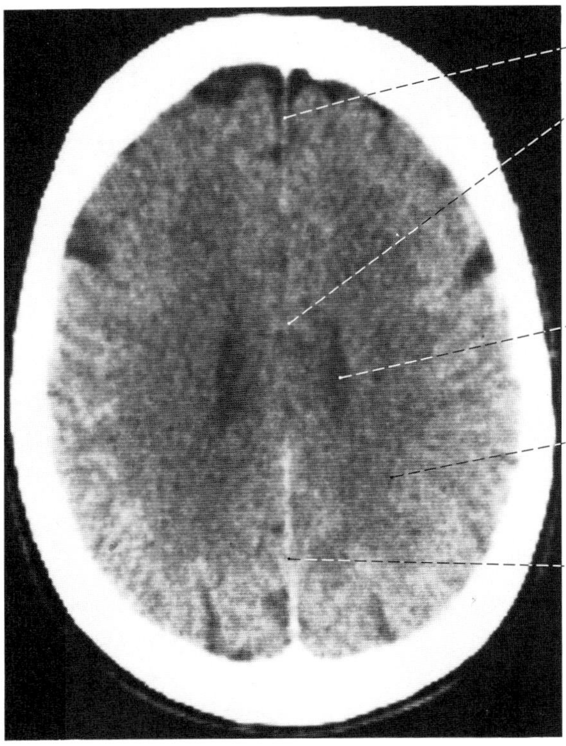

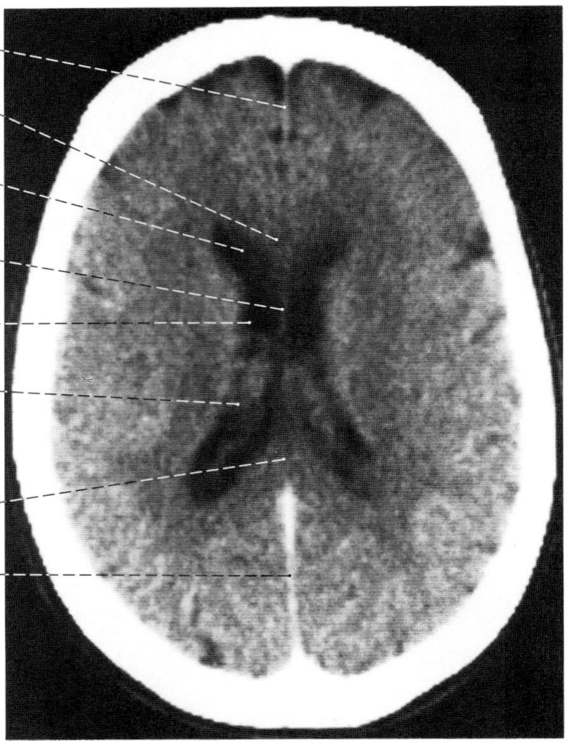

1 2

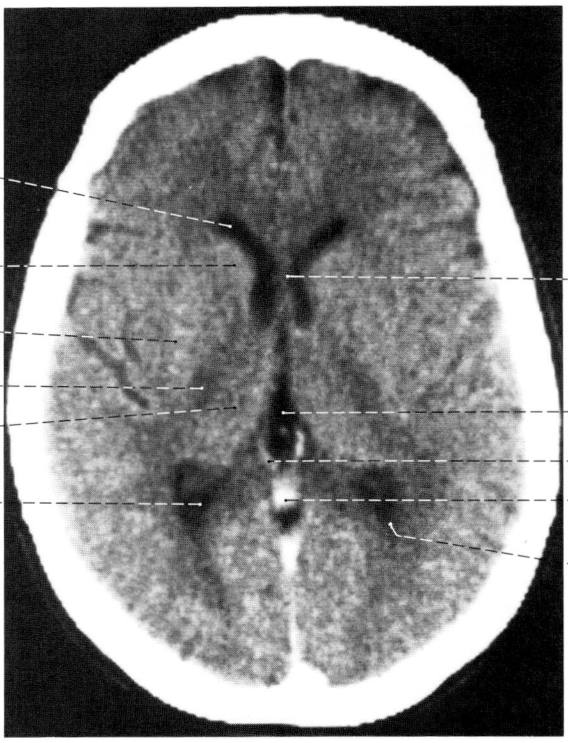

3

The inferior or temporal horn (figure 4) arches first posterolaterally then inferiorly around the pulvinar of the thalamus and then curves anteriorly to within 2–4 cm of the tip of the temporal pole. The tail of the caudate nucleus in the medial portion of the roof ends in the amygdala which indents and limits the antero-medial tip of the temporal horn. The hippocampus and attached fimbria bulge into the medial wall of the temporal horn to give it a "C" shape on coronal section. The choroid fissure and attached choroid plexus are between the fimbria and the tail of the caudate nucleus. More proximally in the temporal lobe lateral to the temporal horns are association tracts anteriorly, and inferior visual radiations (Meyer's loop) posteriorly.

The 3rd ventricle (figures 4, 5) is bounded laterally by the diencephalic and preoptic areas. The membranous lamina terminalis, the anterior commissure, and optic chiasm limit anteriorly. The choroid plexus between the stria medullares forms the roof of the third ventricle, the pineal gland and habenular commissure bound it posterosuperiorly, and the tegmentum of the mesencephalon and posterior commissure form the postero-inferior wall. The floor of the 3rd ventricle is formed by the hypothalamus consisting of, from anterior to posterior, the optic chiasm, infundibulum, tuber cinereum, and the mamillary bodies. Each lateral wall is formed by the thalamus (dorsomedial nucleus) superiorly and hypothalamus and preoptic area inferiorly, separated by the shallow hypothalamic sulcus. A massa intermedia (interthalamic adhesion) of variable size may bridge the 3rd ventricle. The third ventricle communicates with the 4th ventricle through the cerebral aqueduct posteriorly and with the lateral ventricles through the interventricular foramen of Monro antero-superiorly.

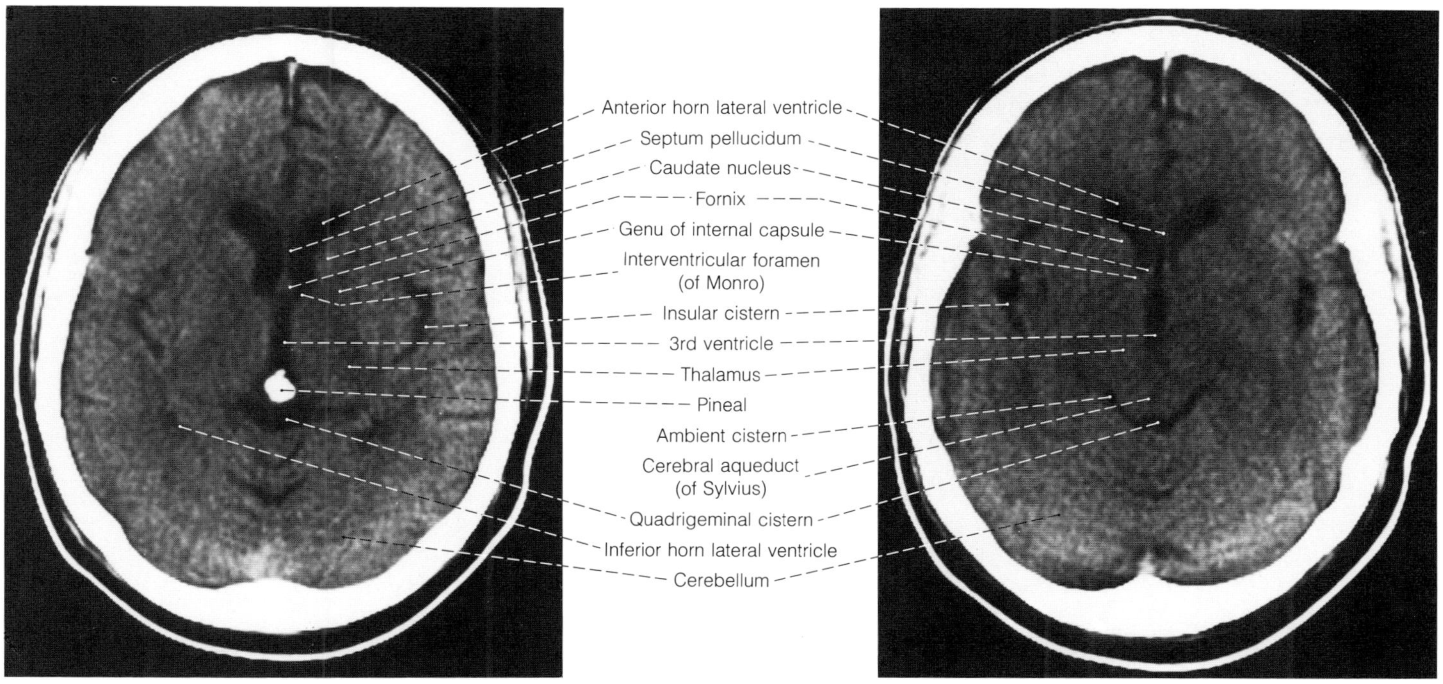

4 5

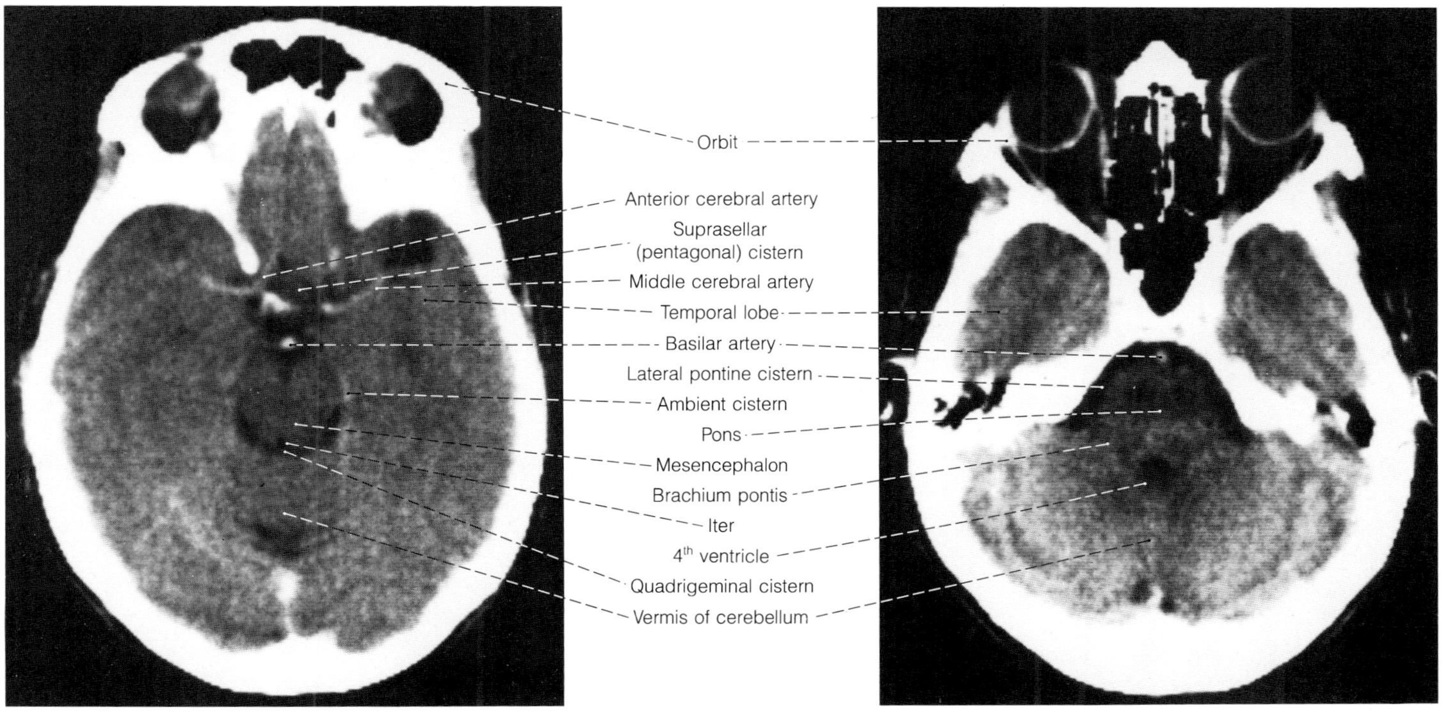

6 7

The slender cerebral aqueduct or iter (figures 5, 6) connecting the 3rd to the 4th ventricle is approximately 15 mm long and runs beneath the tectum of the mesencephalon. The nuclei of the oculomotor and trochlear nerves are just ventral to the aqueduct.

The 4th ventricle extends from the end of the central canal in the mid-medulla to the cerebral aqueduct of the mesencephalon. It is anterior to the cerebellum and dorsal to the pons and the cranial half of the medulla. The 4th ventricle consists of a tent shaped roof, a rhomboid shaped floor (rhomboid fossa), and lateral walls. From the midportion of the ventricle, lateral recesses extend on both sides betwen the inferior cerebellar peduncle and the flocculus of the cerebellum. There are three openings in the 4th ventricle: a midline aperture (foramen of Magendie) in the inferior medullary velum and two lateral apertures (foramina of Luschka) in the lateral recesses. The major nuclei underlying the floor are the hypoglossal (XII) and vagal (X) nuclei inferiorly, the abducens (VI) nuclei just beneath the facial colliculus and the vestibular nuclei in the middle, and the locus ceruleus superiorly. The medial longitudinal fasciculi course on either side of the midline the entire rostrocaudal length of the 4th ventricle. The area postrema lies on either side of the obex inferiorly, the inferior (restiform body) and middle (brachium pontis) cerebellar peduncles form the lateral wall in the middle, and the superior cerebellar peduncle (brachium conjunctivum) constitutes the lateral boundary on either side superiorly. The roof is formed by the inferior (or posterior) medullary velum inferiorly with the nodulus of the cerebellum indenting from below, the cerebellar nuclei and vermis in the middle at the apex, and the superior (anterior) medullary velum superiorly.

Enhancement of the subarachnoid space with positive or negative contrast media (Metrizamide or air respectively) is common practice in studies of the spinal canal and may also be occasionally advantageous in examination of the cerebral cisterns. Figures 1–8 on pages 238–239 are a series of CT scans from below upward in the axial plane. Figures 9–15 on pages 240–241 are a series of CT scans from front to back in the coronal plane with the cisterns enhanced.

A relatively impervious thin arachnoid membrane completely surrounds the CNS between the dura and pia mater and creates a thin subdural space externally and a subarachnoid space of variable size internally. Fibrous strands (trabeculae) extending from the arachnoid to the pia can coalesce to form a membrane; for example, the membrane of Liliequist bridges the right and left oculomotor nerves across the interpeduncular fossa. The size of the subarachnoid space in area depends upon how closely the shape of the brain and cranial vault correlate. In areas where the pia and arachnoid are widely separated (base of the brain and around the brain stem), the expanded subarachnoid spaces are referred to as cisterns. Cisterns tend to enlarge as parenchyma is lost, either generally as in cerebral atrophy or focally as in encephalomalacia.

The subarachnoid space contains CSF, cranial and spinal nerves and major arteries and veins of the brain and spinal cord. The cerebellomedullary subarachnoid cistern (cisterna magna) can be extremely variable in shape and receives CSF produced by the ventricular system through the median and lateral apertures of the fourth ventricle.

When reviewing the subarachnoid cisterns and their contents, it is convenient to think of each cistern as a separate compartment; however, it is important to remember that the cisterns are one large communicating subarachnoid space. Since the subarachnoid cisterns are parts of a continuous space and were of relatively minor anatomical and clinical significance prior to CT imaging, the names applied to its divisions are frequently vague and redundant. We have selected those terms which appear to be most common in current usage.

The subarachnoid cisterns modified from Newton and Potts

Common name	Synonymous names	Location	Contents
Lumbar cistern	Caudal sac	Subarachnoid space between L_1-S_2 vertebrae	Filum terminale and cauda equina (nerve roots L_2-S_5), artery of Adamkiewicz
Cervical cistern	Cavum subarachnoidale medullae spinalis	Subarachnoid space surrounding upper cervical cord, behind dens	Cervical nerve roots, dentate ligaments, spinal arteries and veins, spinal accessory nerves, lower decussation of pyramids
Medullary:			
Cisterna magna	Medullary cistern Cerebello-medullary cistern	Over inferior surface of cerebellum, around medulla oblongata, includes vallecula and fissure between medulla and cerebellum	Posterior inferior cerebellar arteries (PICA) 9th, 10th, 11th, and 12th cranial nerves, vertebral arteries, tonsils of cerebellum
Premedullary cistern	Anterior part of cisterna magna	Between medulla and clivus	Vertebral arteries, 11th and 12th cranial nerves
Lateral medullary cistern	Lateral part of cisterna magna	Lateral to medulla	Vertebral arteries, 9th, 10th, 11th and 12th cranial nerves
Pontine:			
Prepontine cistern	Pontine cistern, pontine portion of basal cistern	Between pons and clivus	Vertebral, basilar, and pontine arteries, 5th and 6th cranial nerves
Lateral pontine cistern	Includes cerebellopontine cistern	Between temporal bone and brachium pontis	Trigeminal nerve, lateral pontine arteries
Cerebellopontine cistern	Part of lateral pontine cistern, cerebellopontine (C-P) angle cistern	Between posterior surface of temporal bone, inferior surface of cerebellum, lateral surface of pons, and tentorium	Anterior inferior cerebellar (AICA) and labyrinthine arteries; petrosal vein; 7th and 8th cranial nerves, lateral recess of 4th ventricle, cerebellar flocculus
Superior cerebellar cistern		Over vermis, upper surface cerebellar hemispheres, below tentorium	Superior cerebellar arteries and veins, superior surface of cerebellum
Interpeduncular cistern	Intercrural cistern, interpeduncular portion of pentagonal cistern	Continuation of pontine cistern from anterior margin of pons to infundibulum; includes interpeduncular fossa	Upper end of basilar artery with terminal branches (posterior cerebral arteries, superior cerebellar arteries), 3rd cranial nerves posterior perforating (thalamic) arteries
Ambient cistern	Posterior-lateral part of "pentagonal cistern"	Ventral and lateral to mesencephalon, communication between pre-pontine and interpeduncular cisterns and quadrigeminal cistern, adjacent to tentorial incisura	Posterior cerebral artery, superior cerebellar artery, mesencephalic veins, 4th cranial nerves, tentorium cerebelli, geniculate bodies, optic tract
Pentagonal cistern	Suprasellar cistern	Contiguous parts of suprasellar, insular, interpeduncular and ambient cisterns	
Quadrigeminal cistern	Cistern of great vein of Galen, dorsal part of ambient cistern, superior cistern	Over and behind quadrigeminal plate of mesencephalon	Pineal body, posterior cerebral arteries, posterior choroidal artery, vein of Galen, basal vein, deep cerebral vein, precentral cerebellar vein, 4th cranial nerve
Cistern of transverse cerebral fissure	Cistern of velum interpositum, cavum velum interpositum, cistern of velum triangulare, lateral wing of ambient cistern, internal subarachnoid channels	Below fornix and corpus callosum and above roof of third ventricle and pulvinar of thalamus; extends lateral to choroid plexus of lateral ventricle, bends around thalamus posteriorly	Anterior, medial, and lateral choroidal arteries; branches to choroid plexus; internal cerebral vein
Callosal cistern	Cistern of corpus callosum, pericallosal cistern	Sweeps along superior surface of corpus callosum from genu to splenium	Pericallosal artery
Suprasellar cistern	Chiasmatic portion of basal cistern, chiasmatic cistern, may include cistern of lamina terminalis, part of "pentagonal cistern"	From infundibulum to posterior surface of frontal lobes, between uncus of parahippocampal gyrus on each side; extends into limen insulae and lateral (Sylvian) fissure; below optic chiasm, above sella	Internal carotid artery and its bifurcation, posterior communicating artery, anterior choroidal artery, ophthalmic artery, anterior perforating arteries, basal vein, optic chiasm, 2nd and 3rd cranial nerves, middle cerebral artery, middle cerebral vein, deep cerebral vein.
Lateral cistern	Cistern of Sylvian fissure, anterior-lateral extension of pentagonal cistern, (cistern of insula)	Between opercula in lateral (Sylvian) fissure	Middle cerebral artery and its branches, frontal, parietal and temporal opercula, transverse temporal gyrus
Insular cistern	Lateral or Sylvian cistern	Over insular lobe (isle of Reil)	Middle cerebral artery and its cortical branches
Interhemispheric cistern	May include cistern of lamina terminalis part of pentagonal cistern	Between cerebral hemispheres on either side of falx cerebri	Anterior cerebral artery anterior, communicating artery, falx cerebri septal area
Subarachnoid spaces over cerebral cortex	Superficial subarachnoid channels	Over surface of hemispheres	Cerebral veins and arteries

Plane of Section

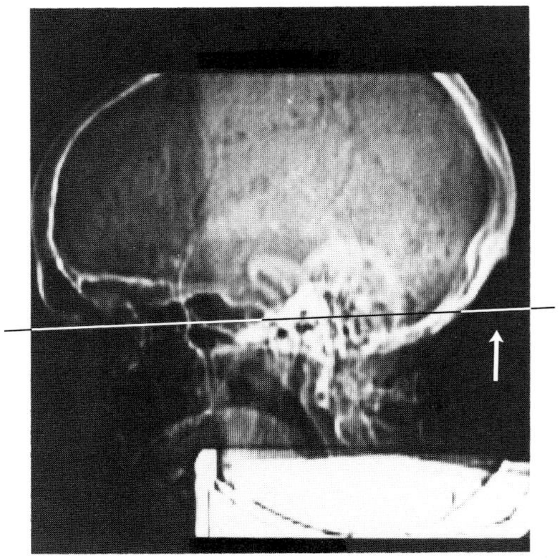

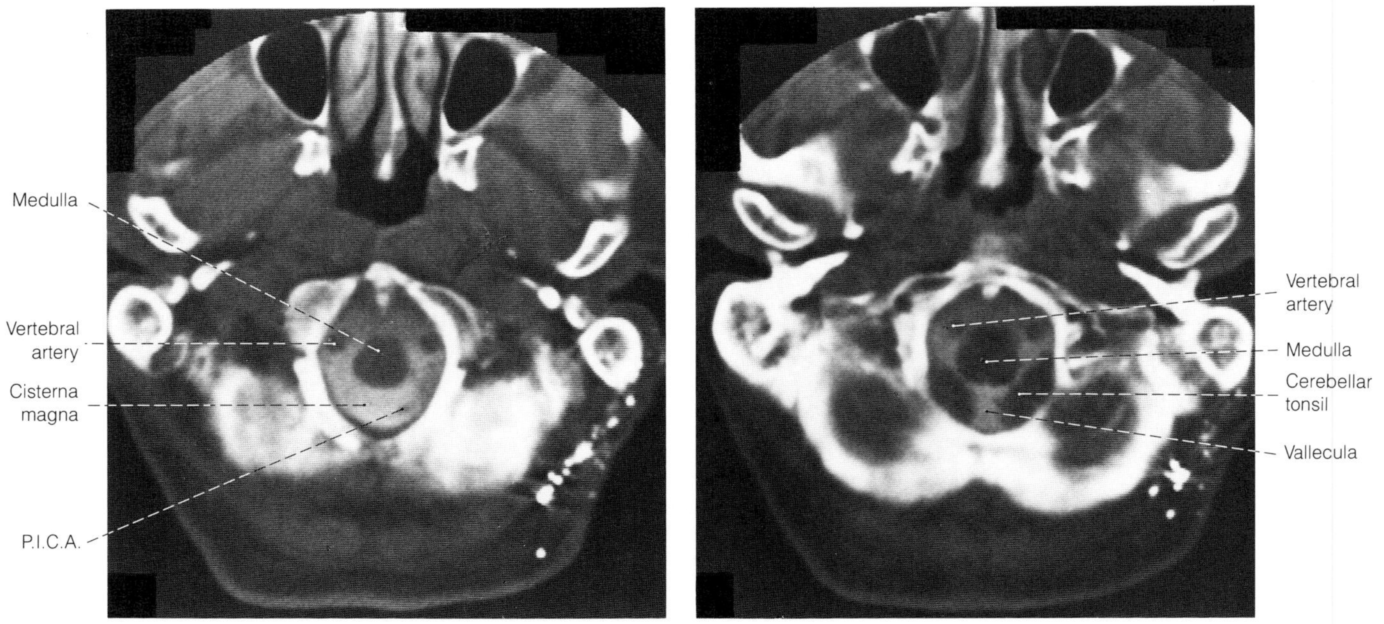

1 2

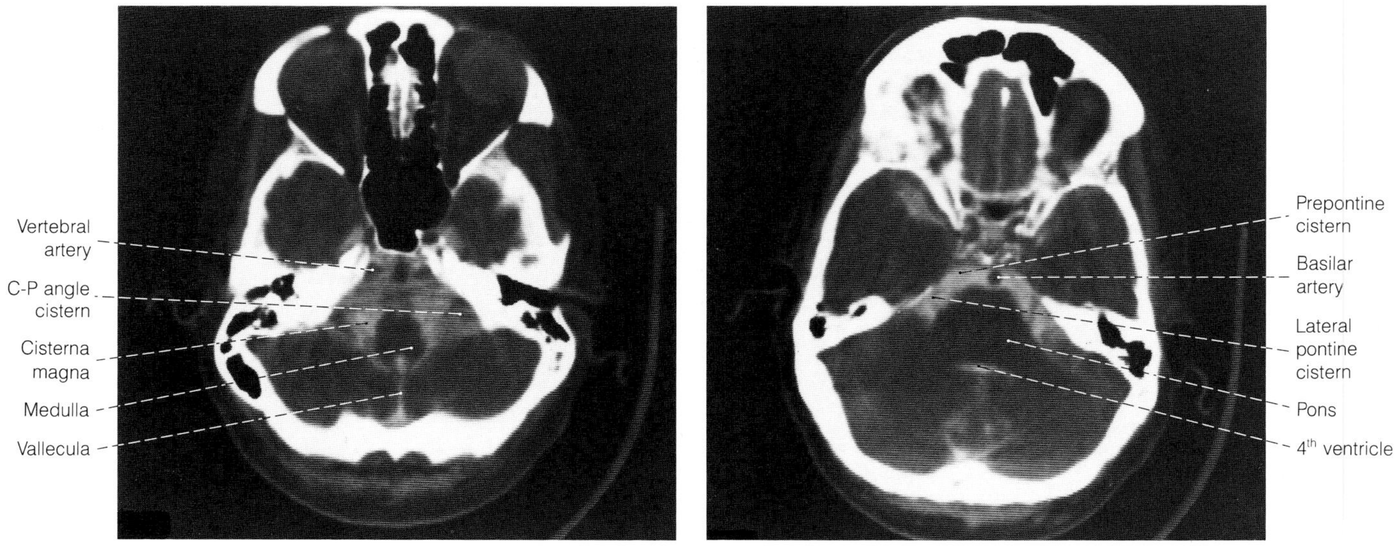

3 4

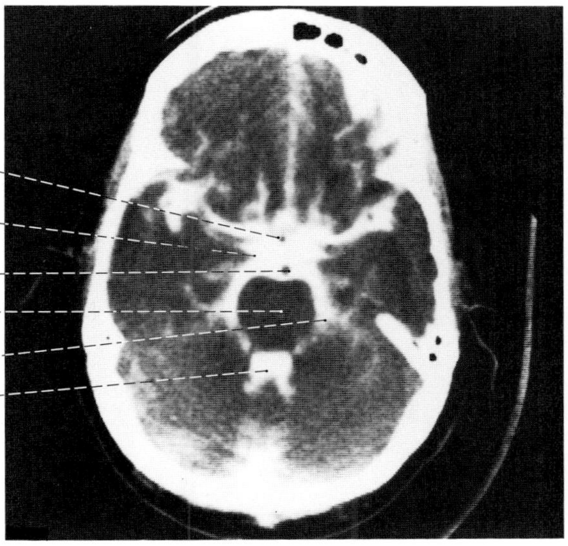

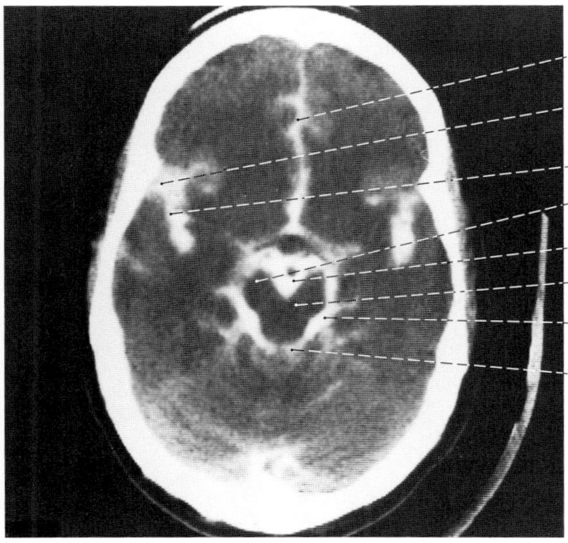

5 6

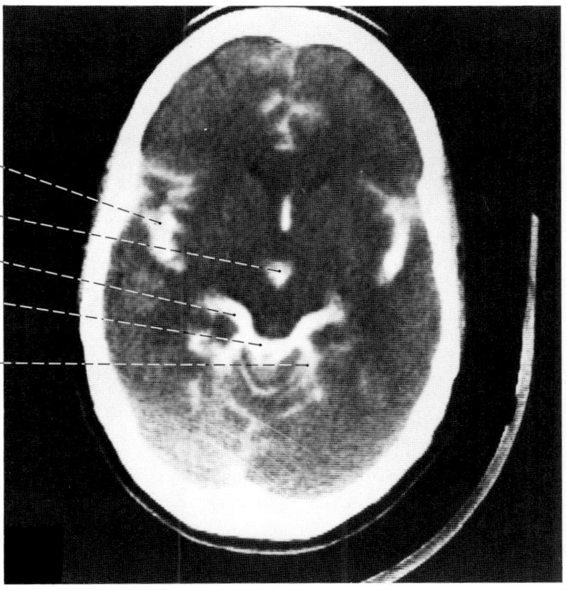

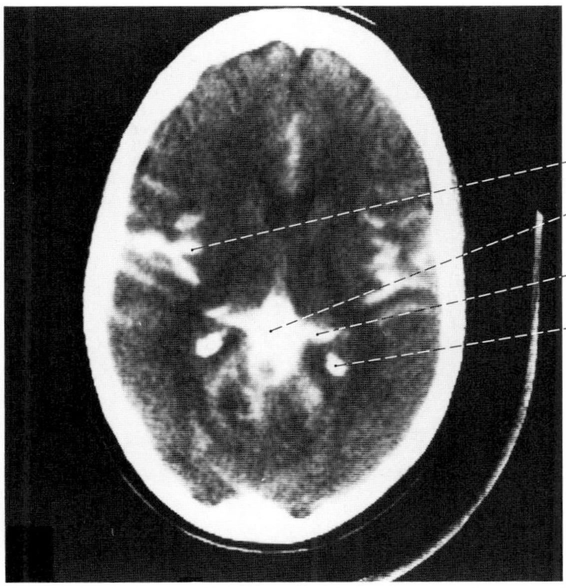

7 8

The ventral and dorsal cisterns communicate laterally around the brainstem via the lateral medullary cistern bordering the medulla, the lateral pontine cistern (figure 5) on either side of the pons, and the ambient cistern (figures 6, 7) lateral to the mesencephalon. These cisterns connect the cisterna magna (figures 1–3) with the pre-medullary, the cerebellar with the pre-pontine (figures 4, 12, 13), and the quadrigeminal (figures 7, 8) with the interpeduncular cistern (figures 6, 12) respectively. Ventrally, CSF flows from the pre-medullary superiorly to the suprasellar cistern (figure 11) through the pre-pontine (figures 4, 12, 13) and interpeduncular cisterns (6, 7, 12, 13). From the suprasellar cistern, CSF can pass superiorly into the interhemispheric cistern (figures 6, 9, 10) or laterally into the lateral (figures 6, 10) and insular (figures 6, 10) cisterns. Dorsally, CSF flows from the cisterna magna (figures 1–3) superiorly over the cerebellar hemispheres (figure 15) and through the tentorial notch to cover the cerebral cortex dipping into the sulci. Inferiorly, the cisterna magna and medullary cistern communicate with the subarachnoid space around the spinal canal. CSF returns to the vascular system by arachnoid granulations in the superior sagittal and other sinuses, granulations in the basal cisterns, and the dural sleeves of the nerve roots by a process of transmigration of fluid which depends for proper flow upon a pressure gradient from the CSF spaces to the venous system.

Plane of Section

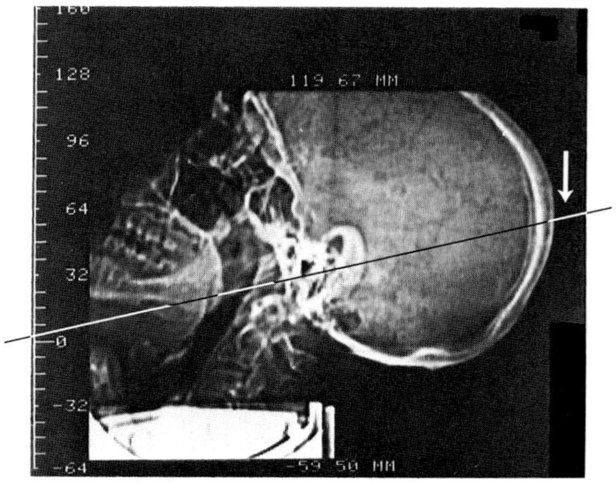

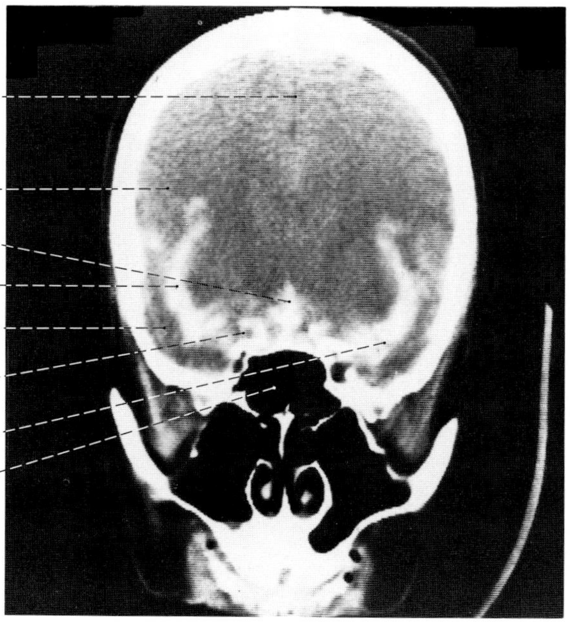

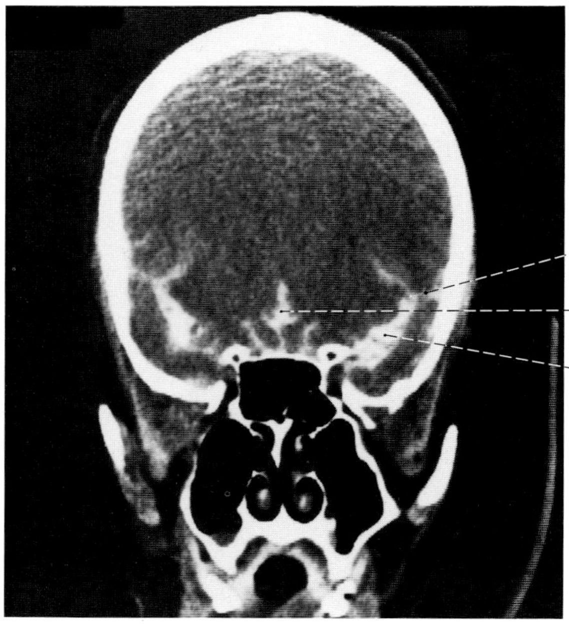

9 10

The cisterna magna or medullary cistern surrounds the medulla, having rough divisions ventral (premedullary), lateral (lateral medullary) and dorsal (vallecula, figure 2) to the medulla oblongata. The right and left vertebral arteries (figure 1) lie ventral to the medulla and their branches, the posterior inferior cerebellar arteries (PICA, figure 1), traverse the lateral medullary cistern and cisterna magna to reach the cerebellum. The ninth, tenth, eleventh, and twelfth cranial nerves pass through the premedullary cistern on their way to the jugular foramen and hypoglossal canal. The cerebellar tonsils (figure 2) occupy a variable amount of the dorsolateral cisterna magna.

The vertebral arteries unite to form the basilar artery (figures 4, 5, 13) in the pre-pontine cistern. The basilar artery gives off the anterior inferior cerebellar and labyrinthine arteries which traverse the cerebellopontine cistern (figure 3) along with the seventh and eighth cranial nerves to reach the internal auditory meatus. The fifth (trigeminal) and sixth (abducens) cranial nerves pass through the prepontine cistern (figure 4) on their way to the semilunar ganglion and cavernous sinus.

The basilar artery ends in the interpeduncular cistern (figure 6, 7) ventral to the mesencephalon. Its terminal branches, the superior cerebellar and posterior cerebral arteries, pass lateral to the mesencephalon through the ambient cistern (figures 6, 7, 14) into the quadrigeminal cistern (figures 6, 7, 14) and on to the cerebrum above the tentorium and to the cerebellum below the tentorium. The quadrigeminal cistern also contains the great vein of Galen and its tributaries as it runs into the straight sinus. The trochlear nerve, arising from the dorsal surface of the brain stem, traverses the ambient cistern and joins the oculomotor nerve passing through the interpeduncular cistern on their way to the wall of the cavernous sinus.

The suprasellar cistern (figure 11) lies above the diaphragma sellae and below the hypothalamus and contains the optic chiasm and the bifurcation of the internal carotid arteries (figure 11) into anterior and middle cerebral arteries. The middle cereberal artery courses laterally through the Sylvian cistern into the insular cistern. The pentagonal cistern includes the suprasellar cistern (figure 5) and is a combination of the suprasellar and interhemispheric cisterns anteriorly, the lateral cistern anteriolaterally, the interpeduncular cistern posteriorly, and the ambient cistern posterolaterally. In practice, suprasellar cistern and pentagonal cistern can be used interchangeably.

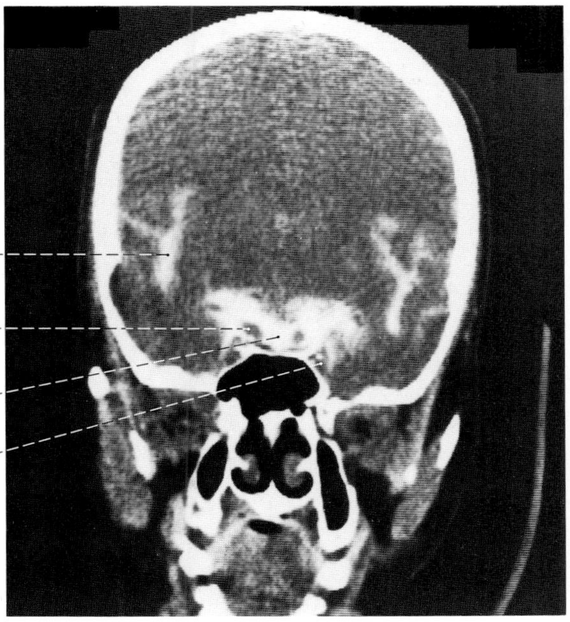
Insular
cistern
Internal
carotid
artery
Suprasellar
cistern
Cavernous
sinus

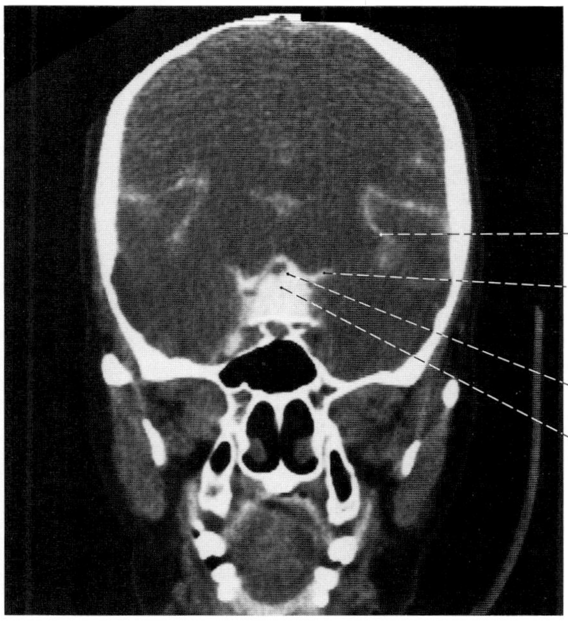
Insular
cistern
Ambient
cistern
Interpeduncular
cistern
Prepontine
cistern

11 12

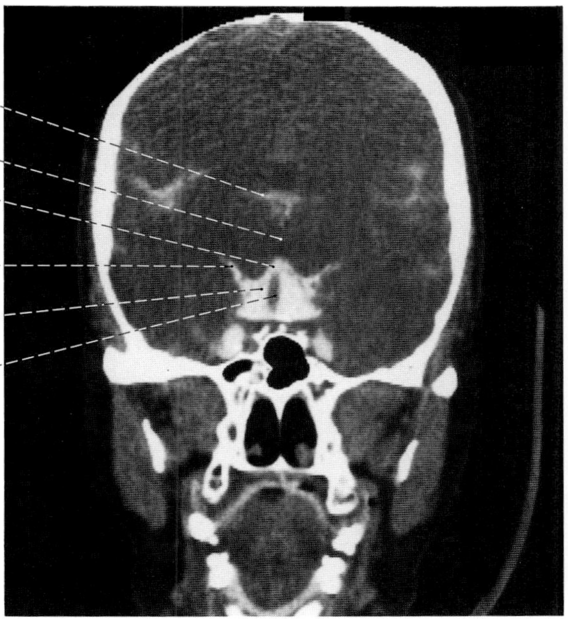
Transverse
cerebral
cistern
Mesencephalon
Interpeduncular
cistern
Ambient
cistern
Prepontine
cistern
Basilar
artery

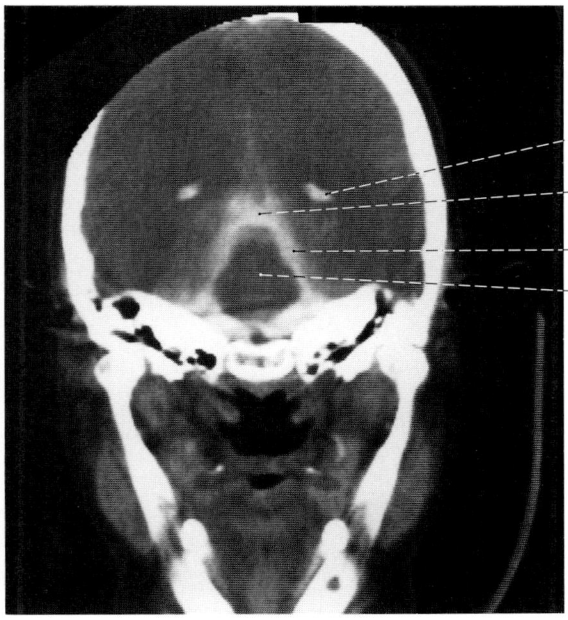
Glomus
Quadrigeminal
cistern
Ambient
cistern
Pons

13 14

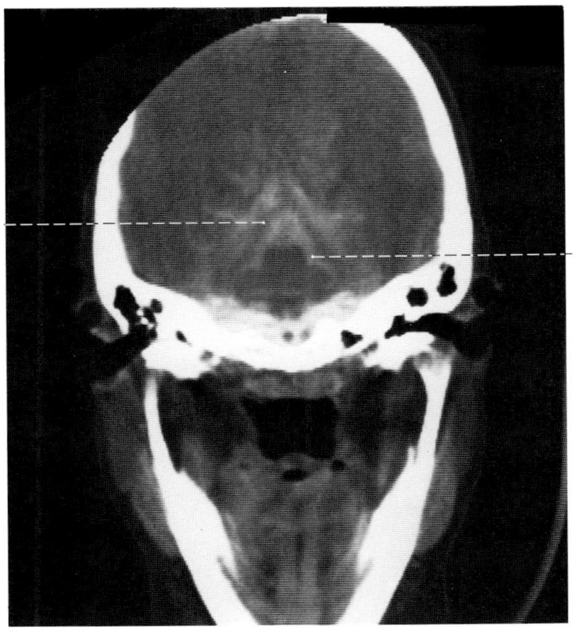
Tentorium
Superior
cerebellar cistern

15

Selected Bibliography

Carpenter, M. B., and Sutin, J. *Human Neuroanatomy,* 8th Edition, Williams & Wilkins, Baltimore, 1983.

Harwood-Nash, D. C. and Fitz, C. R., eds. *Hydrocephalus in Neuroradiology of Infants and Children*. C. V. Mosby Co., St. Louis, 1976.

Milhorat, T. H. The third circulation revisited. *J. Neurosurg*. 46: 628–654, 1975.

Naidich, T. P., Schott, L. H., and Baron, R. L. Computed tomography in evaluation of hydrocephalus. *Rad Clin North Amer.* 20: 143–168, 1982.

Newton, T. H., and Potts, D. G., eds. *Radiology of the Skull and Brain. Volume 4: Ventricles and Cisterns*. C. V. Mosby Co., St. Louis, 1978.

Warwick, R., and Williams, P. L., eds. *Gray's Anatomy.* 36th British Edition, W. B. Saunders Co., Philadelphia, 1981.

Vasculature of the Brain

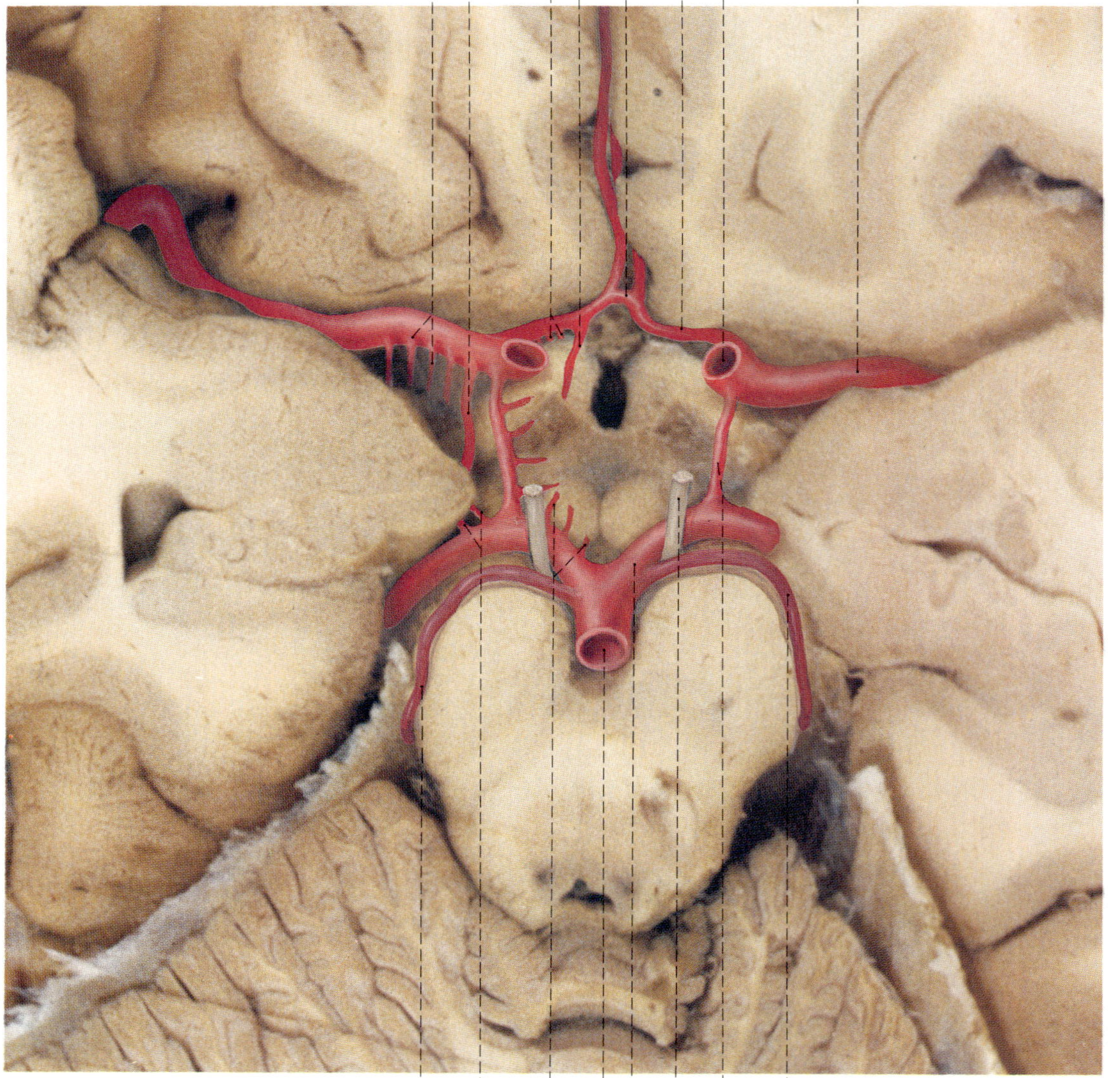

The base of the brain through the suprasellar cistern (see also page 38). A drawing of the arteries forming the circle of Willis has been superimposed on an axial section of the head. On the opposing page, the branches of the internal carotid and vertebral arteries have been superimposed on a tracing of the lateral radiograph of the head. The blood supply of the dura (not illustrated) is from the middle meningeal branch of the external carotid system *except* for the anterior falx, which is variably perfused by a branch of the ophthalmic artery and the falx cerebelli, which can be variably supplied by a posterior meningeal branch of a vertebral artery, and the dura of the cavernous sinus and tentorium which is supplied by branches of the internal carotid.

The configuration of the circle of Willis (circulus arteriosus cerebri) conforms to the shape of the pentagonal (suprasellar) cistern as noted in axial sections. The circle of Willis, in fact, forms the borders of that cistern. Important relationships are the close proximity of the uncus to the posterior communicating artery and to the oculomotor (3rd cranial) nerve which courses just medial to the artery. Aneurysms of the supraclinoid internal carotid artery at the origin of the posterior communicating artery may impinge on the oculomotor nerve and produce ipsilateral pupillary dilatation. The almost invariable path of the oculomotor nerve between the posterior cerebral artery and the superior cerebellar artery is illustrated. The latter arteries partially encircle the brainstem in the ambient cistern but the posterior cerebral is above the tentorium while the superior cerebellar courses beneath it.

The supraclinoid carotid is shown bifurcating on either side into anterior and middle cerebral arteries. The "A-1" segment of the

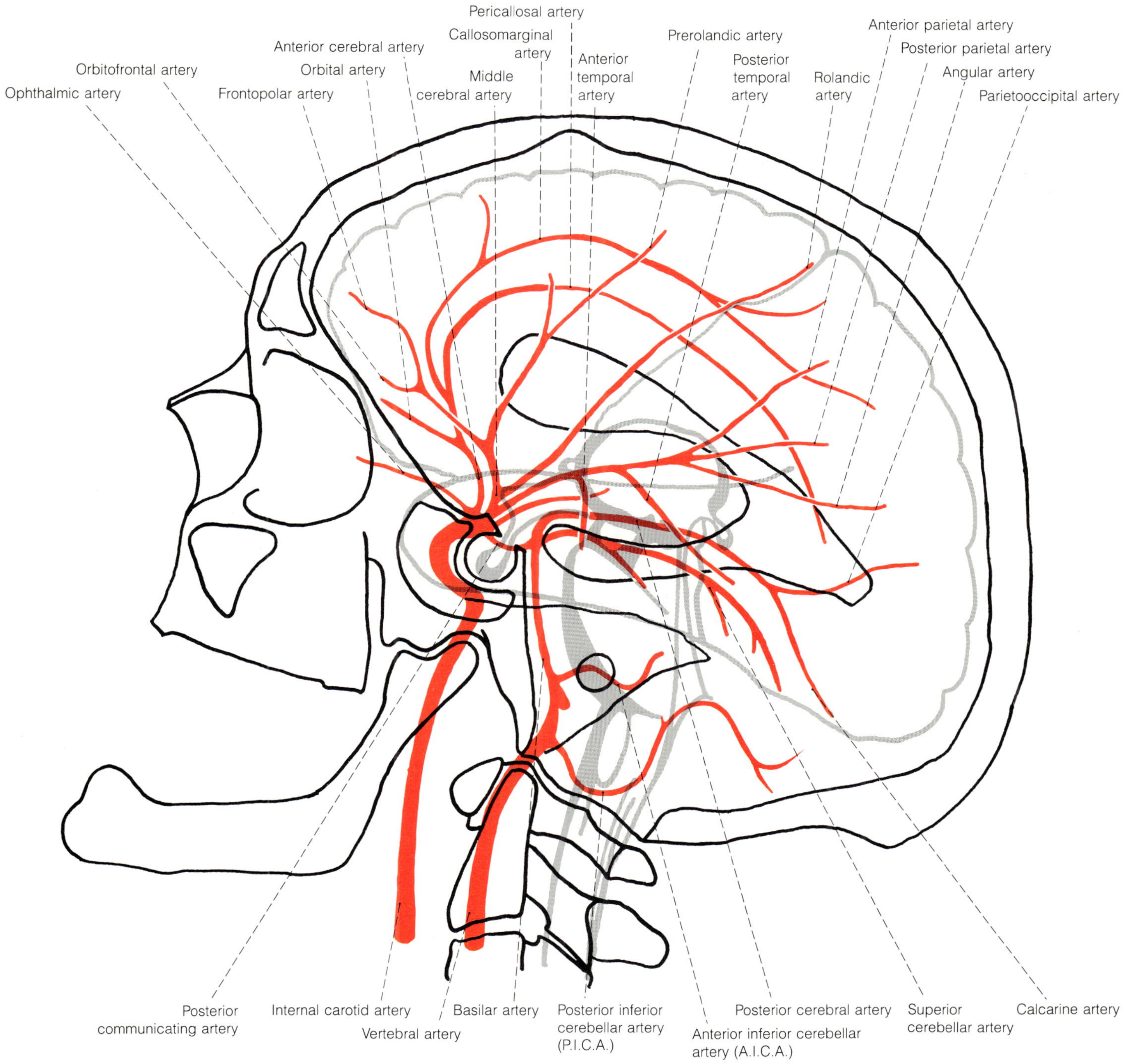

anterior cerebral artery runs from the supraclinoid carotid to the anterior communicating artery where it becomes pericallosal. The anterior cerebral artery bifurcates terminally into pericallosal and callosomarginal branches with multiple tributaries to the medial cerebral cortex. The middle cerebral artery is, in most patients, the most direct continuation of the internal carotid artery. The "M-1" segment of the middle cerebral artery extends from carotid bifurcation to the bifurcation or trifurcation of the middle cerebral artery into its Sylvian branches in the insular cistern. Arising from the M-1 segment are the lenticulostriate arteries which are of small caliber and fragile. These vessels supply the major mass of the basal ganglia (globus pallidus, putamen and head of the caudate nucleus) as well as the anterior limb and genu of the internal capsule. These lenticulostriate (or antero-lateral perforating) arteries are prone to rupture with high blood pressure. The genu of the internal capsule and the anterior part of the thalamus may also be supplied by these small perforating arteries. Similar tiny perforating vessels supply the major mass of the thalami but they arise from the tip of the basilar artery and initial segments of the posterior cerebral artery. The posterior cerebral artery from the basilar bifurcation to the posterior communicating artery is known as the "P-1" segment.

The brainstem and cerebellum in the posterior fossa are perfused by the vertebral-basalar system. These vessels not only also supply the medial temporal and occipital lobes above the tentorium but contribute to the arterial supply of the cervical spinal cord.

The venous drainage of the brain can be roughly divided into a larger superficial system covering the cerebral hemispheres and a smaller deep system, which is in a subependymal relationship to the ventricles.

The superficial veins of the cortex are highly variable. Several cortical veins of differing sizes drain the bulk of the surface cortex, flowing superiorly and posteriorly until just before entering the superior sagittal sinus, where they turn abruptly anteriorly to actually join the flow of that sinus. Temporal veins carry venous drainage from the temporal lobe into either the sphenoid dural sinus anteriorly or the transverse dural sinus posteriorly. Like the veins of the vertex, these are highly variable in size and shape. If dominant drainage is superiorly into the superior sagittal sinus, there is often a single large vein at the postcentral gyrus area which can be designated a "vein of Trolard". Inferior-posterior drainage can often produce a dominant vein designated as the "vein of Labbé" which drains into a transverse sinus.

Deep drainage is through a system of small veins which travel through the white matter pathways known as medullary veins. These are microscopic and usually not appreciated on angiograms unless they are congenitally dilated and are then referred to as "venous angiomata". Medullary veins drain into subependymal veins which are bilaterally symmetrical in the midline. Septal and caudate veins on either lateral ventricle course in the septum pellucidum and head of the caudate nucleus respectively, joining at about the foramen of Monro with the thalamostriate vein which drains the postero-lateral wall of the lateral ventricle and thalamus. These three or more vessels are somewhat variable but join together to form the internal cerebral vein. An internal cerebral vein runs on each side of midline in the roof of the 3rd ventricle or tela choroidea in a posterior direction until it joins with its twin to form the vein of Galen. Other large paired veins draining the uncal region have coursed dorsally around the brainstem in the ambient cistern and are designated the basal veins of Rosenthal. The basal veins drain into the vein of Galen or sometimes into the internal cerebral veins and the flow of blood then passes into the straight sinus at the apex of the tentorium. The straight sinus runs dorsally and caudally to join the superior sagittal sinus at the confluence of sinuses (torcular Herophili) where it is joined by blood draining via the superior sagittal sinus. Blood then runs around the inner surface of the occiput in the transverse sinus on either side to the sigmoid sinus, jugular bulb, and out of the skull via the internal jugular vein. Dominant drainage is more often asymmetric, greater on the right than on the left.

Veins draining the base of the brain are not as variable and consist mainly of the superior and inferior petrosal sinuses running along the petrous ridges and petrous bones respectively. These collect blood from the cavernous sinuses and venous plexuses along the sphenoid ridge and the sella and along the dorsum sella as well. Drainage is then laterally via the superior and inferior petrosal veins to the jugular system.

In addition to the major drainage from within the skull via the internal jugular vein, numerous smaller channels traverse the bone either directly or through the diploë. These include communications with the occipital veins, through the rete hypoglossi in the hypoglossal foramen, communications with the pterygoid plexus through the foramen lacerum, and anastomoses with the facial veins by the ophthalmic veins. These communicating veins are rarely visualized in CT scans because of their relationships to bone and their diminutive size.

In the posterior fossa multiple variable veins drain the brainstem forming a capillary network, which can sometimes be seen rather well on angiography, known as the pre-pontine plexus. A lateral anastomatic mesencephalic vein may exist and supply drainage around the midbrain.

Drainage of the cerebellar hemispheres is similar to the drainage of the cerebral hemispheres with cortical veins draining toward the transverse and straight sinuses. Many veins drain medially forming larger midline channels known as vermian veins since they overlie the cerebellar vermis. Superior and inferior vermian veins will drain directly into the straight sinus. A rather constant vessel, the pre-central cerebellar vein, marks the anterior-superior extent of the vermis and drains usually into the vein of Galen. Cortical veins over the anterior half of the cerebellar hemispheres may coalesce and form petrosal vein complexes which drain across the subarachnoid space into the superior petrosal sinus bilaterally.

The large cavernous sinuses on either side of the sella turcica are traversed by numerous trabeculae so that there is no single central cavity. These sinuses transmit the internal carotid arteries and all the nerves (except the optic) entering the orbit. On coronal CT with contrast each of these can be identified.

The cavernous sinuses intercommunicate through channels anterior and posterior to the pituitary. The ophthalmic and sphenoparietal sinuses enter it anteriorly and the superior and inferior petrosal sinuses drain posteriorly. A Vesalian vein may perforate the great wing of the sphenoid to communicate with the pterygoid plexus of veins but more constant communications are through a venous rete in the foramen ovale and small veins penetrating the foramen lacerum.

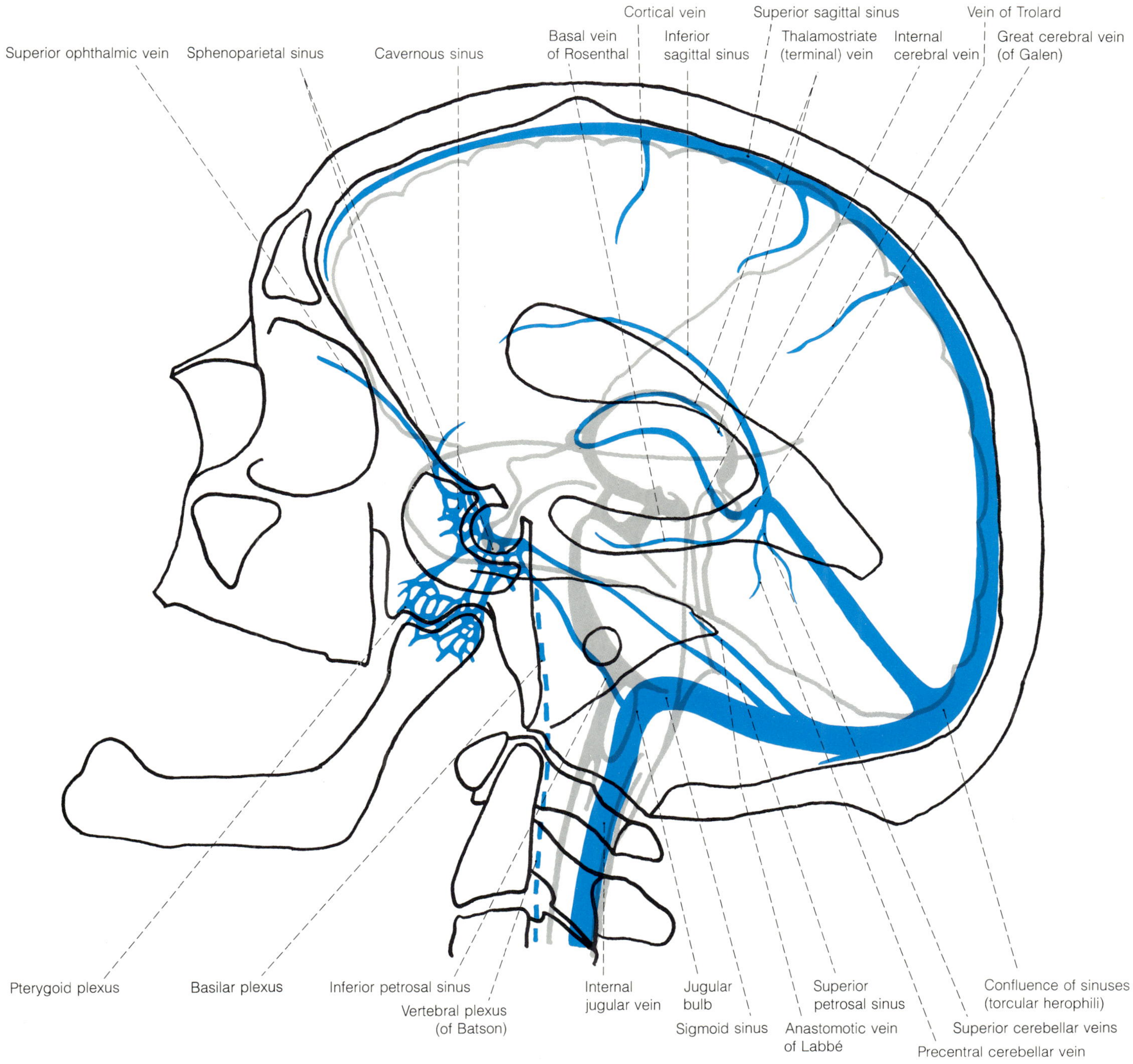
Superior ophthalmic vein
Sphenoparietal sinus
Cavernous sinus
Basal vein of Rosenthal
Cortical vein
Inferior sagittal sinus
Superior sagittal sinus
Thalamostriate (terminal) vein
Internal cerebral vein
Vein of Trolard
Great cerebral vein (of Galen)
Pterygoid plexus
Basilar plexus
Inferior petrosal sinus
Vertebral plexus (of Batson)
Internal jugular vein
Jugular bulb
Sigmoid sinus
Superior petrosal sinus
Anastomotic vein of Labbé
Confluence of sinuses (torcular herophili)
Superior cerebellar veins
Precentral cerebellar vein

Selected Bibliography

Adachi, B., and K. Hasebe. *Das Arteriensystem der Japaner.* Bd. 1, Bd. 2, Kenkyusha, Tokio, 1928.

Berman, S. A., L. A. Hayman, and V. C. Hinck. Correlation of C. cerebral vascular territories with function: I. Anterior cerebral artery. *AJNR* 1: 259–26, 1980.

Carpenter, M. B., and J. Sutin. *Human Neuroanatomy, 8th ed.* Williams & Wilkins, Baltimore, 1983.

Dandy, W. E. *The Brain* (Reprint). Hueber Division of Harper and Row, New York, 1969.

Ferner, H. *Eduard Pernkopf Atlas of Topographical and Applied Human Anatomy, 2nd ed.* Urban & Schwarzenberg, Baltimore and Munich, 1980.

Ferner, H., and J. Staubesand. *Sobotta Atlas of Human Anatomy, 10th English ed.,* Translated by W. Hild. Urban & Schwarzenberg, Baltimore and Munich, 1983.

Hayman, L. A., S. A. Berman, and V. C. Hinck. Correlation of CT cerebral vascular territories with function: II. Posterior cerebral artery. *AJNR* 2: 219–225, 1981.

Lang, J. *Clinical Anatomy of the Head, Neurocranium, Orbit, Craniocervical Regions.* Trans. by R. R. Wilson and D. P. Winstanley. Springer-Verlag, Berlin, Heidelberg, N.Y., 1983

Newton, T. H., and D. G. Potts. *Radiology of the Skull and Brain, Vol. 2: Angiography.* C. V. Mosby Co., S. Louis, 1974.

Siekert, R. G. *Cerebrovascular Survey Report (revised) for the Joint Council Subcommittee on Cerebrovascular Disease.* NINCDS and National Heart and Lung Institute, 1980.

Taveras, J. M., and E. H. Wood, *Diagnostic Neuroradiology, 2nd ed. Vols. I* and *II.* Williams & Wilkins, Baltimore, 1976.

Wackenheim, A., and J. P. Braun. *The Veins of the Posterior Fossa.* Springer-Verlag, Berlin, Heidelberg, N.Y., 1978.

Larynx

Carlos R. Martinez, M.D.

We have used a twelve section approach to the cross-sectional anatomy of the larynx as shown by computed tomography. Sections displayed here were obtained with a third generation unit, with a scanning time of 4.7 seconds. The scanning plane is nearly parallel to the true vocal cords. These adjacent sections are 4 mm in thickness. Since the average height of the adult larynx is 44 mm in males and 36 mm in females, these sections afford cross-sectional display of the entire larynx in most individuals. It should be noted that the position of the larynx in relation to the cervical vertebrae is variable; it occupies a higher position in children and women.

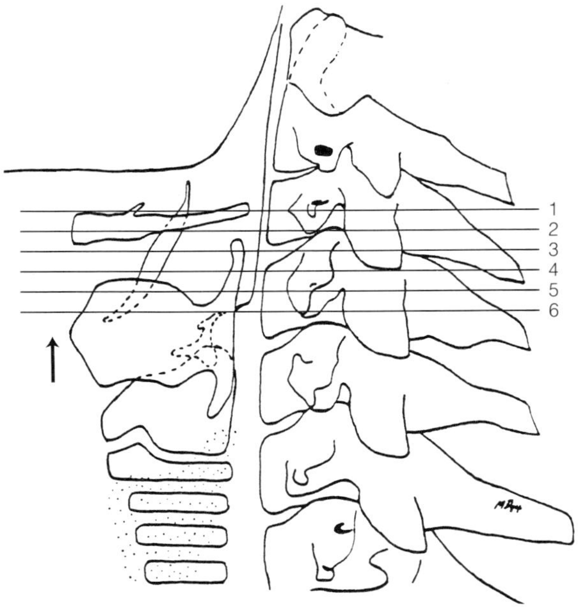

Sections 1–2

In sections 1–2 the tip (free margin) of the epiglottis is visualized in the middle of the airway. The valleculae separate the base of the tongue from the epiglottis. The upper part of the anterior surface of the epiglottis is covered by mucosa which reflects laterally onto the lateral wall of the pharynx as the pharyngoepiglottic fold and in the midline to the base of the tongue as the median glossoepiglottic fold. The lower part of the anterior surface of the epiglottis lies behind the hyoid bone and is separated from it by the predominantly fatty tissue that comprises the pre-epiglottic space. The body of the hyoid and its greater horns are well seen. The common carotid artery bifurcates at these levels in most individuals.

Sections 3–6

Sections 3–6 are at the level of the laryngeal inlet, bound anteriorly by the epiglottis, laterally and posterolaterally by the aryepiglottic folds. At these levels the epiglottis is separated from the thyrohyoid membrane and the upper thyroid cartilage by fatty tissue (lower pre-epiglottic space). The aryepiglottic folds are best visualized by CT during E-phonation or modified valsalva maneuver. They separate the laryngeal inlet from the pyriform sinuses. Aryepiglottic folds are made up of mucosa covered quadrangular membrane which extends from the lateral margin of the epiglottis superiorly to the vestibular fold (false cord) inferiorly.

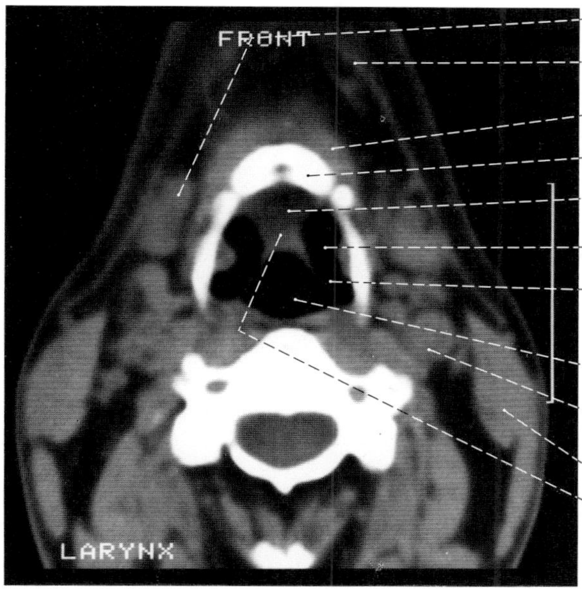

1 Left

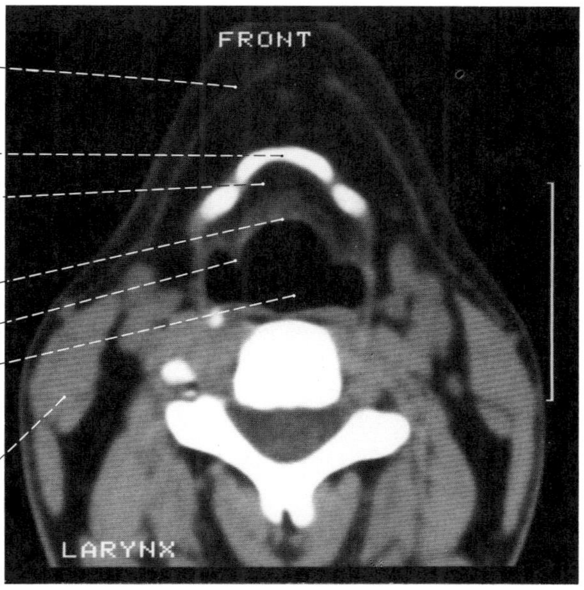

2 Left

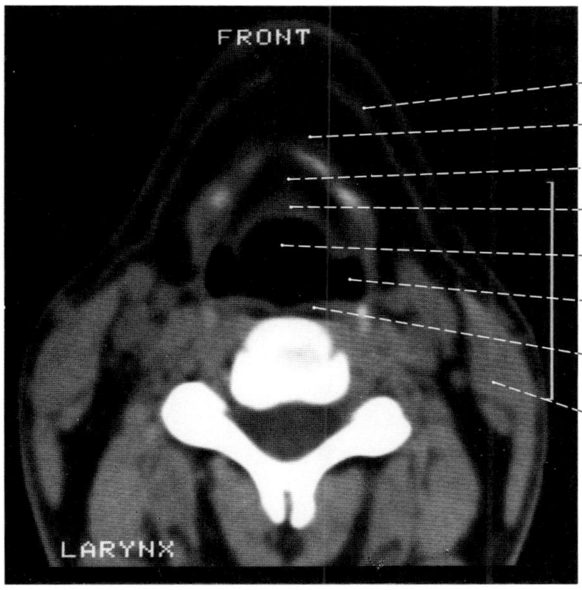

3 Left

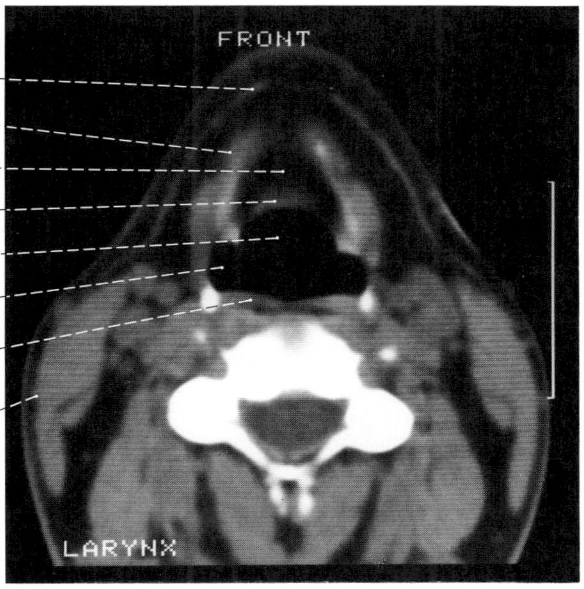

4 Left

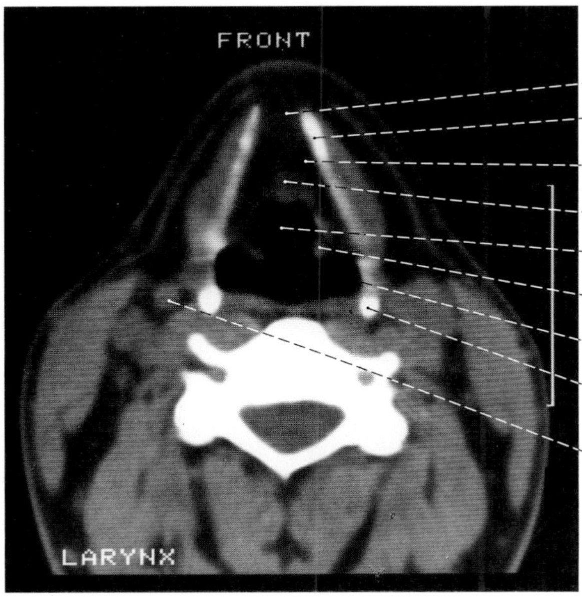

5 Left

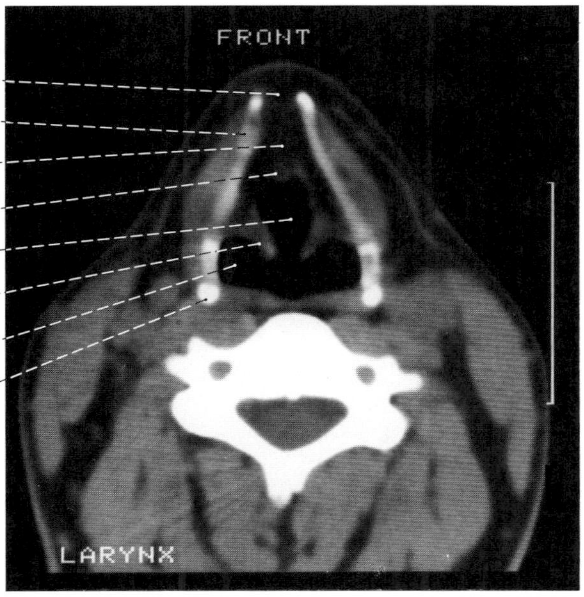

6 Left

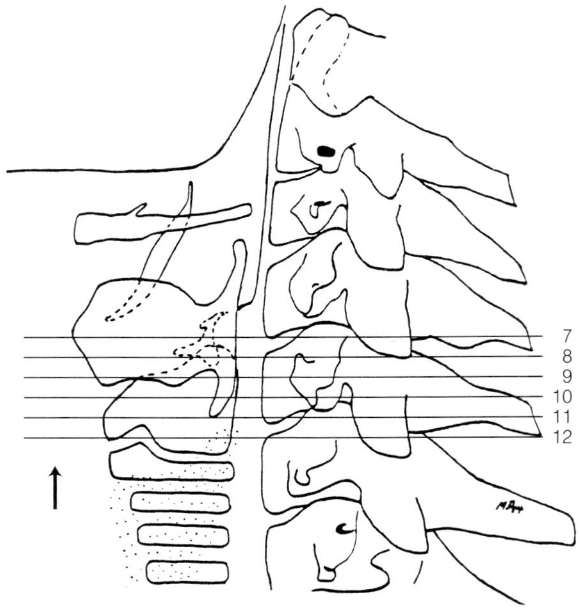

Levels 7–8

Sections 7–8 are at the level of the laryngeal vestibule. Key structures visualized include the ossified thyroid cartilage, the lower-most portion of aryepiglottic folds and pyriform sinuses, and the vestibular folds (false cords). The thyroid cartilage consists of two quadrilateral laminae that are fused anteriorly forming an angle of about 90° in men and 120° in women. Posteriorly the laminae diverge and the posterior border of each projects inferiorly and superiorly as the lesser and greater horns respectively. The pattern of ossification of the thyroid cartilage is variable but usually symmetric from side to side. The thyroid cartilage may ossify as a solid sheet of bone or there may be ossification of the margins of the laminae leaving an uncalcified marrow space. The false cords (vestibular folds) are two thick folds of mucosa surrounding a fibrous band called the vestibular ligament which extends from the thyroid cartilage to the anterolateral surface of the arytenoid cartilage. The lower-most portion of the epiglottis (petiole) is also seen at this level projecting posteriorly as a small tubercle just above the attachment of vestibular folds. The petiole is connected to the thyroid laminae angle by the thyroepiglottic ligament. Cuneiform and corniculate cartilages are present at these levels but rarely distinctly visualized by CT due to their small size and lack of ossification.

Sections 9–10

Sections 9–10 are at the level of the glottic space. The true vocal cords (vocal folds) are well seen stretching from the angle of the thyroid cartilage to the vocal process of the arytenoid cartilage. Each vocal cord consists of a tough band of elastic tissue (vocal ligament) covered by stratified squamous epithelium and bound laterally by a muscular bundle, the vocalis muscle, which extends from the vocal process of the arytenoid cartilage to the anterior commissure at the inner surface of the thyroid cartilage. The laryngeal ventricles may be visualized at these levels as air-filled recesses which lie between the anterior half of the true and false cords. The space between the true cords is usually referred to as the rima glottidis, extending between the vocal cords anteriorly and the vocal processes of the arytenoid cartilages posteriorly. The true cords are distinguished from the false cords by localizing the upper portion of the cricoid lamina, the vocal process of the arytenoid and by the close apposition of the anterior commissure to the thyroid cartilage.

Sections 11–12

Sections 11–12 are at the level of the subglottic space. The cricoid cartilage is shaped like a signet ring, comprised of a quadrate posterior lamina and a narrow anterior arch which measures 5–7 mm in height. The cricoid lamina measures 2–3 cm in height and serves as support for the arytenoid cartilages. The cricothyroid joint is seen posteriorly. Note the smooth sharply defined internal surface of the subglottic space, the mucosa being closely applied to the cricoid cartilage. The subglottic space extends from the under surface of the true cords to the lower border of the cricoid cartilage. The upper poles of the thyroid gland are usually seen at these levels and readily identified by the characteristically high density of the normal thyroid tissue.

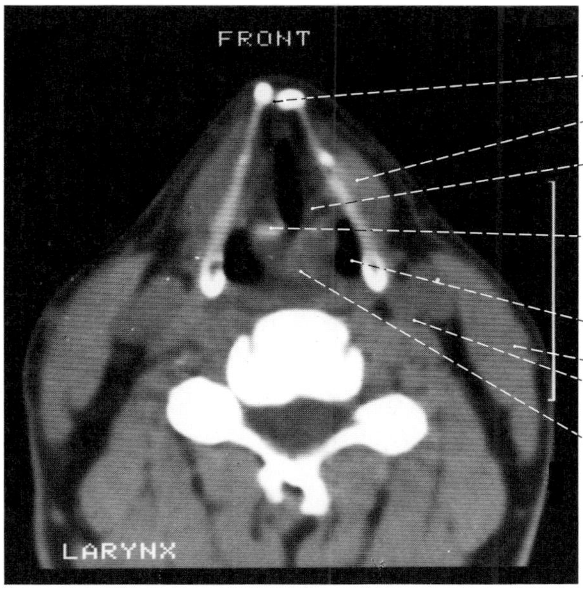

7 Left

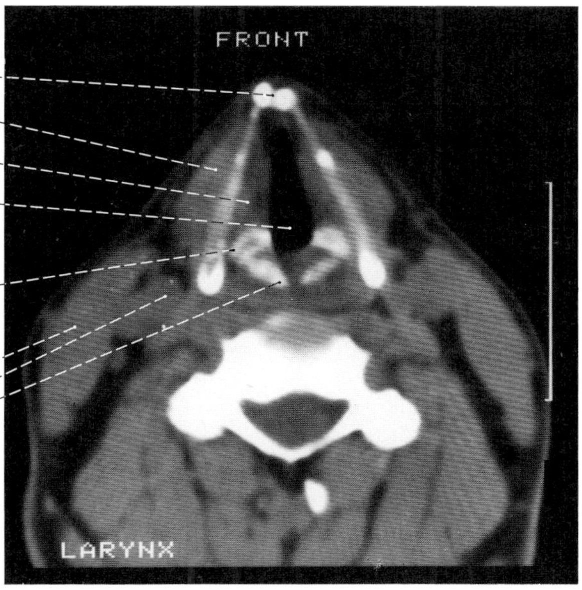

8 Left

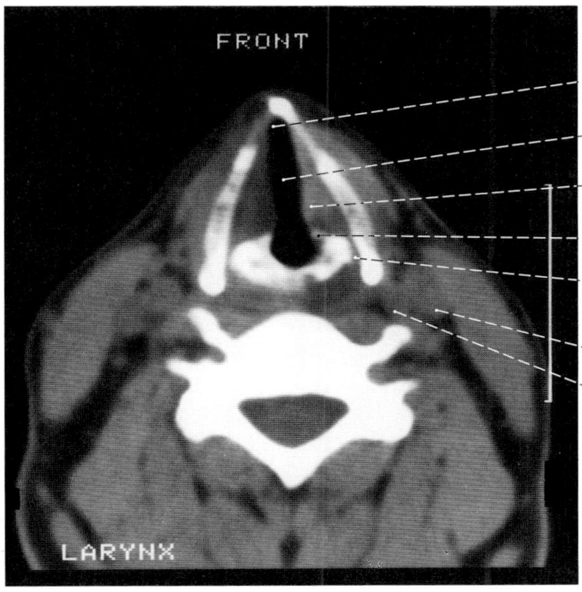

9 Left

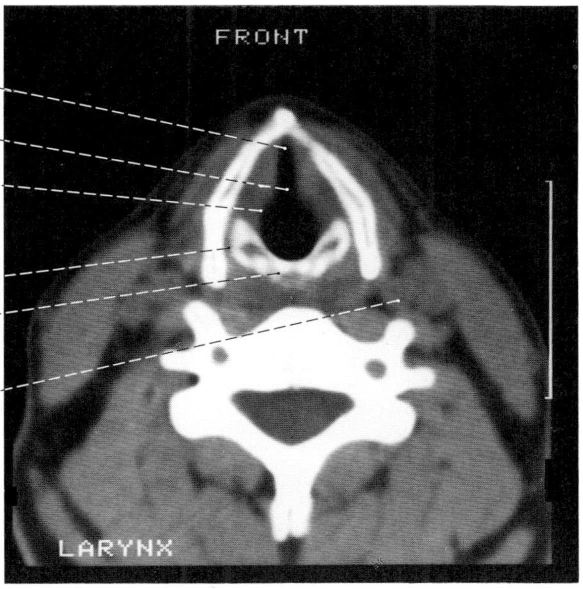

10 Left

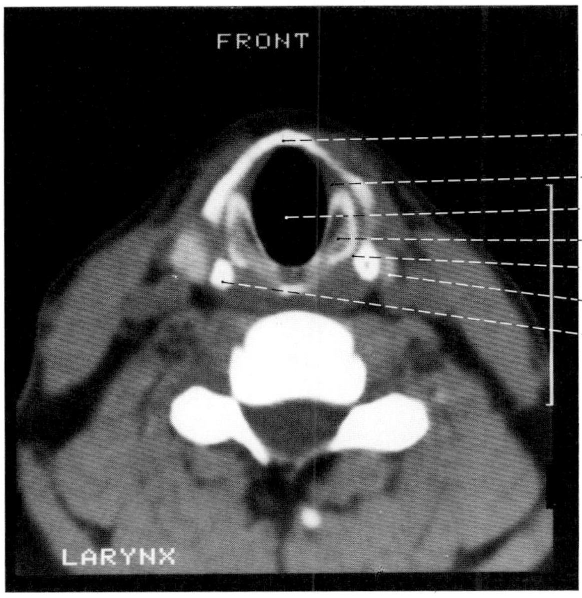

11 Left

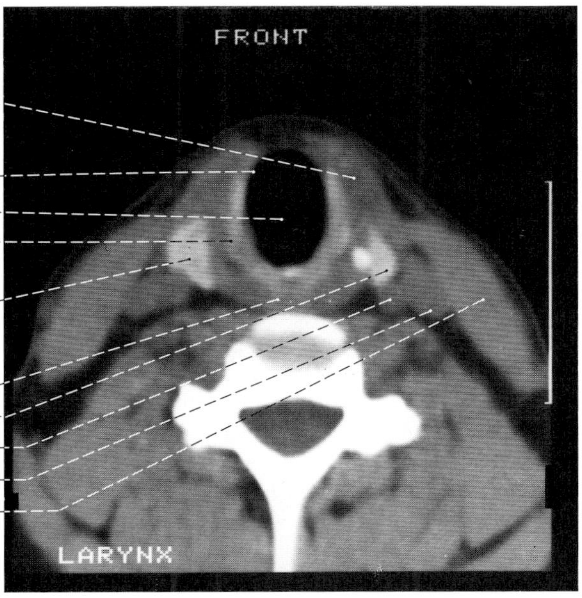

12 Left

Selected Bibliography

Gamsu, G., A. S. Mark, and W. R. Webb. Computed Tomography of the Normal Larynx During Quiet Breathing and Phonation. *J. Comp. Assist. Tomog.* 5: 353, 1981.

Mancuso, A. A., and W. N. Hanafee. *Computed Tomography of the Head and Neck.* Williams & Wilkins, Baltimore, 1982.

Reede, D. L., M. A. Whelan, and R. T. Bergeron. Computed tomography of the infrahyoid neck: Part I, normal anatomy. *Radiology* 145: 389, 1982.

Archer, C. R., V. L. Yeager, W. H. Friedman, and G. P. Katsantonis. Computed tomography of the larynx. *J. Comp. Assist. Tomog.* 2: 404, 1978.

Bergeron, R. T., A. G. Osborn, and P. M. Som. *Head and Neck Imaging: Excluding the Brain.* C. V. Mosby, St. Louis, 1983.

Martinez, C. R., H. Kashima, B. W. Gayler, and S. S. Siegelman. Computed tomography of the neck. *Ann. Otol. Rhinol. Laryngol.* (Suppl.) 99: 1, 1982.

Silverman, P. M., M. Korobkin, W. M. Thompson, J. A. Johnson, T. B. Cole, and S. R. Fisher. High resolution, thin section computed tomography of the larynx. *Radiology* 145, 723, 1982.

Hately, W., G. Evison, and E. Samuel. The pattern of ossification in the laryngeal cartilages: A radiological study. *Brit. J. Radiol.* 38: 585, 1965.

Reede, D. L., R. T. Bergeron, M. A. Whelan, N. L. Cohen, and M. S. Persky. Computed tomography of the cervical lymph nodes. *Radiograph.* 3: 339, 1983.

Cervical Spine

Carlos R. Martinez, M.D.

The availability of cross-sectional images of the body as depicted by computed tomography imaging (CT) revolutionized the learning and practice of neuroradiology. In the past, plain radiography, conventional tomography and/or myelography were the main diagnostic techniques used in the evaluation of the cervical spine and its contents. At the present time, CT has replaced to some extent conventional tomography and has gained more and more acceptance in the evaluation of the spinal cord, surrounding bony structures and paraspinal soft tissues. More recently, magnetic resonance imaging (MRI) has provided the means for imaging of the cervical cord and surrounding structures with the ability to obtain sections in multiple planes without loss of resolution. Experience to date suggests that the cord and cerebrospinal fluid are best seen with MRI techniques while bony structures are best imaged with computed tomography. This section has been designed to provide a better understanding of images of the cervical spine as depicted by sectional imaging techniques, predominatly by CT.
In preparing this chapter we took the following steps:

a) Cadaver axial sections were obtained using a GE 8800 CT scanner. Sections were 5 mm thick, 5 mm apart. Each section was photographed using soft tissue and bone settings. Since we used a torso, air occupies vascular and subarachnoid spaces and some fascial planes.

b) The cadaver torso was then embedded in gelatin, frozen, and later sectioned in the same axial plane using a commercial band saw. Each section is approximately 8–10 mm thick. The caudal inferior surface of each section was photographed so that the cadaver and CT sections would be displayed with the same orientation (cadaver's left side to viewer's right).

c) Cadaver anatomic sections were labeled with particular emphasis on those structures that are identifiable on current generation CT images.

d) Cadaver CT and anatomic sections were then matched as closely as possible with normal cervical spine CT images obtained from a patient volunteer who had had lumbar myelography with water soluble contrast material 4 hours earlier. Opacification of the subarachnoid space with contrast material makes the CT delineation of the cord more precise and more reliable. Because relationships of certain pre-vertebral structures (such as the larynx) to the cervical spine are variable, there is some discrepancy between cadaver and patient sections.

e) Finally, the captions that accompany each set of images are intended to emphasize clinically important anatomic facts or relationships.

Patient CT Scan

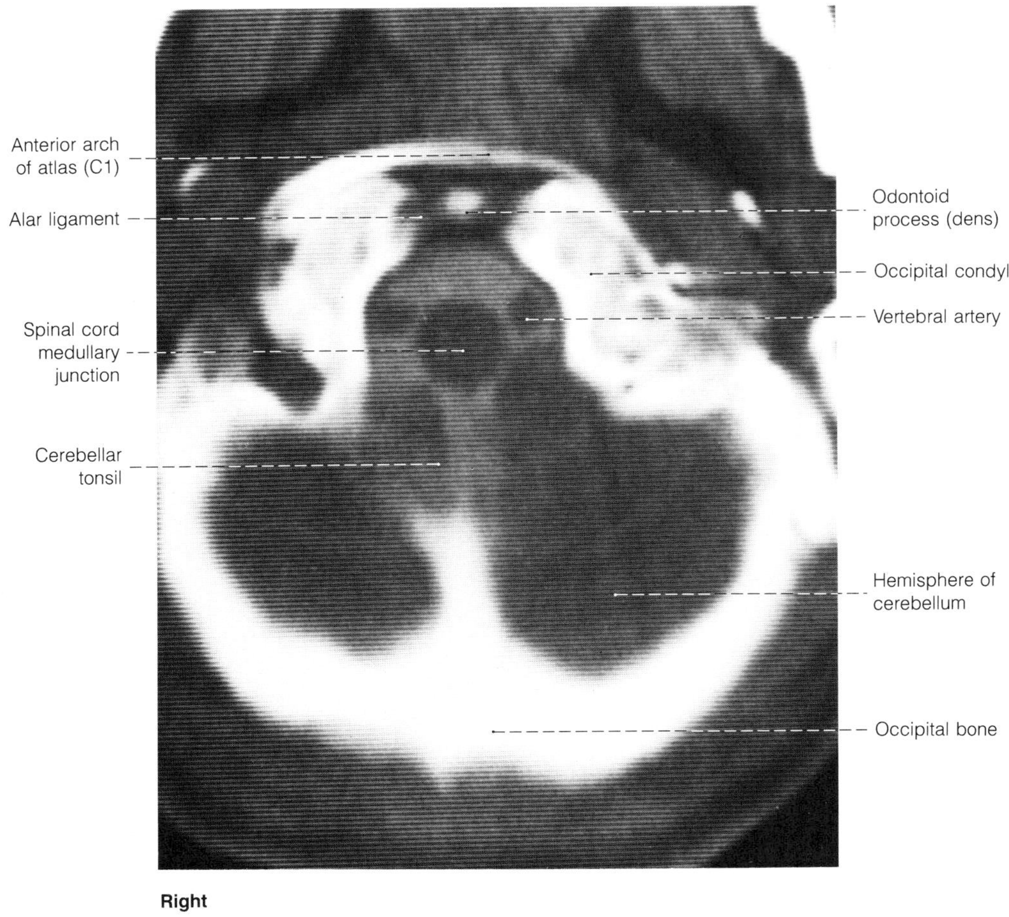

Cadaver CT Scan

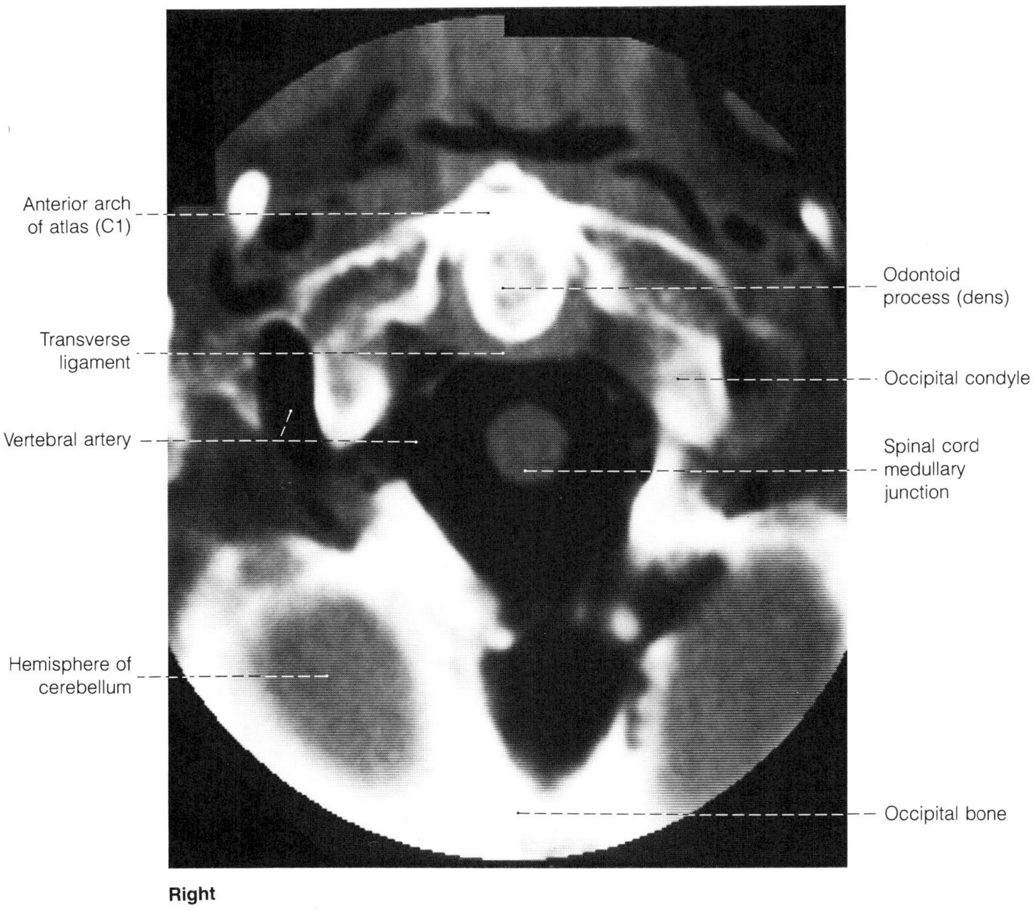

The CT anatomy displayed at this level varies according to the degree of flexion/extension of the cervical spine and also with the angulation of the plane of scanning. The scan of the cadaver is approximately 5 mm inferior to the patient scan. The atlanto-occipital joint is not well visualized on axial sections due to its shape (deeply concave superior articular surface of C1) and orientation (converging inferior-medially). Thus, only a portion of this narrow joint can be seen on a given axial section, the occipital condyle being found slightly posterior and medial to the lateral mass and superior articular surface of C1. The alar ligaments are visualized on scans at this level as soft tissue bands that extend from the tip of the odontoid process to the inferomedial aspect of the occipital condyles.

The size of the subarachnoid space which surrounds the cervico-medullary junction is variable but is usually about twice the diameter of the cord at this level. The cerebellar tonsils are usually

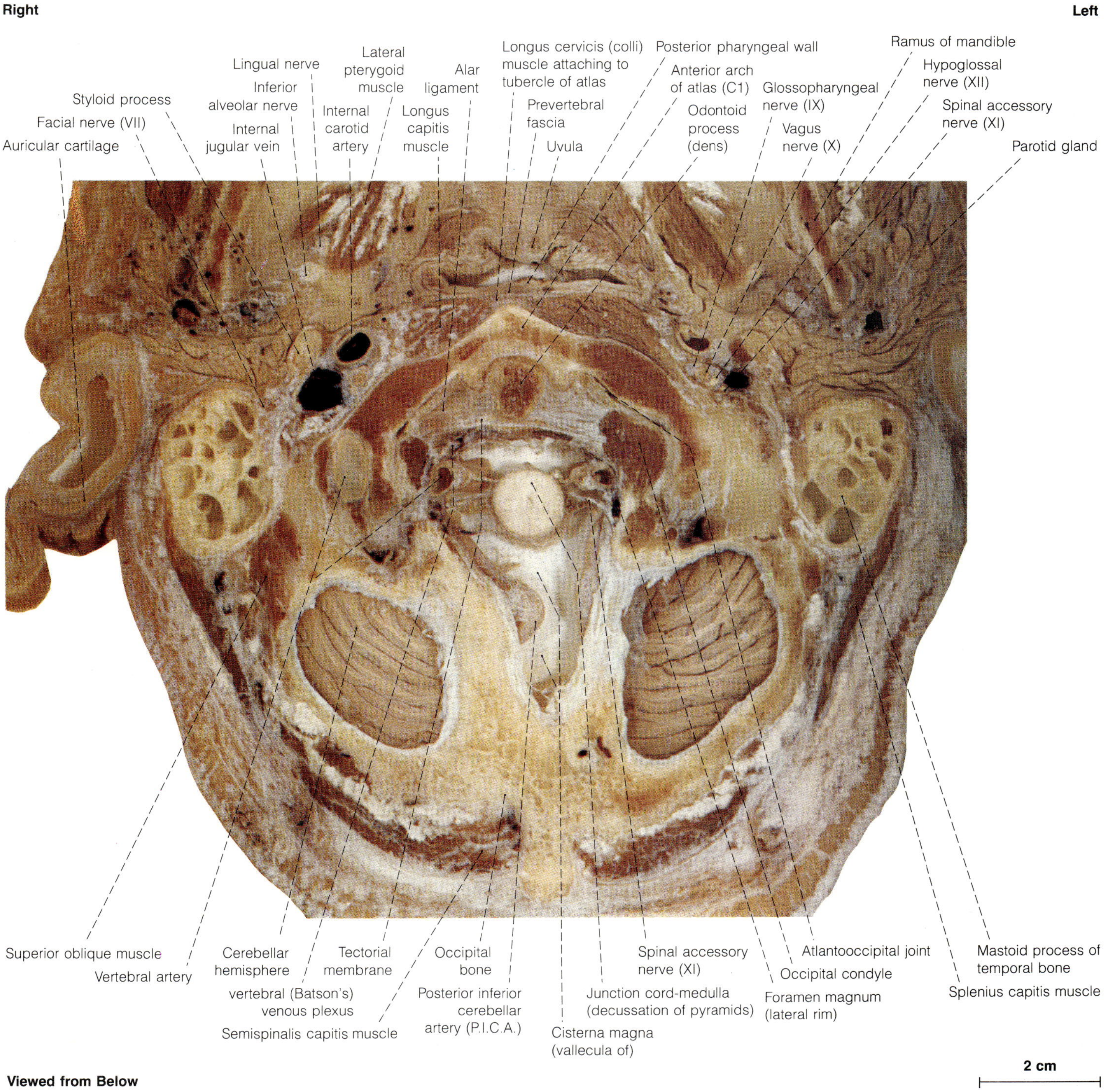

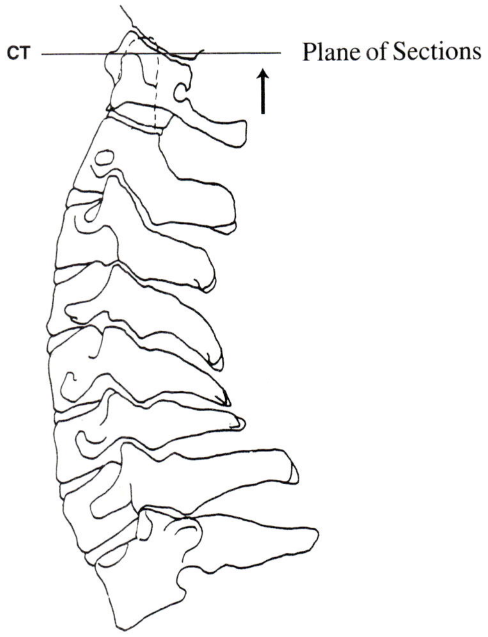

found just above the posterior lip of the foramen magnum, but can occasionally extend just below the foramen magnum in asymptomatic patients. A variable degree of inferior displacement of the tonsils, usually to the C1-C2 level is one of the hallmarks of the adult type of Arnold-Chiari malformation.

These sections demonstrate well the relationships of the vertebral arteries, ventro-lateral to the cervico-medullary junction. The cadaver CT scan, corresponding to the photograph of the cadaver, shows the right vertebral artery as it loops posterio-medially from the transverse foramen of C1 to enter the intradural (subarachnoid) space after piercing the posterior atlantooccipital membrane. The posterior inferior cerebellar arteries, quite evident in this figure, usually arise from the vertebral arteries just above the foramen magnum.

Patient CT Scan

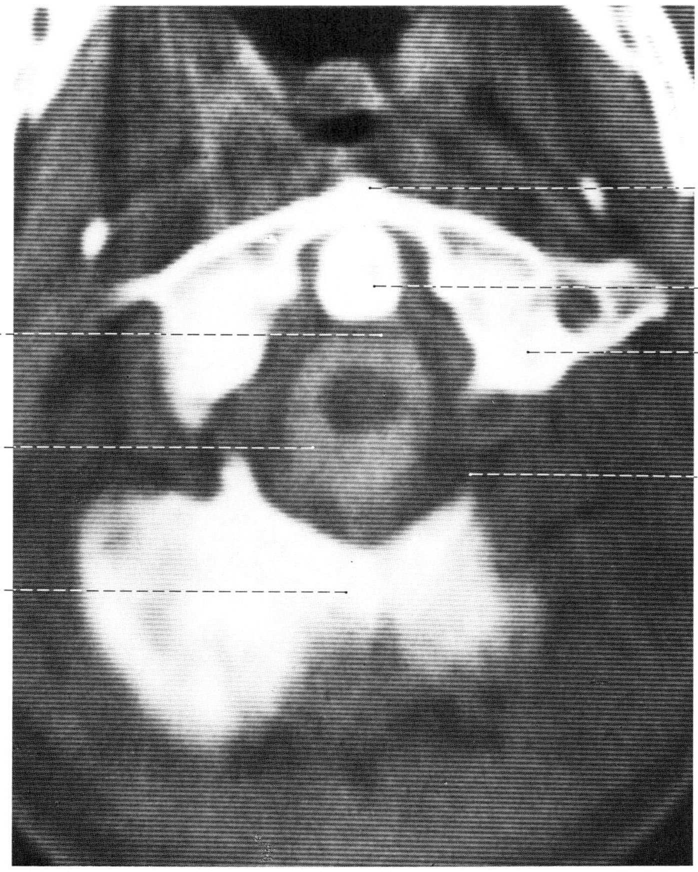

Cadaver CT Scan

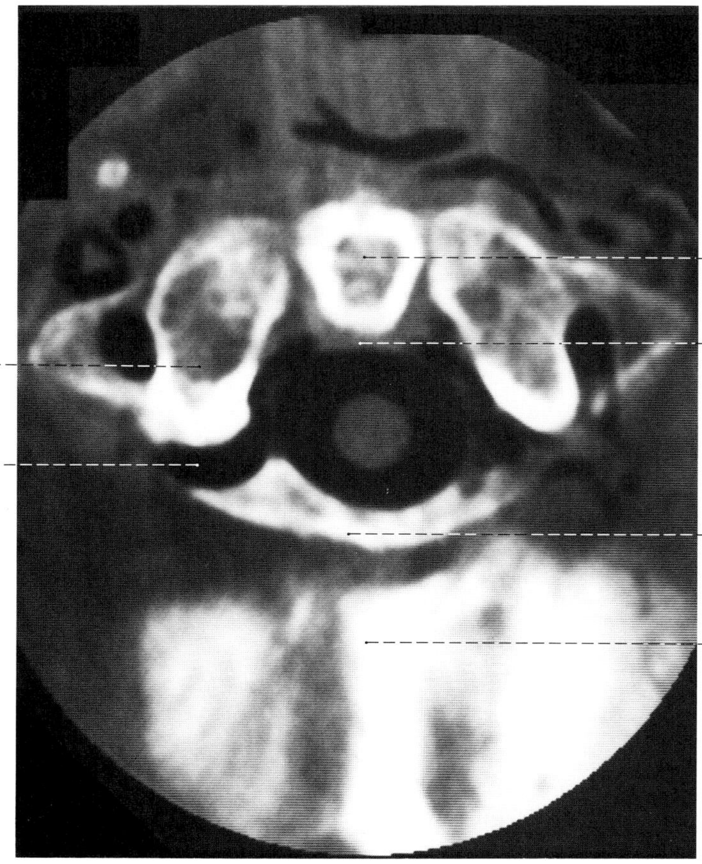

The plane of the two CT sections is through the lateral mass of C1. The image above of a patient is approximately 5 mm cephalad to that of the cadaver.

The atlanto-dental joint space is rather small and best resolved on CT sections by viewing the image with bone window setting. The articular surfaces of the odontoid anteriorly and posteriorly are lined by articular fibrocartilage. The space between the odontoid process medially and the axis laterally is filled by strong bands of connective tissue that form the atlanto-dental articular capsule. The transverse ligament is attached bilaterally to a small tubercle of

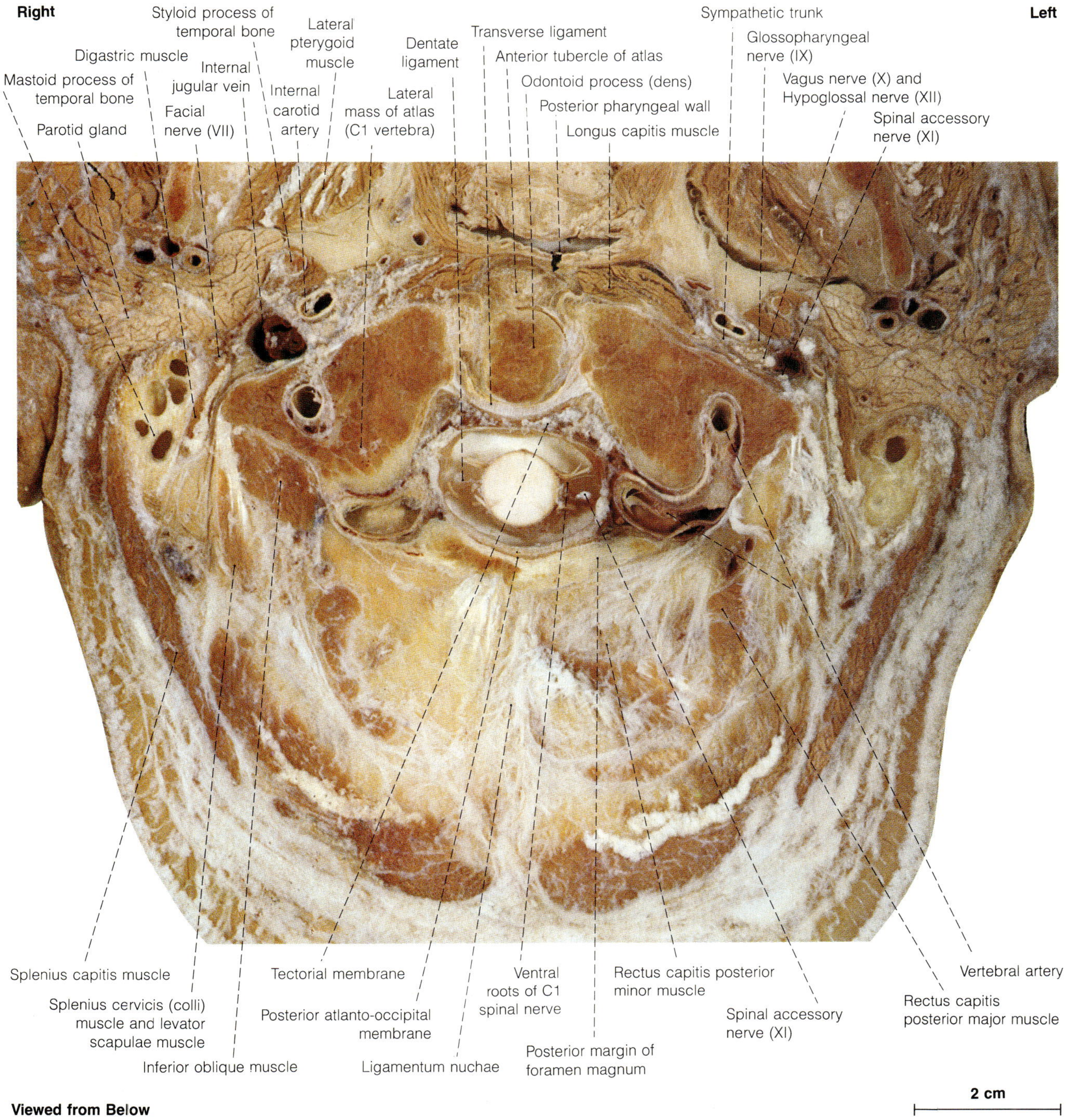

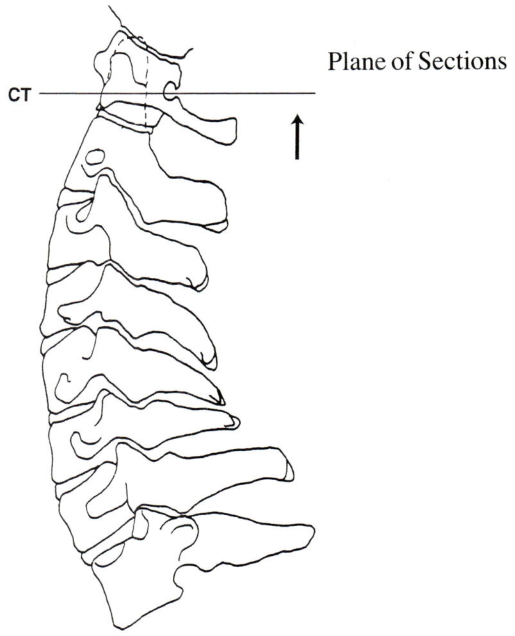

the medial surface of the lateral mass, which may be avulsed in C1 fractures, especially those associated with axial loading (Jefferson's fracture).

In this plane and those immediately caudal, the vertebral artery is quite close to the internal carotid artery and internal jugular vein. The glossopharyngeal (IX), vagus (X), spinal accessory (XI), and hypoglossal (XII) cranial nerves are found adjacent to the internal carotid artery and internal jugular vein, contained within the carotid sheath. There is a deep vertebral artery groove on the upper surface of the posterior arch of C1 just posterior to its junction with the lateral mass of C1. This groove could be mistaken for a fracture during CT examination.

CT has proved most valuable in delineating the extent of C1, C2 fractures, their displacement, and the degree of impingement on the subarachnoid space.

Patient CT Scan

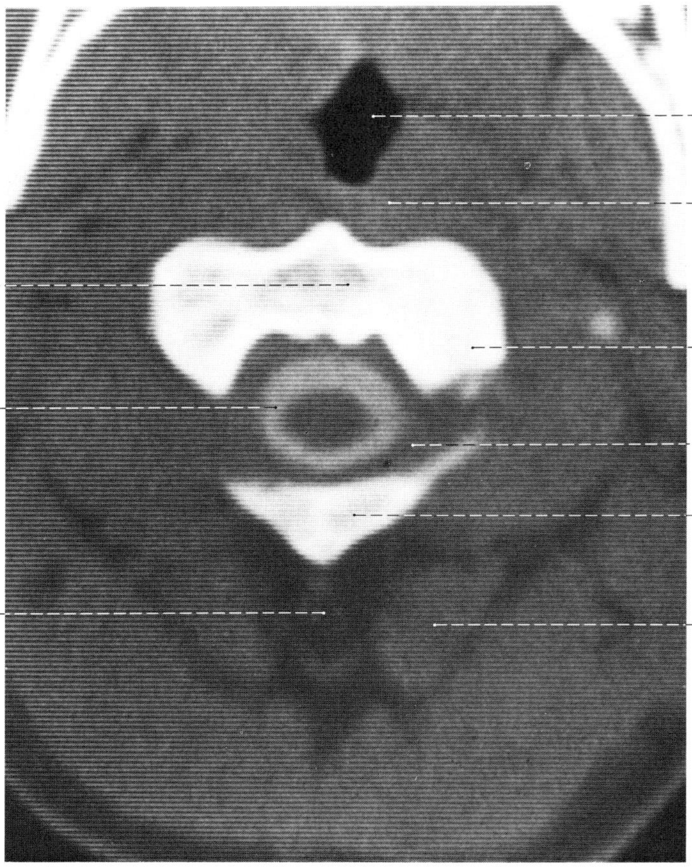

Cadaver CT Scan

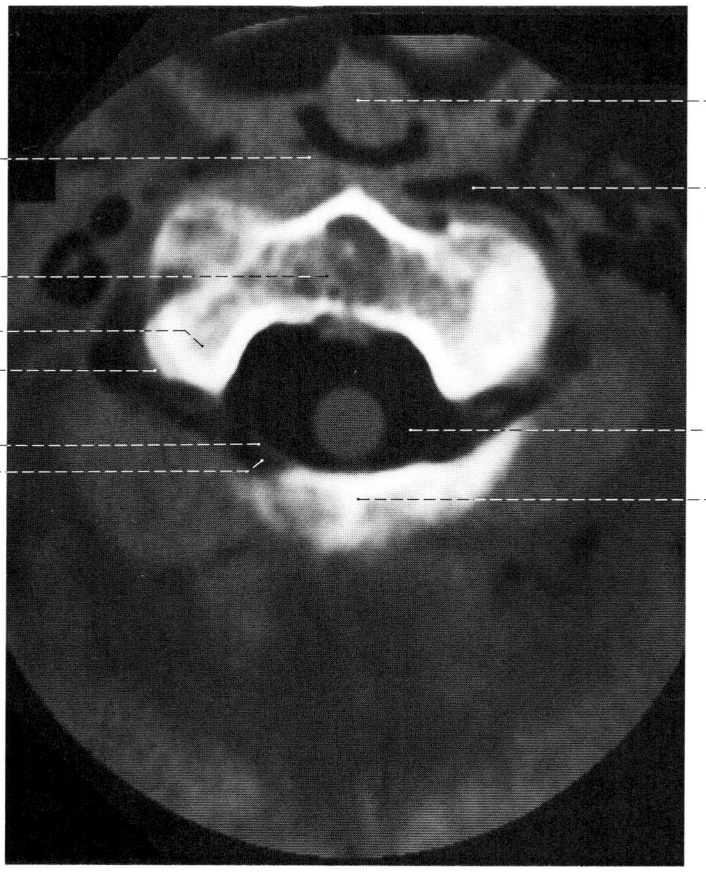

The upper portion of the vertebral body of C2 frequently has a small tuberosity anteriorly. Fibers of the anterior longitudinal ligament and the anterior atlanto-axial ligament attach to the ventral surface of the axis. The atlanto-axial facet joints are oval in shape, and slope laterally with a downward convexity. Consequently, only portions of these joints are visualized on a given thin axial CT section, the superior articular process of C2 being medial to the joint. The atlanto-axial facet joints are more anteriorly placed than similar articulations in the succeeding cervical vertebra. The dorsal root ganglion of C2 is located posterior to the C1-C2 articulation (retroarticular). A true intervertebral foramen does not exist between the atlas and the axis. At this level the spinal cord has a near round appearance in cross section and the mean antero-posterior diameter is 8–9 mm in adults, which is usually about one

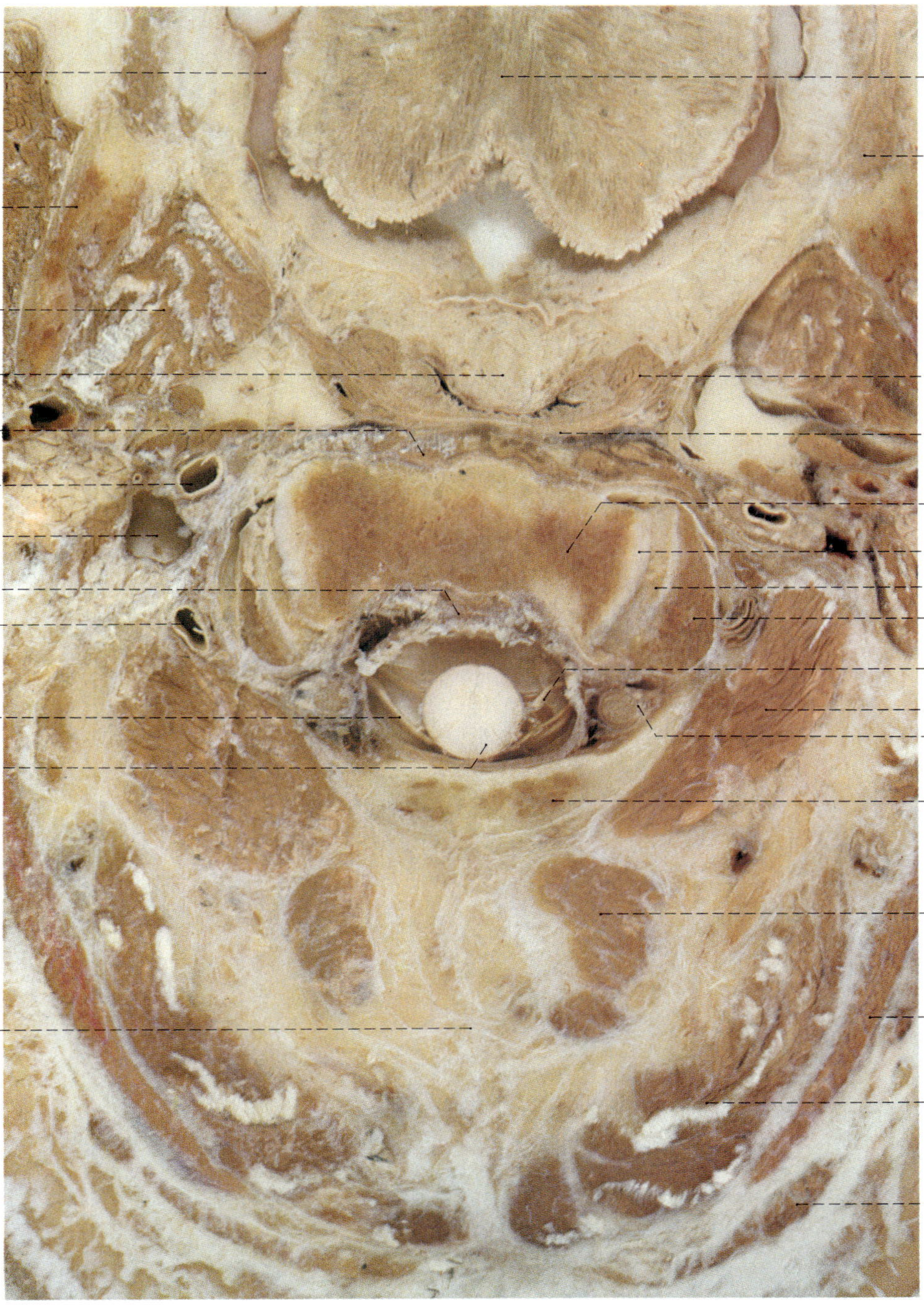

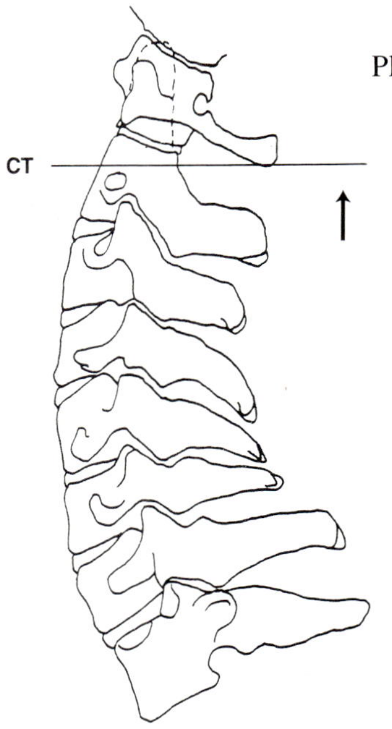

half of sagittal diameter of the spinal canal at this level. For this reason, traumatic cord compression at C1-C2 is less common than it is at lower cervical segments.

The longus cervicis (colli) muscle and the superior pharyngeal constrictor and related fascia separate the body of the axis from the pharynx. Enlargement of the retropharyngeal (prevertebral) space, due to hemorrhage and/or soft tissue swelling, frequently accompanies fracture/dislocations of the cervical spine. Conversely retropharyngeal inflammatory process may affect adjacent vertebral bodies and articulations. The parapharyngeal space is seen here as a triangularly shaped area filled with fatty tissue and bound antero-medially by the pharyngeal musculature, postero-laterally by the carotid sheath and longus colli muscle and laterally by the medial pterygoid muscle.

Middle of Axis (C2 Vertebra)

Patient CT Scan

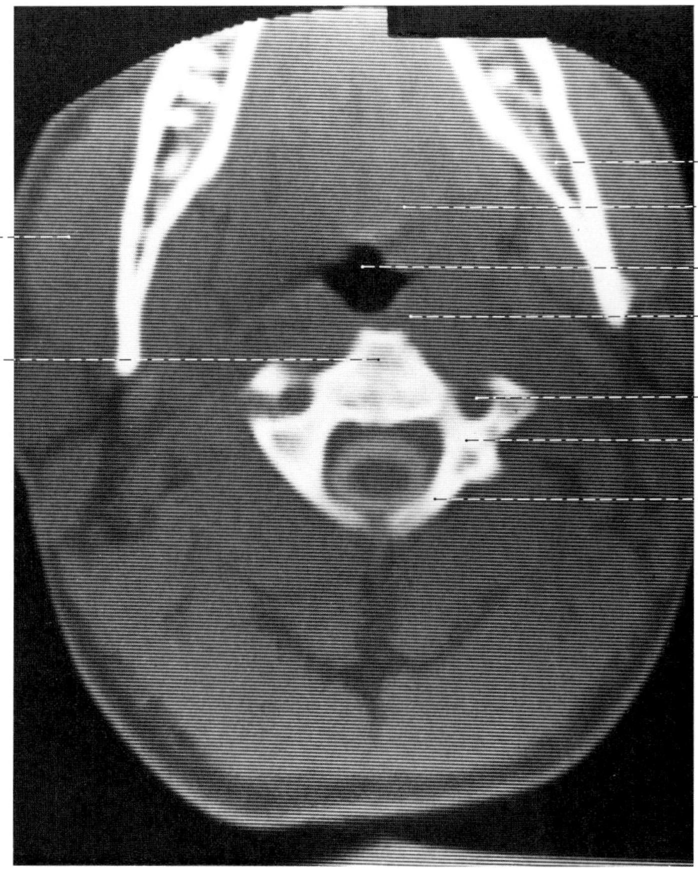

Cadaver CT Scan

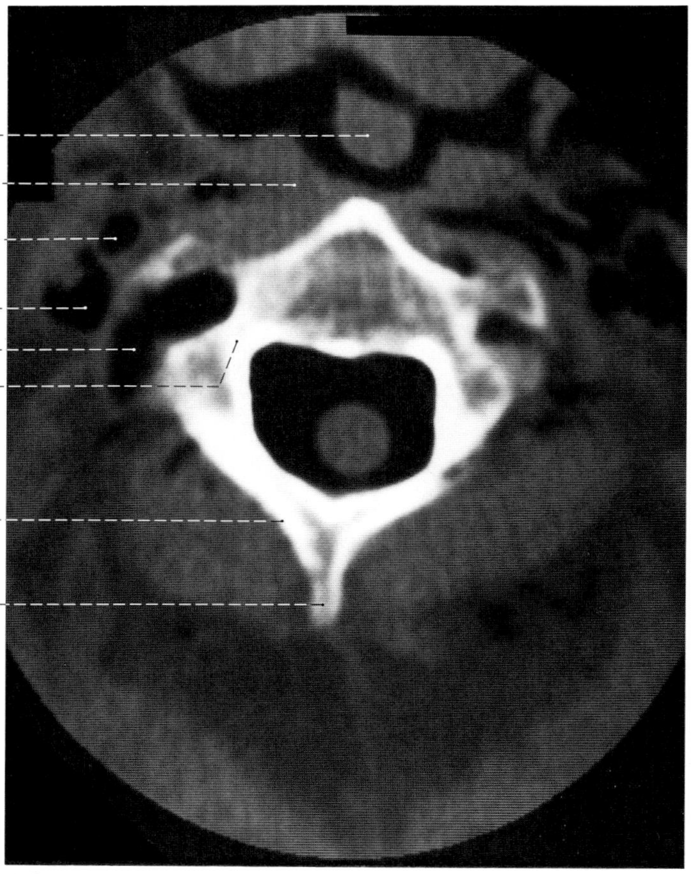

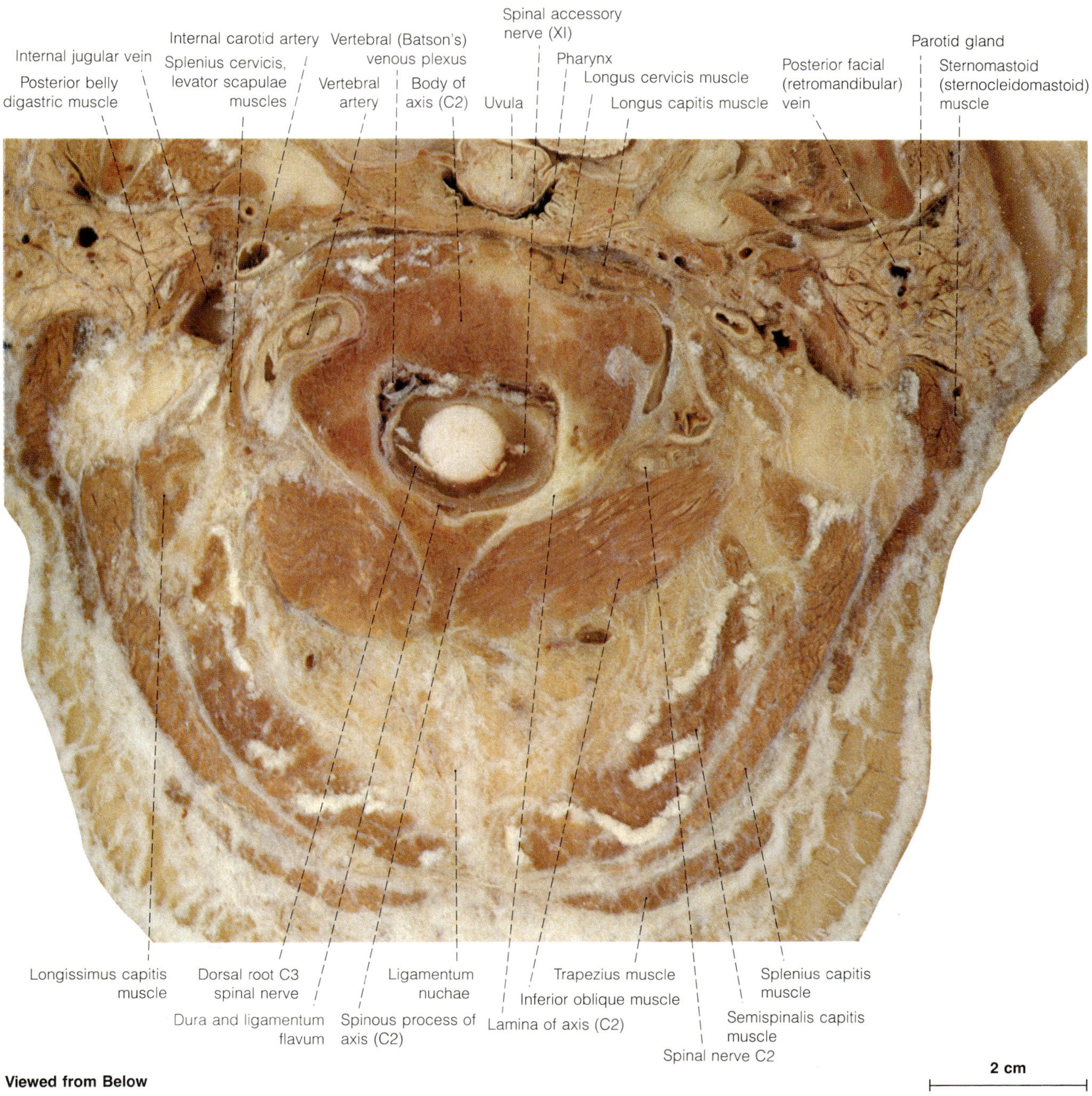

The characteristic central ridge on the ventral surface of the body of C2 (also evident on page 260) may be noted. This ridge is created by two lateral shallow grooves where the longus colli attach.

The transverse foramen of C2 is slightly more anterior than the succeeding foramina. Note the close proximity of the internal carotid artery and the internal jugular vein to the vertebral artery. The posterior belly of the digastric separates the carotid sheath (and related glossopharyngeal, vagus, spinal accessory and hypoglossal nerves) from the deep lobe of the parotid. Major vascular structures of the neck such as the carotid artery and jugular vein can be visualized on CT images when contrast material is administered rapidly during the CT examination. The prominent epidural venous plexus may explain the enhancement in the epidural space observed on CT images when contrast material has been given.

The pharynx is immediately anterior to the prevertebral musculature. Pharyngeal tumors extend into the lateral pharyngeal and retro-pharyngeal spaces and may invade the longus colli muscles or cause vertebral body erosion. Deep muscle or vertebral body invasion may preclude complete surgical resection of pharyngeal tumors.

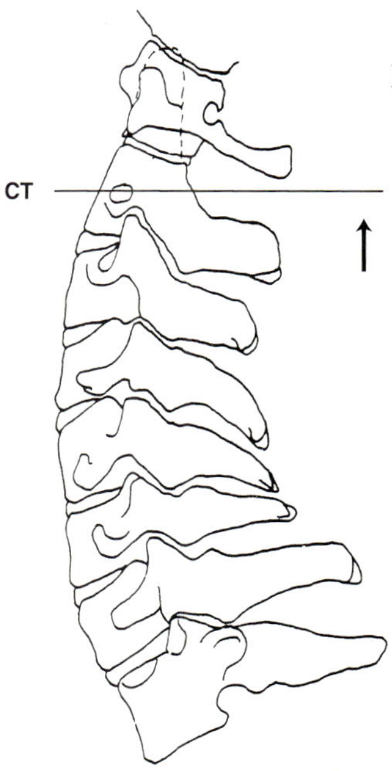

Plane of Sections

Lower C2 Vertebra – C2-3 Disc

Patient CT Scan

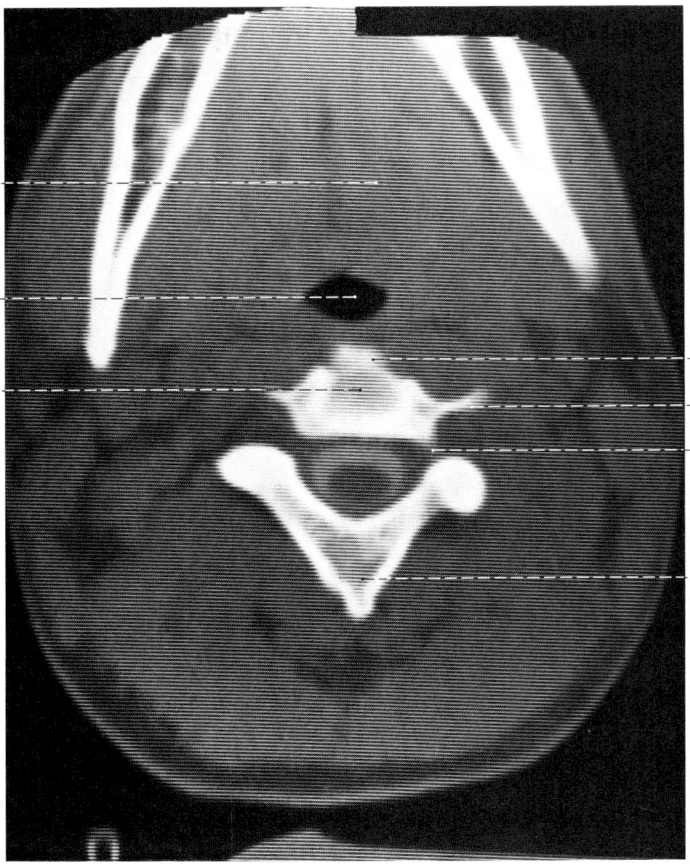

Cadaver CT Scan

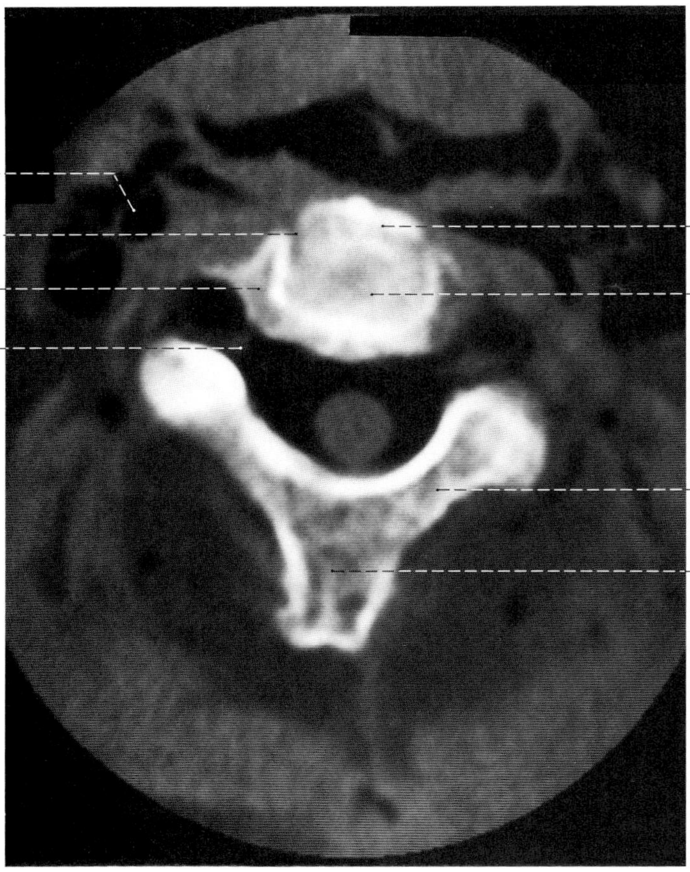

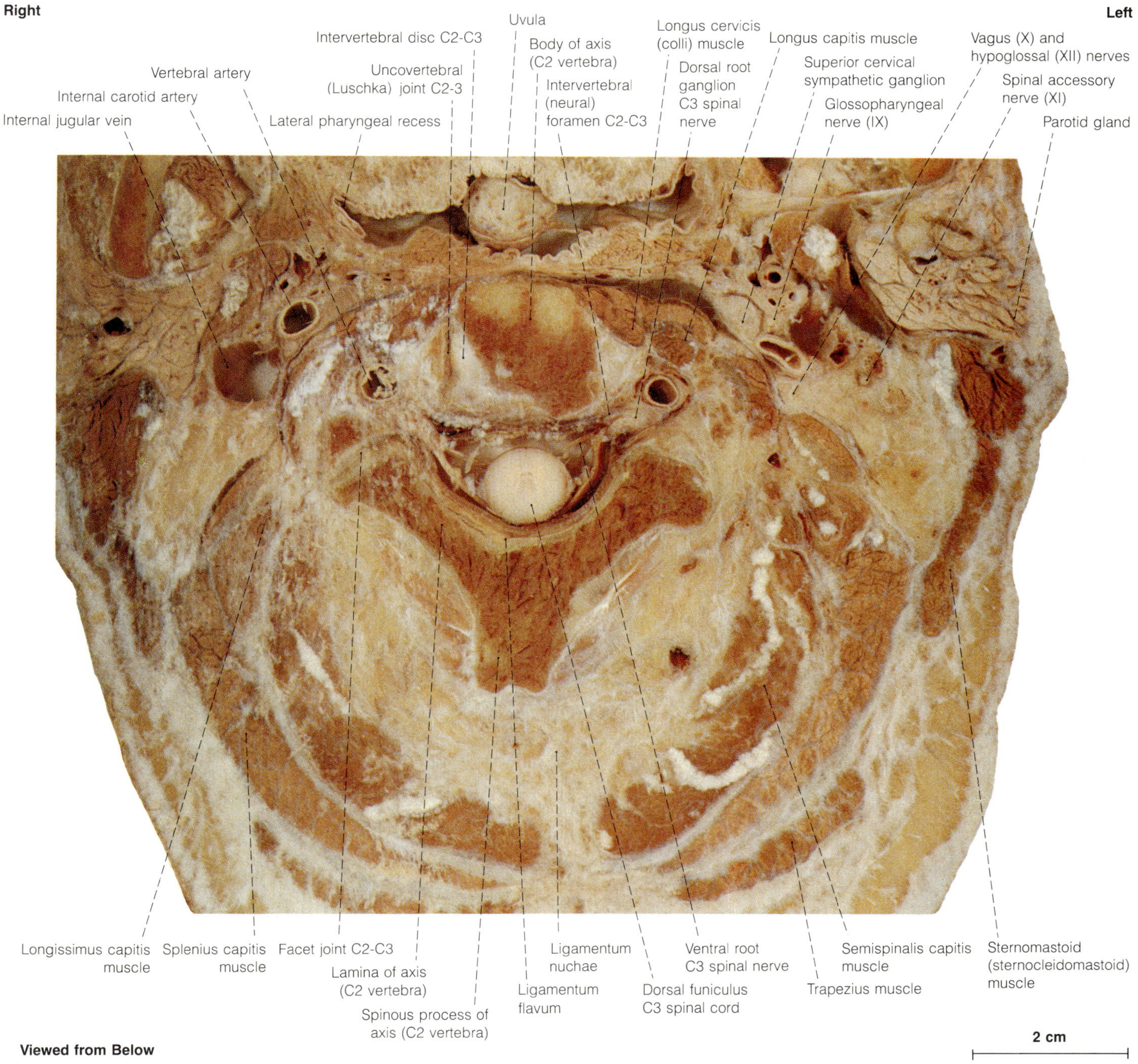

The C2-3 intervertebral disc space and disc have a forward slope and downward convexity. Sections in the axial plane, parallel to the orbito-meatal line will demonstrate only a portion of the disc. The synovial unco-vertebral (Luschka) joints are well seen since they are oriented in the sagittal plane. The spinous process of C2 is characteristically shorter but wider and frequently bifid. The laminae of C1 are thicker than at lower levels. These sections also illustrate well the relationship of the dorsal root ganglion and the vertebral body, the vertebral artery and the neural foramen. Hypertrophic osteophytes secondary to degenerative arthritis of the articular facets or the unco-vertebral joints may result in narrowing of the neural foramen and compression of the root and/or ganglion. The posterior longitudinal ligament is just posterior to the vertebral body and disc. It extends completely across the vertebral body and widens slightly at the level of the intervertebral disc.

The spinal cord retains its near rounded cross-sectional shape; at this level the transverse diameter is slightly greater than the antero-posterior diameter. Individual nerve roots can be seen with CT when the subarachnoid space has been rendered visible with non-ionic contrast materials such as metrizamide (Amipaque ®).

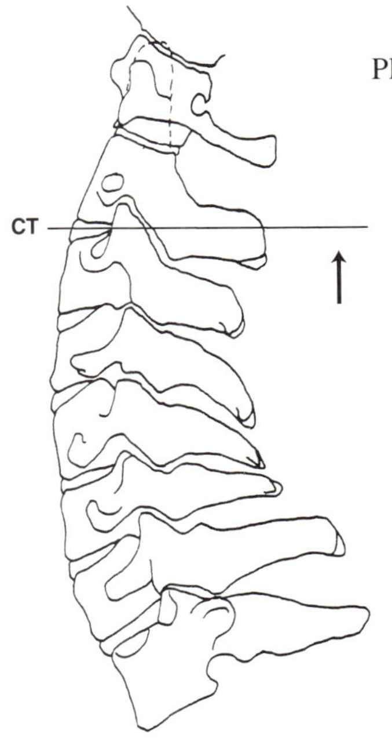

Plane of Sections

Upper C3 Vertebra

Patient CT Scan

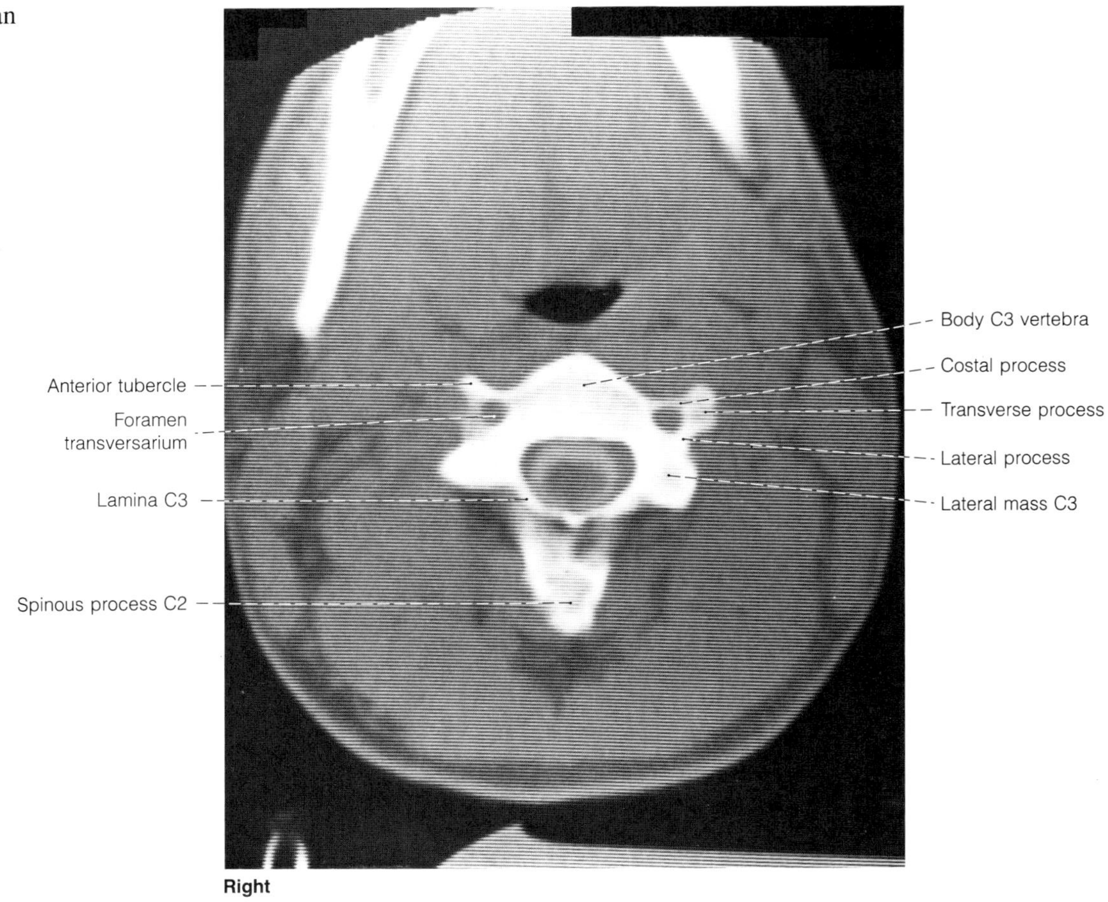

Cadaver CT Scan

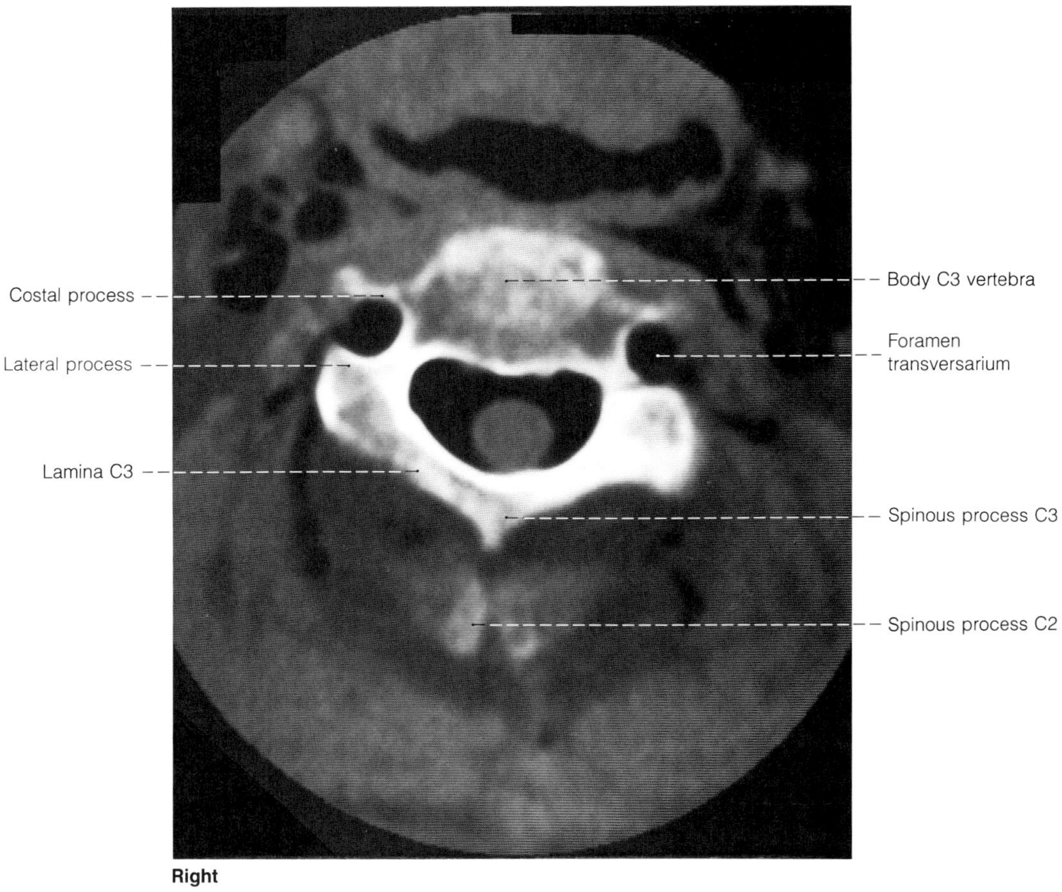

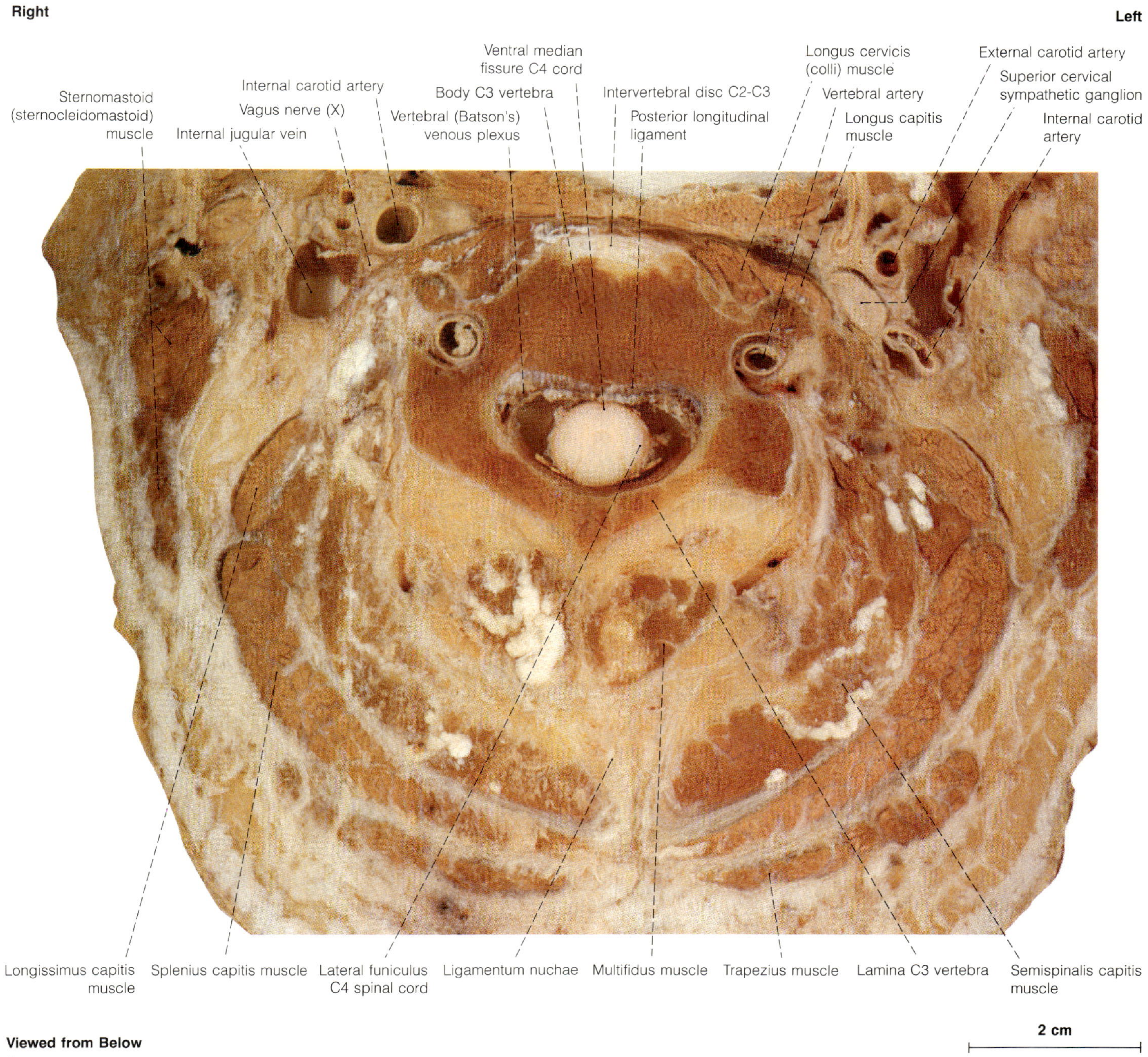

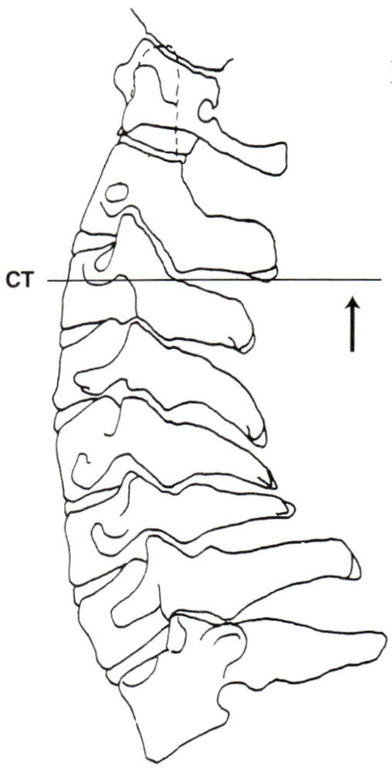

Plane of Sections

The longus cervicis (colli) muscle, attaches more laterally at this level than at higher levels on the ventral surface of the vertebral body. The longus capitis muscle inserts slightly more laterally, at the costal process. These muscles bend the neck forward, help in rotation and prevent hyperextension. The superior cervical (sympathetic) ganglion lies just antero-medial to the internal carotid artery. It frequently extends cephalad to reach the carotid foramen. The transverse foramen is bound anteriorly by the costal process, laterally by the transverse (costo-transverse lamella) and posteriorly by the lateral process. The vertebral artery and veins and some sympathetic fibers occupy the transverse foramen.

The spinal cord is nearly of the same size and shape as in higher levels, but the spinal canal, especially the anterior-posterior diameter, is smaller than it is at C1 or C2. The epidural space contains fat and Batson's plexus of veins. Note that the epidural plexus is more easily seen ventro-lateral to the thecal sac.

Body of C3 Vertebra

Patient CT Scan

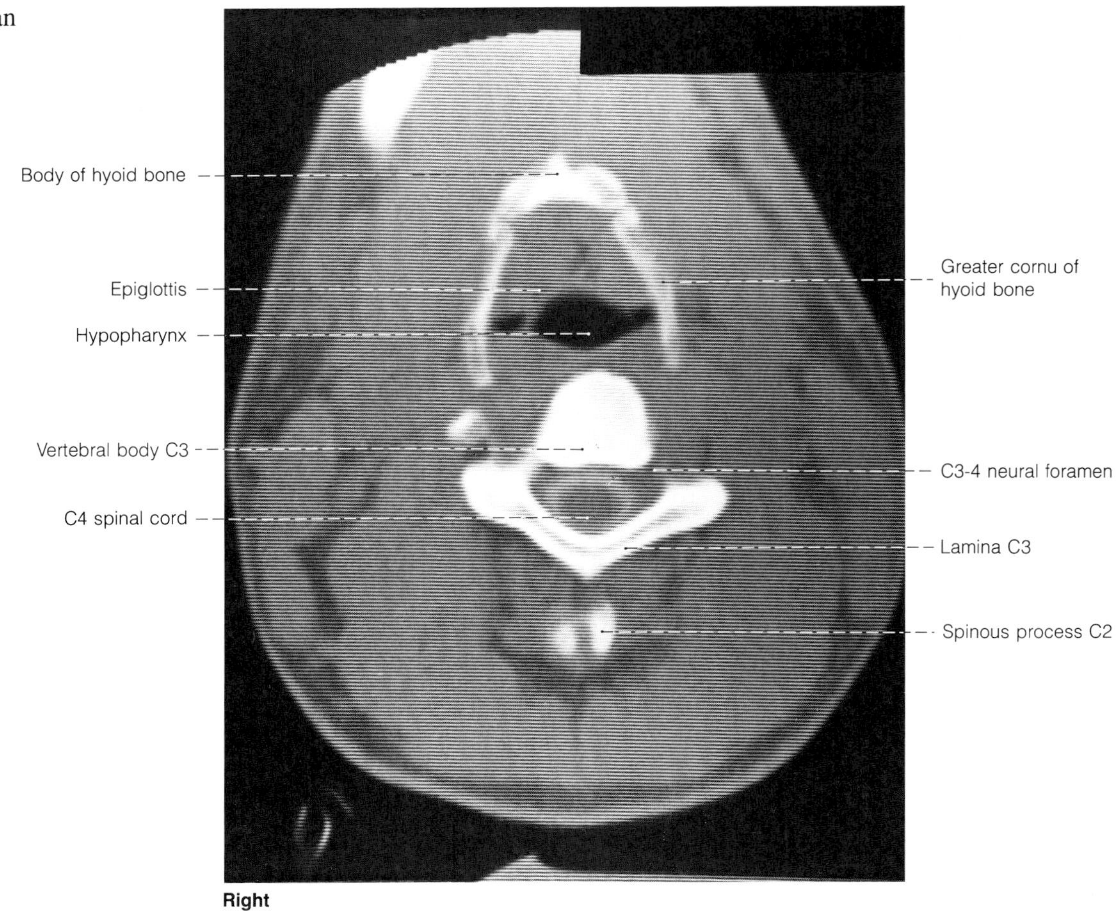

Cadaver CT Scan

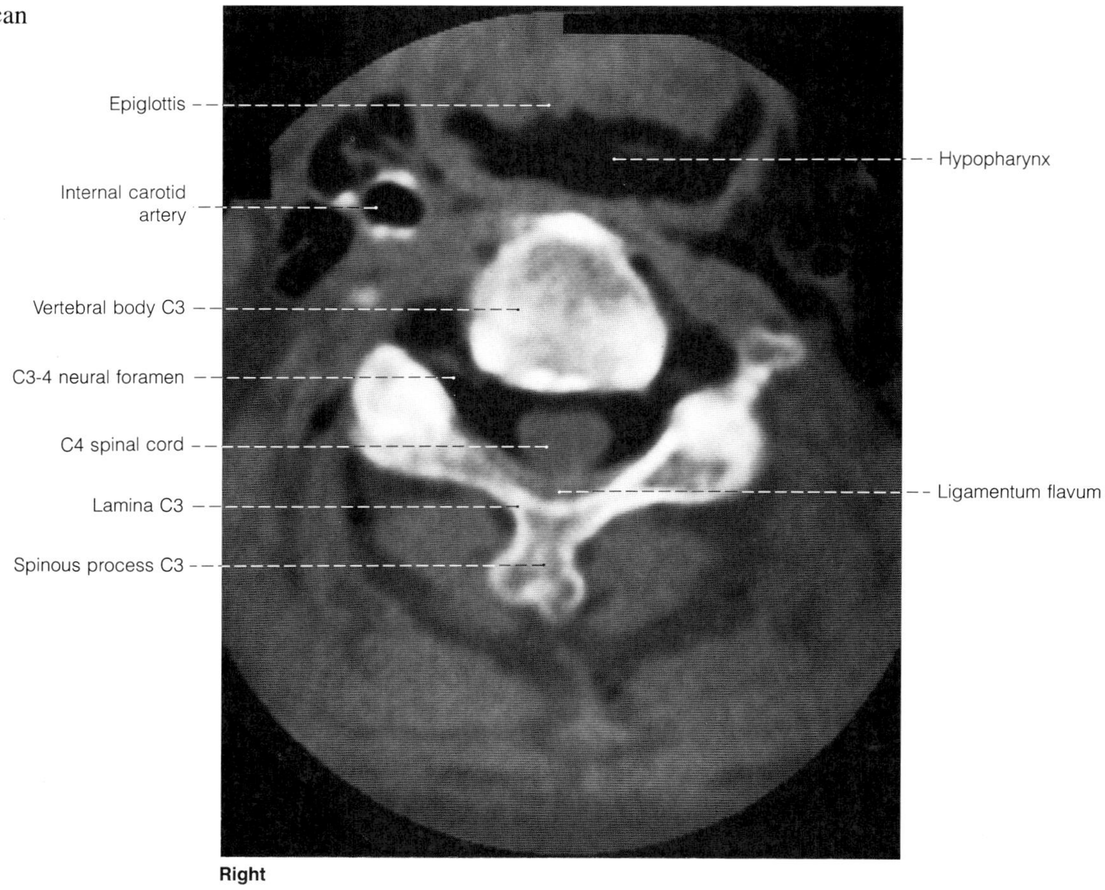

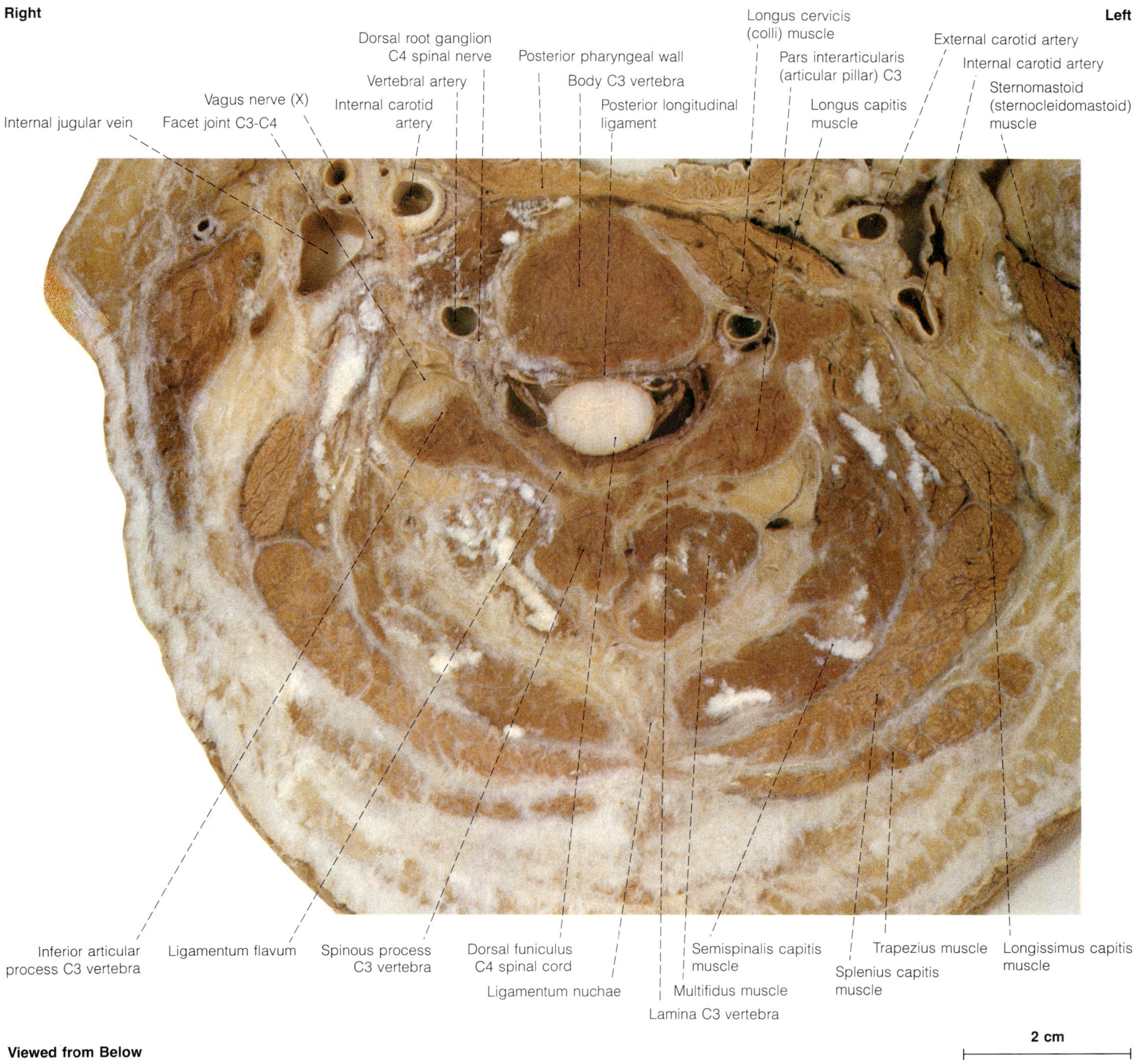

This level marks the most cephalad portion of the cervical enlargement of the spinal cord which extends from C3 to T1. Consequently, the cross-sectional appearance of the cord changes from rounded to a more elliptical shape. The nerve roots of C4 are seen at the C3-4 neural foramen. The dorsal root ganglion is just posterior to the vertebral artery at the lateral aspect of the neural foramen. Although the C4 nerves contribute only minimally to the brachial plexus, the phrenic nerves arise primarily from these C4 roots.

The ligamenta flava (yellow ligaments) are bands of fibroelastic tissue extending from the inferior margin of the lamina above to the cranial border of the lamina below. Antero-laterally the ligamentum flavum extends to the posterior margin of the neural foramen and the medial edge of the articular facet. Since they are made of elastic tissue, the shape and thickness of the ligamentum flavum changes with flexion and extension of the cervical spine. Chronic degenerative disc disease of the cervical spine is accompanied by loss of elasticity and thickening of the ligamentum flavum. These ligaments may produce a corrugated extra-dural impression on the posterior aspect of the subarachnoid space, thus contributing to the spinal stenosis seen in cervical spondylosis.

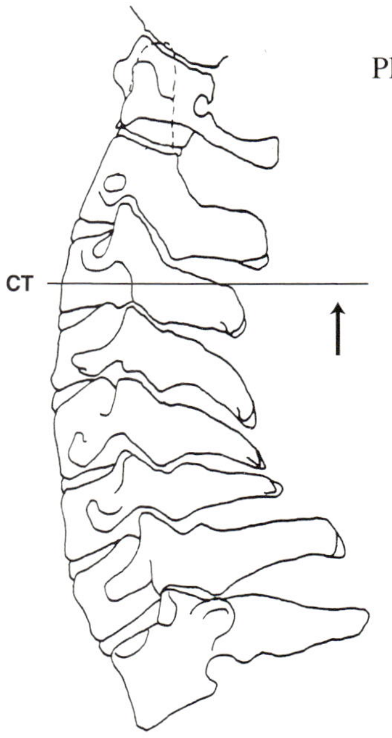

Patient CT Scan

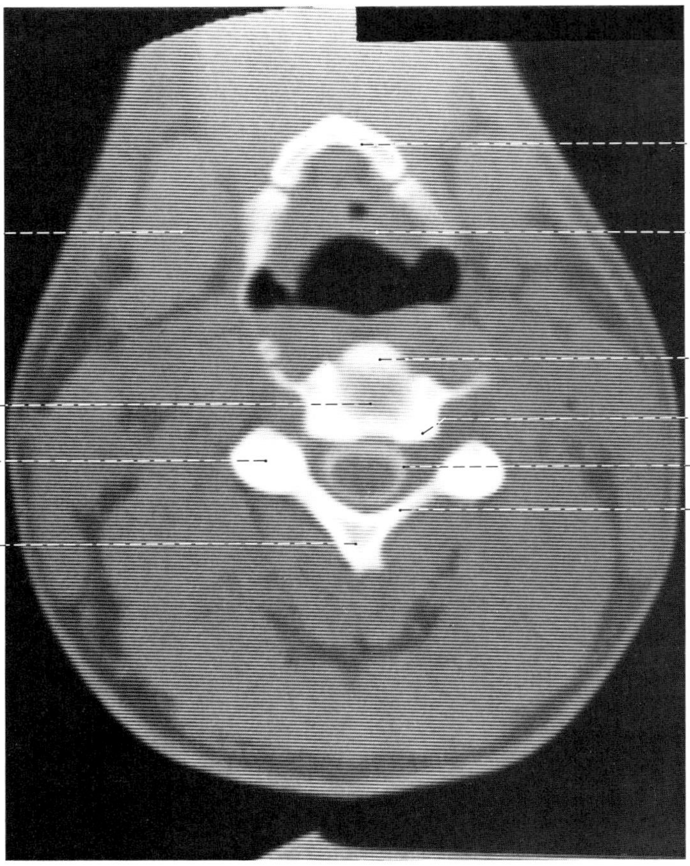

Cadaver CT Scan

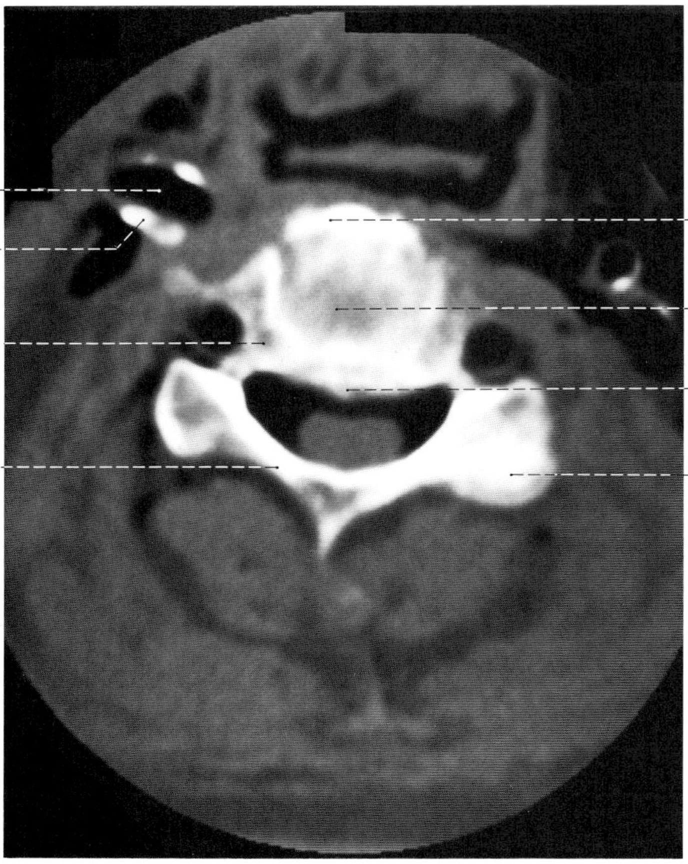

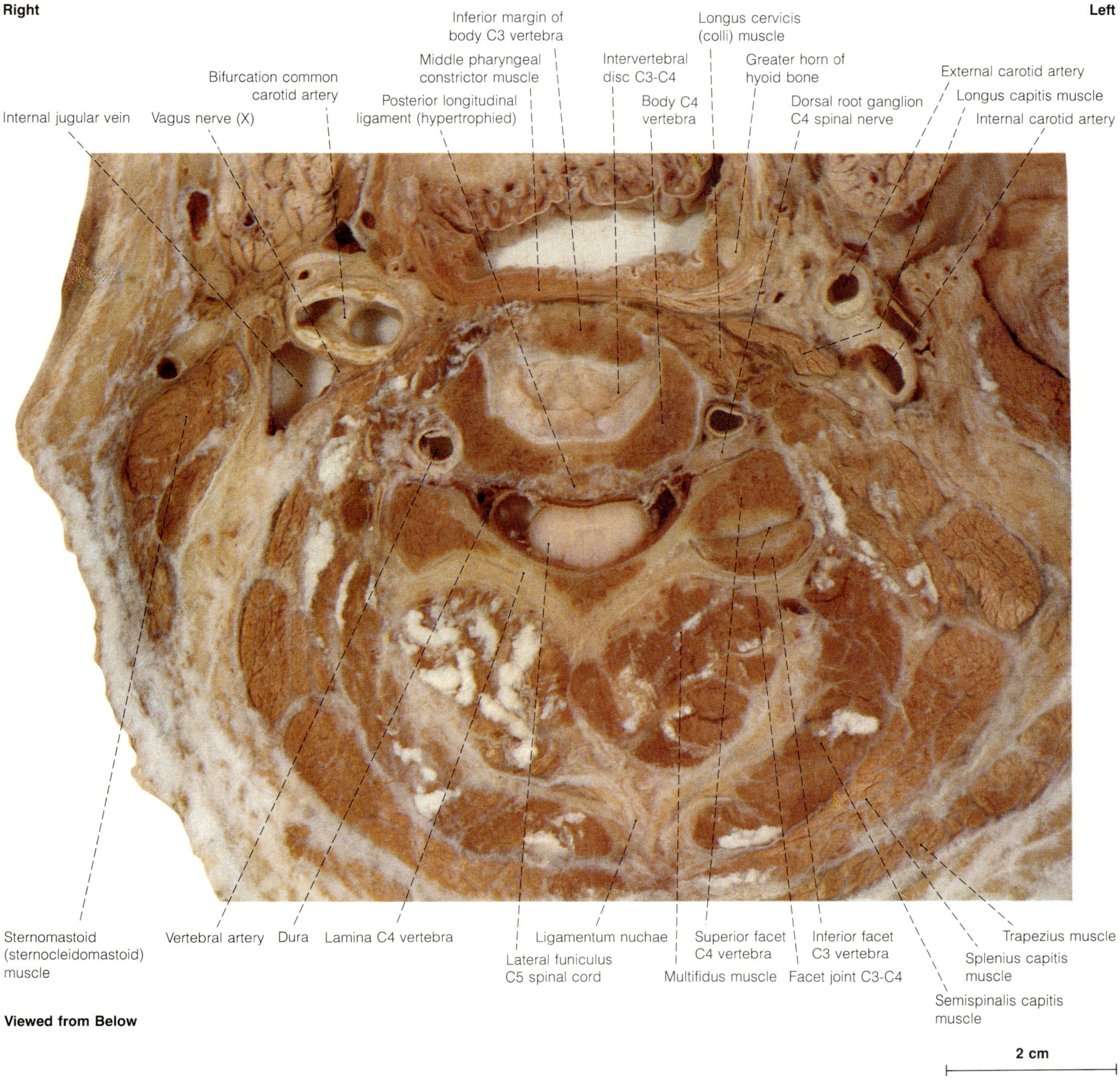

This section nicely illustrates normal anatomic relationships at the C3-4 intervertebral disc level on axial section. The anterior-inferior portion of the vertebral body above projects anterior to the disc. On this anatomic slice of an elderly male note should be made of the hypertrophic ridge that projects into the spinal canal reducing the size of the adjacent subarachnoid space and flattening the ventral surface of the cord. This ridge is formed by a combination of bony osteophyte, bulging disc anulus and hypertrophied posterior longitudinal ligament. In some cases, flexion-extension injuries to the spine may cause disruption of this posterior longitudinal ligament. As also illustrated on the anatomic section, adjacent laminae can overlap, especially if the lordotic curvature of the cervical spine is accentuated.

At the C5 spinal cord level shown here, the cord has an oval shape. Where the upper fibers of the brachial plexus arise the transverse diameter of the spinal cord is slightly larger when compared to the C1 or C2 levels. There is less subarachnoid space surrounding the cord at the levels of the cervical enlargement. In most individuals, the common carotid bifurcation is found at the C3-4 level which also corresponds to the level of the hyoid bone, an easily palpable anatomic landmark.

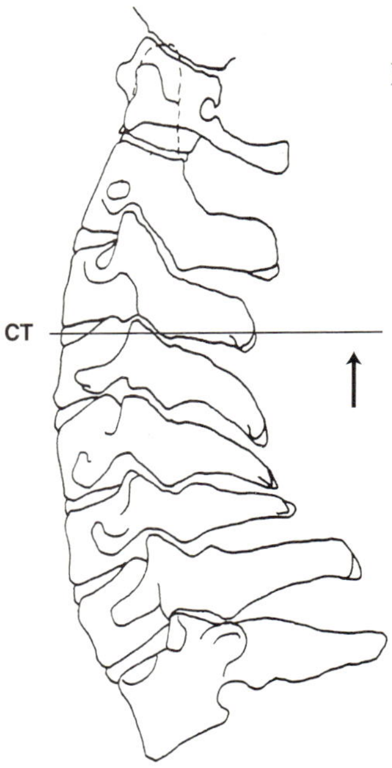

Plane of Sections

Patient CT Scan

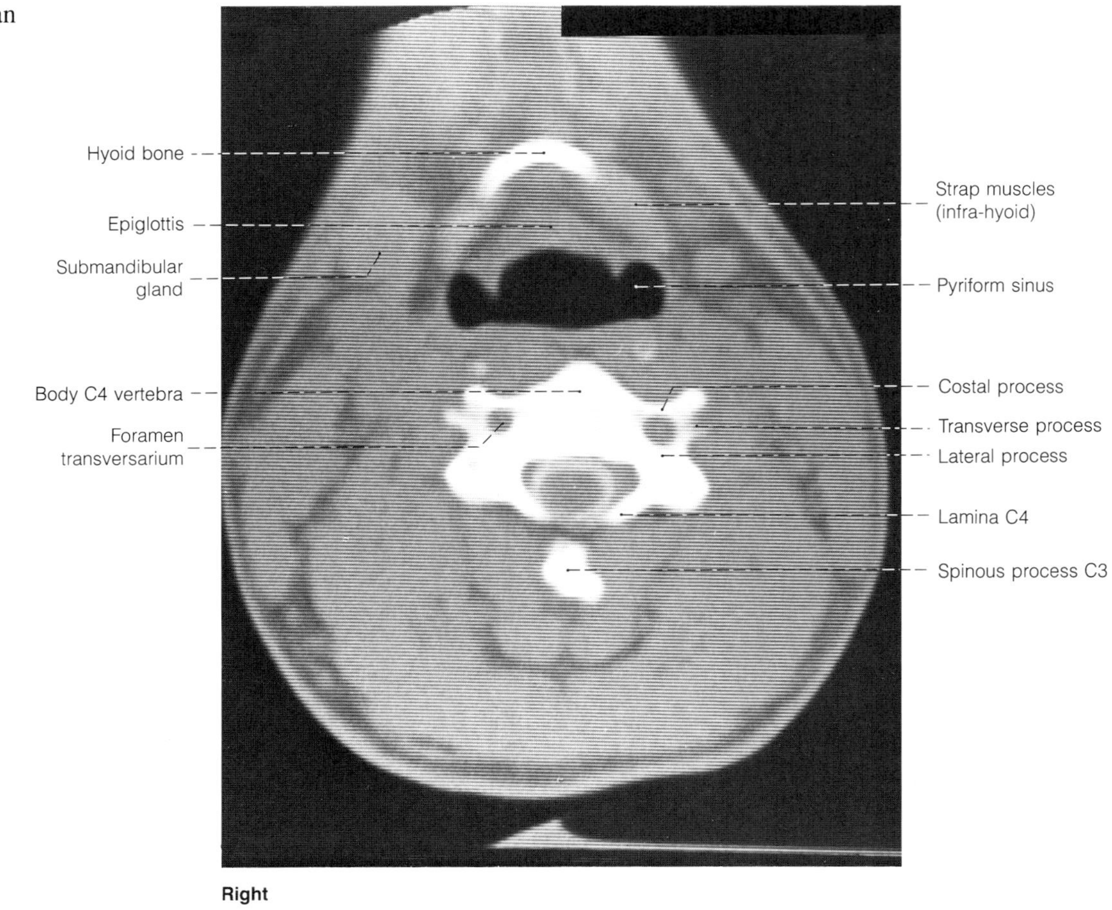

Cadaver CT Scan

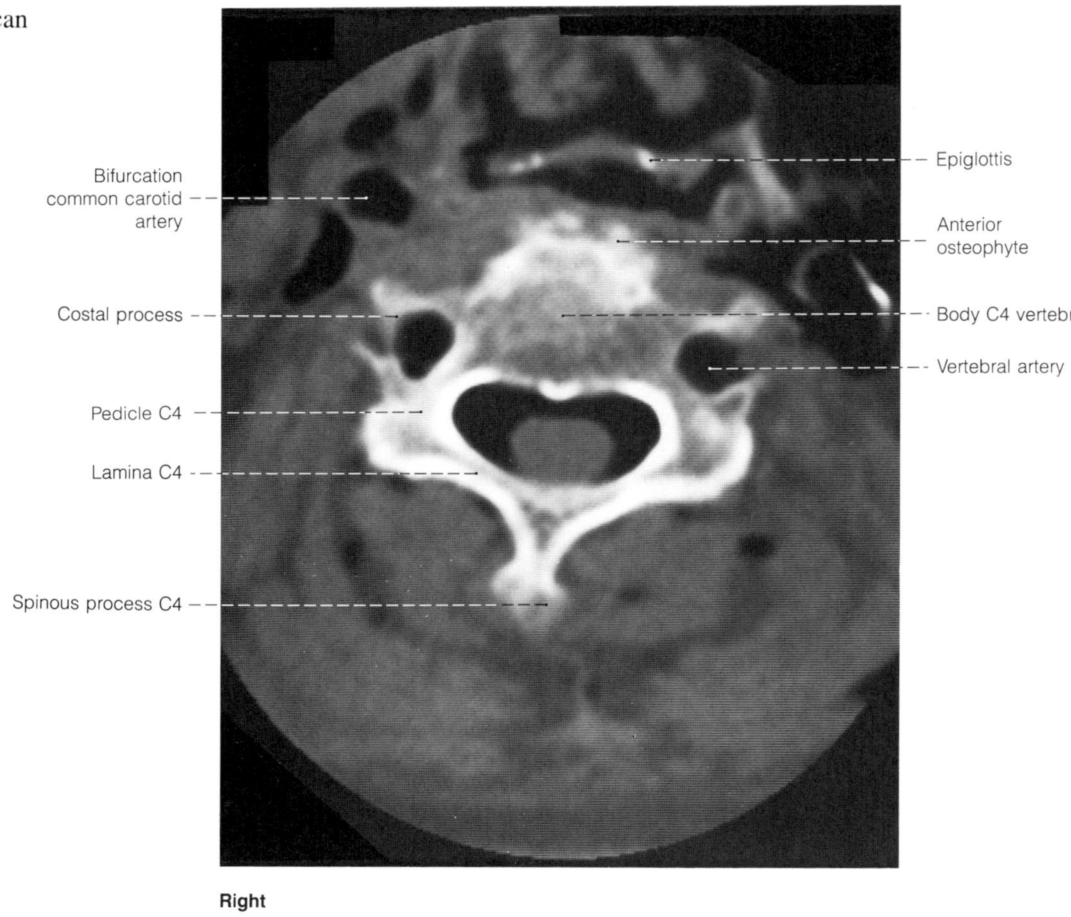

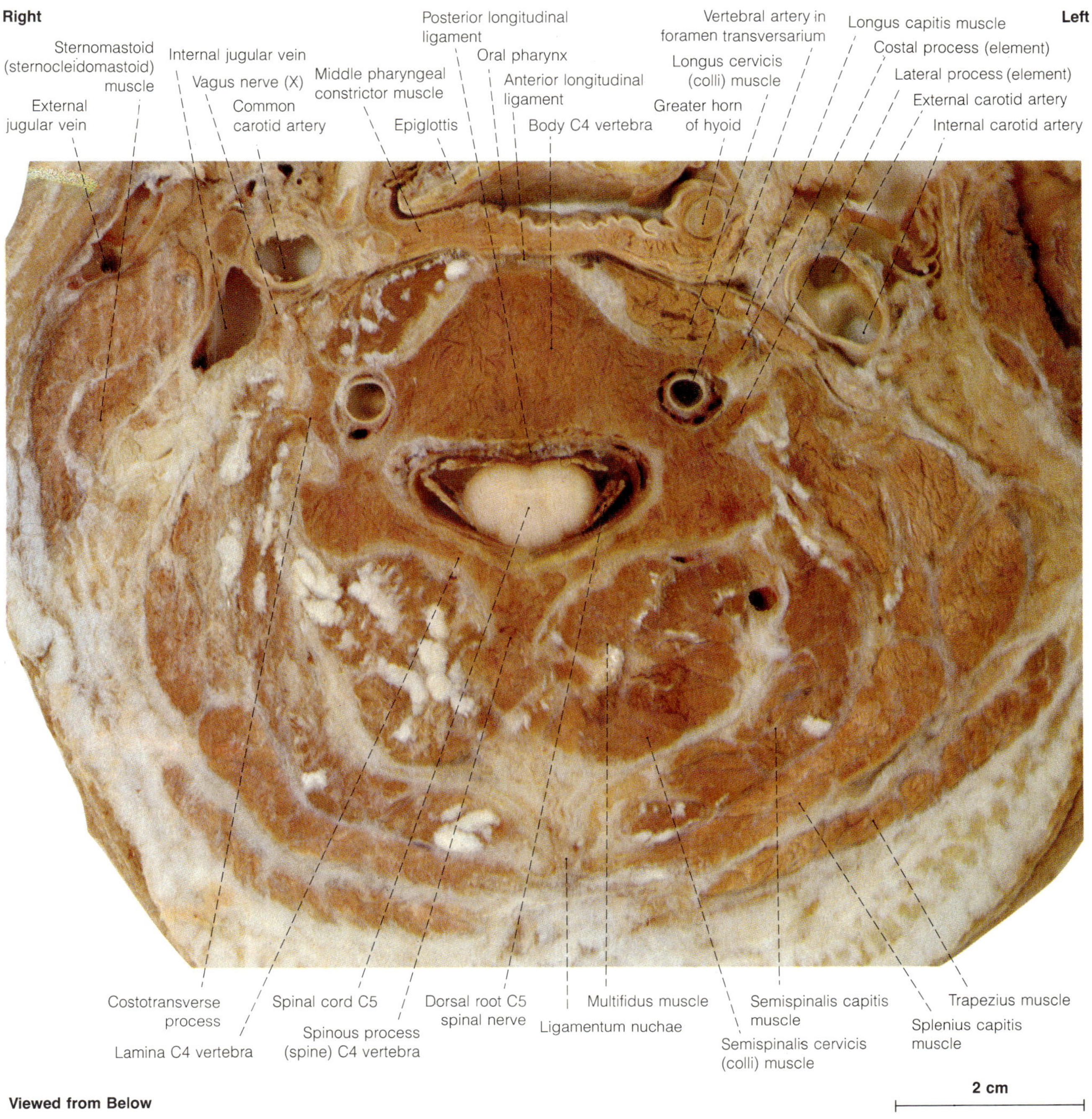

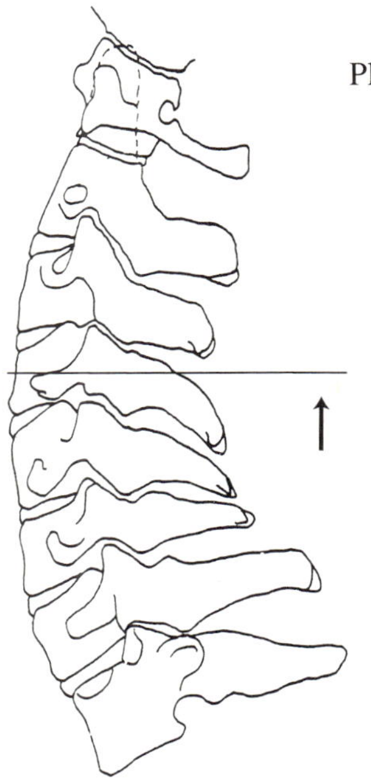

The bodies of the mid-cervical vertebrae have a trapezoid or truncated cone cross-sectional appearance, the side of the cone serving as attachment for the longus cervicis muscles. The anterior longitudinal ligament lies anteriorly attached to the anterior margins of the vertebral bodies. Anterior hypertrophic spurs blend with the anterior longitudinal ligament.

This section demonstrates well the boundaries of the transverse foramen (foramen transversarium), the size of which is related to the size of the vertebral artery. In most individuals (80%) the left vertebral artery is larger or as large as the right. A good portion of the bony spinal canal is occupied by epidural soft tissues, vessels, ligaments (posterior longitudinal ligament) and ligamentum flavum. Fractures and/or dislocations of the C4 vertebra are not uncommon and are frequently associated with severe neurologic deficit. Fractures of the vertebral bodies are often accompanied by fractures of the pedicles and/or laminae, compromise of the spinal canal and cord compression.

Patient CT Scan

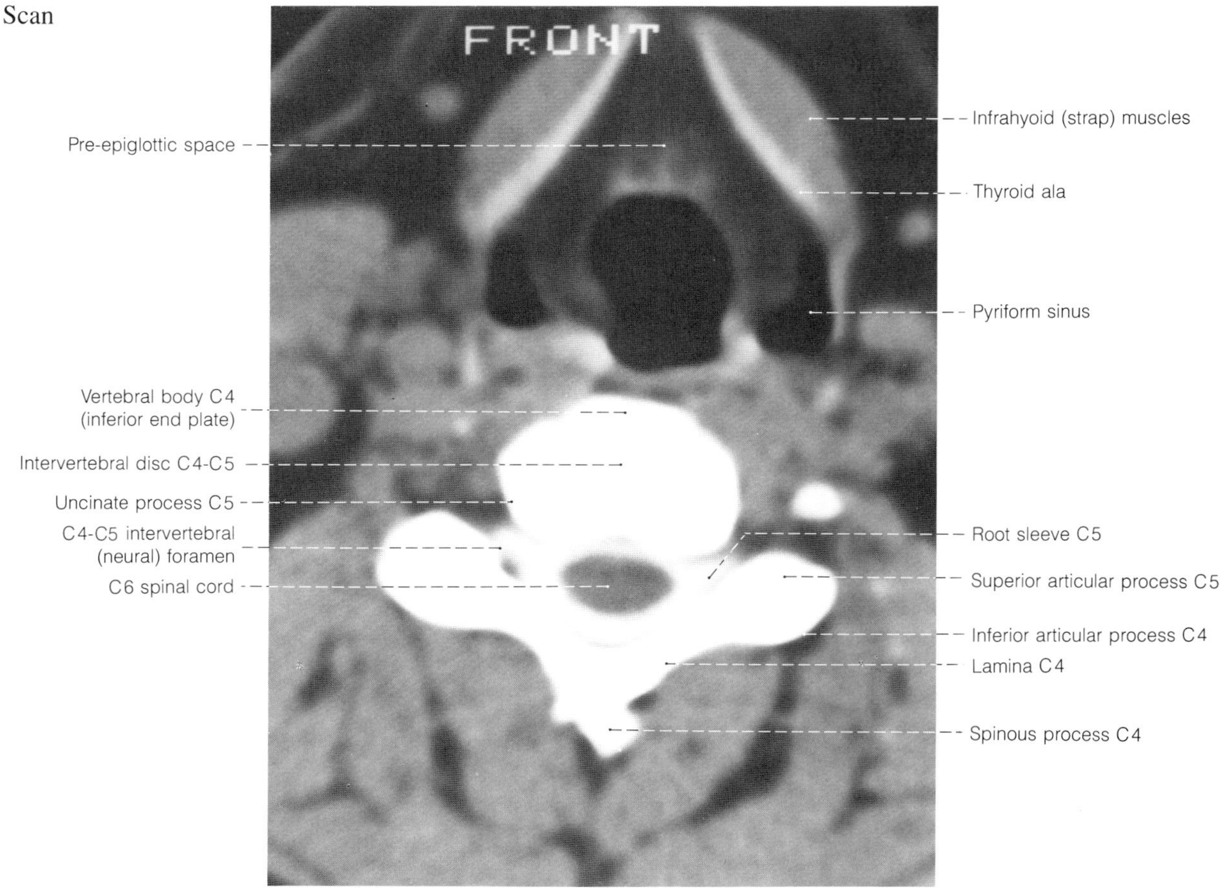

Right

Cadaver CT Scan

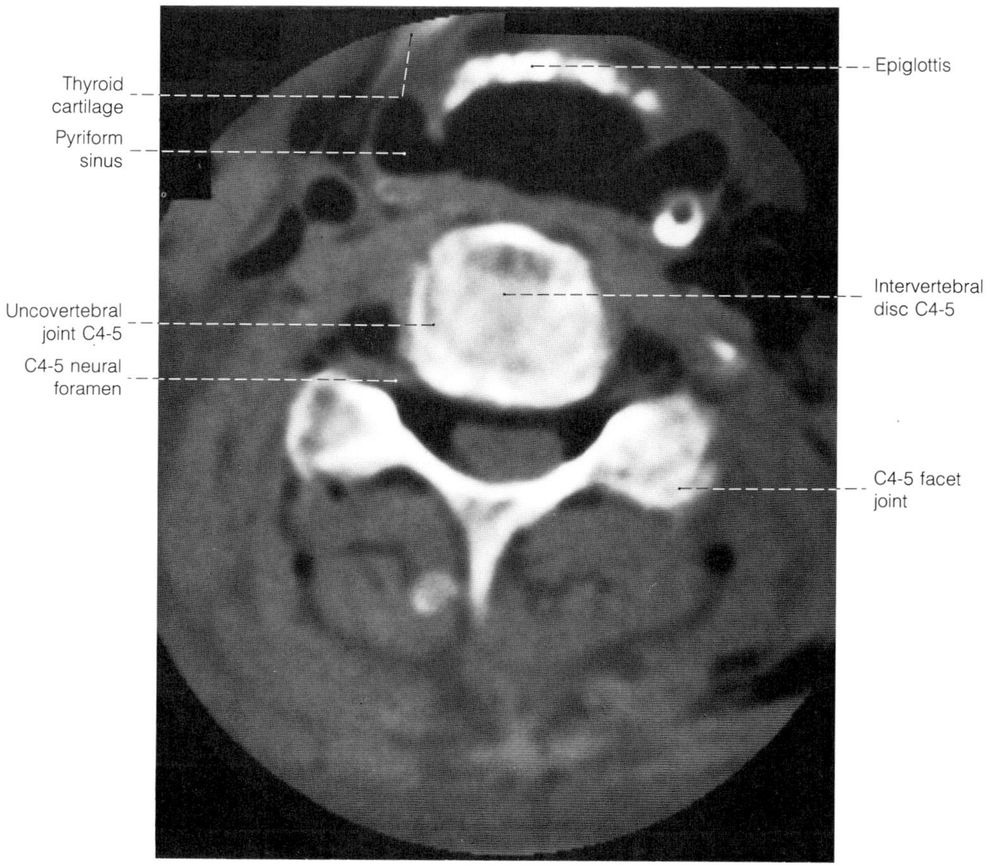

Right

At this level the sections illustrate well the relationships of the intervertebral disc, the uncovertebral joints and the neural foramina. Note the difference in the relationship of vertebral bodies and larynx. On the patient CT, the C4-5 disc is at the level of the false vocal cords while on the anatomic specimen it is at the level of the mid-portion of the epiglottis. The epiglottis, composed predominantly of elastic cartilage, does not usually calcify.

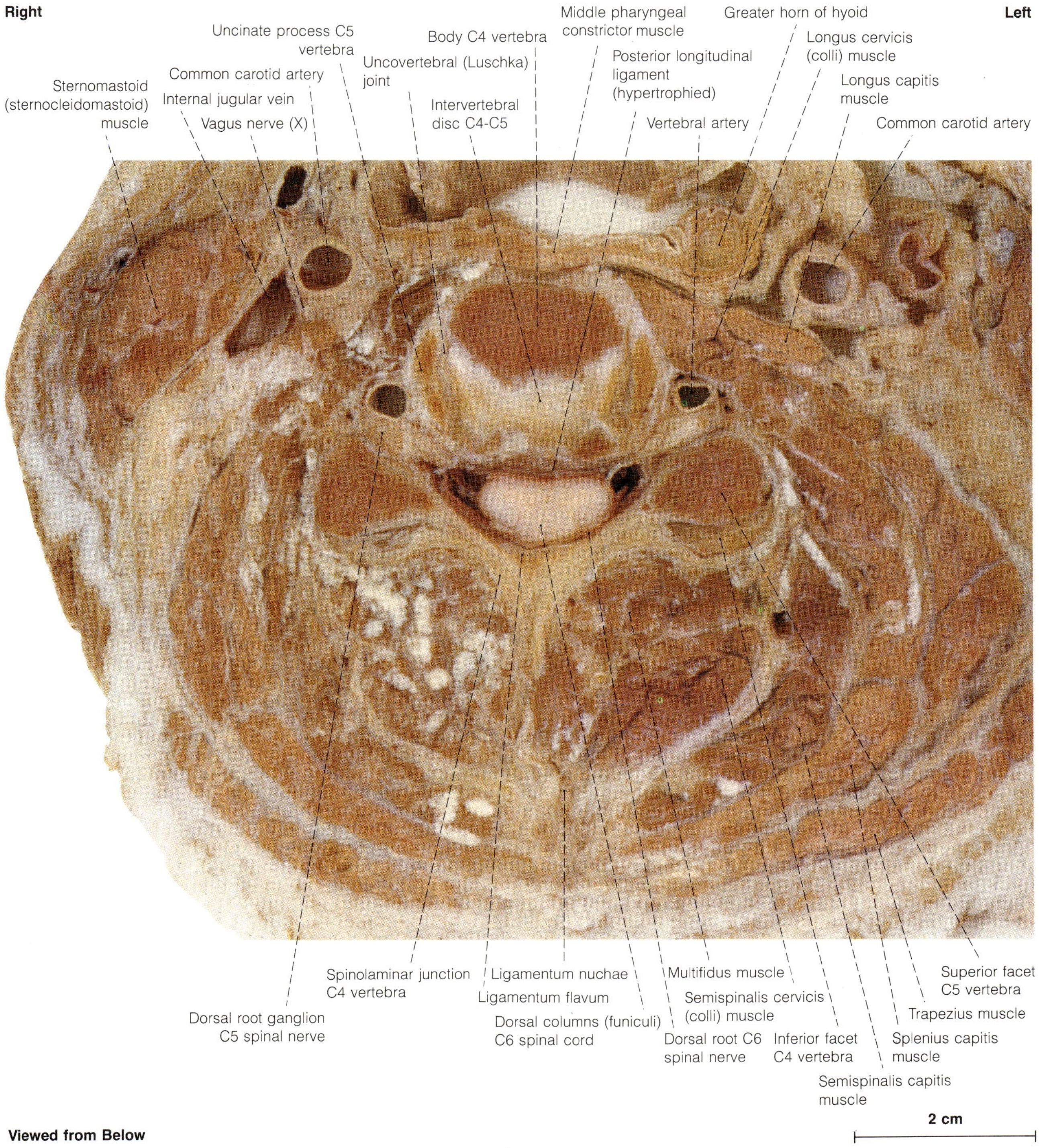

The uncovertebral joints, characteristic of cervical vertebra, are diarthrodial joints placed on each side of the intervertebral fibrocartilage (disc). Degenerative arthritis of these joints is usually seen in conjunction with degenerative disc disease. Osteophytes projecting postero-laterally from the uncinate process can produce narrowing of the neural foramen and compression of the exiting nerve roots. Similarly, lateral osteophytes can produce extrinsic compression on the vertebral artery. The facet joints are also frequently involved with age related and/or post-traumatic degenerative changes that result in narrowing of the joint space, laxity of the joint ligamentous support and osteophyte formation. Note that the normal facet joint is a very narrow space; widening should alert one to the presence of post-traumatic changes or ligamentous laxity.

The cadaver specimen has a narrow spinal canal due to cervical spondylosis. Note the flattening of the cord and lack of subarachnoid space ventral or dorsal to the cord. Radiculopathy and/or compressive myelopathy are frequent complications of cervical spondylosis.

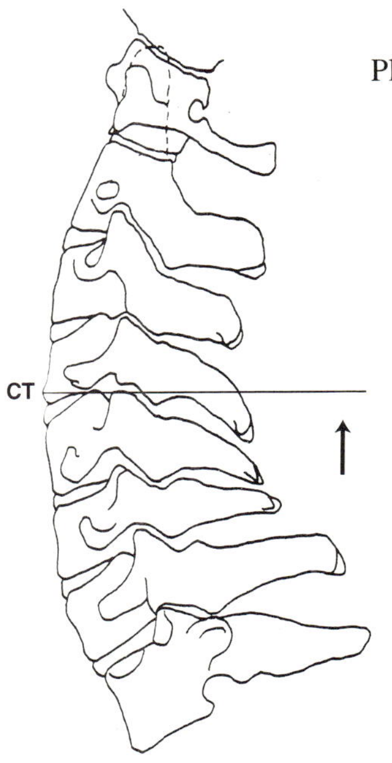

Plane of Sections

Patient CT Scan

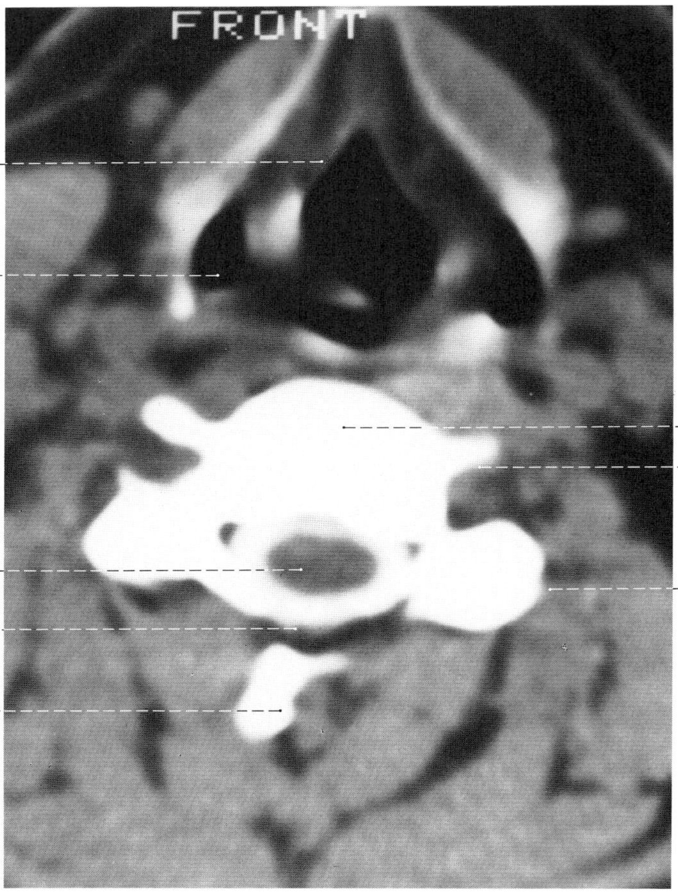

Cadaver CT Scan

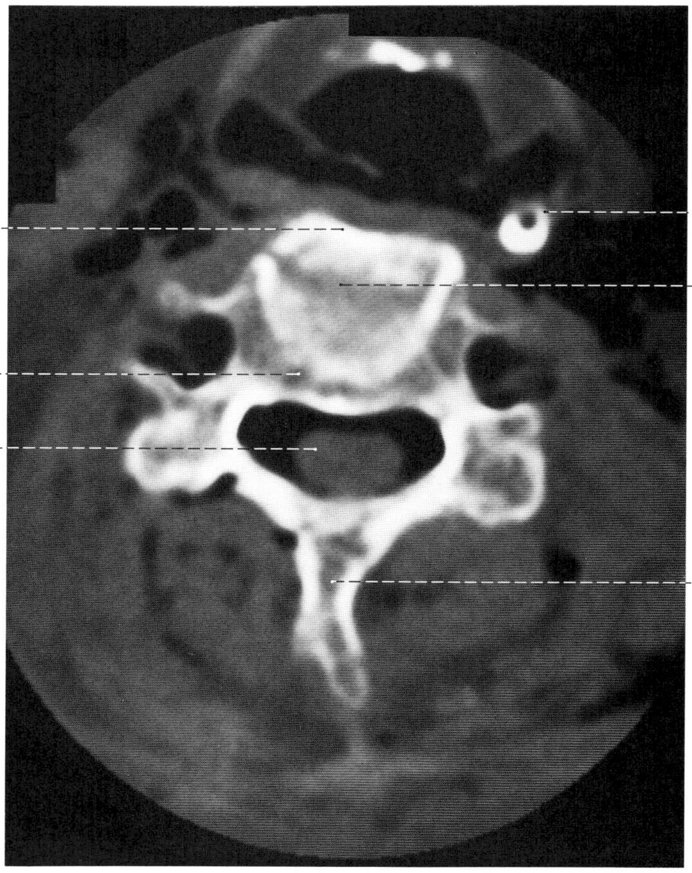

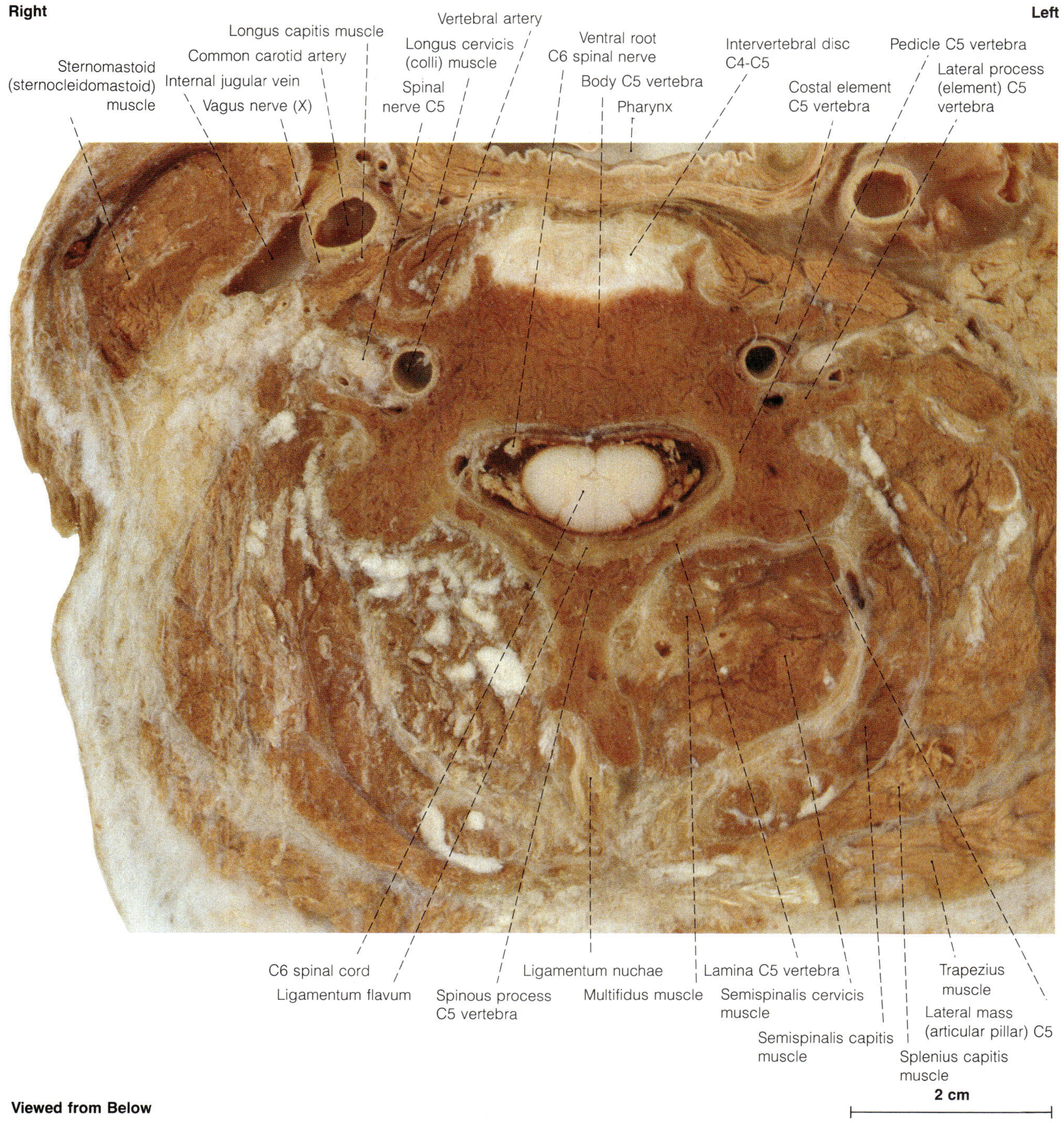

The spinal cord attains its maximal transverse diameter at the level of the vertebral body of C5. This corresponds to the level of the C6-C7 nerve roots. The sagittal diameter of the cord at this level is approximately 7–8 mm and the transverse diameter about 12 mm. The ventral surface of the cord can be flat or slightly convex. The anterior median fissure may be visualized with high resolution scanners when the subarachnoid space is opacified with water soluble myelographic contrast medium. Cord compression associated with spondylosis or cervical fractures is more common in the lower cervical region since the spinal canal is relatively narrow in relation to the size of the cord. As seen on this section the anterior and posterior elements of the cervical vertebra form a ring; thus vertebral body fractures are commonly associated with fracture of the laminae or pedicles or disruption of the articular facets. The cricoid cartilage is like a signet ring taller posteriorly. Note the close proximity of the cricoid to the vertebral bodies. Crush injuries of the neck may result in a fracture of the cricoid as it becomes compressed against the vertebral body.

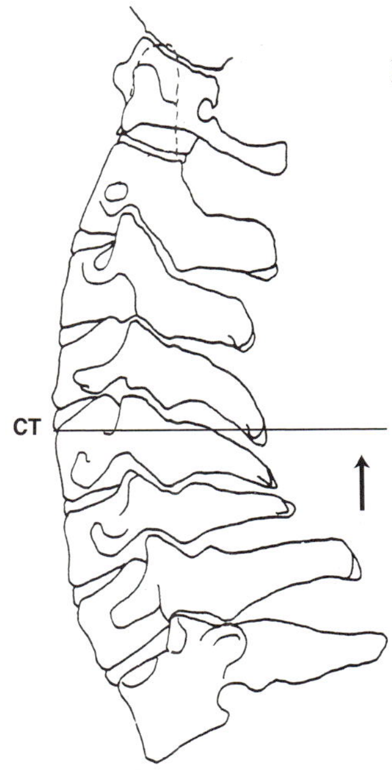

Plane of Sections

Patient CT Scan

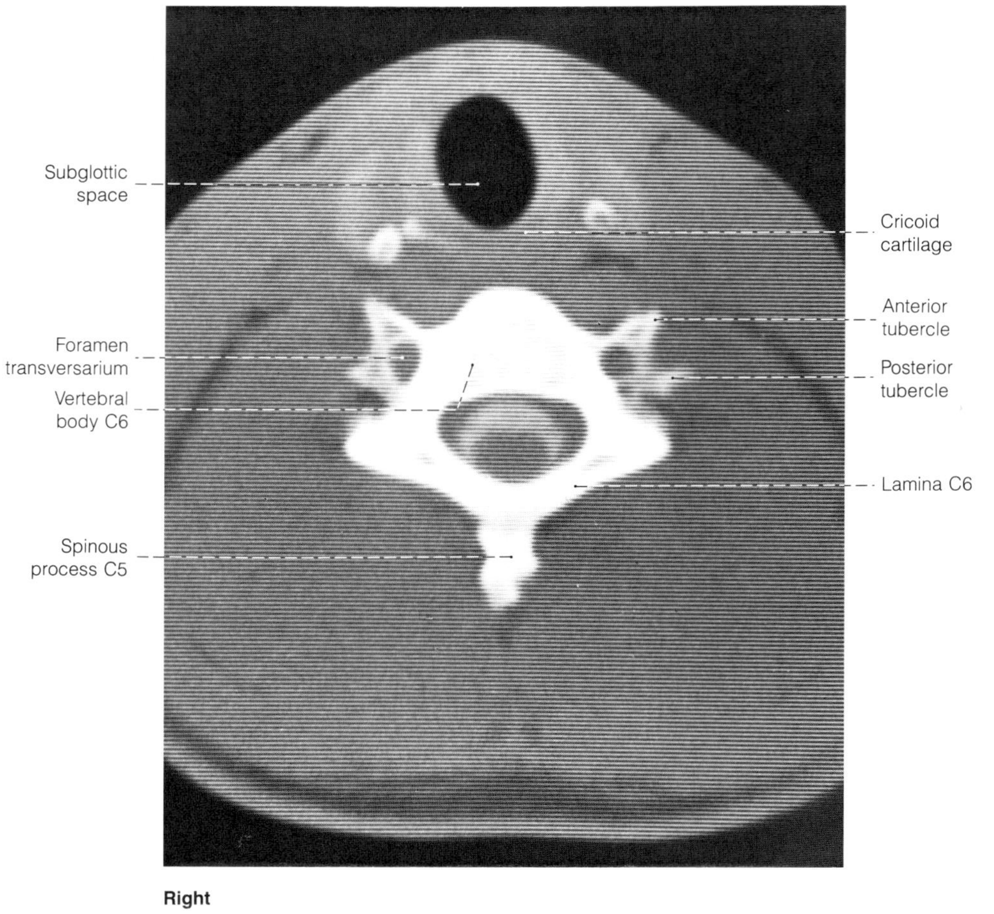

Cadaver CT Scan

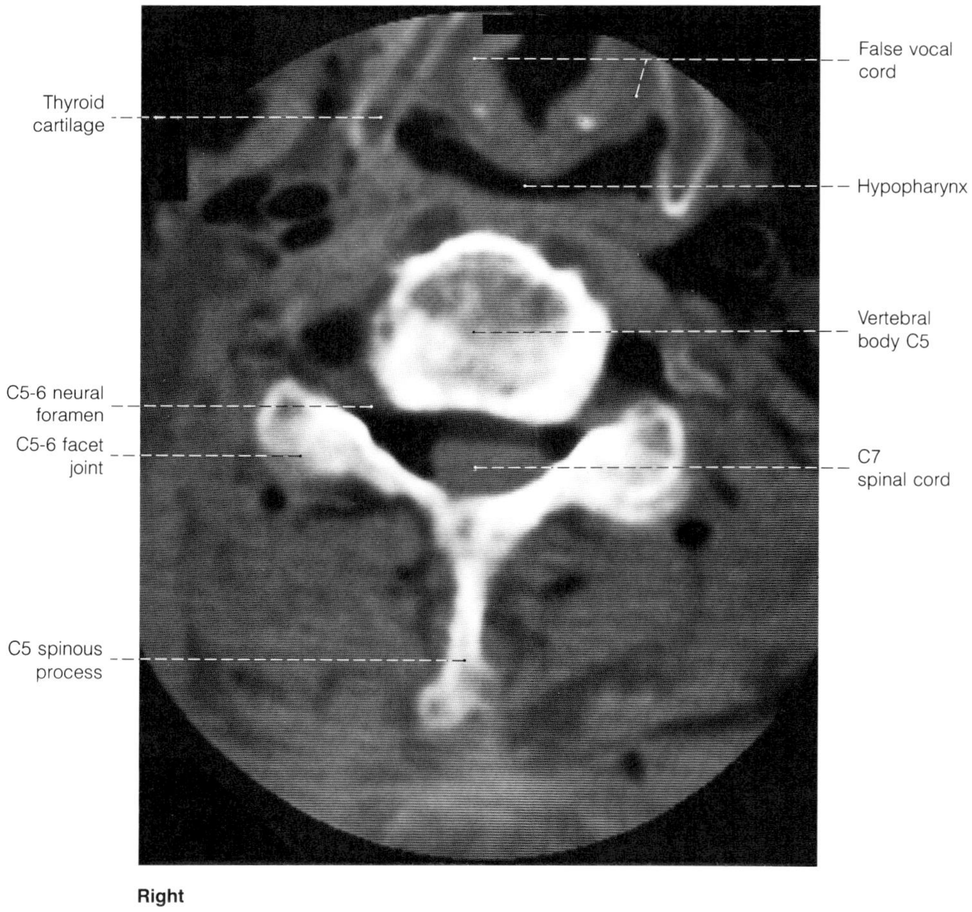

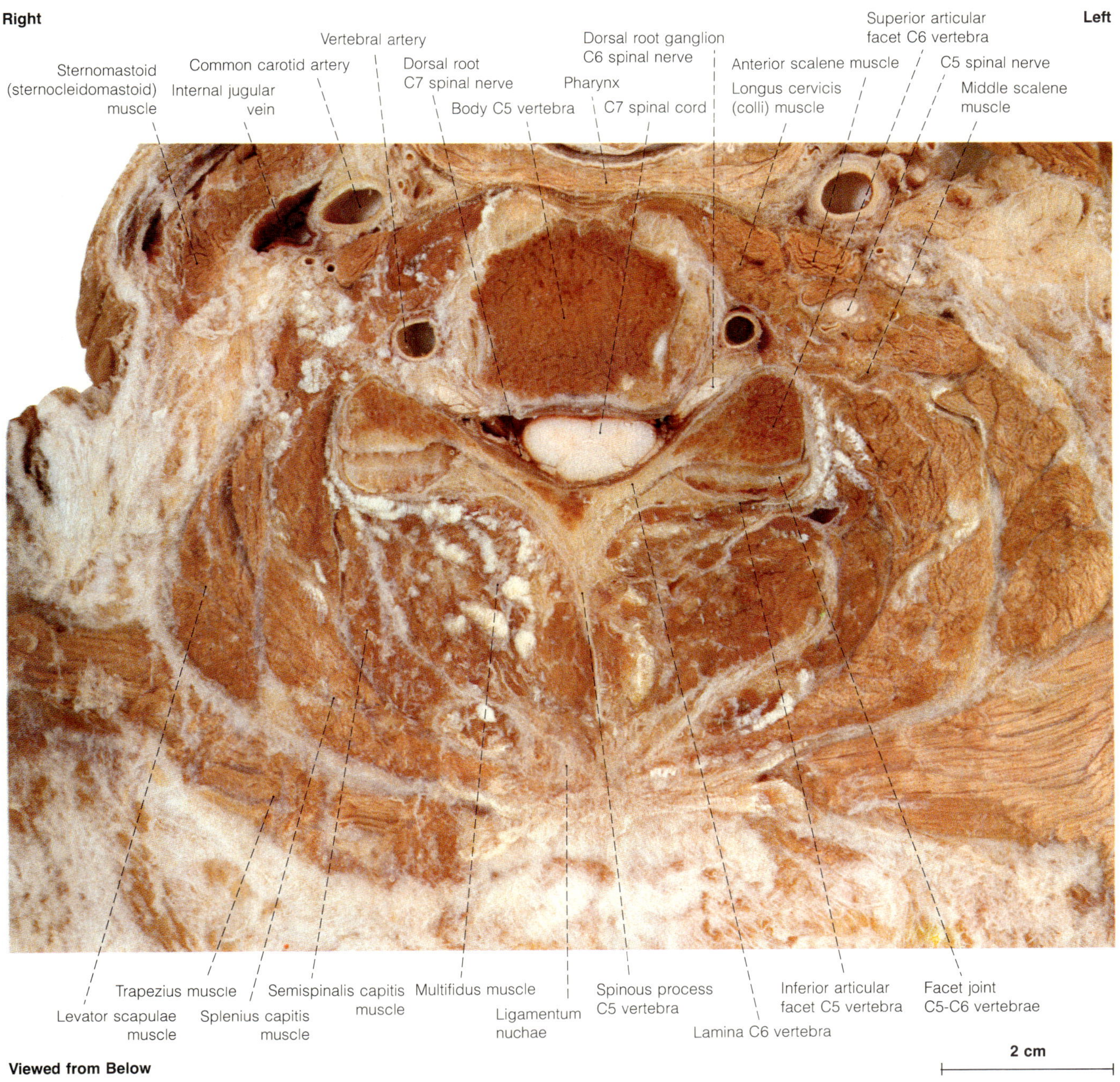

The strap muscles (sterno-thyroid, sterno-hyoid) are seen on CT as a thin band located just anterior to the trachea and the thyroid gland. These muscles are part of the infra-hyoid musculature which fixes or depresses the hyoid bone during laryngeal motion. The normal thyroid gland is well seen because of its greater density when compared to adjacent soft tissue. The density of the thyroid reflects both its vasculature and high iodine content.

The upper cervical esophagus is seen either at or just to the left of the midline. The close anatomical relationship of the posterior pharyngeal wall and upper cervical esophagus to cervical vertebral bodies is apparent. Large anterior osteophytes may impinge upon the upper cervical esophagus and hypopharynx but rarely cause dysphagia. The parathyroid glands are usually found just posterior to the thyroid lobes, medial to the carotid sheath and anterior to the longus colli and anterior scalene muscles.

The intimate relationship of the vertebral arteries to the cervical vertebral bodies may explain occasional vertebral arterial injuries (occlusion, intimal injuries) that may occur after manipulation of cervical spine or following rotational injuries of the neck with or without fracture dislocation. The position of the dorsal root ganglia and emerging spinal nerves just posterior to the vertebral arteries is quite apparent in the photograph of the cadaver.

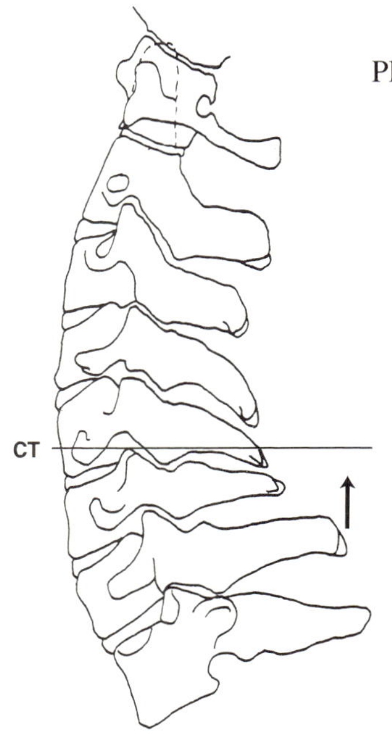

Plane of Sections

Patient CT Scan

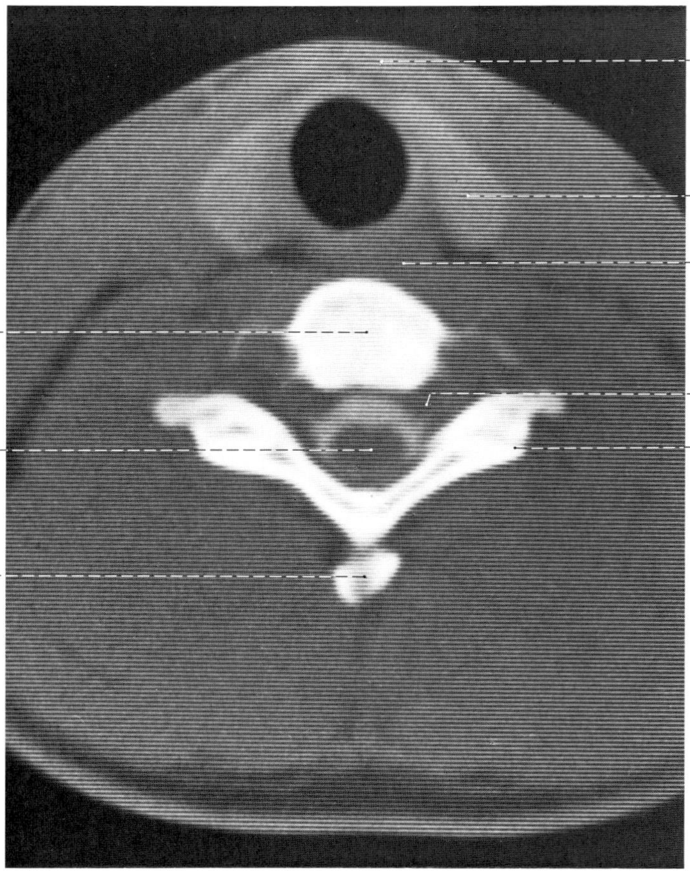

Right

Cadaver CT Scan

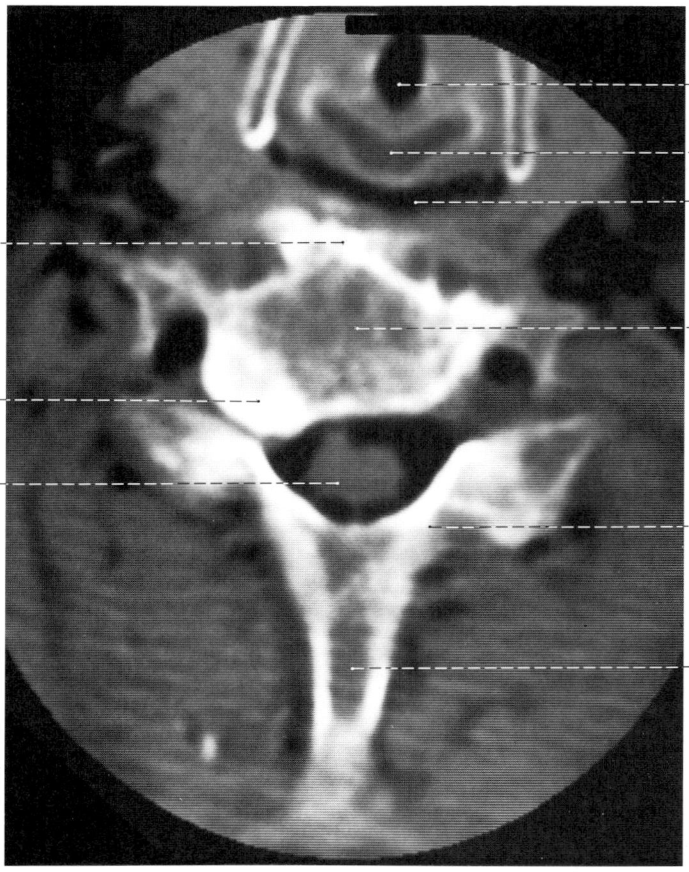

Right

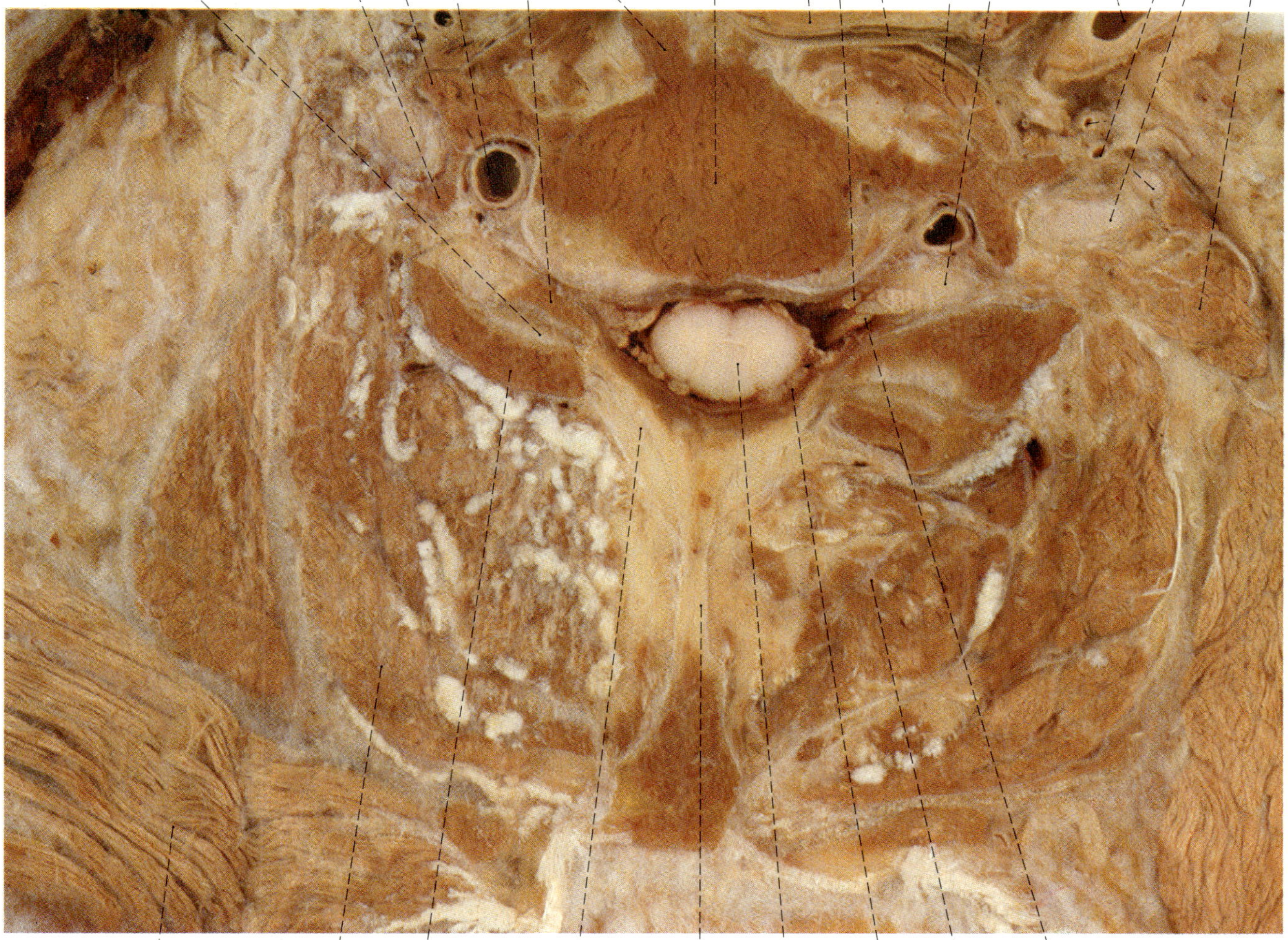

The anatomic specimen has typical spondylotic changes seen in association with chronic degenerative disc disease not present on the patient CT. Note the large osteophytes that project anteriorly and displace the posterior hypopharyngeal wall, thereby displacing the prevertebral fascia and longus colli muscle. In addition, there is moderately severe narrowing of the C6-7 neural foramen on the right caused by osteophytes arising from posterior-lateral portion of the vertebral body as well as from the uncinate process (uncovertebral joint). Such narrowing of neural foramen may produce the radicular symptoms which are often found in patients with cervical spondylosis. The CT evaluation of the neural foramen requires sequential 2 mm sections through the foramen. The use of high spatial resolution reconstruction algorithm affords excellent visualization of bony detail.

The cricoid cartilage ossifies in adulthood with a cortical bony margin of variable thickness and a central marrow space.

Note the close proximity of the carotid sheath to the upper trunks of the brachial plexus. Occasionally, metastatic adenopathy along the internal jugular chain may result in brachial plexus symptoms.

The amount of fat found between various muscle groups of the neck is quite variable, usually minimal in young, lean, athletic individuals.

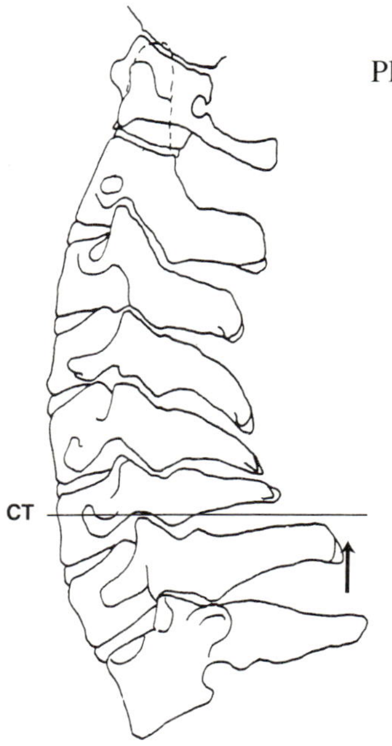

Plane of Sections

Patient CT Scan

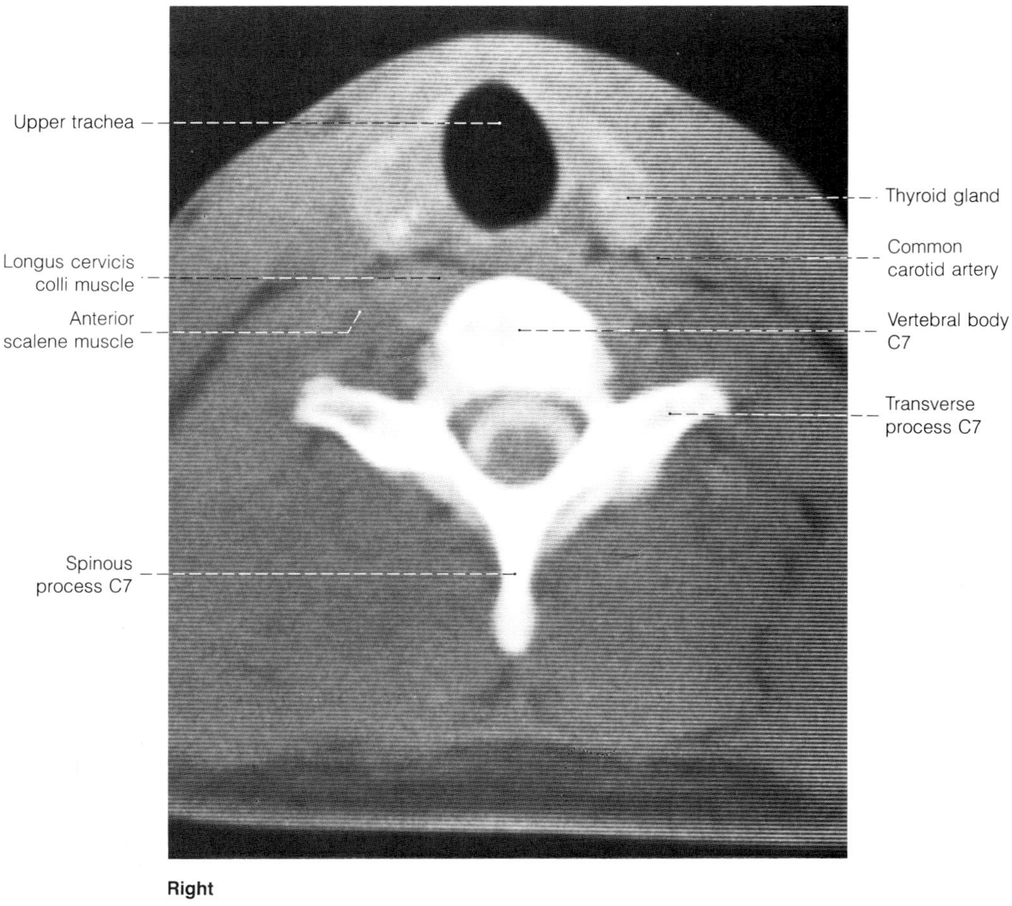

Cadaver CT Scan

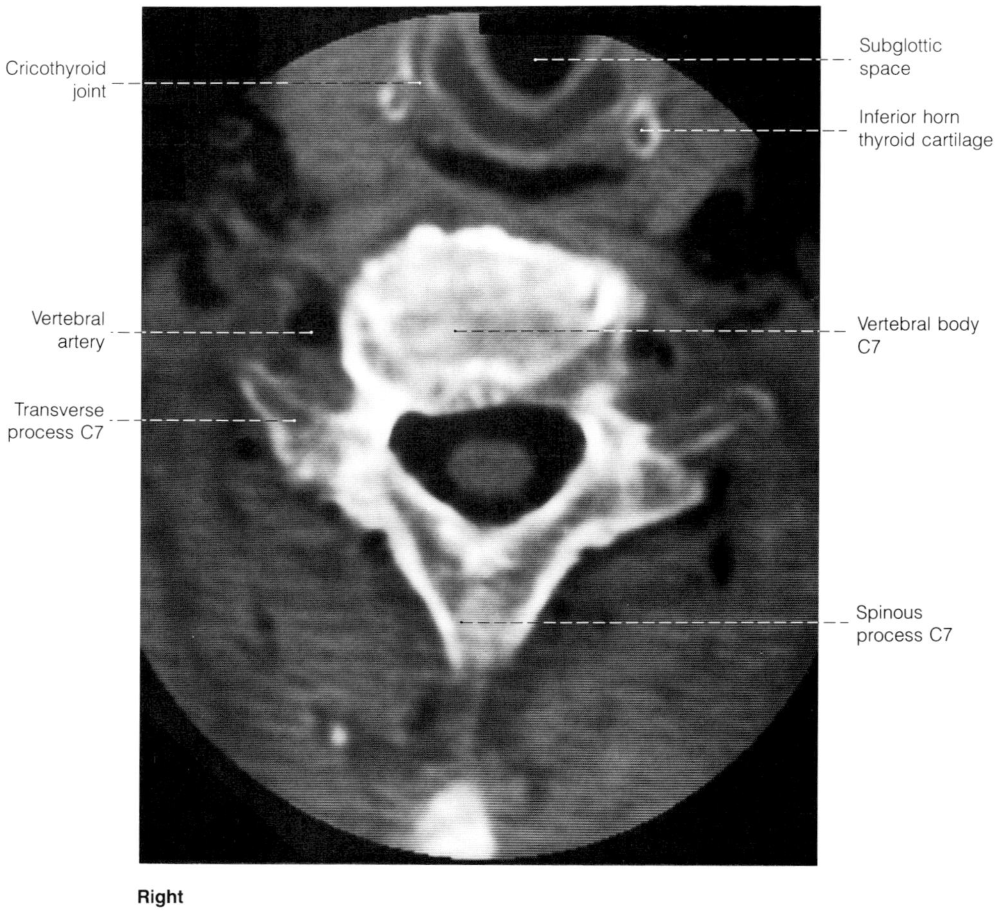

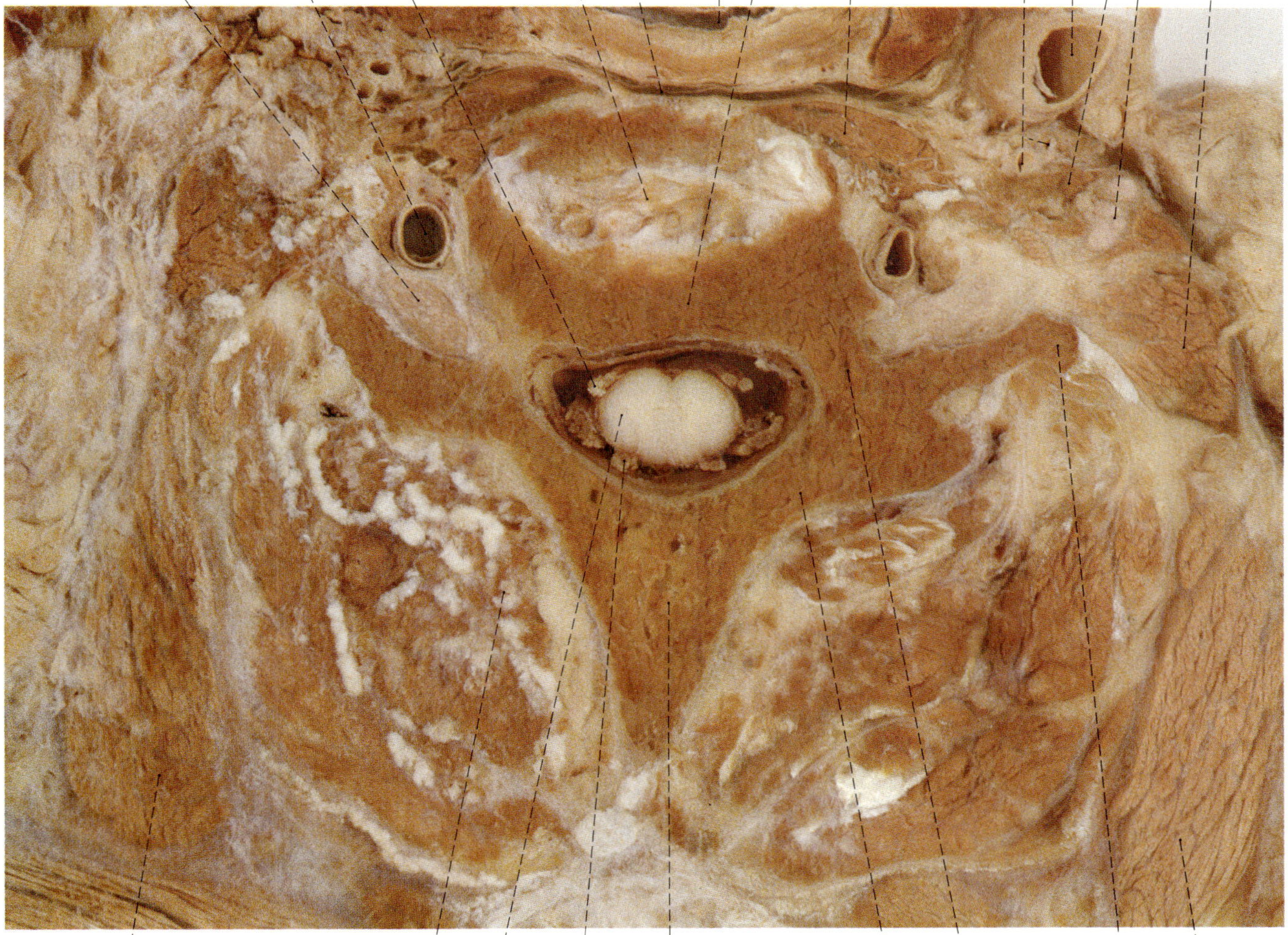

The subarachnoid space is slightly larger at this level and the cord somewhat rounder since this is the lower level of the cervical enlargement. C7 is a transitional vertebra; the costal process is very small while the lateral process is rather large and is more like the transverse process of thoracic vertebrae. The spinous process is larger and broader than other spinous processes in the cervical spine. The vertebral arteries usually enter the transverse foramina at the level of C6. Consequently, the transverse foramina at C7 can be absent.

The upper trunk of the brachial plexus, formed by fifth and sixth cervical rami, is seen at this level between the anterior and middle scalene muscles. These nerves supply the shoulder and arm flexors as well as the serratus anterior.

There is variation in the relationship of the laryngeal structures and the vertebral bodies. This in part depends on the length of the neck and, in part, to normal upward/downward motion of the larynx during respiration, swallowing, etc. This explains the variable relationship of C7 vertebral body to the lower larynx and upper trachea.

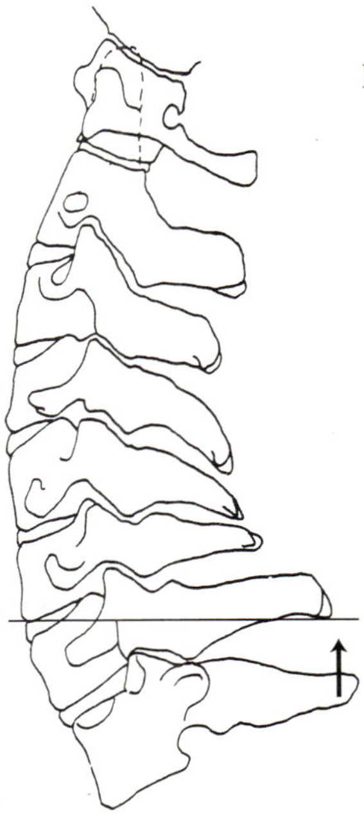

Plane of Sections

Patient CT Scan

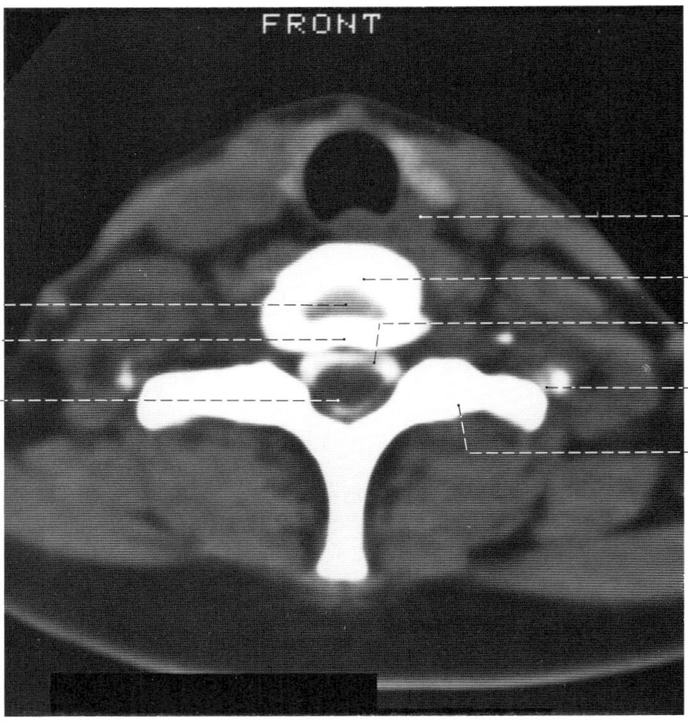

Patient CT Scan

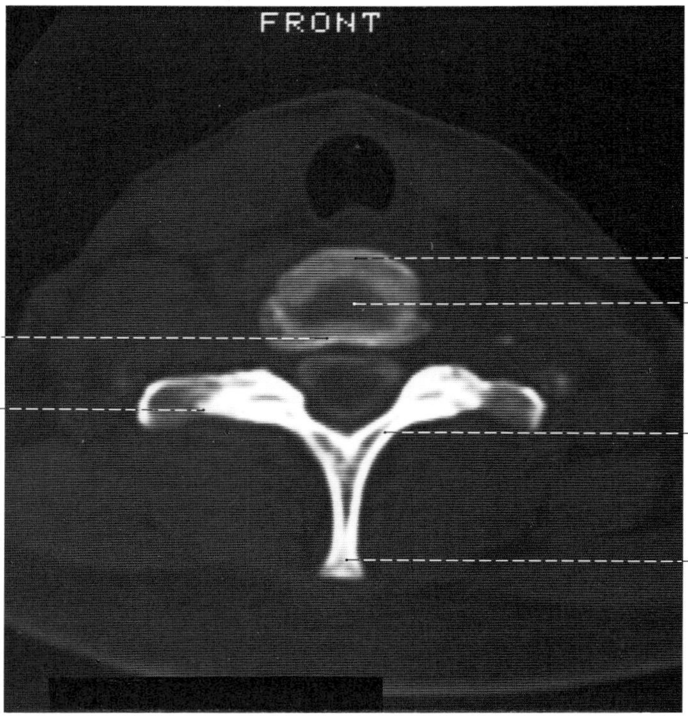

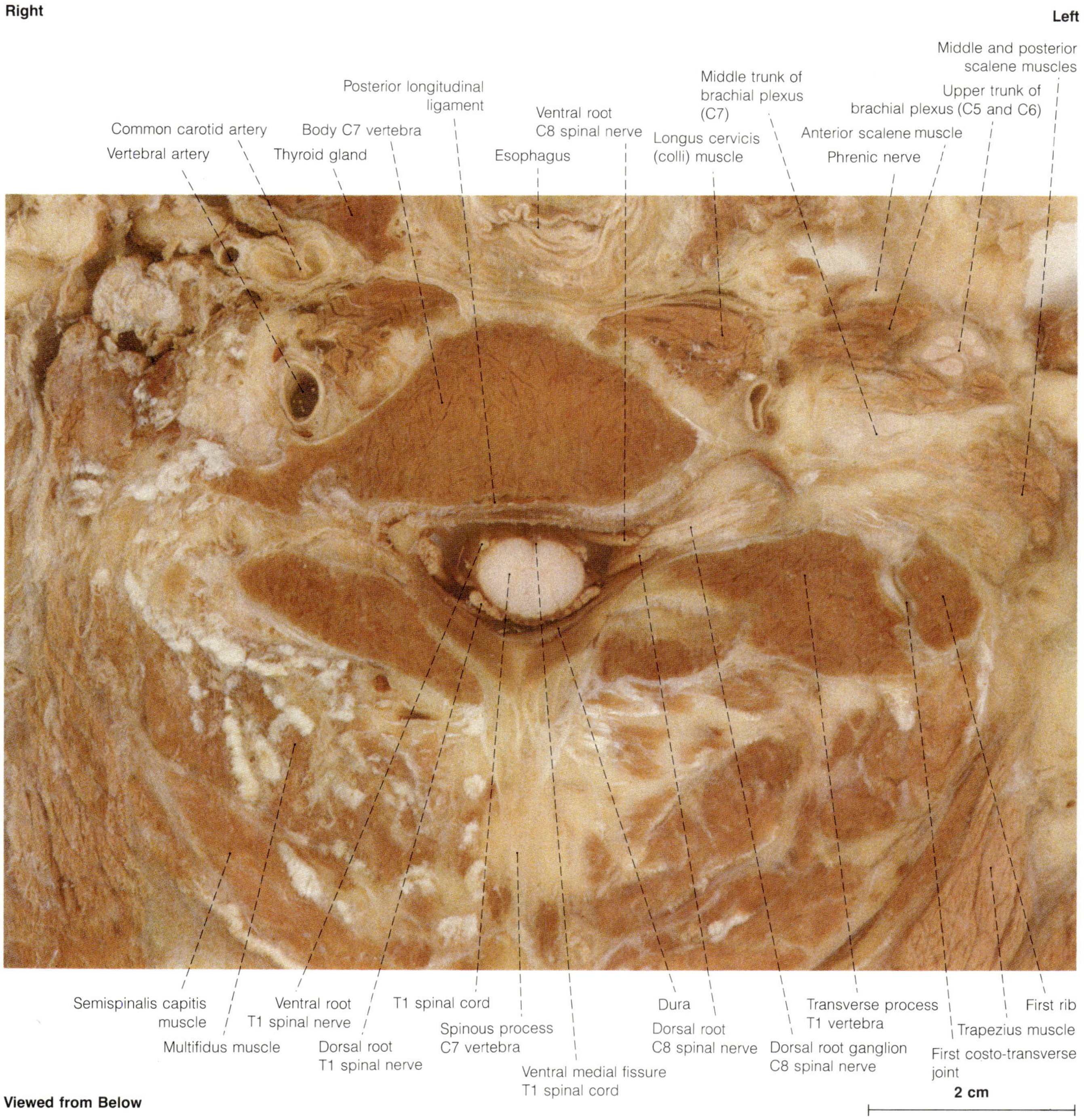

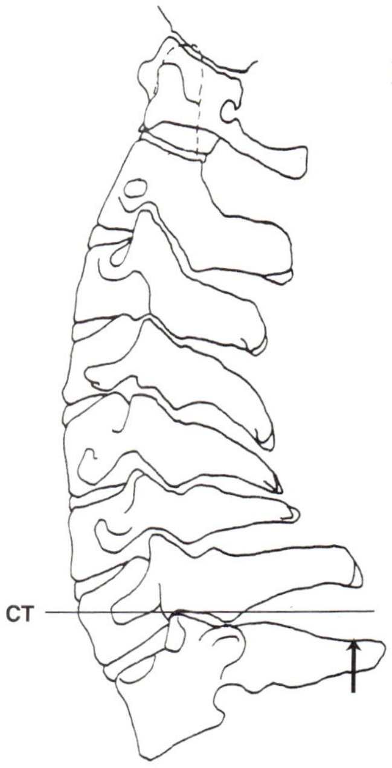

Plane of Sections

This section through the lower portion of the vertebral body of C7 also includes the transverse process of T1 and the first costo-transverse joint due to the transitional curvature of the spine at the cervico-thoracic junction.

The image on the top is the same as the one below it. The only difference is that one (top) has been displayed with emphasis on soft tissues while the one below it is displayed with a wide window for better bone detail.

The vertebral artery lies anterior to the transverse process of C7. It is at this level where the vertebral artery can be occluded by manual external compression. The longus cervicis (colli) muscle is rather bulky at this level and separates the carotid sheath structures from the vertebral arteries. The upper trunk of the brachial plexus lies lateral to the anterior scalene while the middle trunk formed primarily by C7 roots is seen medially between the anterior scalene and middle/posterior scalenes.

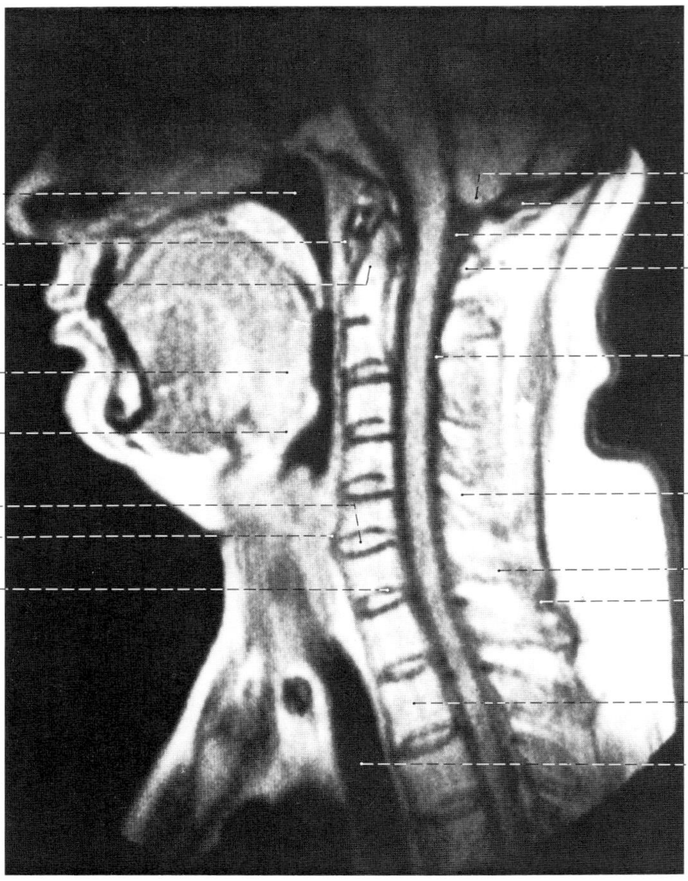

A midline sagittal section through the cervical spine permits better understanding of the relationships between the spinal cord and its surroundings. The cadaver section is that of an elderly male. Note the narrowing of the intervertebral disc spaces that accompanies age-related disc degeneration. There is prominent bulging of disc material posteriorly and osteophyte formation at C5-6 resulting in a ridge that narrows the subarachnoid space. If sufficiently large, spondylotic ridges can compress the spinal cord.

The MRI image is that of a younger patient. It is normal except for minimal anterior osteophyte formation at C5, not associated with adjacent disc space narrowing.

It is important to note how the ratio of subarachnoid space to cord varies from upper cervical levels (C1, C2) to lower levels (C3 to C7). The mean sagittal diameter of the spinal canal at C1 is about 19 mm and about 15 mm at C4. The sagittal diameter of the cervical cord varies minimally as can be appreciated in both cadaver and MRI images. The mean sagittal diameter of the adult cord is 8–9 mm at C1 and 7-8 mm at C5, one standard deviation being approximately 1 mm.

Direct sagittal sections of the cervical spine and cord cannot be obtained with computed tomography but are relatively easily obtained with MRI. Furthermore, improved low contrast resolution afforded by MRI makes it ideal for visualization of cord and surrounding cerebro-spinal fluid. On the other hand, bone detail is better demonstrated by CT imaging techniques.

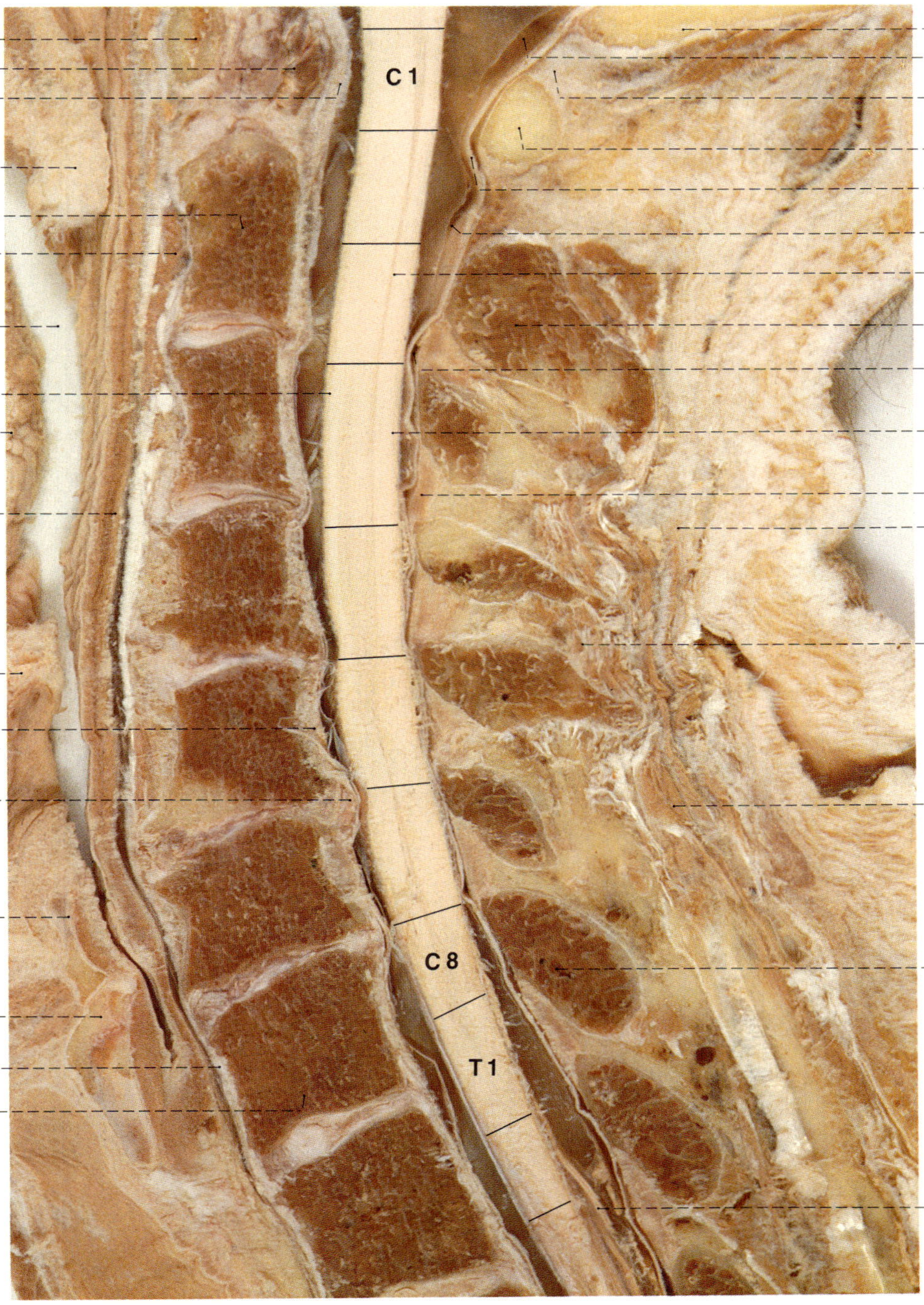
Anterior arch of atlas (C1)
Odontoid process (dens)
Transverse ligament
Soft palate
Vertebral body of axis (C2)
Longus colli (cervicis) muscle
Oropharynx
Ventral (anterior) funiculus
Base of tongue
Pharyngeal constrictor muscle
Epiglottis
Posterior longitudinal ligament
Degenerated disc and hypertrophic spur C5-6
Arytenoid cartilage
Cricoid cartilage
Anterior longitudinal ligament
Vertebral body C7
C1
C8
T1
Occipital bone
Cisterna magna
Posterior atlanto-occipital membrane
Posterior arch atlas (C1)
Dura
Arachnoid
Dorsal horn of spinal gray
Spinous process axis (C2)
Epidural space
Posterior column (dorsal funiculus)
Ligamentum flavum
Ligamentum nuchae
Interspinalis muscle
Multifidus muscle
Spinous process C7
Dorsal root T2

Selected Bibliography

Cunningham, D. J., *Cunningham's Textbook of Anatomy,* 12th Edition, ed. G. J. Romanes, London: Oxford University Press, 1981.

Di Chiro, G., and Schellinger, D., "Computed Tomography of the Spinal Cord after Lumbar Intrathecal Introduction of Metrizamide (Computer Assisted Myelography)", *Radiology* 120: 101–104, 1976.

Elliot, H. D., "Cross Sectional Diameters and Areas of the Human Spinal Cord", *Anat. Rec.* 93: 287, 1945.

Epstein, B. S., *The Spine: A Radiological Text and Atlas,* Philadelphia, Lea and Febiger, 1976.

Han, J. S., Kaufmann, B., El Yousef, S.-J., Benson, J. E., Bonstelle, C. T., Alfidi, R. J., Haaga, J. R., Yeong, H., and Huss, R. G., "N. M. R. Imaging of the Spine", *AJNR* 4: 1151–1159, 1983.

Haughton, V. M., and Williams, A. L., "C. T. Anatomy of the Spine", *CRC Crit. Ref. Diagn. Imaging* 15 (2) 173–192, 1981.

Koehler, P. R., Anderson, R. E., Baxter, B., "The Effect of Computed Tomography Viewer Controls on Anatomic Measurements", *Radiology* 130: 189–194, 1979.

Lamont, A. C., Zachary, J., and Sheldon, P. W. E., "Cervical Cord Size in Metrizamide Myelography", *Clinical Radiology* 32: 409–412, 1981.

Lowman, R. M., and Finkelstein, A., "Air Myelography for Demonstration of the Cervical Spinal Cord", *Radiology* 39: 700–706, 1942.

Modic, M. T., Weinstein, M. A., Pavlicek, W., Boumphrey, F., Starnes, D., and Duchesneau, P. M., "Magnetic Resonance Imaging of the Cervical Spine: Technical and Clinical Observations", *AJNR* 1: 15–24, 1984.

Newton, T. H. and Potts, D. G., eds., *Computed Tomography of the Spine and Spinal Cord,* Vol. I, Chapter 4, "Normal Cervical Spine", 1983, Clavadel Press, San Anselma, Ca.

Nordquist, L., "The Sagittal Diameter of the Spinal Cord and Subarachnoid Space in Different Age Groups: A Roentgen Post-mortem Study", *Acta Radiol.* (suppl.) (Stockh.) 227: 1–96, 1964.

Norman, D., Mills, C. M., Brant-Zawadzki, M., Yeates, A., Crooks, L. E., and Kaufman, L., "Magnetic Resonance Imaging of the Spinal Cord and Canal: Potentials and Limitations", *AJNR* 1: 9–14, 1984.

Parke, W. W., "The Vascular Relations of the Upper Cervical Vertebrae", *Orthop. Clin. North Am.* 9 (4) 879–889, 1978.

Payne, E. E., and Spillane, J. D., "The Cervical Spine: An Anatomic-Pathological Study of 70 Specimens with Particular Reference to the Problem of Cervical Spondylosis", *Brain* 80: 571–596, 1957.

Rothman, R. H., and Simeone, F. A., *The Spine,* Philadelphia: W. B. Saunders, Co., 1975.

Seibert, L. E., Barnes, J. E., and Dreisbach, J. N., "Accurate CT Measurement of the Spinal Cord Using Metrizamide: Physical Factors", *AJNR* 2: 75–78, 1981.

Skalpe, I. O. and Sortland, O., "Cervical Myelography with Metrizamide", *Neuroradiology* 16: 275–278, 1978.

Taiz, C., Nathan, H., and Arensburg, B., "Anatomical Observations of the Foramina Transversaria", *J. Neurol. Neurosurg Psychiatry* 41: 170–176, 1978.

Thijssen, H. O. M., Keyser, A., Horstink, M. W. M., and Meijer, E., "Morphology of the Cervical Spinal Cord on Computed Myelography", *Neuroradiology* 18: 57–62, 1979.

Warwick, R., and Williams, P. L., eds. *The Gray's Anatomy,* W. B. Saunders, Co., Philadelphia, 1981.

Thoracic and Lumbar Spine

Ascending Fiber Tracts of the Spinal Cord

Name of tract	Crossed (×) or uncrossed (–)	Termination	Function
Fasciculus gracilis	–	Nucleus gracilis	Primary afferent for proprioception from muscles, tendons, joints, deep pressure, 2 point tactile localization, vibration; essential for recognition of stereognosis
Fasciculus cuneatus	–	Nucleus cuneatus (Acc. cuneate nuc.)	
Fasciculus dorsolateralis (Lissauer's tr.)	–	Dorsal funicular gray (Substantia gelatinosa)	Pain and temperature
Dorsal spinocerebellar	Mostly – (few ×, about level of origin)	Cerebellum (homolateral)	Proprioception, etc. to cerebellum for coordination of muscle action, maintenance of balance and equilibrium; dorsal tract for trunk and lower extremity primarily; ventral tract especially for extremities (particularly upper)
Ventral spinocerebellar	Mostly × in cord (about level of origin), some –	Cerebellum (most recross to side of origin)	
Lateral spinothalamic	× (about level of origin)	Thalamus, V.P.L.	Pain and temperature from cord levels to thalamus
Spinotectal	× (about level of origin)	Superior colliculus	Pain, temperature, and gen. tactile; part of path for pupillary dilation to pain
Ventral spinothalamic	× (about level of origin)	Thalamus, V.P.L.	General tactile or light touch from cord levels
Secondary ascending visceral tract (ventrolateral fasciculus proprius)	× and – (many multisynaptic)	Diencephalon, Mesencephalon	Visceral sensations, particularly disagreeable; poorly localized
Spinovestibular	× and –	Inferior vestibular nucleus	Orientation of head movements and eye position in response to movements of neck
Fasciculus proprius	× and –	Spinal cord gray	Intersegmental spinal cord reflexes

Descending Fiber Tracts of the Spinal Cord

Name of tract	Crossed (×) or uncrossed (–)	Termination	Function
Lateral corticospinal	× motor decussation at medulla	Internuncials, Alpha motor neurons	Fine voluntary muscular control especially for extremities; voluntary micturition
Ventral corticospinal	Uncrossed (some × at termination)	Internuncials, Alpha motor neurons	Voluntary control, especially of neck and trunk
Rubrospinal and Tegmentospinal (Caudal rubrospinal)	× at origin (Vent. teg. dec.) × and – at origin	Internuncials, Motor neurons, Cervical cord Internuncials, Motor neurons	Part of path for impulses from extrapyramidal cerebral cortex, basal ganglia and cerebellum; related to muscular coordination (cerebellum), gross movements, and tonus
Medial tectospinal	× at origin	Internuncials, Motor neurons	Part of reflex pathway for movements of head and neck to visual and auditory stimuli
Medial vestibulospinal (med. long fasc.)	Mostly × at origin, few –	Internuncials, Motor neurons	Reflex changes in position of head and upper extremity in response to vestibular stimulation
Lateral (ventrolat.) vestibulospinal		Internuncials, Motor neurons	Reflex movements of trunk and extremities in response to vestibular stimulation
Lateral tecto-tegmentospinal	Few × at origin, mostly –	Internuncials, Motor neurons, Sympathetic preganglionics	Pupillary dilation; part of reflex path for movements in response to visual and auditory stimuli
Lateral reticulospinal	Mostly –	Pregang. sympathetic cell column, Sacral parasympathetic nucleus	Part of path for sweating on face and scalp; bladder tone
Ventral reticulospinal	× and – at origin	Pregang. sympathetic cell column	Part of path for bilateral sweating on trunk and extremities related to temperature regulation
Ventrolateral reticulospinal	Mostly –	Internuncials, Ventral horn neurons, Phrenic nuc.	Regulation of respiration
Medial reticulospinal	× and – at origin	Intermediolateral pregang. sympathetic cell column, Internuncials	Part of path for salivary gland, blood vessel, and heart regulations

T3 Spinal Cord

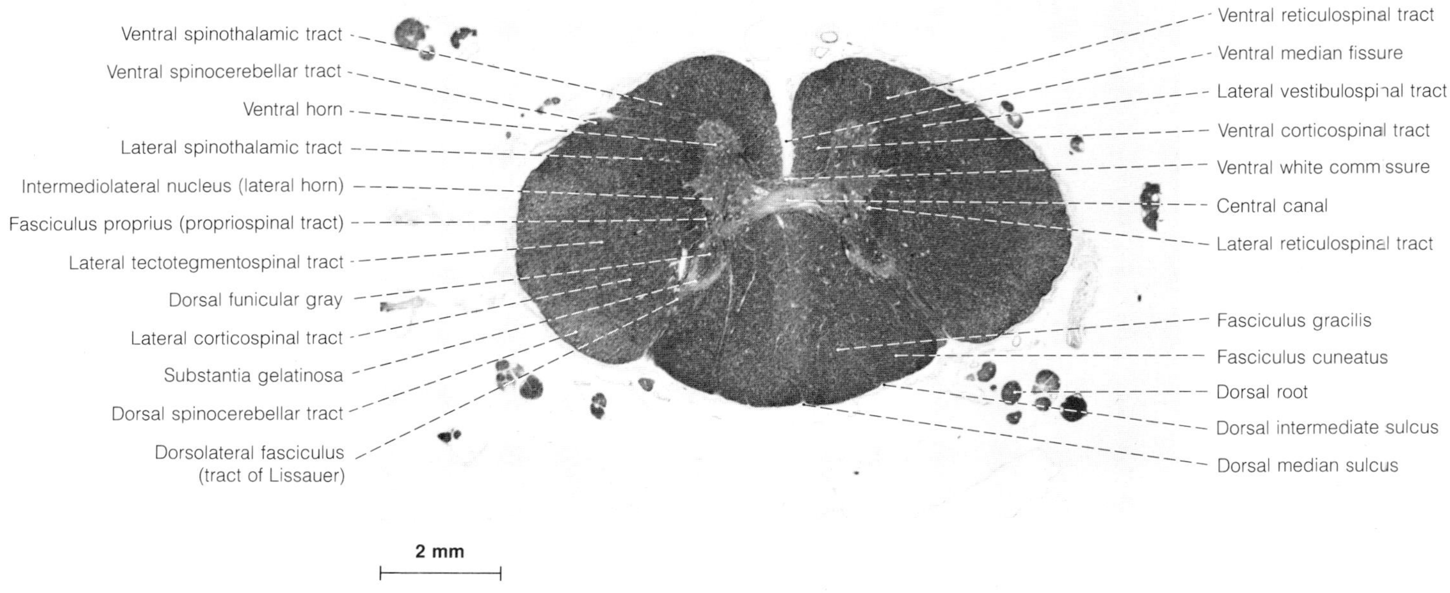

Patient CT Scan of the T2 Vertebra

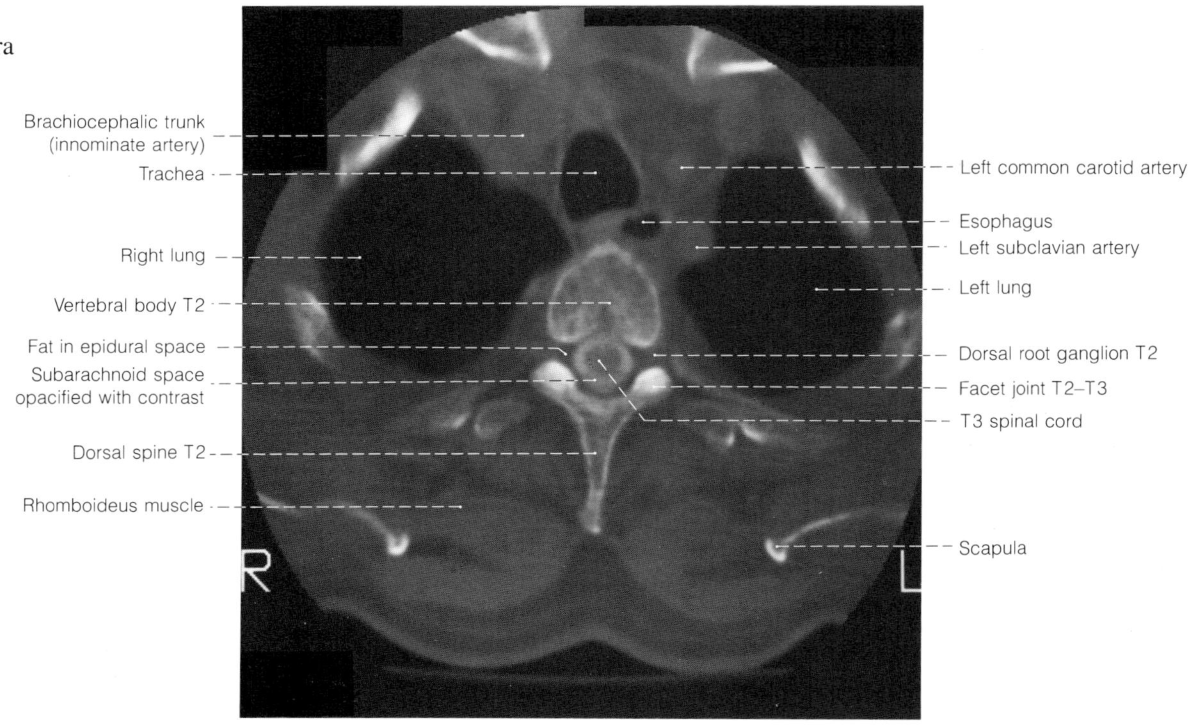

Right

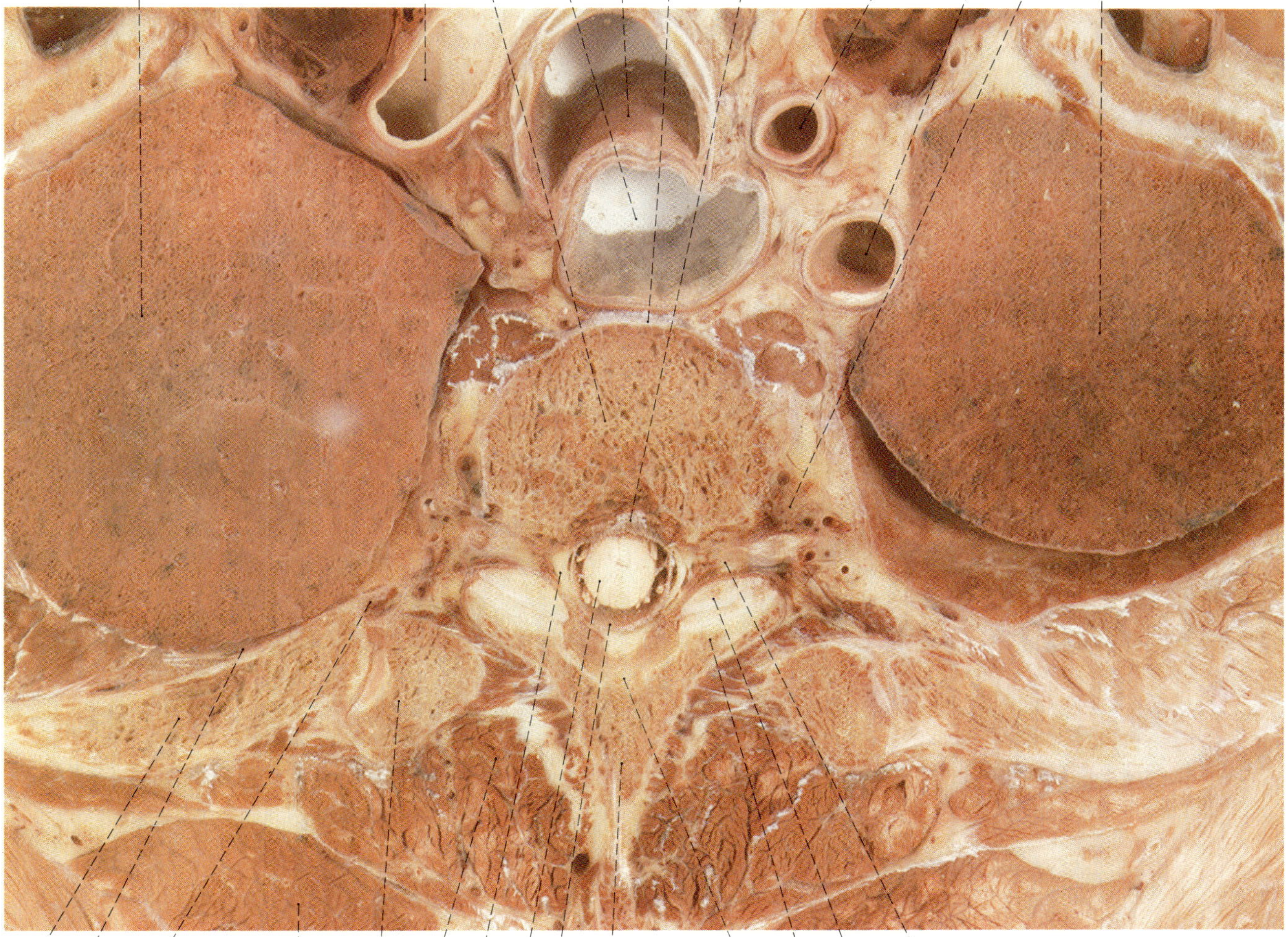

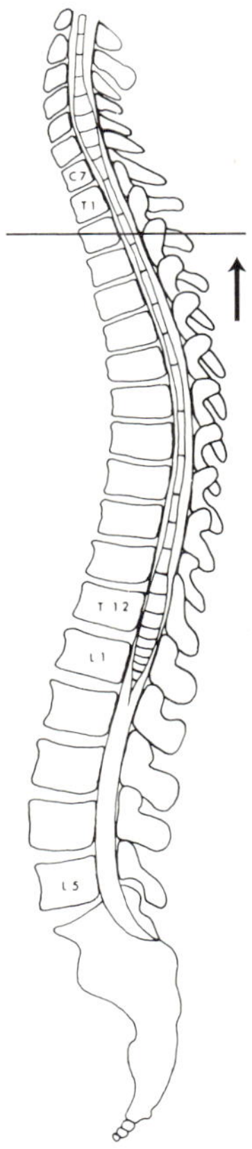

The gross anatomical section passes through the upper thoracic cavity, apices of the lungs, and superior mediastinum. The esophagus is open in this cadaver specimen, but it is not unusual for it to be collapsed and not directly visualized. The T2 vertebral level is below the cervical enlargement of the spinal cord, and the smaller thoracic cord is evident radiographically with Metrizamide® in the canal. The facet joints between the vertebrae become oriented more coronally as one moves caudally through the thoracic levels.

At this level the ventral horns of the spinal cord are small, containing anterior horn cells that only supply axial musculature (back and intercostal muscles). The sympathetic contributions to the head (by way of the cervical sympathetic trunk) and to the heart arise from the intermediolateral nuclei or cell columns of the upper five thoracic segments. Visceral afferents accompany the sympathetic nerves to the thorax. The cutaneous sensory distribution is to a segment of the upper thorax.

T10 Spinal Cord

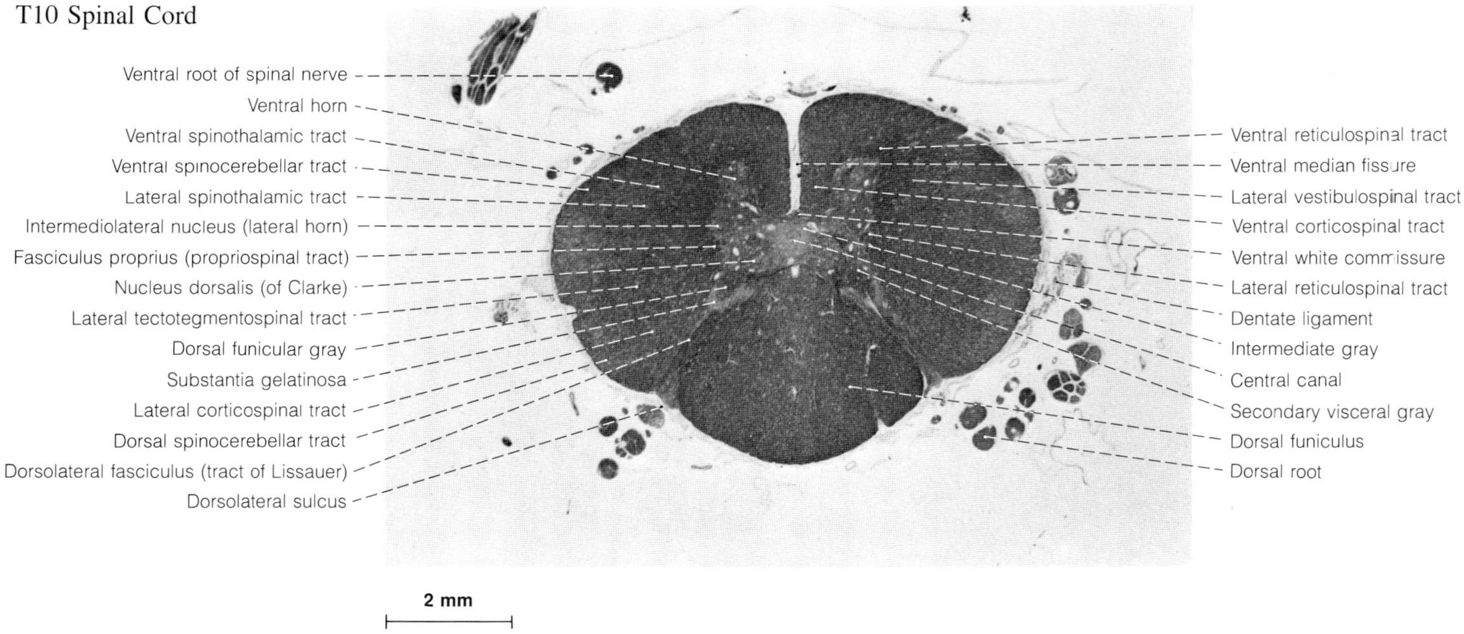

Patient CT Scan of the T8–T9 Vertebra

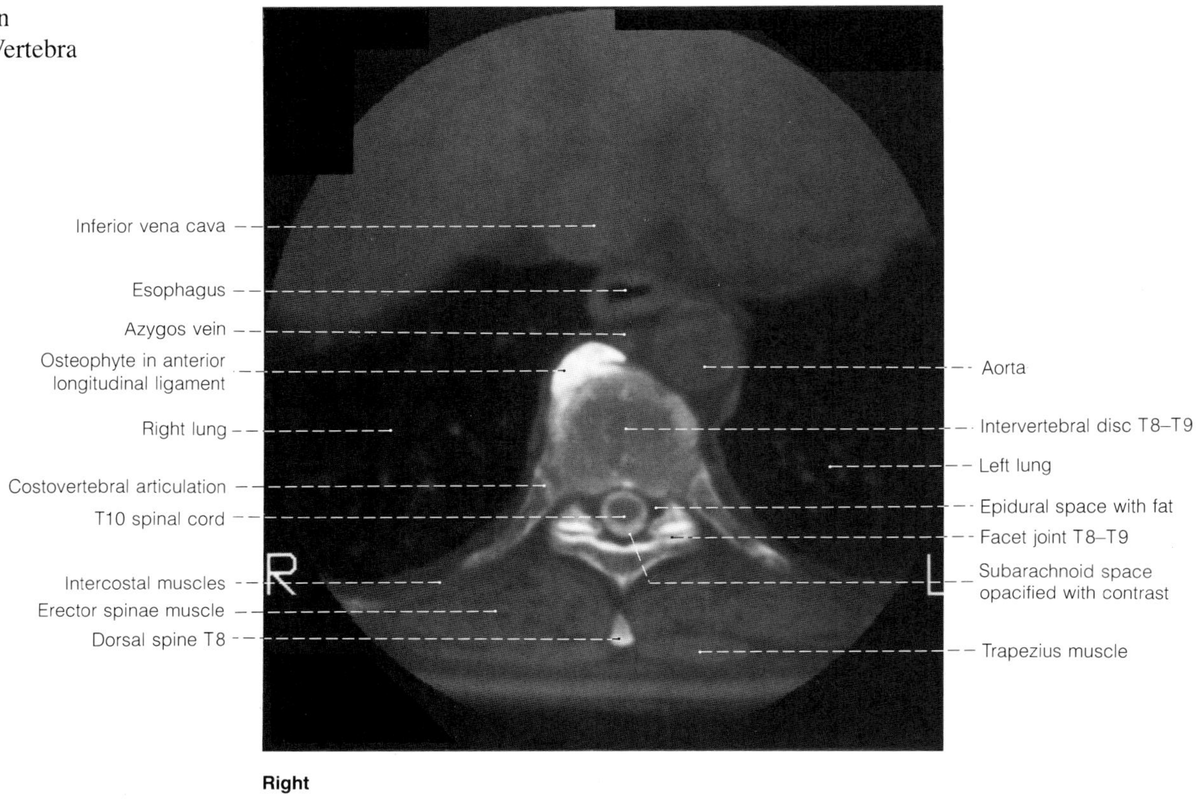

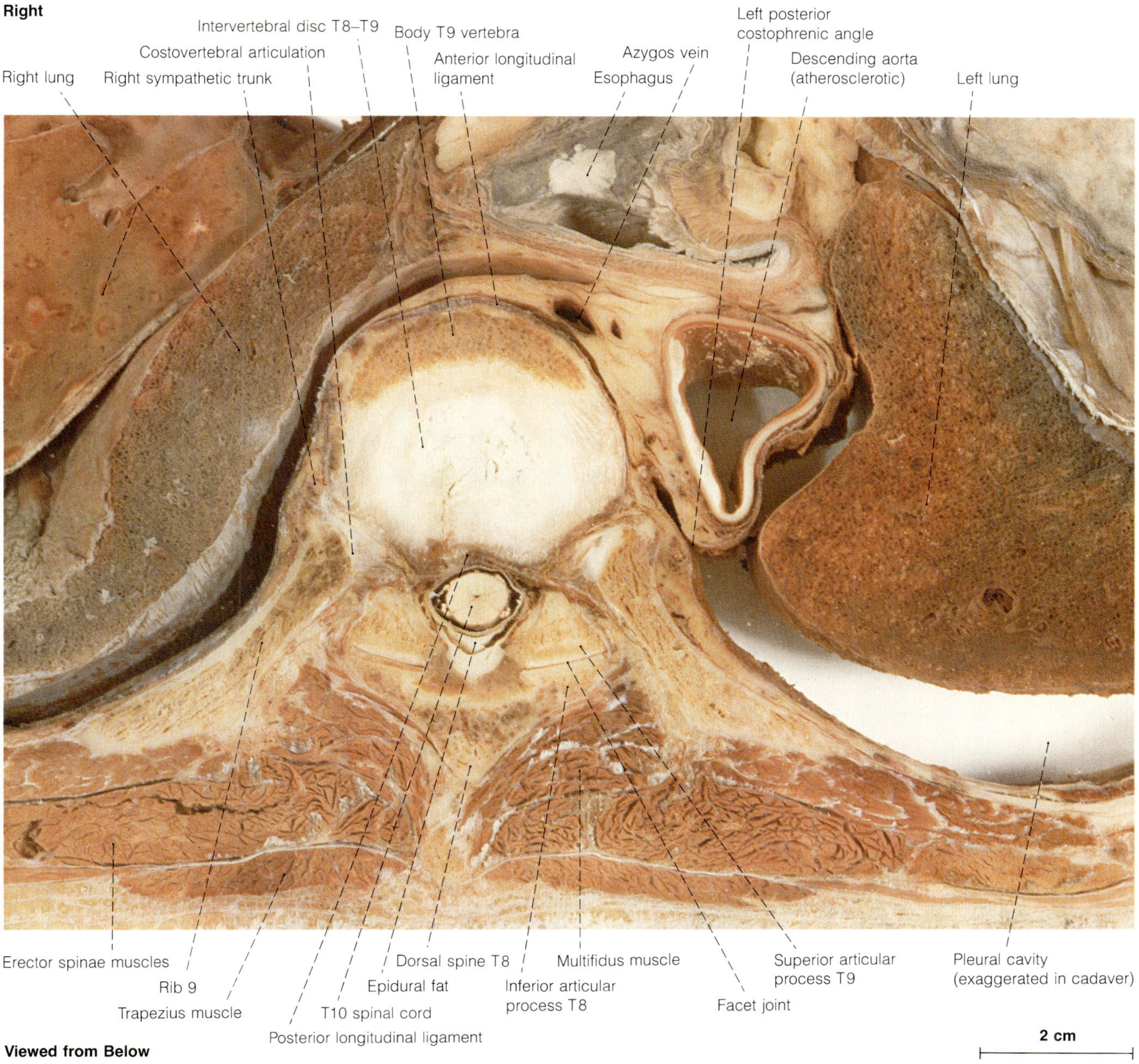

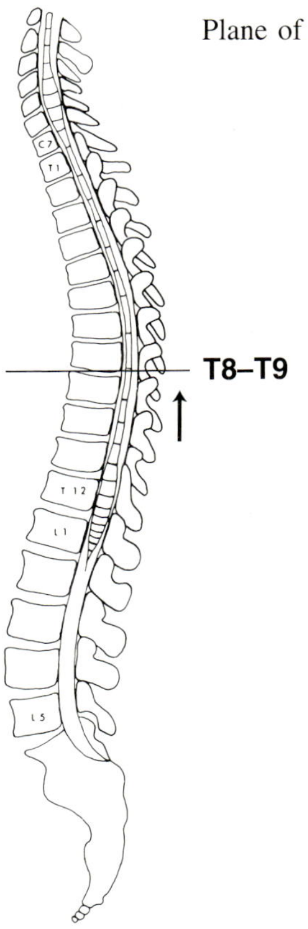

The transverse plane of the gross section includes the T8–T9 intervertebral disc. In the anatomical and CT sections the dome of the patient's diaphragm is below the plane of the cut; however, it may extend to this level. The visceral relationships will obviously change with respiration, posture, and the amount of abdominal fat.

The size of the cord and of the spinal canal remains relatively uniform through the thoracic levels. The facet joints of the thoracic spine are oriented in the coronal plane, whereas in the cervical area they are in the axial-transverse plane, and in the lumbar area they are oblique (approximately 45°) to the coronal or sagittal planes. Because of this orientation, facet osteophyte formation in the thoracic area does not necessarily encroach upon the neural canal.

The cutaneous nerves arising from the T9 spinal nerve supply the segment of skin superior to the umbilicus. Branches of the visceral nerves from the T9 spinal nerve are distributed in part by way of the greater splanchnic nerves to the celiac ganglion. Transection of the spinal cord at the level of T10 will result in a loss of sensation below the T12 dermatome (inguinal region).

L2 Spinal Cord

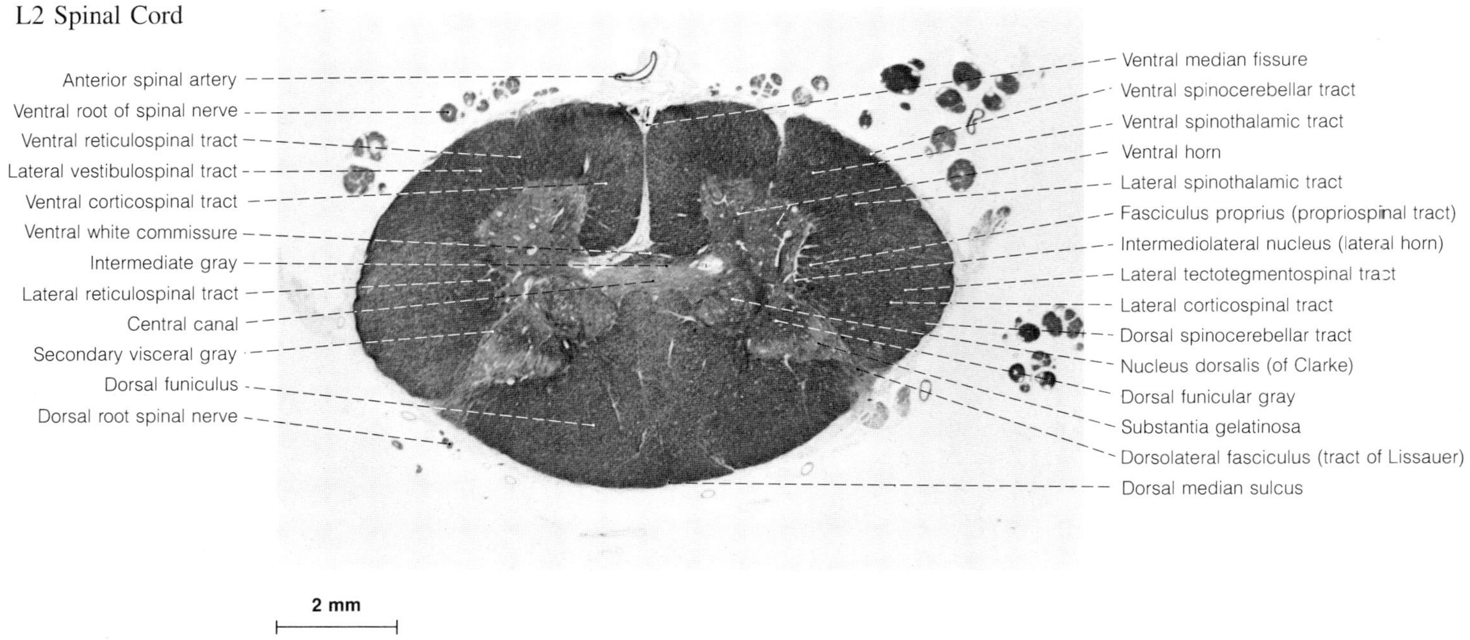

Patient CT Scan of the T11–T12 Disc

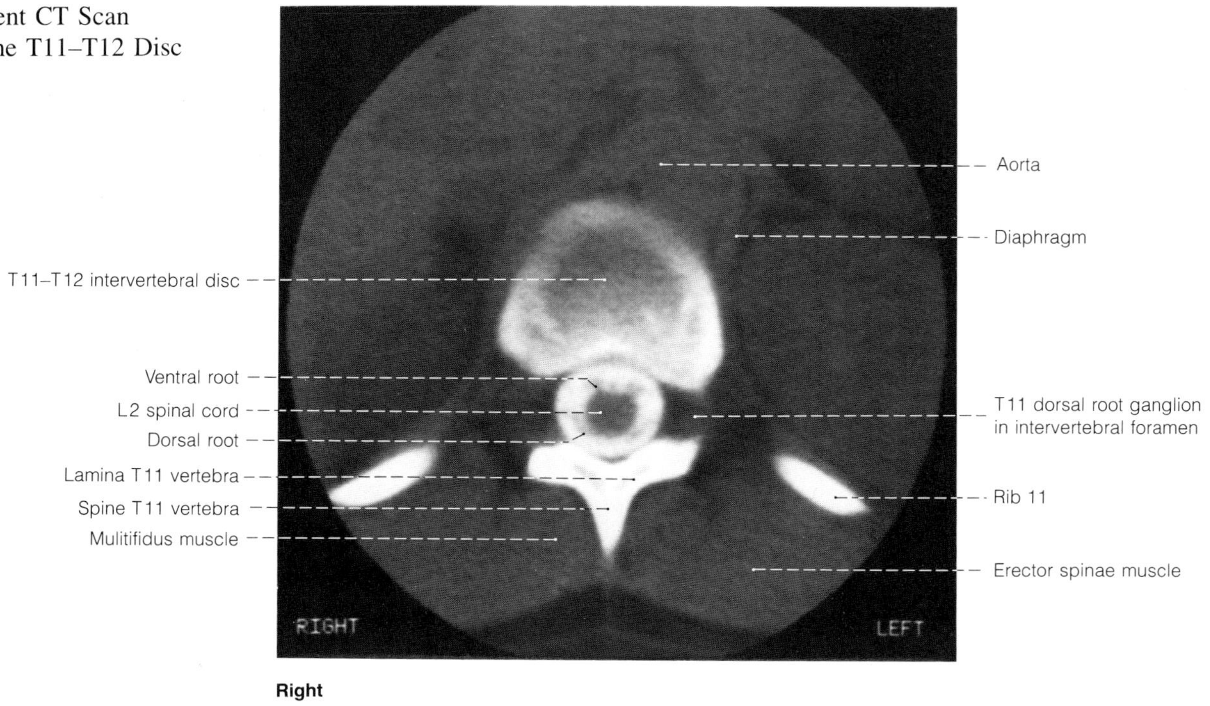

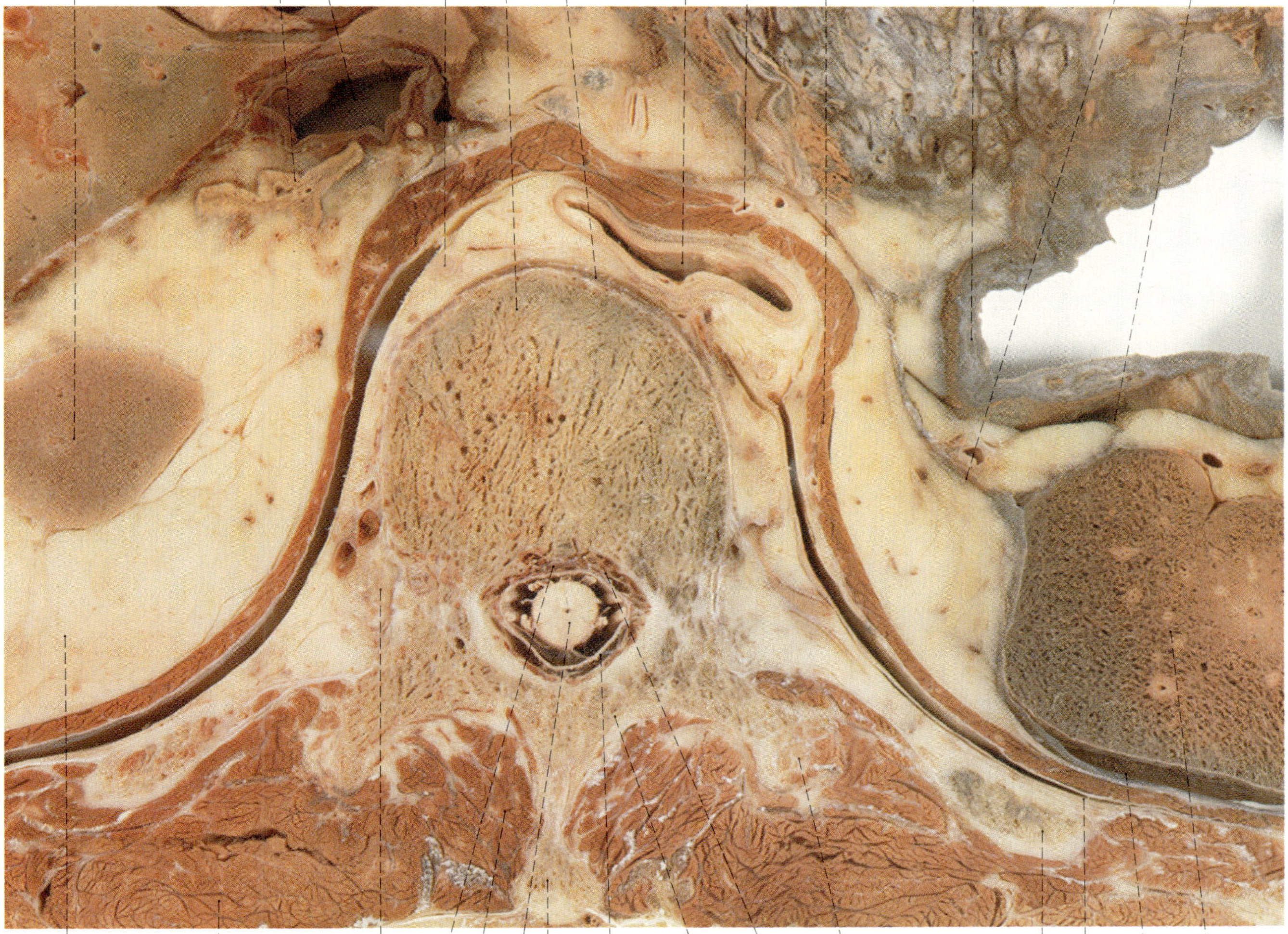

Viewed from Below

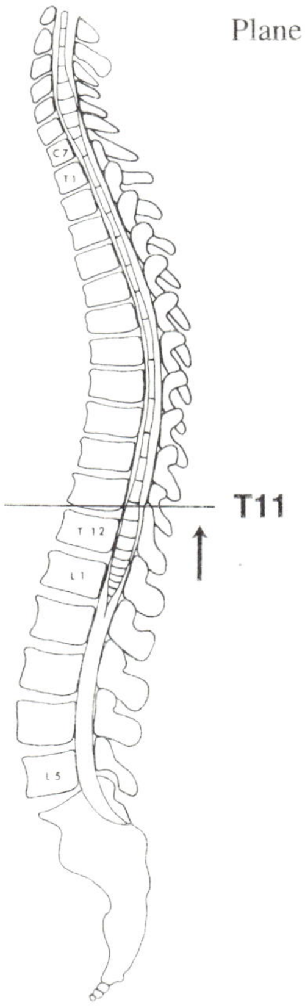

Plane of Section

The lower thoracic vertebrae are transitional between the "typical" thoracic and the "typical" lumbar. The facet joint illustrated in the CT scan is oriented in a plane between the coronal thoracic and the sagittal lumbar.

Although the aortic hiatus of the diaphragm is below this level, the abdominal viscera anterior to the posterior part of the diaphragm are quite variable depending on respiration, the position of the patient, and the amount of abdominal fat. In the somewhat obese cadaver illustrated, the upper pole of the right kidney and the related adrenal gland are illustrated at a higher location than usual along with the stomach and spleen.

The L2 segment of the spinal cord is the highest level of the lumbar enlargement providing motor innervation to the lower extremity (contributing to the femoral and obturator nerves). It is also the lowest level of preganglionic sympathetic neurons (intermediolateral nucleus) influencing the pelvic viscera and the sweat glands and blood vessels of the lower extremity, and the lowest (and largest) appearance of the nucleus dorsalis (Clarke's nucleus).

Body T12 Vertebra

L4 Spinal Cord

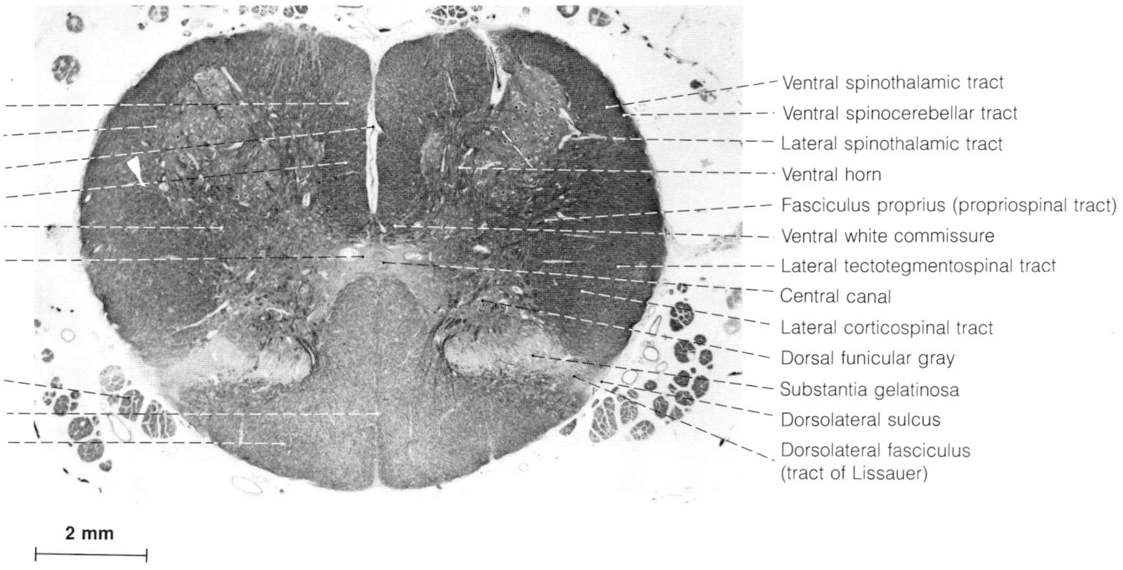

Patient CT Scan of the T12 Vertebra

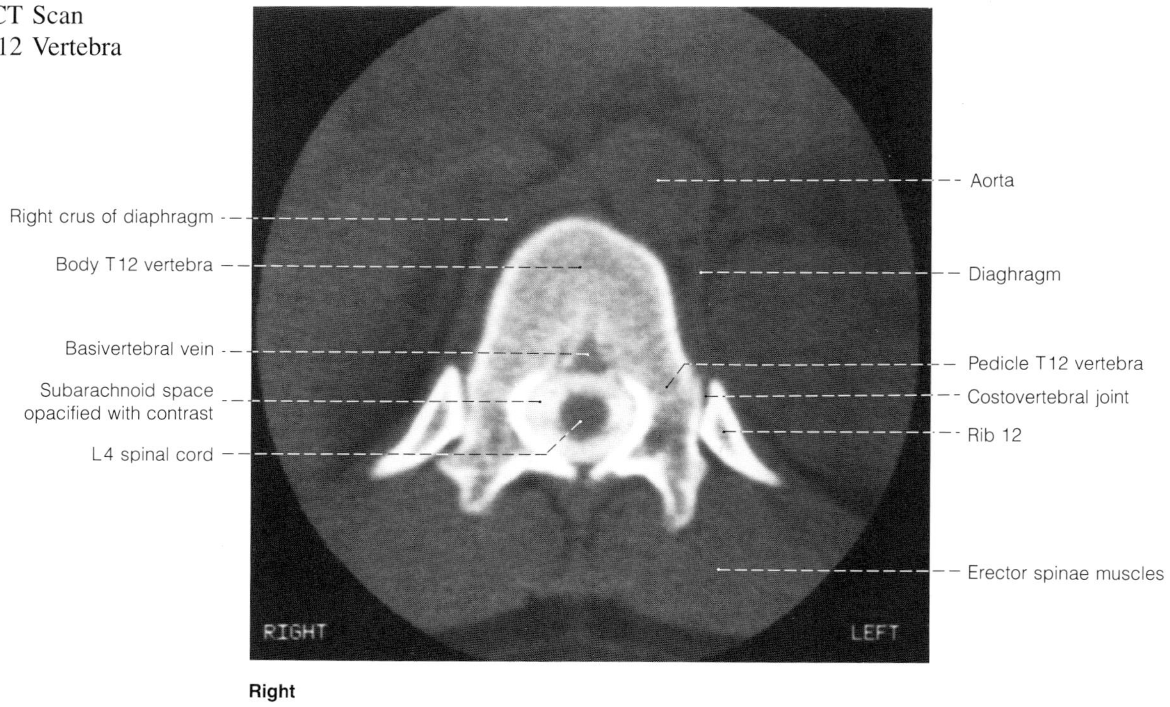

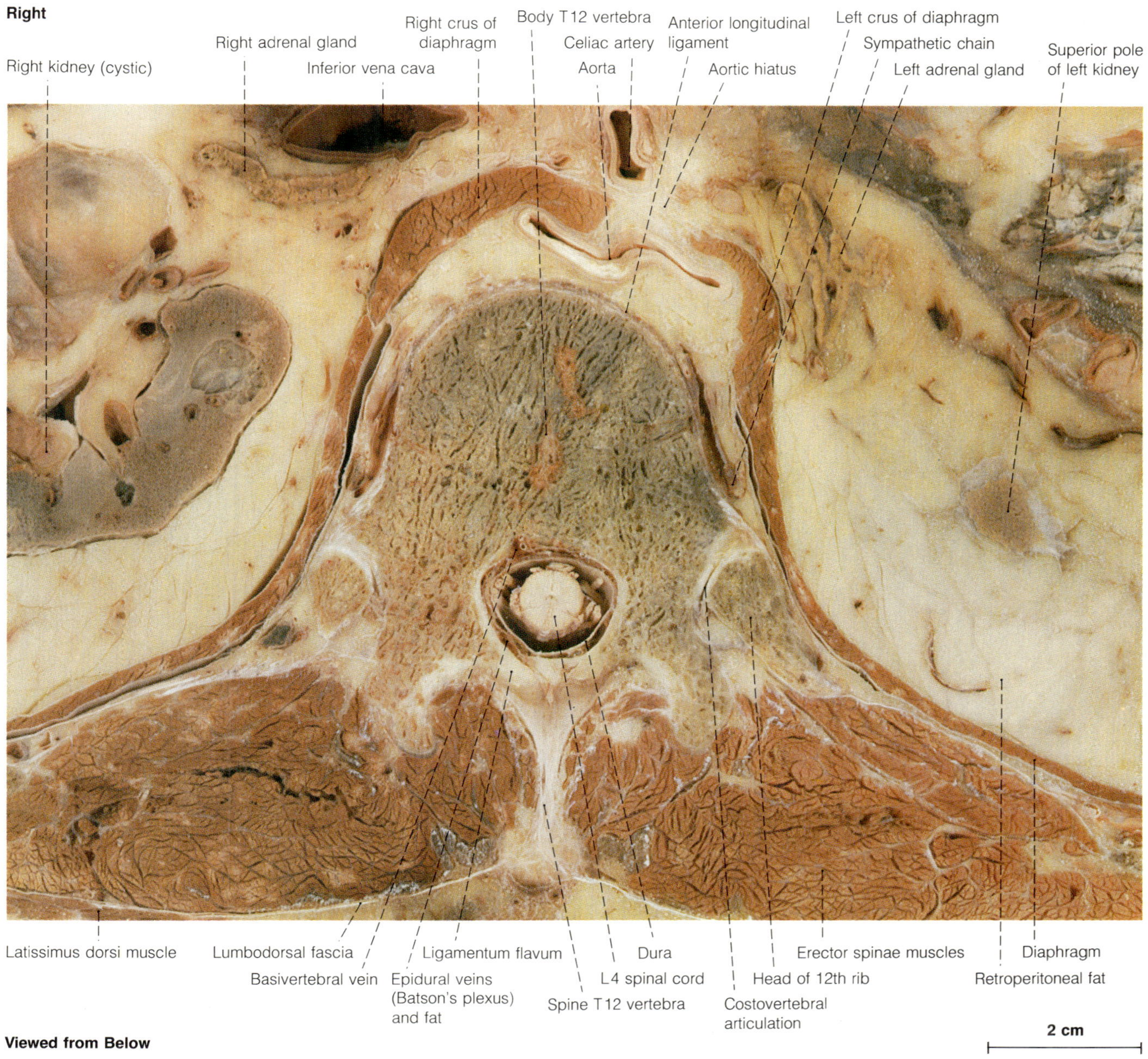

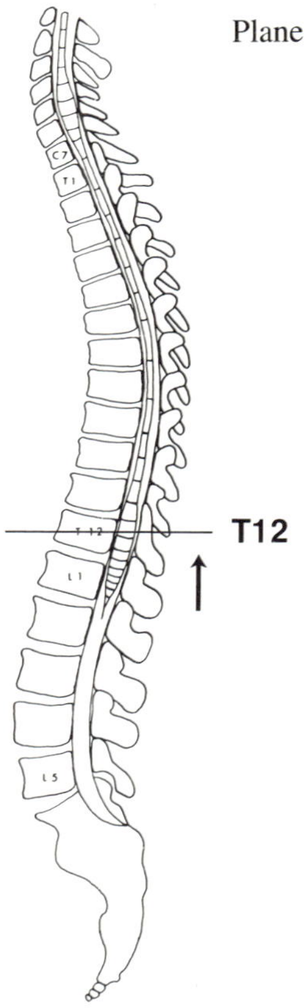

The lower lumbar spinal cord is located near the inferior body of the T12 vertebra. The gray matter is increased within the lumbar enlargement of the spinal cord, and the lateral corticospinal tract extends to the pial surface below the second lumbar cord segment. The subarachnoid space at this level contains the dorsal and ventral roots of T12, L1, L2, L3, and L4. The distribution of L2, L3, and L4 to the thigh is via the femoral and obturator nerves.

This CT slice is in a patient with Metrizamide® in the caudal sac to demonstrate the contents of the dural envelope (subarachnoid space, nerve roots, and spinal cord). The basivertebral veins of the spine may be compared to the sinus of the dorsum sellae in the basisphenoid (page 221).

S2 Spinal Cord

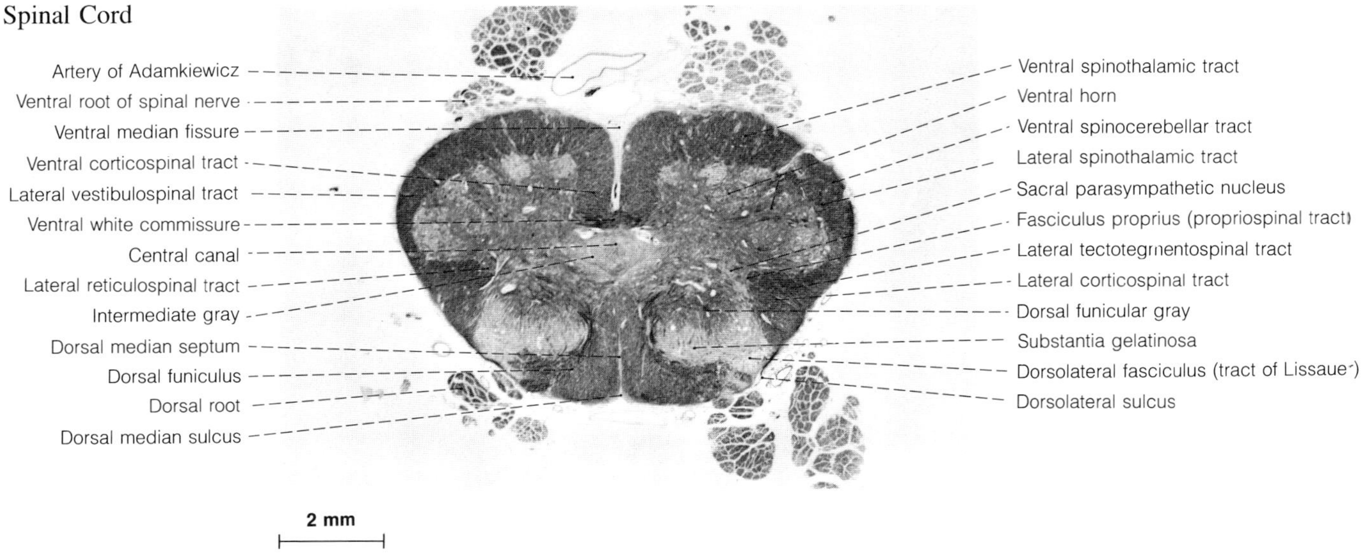

Patient CT Scan of the L1 Vertebra

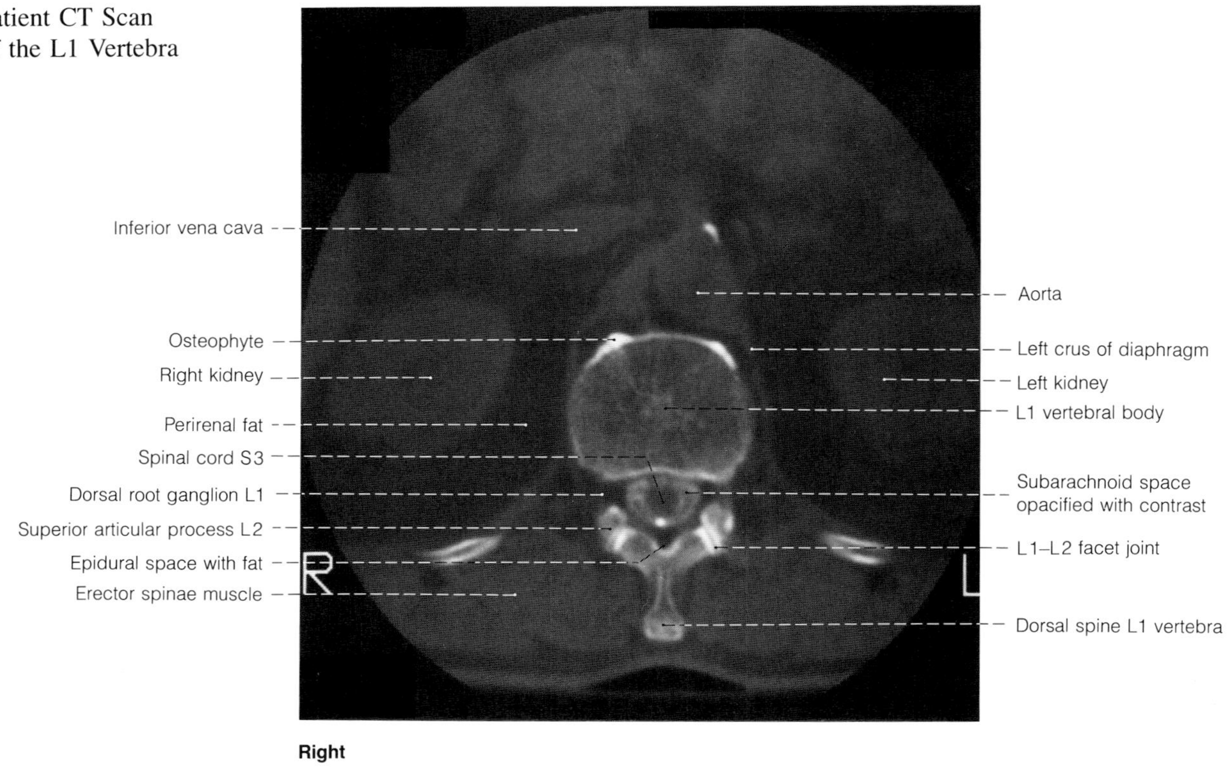

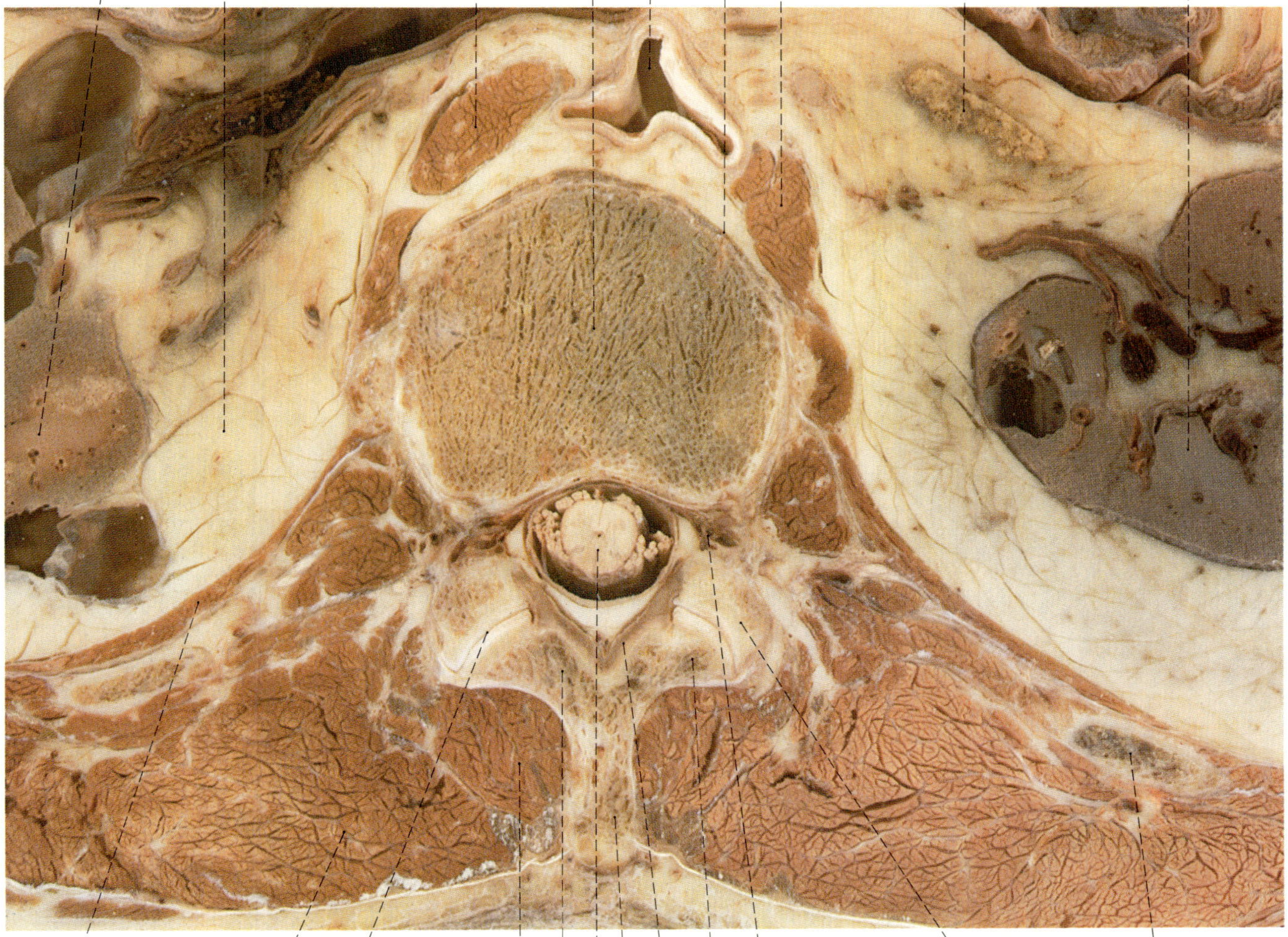

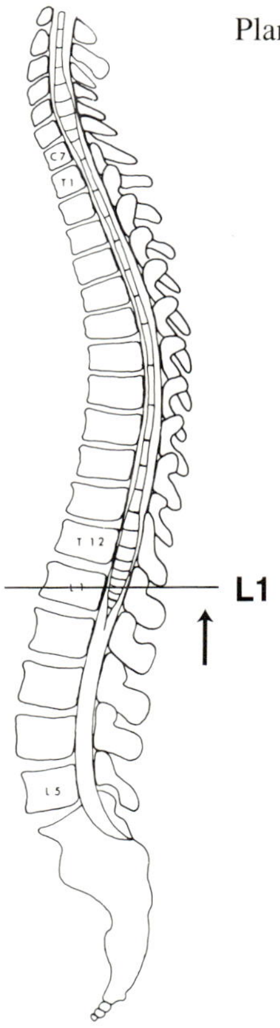

The S2 spinal cord and surrounding lumbar roots are posterior to the upper portion of the body of the L1 vertebra. This segment of the cord and the short S3 and S4 segments of the conus medullaris give rise to the parasympathetic innervation of the urinary bladder and other pelvic viscera. The slight caudal enlargement tapers to an end at the tip of the conus medullaris, with a continuing fibrous band, the filum terminale, always present and sometimes visualized on caudal slices. On the CT scan with Metrizamide®, one filling defect pattern (given by the dorsal and ventral nerve roots emerging from the sacral cord levels) resembles the symbols seen on certain video games, giving rise to the "space invader sign" designating this pattern.

L1–L2 Intervertebral disc

Patient CT Scan

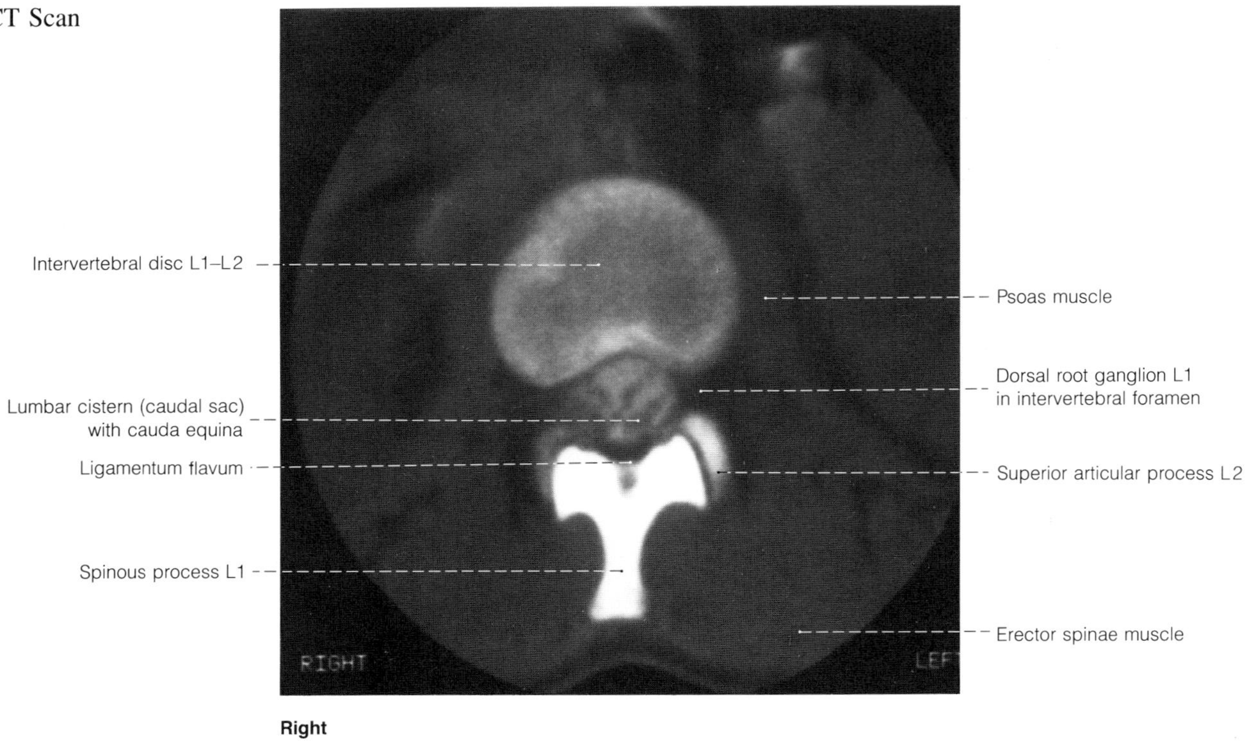

Patient MRI Scan

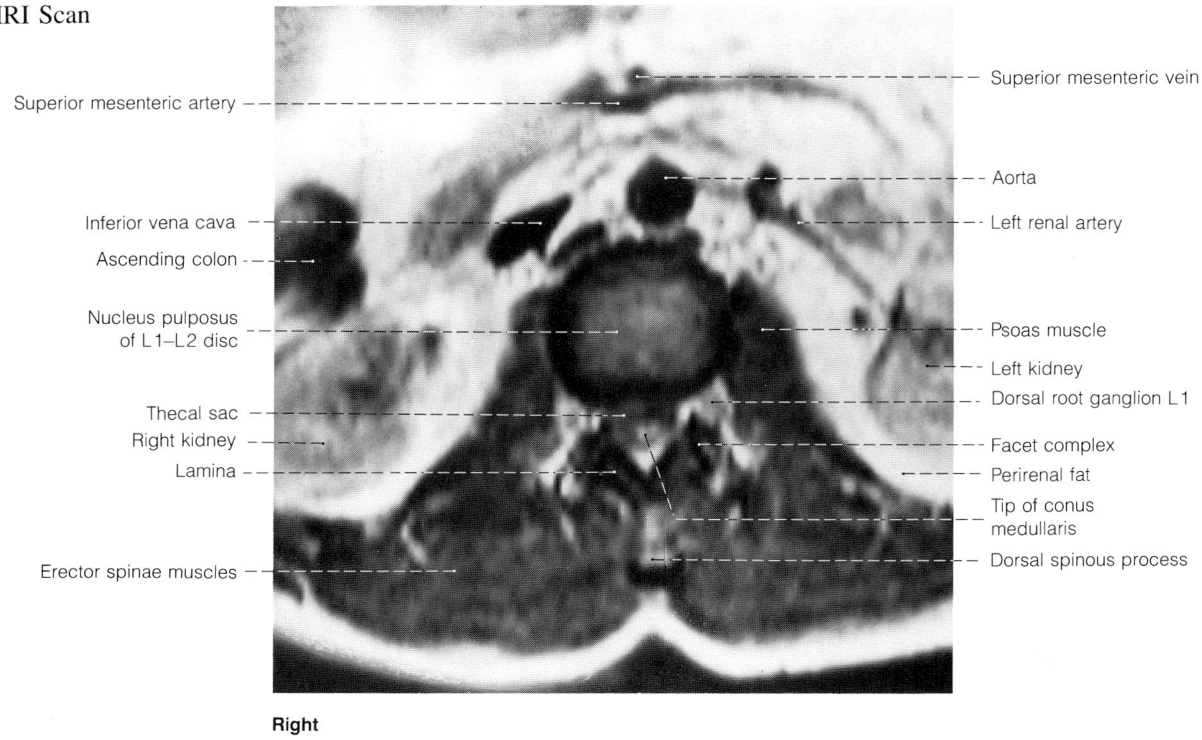

The gross specimen illustrates the position of the dorsal root ganglion of L1 in the intervertebral foramen and its relationship to the dura. The roots of the lumbar and sacral nerves carry a sleeve of dura and CSF space inferiorly which ends proximal to the ganglion. The ganglion is encased in fat which aids in its identification in both CT and MRI. The spinal cord in the adult may end (conus medullaris) at the L1–L2 disc or may extend somewhat lower as in the cadaver specimen. The nerve roots constituting the cauda equina may be delineated with contrast media on CT.

The S2, S3, and S4 segments of the spinal cord contain the tiny but important sacral parasympathetic nucleus providing preganglionic innervation for the pelvic viscera. The coccygeal spinal cord, with the lower sacral segments, also distributes to the perianal region and is involved in the perianal "wink" reflex.

On the CT scan the position of nerve roots is imaged as negative or black dots in the Metrizamide®-enhanced CSF. These roots come to lie dorsally in the sac. Metrizamide® concentration decreases steadily with time after injection, as illustrated in this very faint example scanned 6 hours after injection.

Right

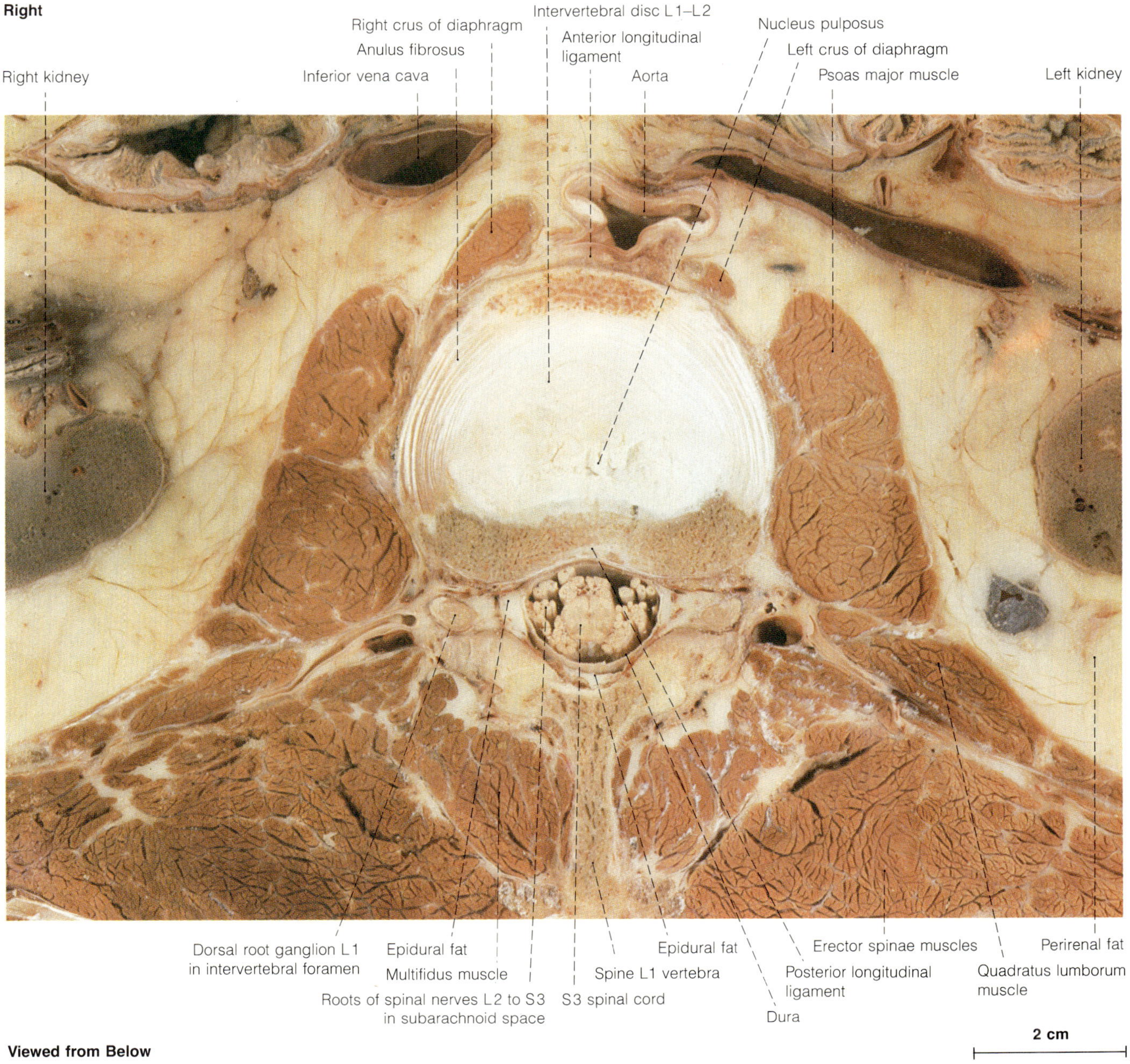

Viewed from Below

Plane of Section

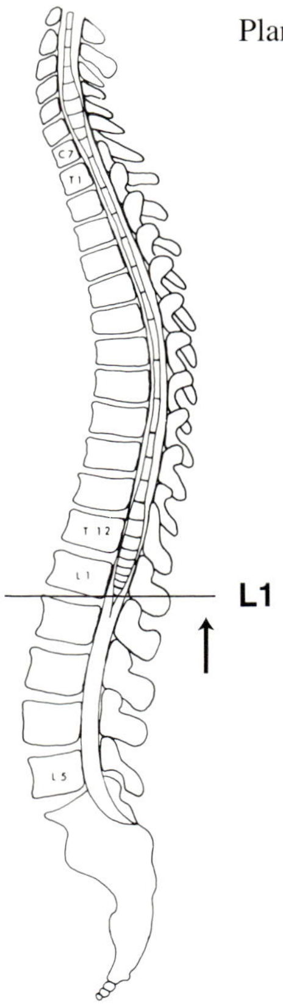

The MRI, CT, and gross anatomical sections may be rather nicely compared in this series. The information displayed on the MRI closely parallels that available on the CT even though mineralized bone is not directly imaged. The lack of signal from cortical bone, imaged here as a black line, on the MRI may be most helpful. Signals from the marrow in the laminae and facets in the MRI are adequate to determine the location of bone overgrowth or canal encroachment. The marrow containing spaces are clearly seen on the gross specimen. In the MRI illustrated, the anulus fibrosus gives less signal than the more fluid nucleus pulposus. Fat is quite evident in these obese specimens in both the subcutaneous and mesenteric regions.

Patient CT Scan

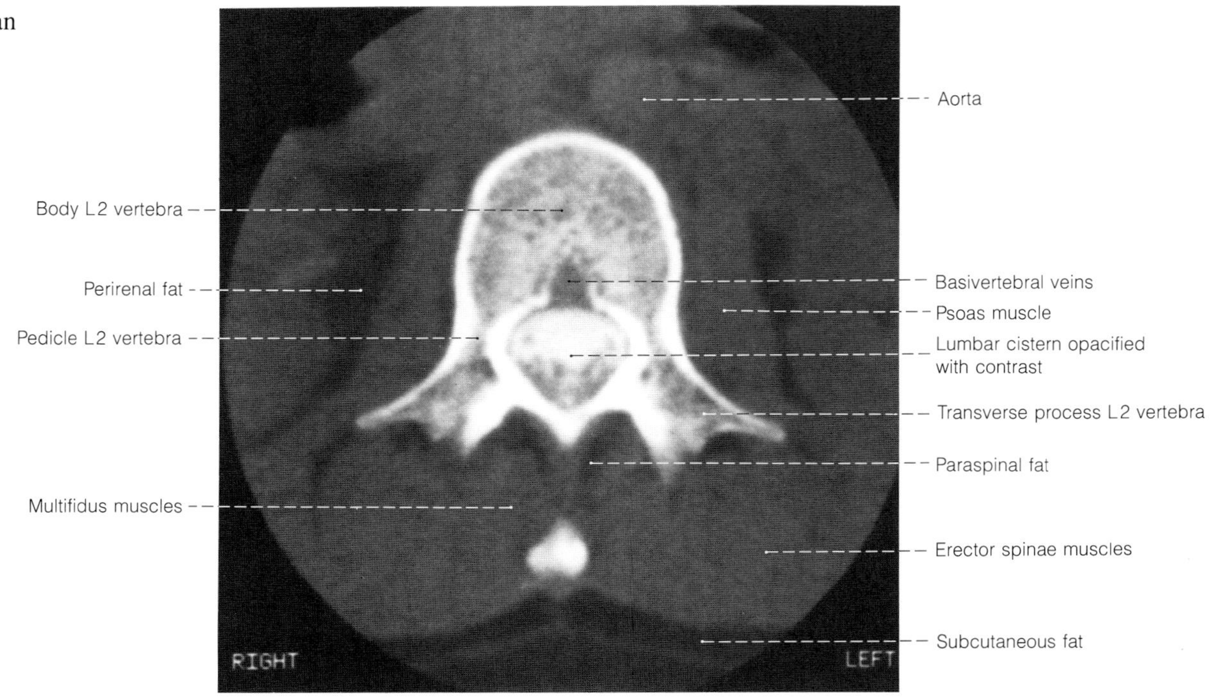

Right

Patient MRI Scan

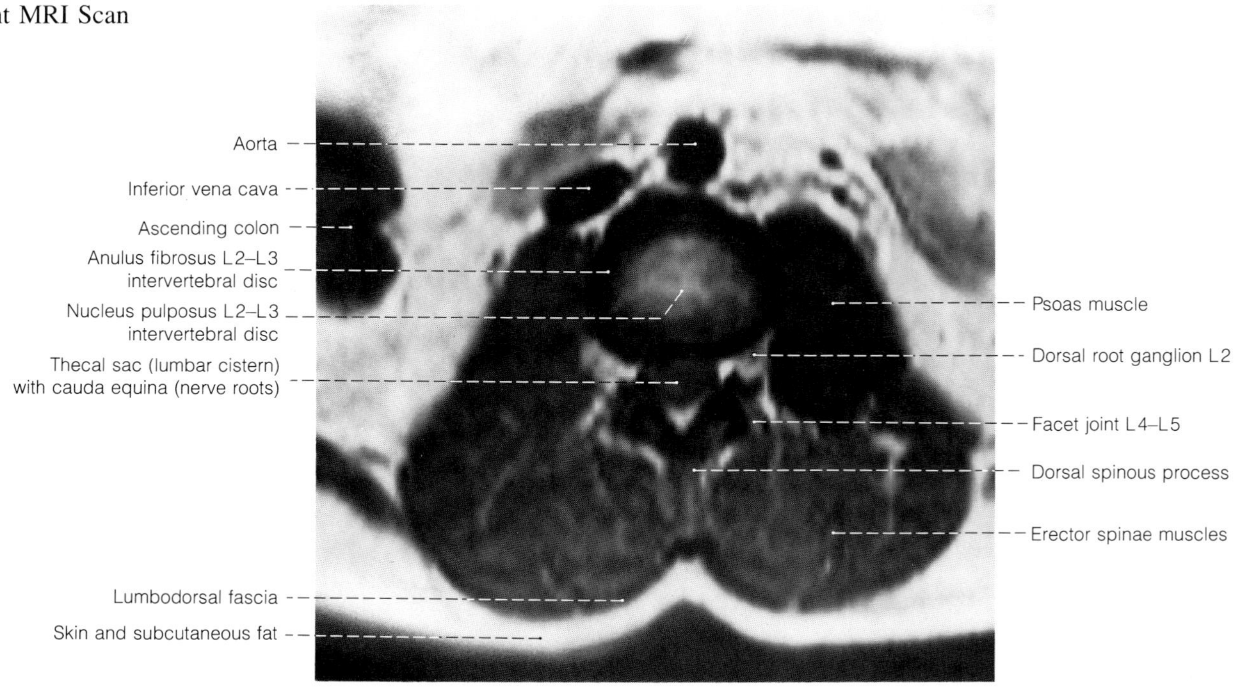

Right

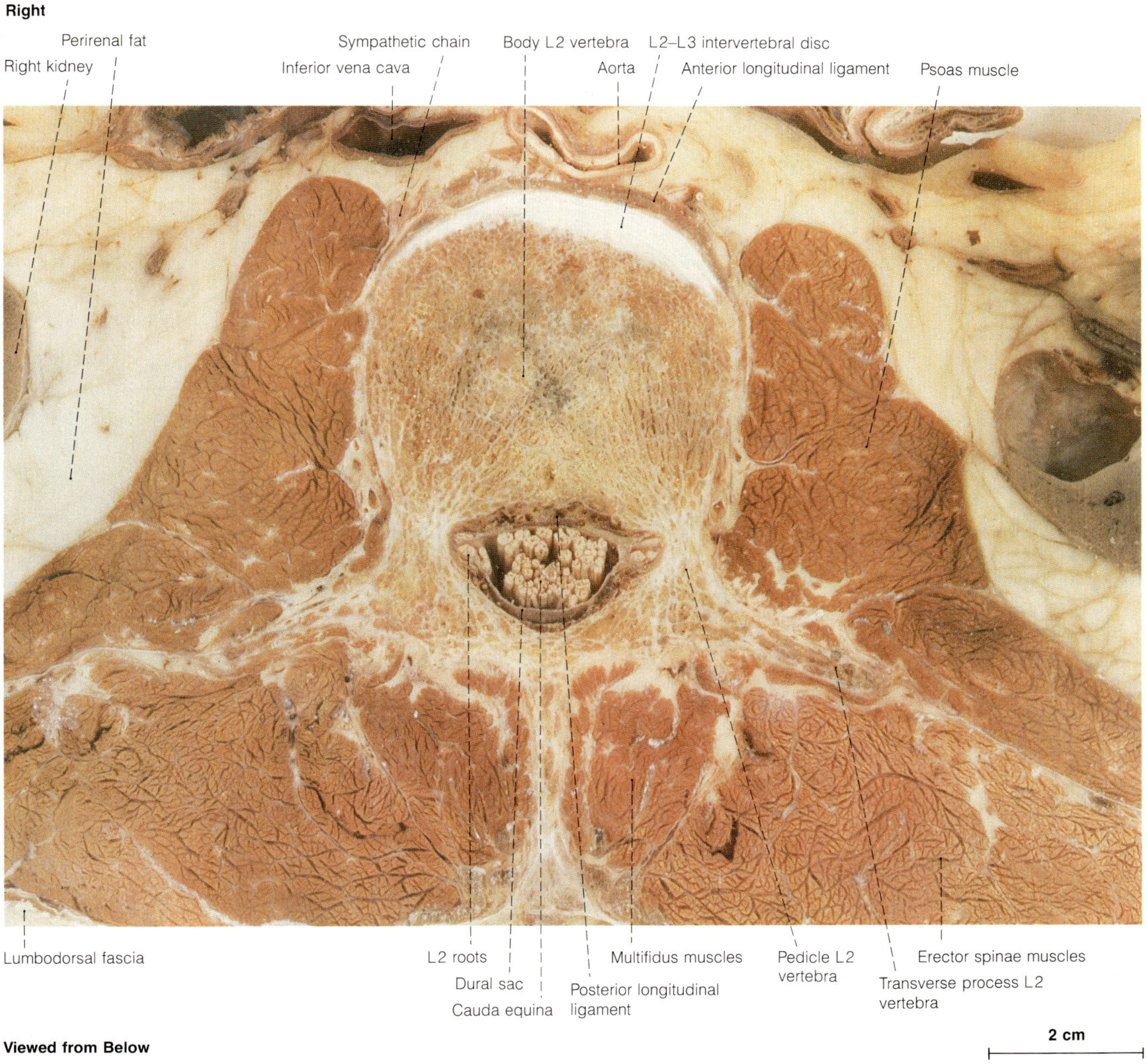

Plane of Section

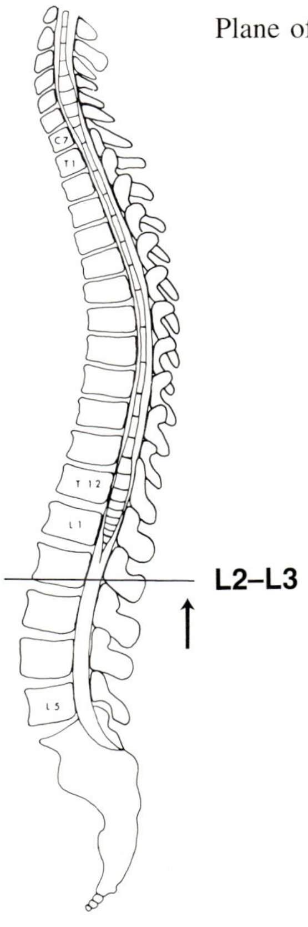

Only nerve roots of the cauda equina and the filum terminale are present in the subarachnoid space at this vertebral level, but Metrizamide® delimitation of the exact inner dimensions of the meningeal envelope is sometimes critical in visualizing impingement by herniated intervertebral discs with CT. With narrow CT slices (1–3 mm) at just the right levels, the dorsal root ganglion can be visualized. These ganglia can also be identifed with MRI as well as with CT because of the fat surrounding them in the intervertebral foramina.

The MRI is through the L2–L3 intervertebral disc where the anulus fibrosus and nucleus pulposus are differentiated extremely well. It will theoretically be possible to differentiate normal healthy disc material from a degenerative disc very early in the course of the disease and perhaps modify its course with this information. Soft tissue elements in the thecal sac are better seen on MRI than on CT (without Metrizamide®) because of the lack of interference of the surrounding bony canal with the former modality.

Patient CT Scan

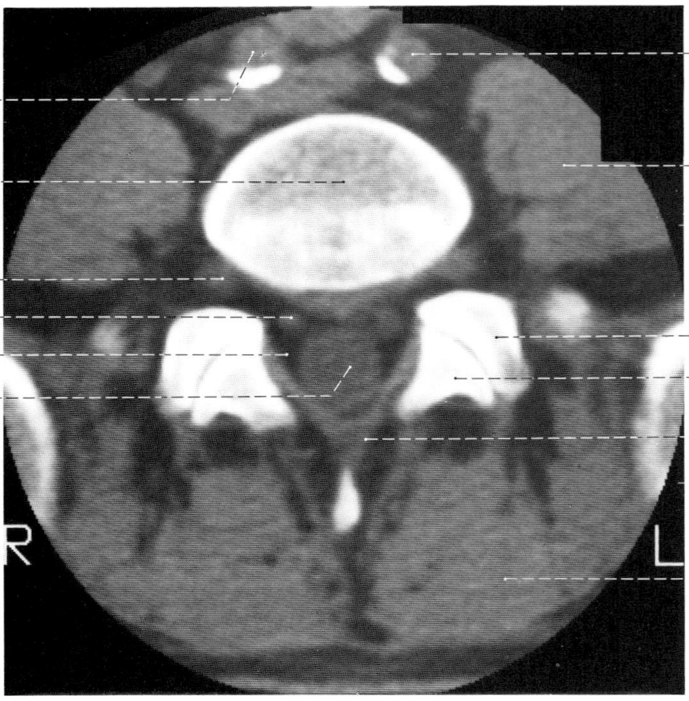

Right

Patient MRI Scan

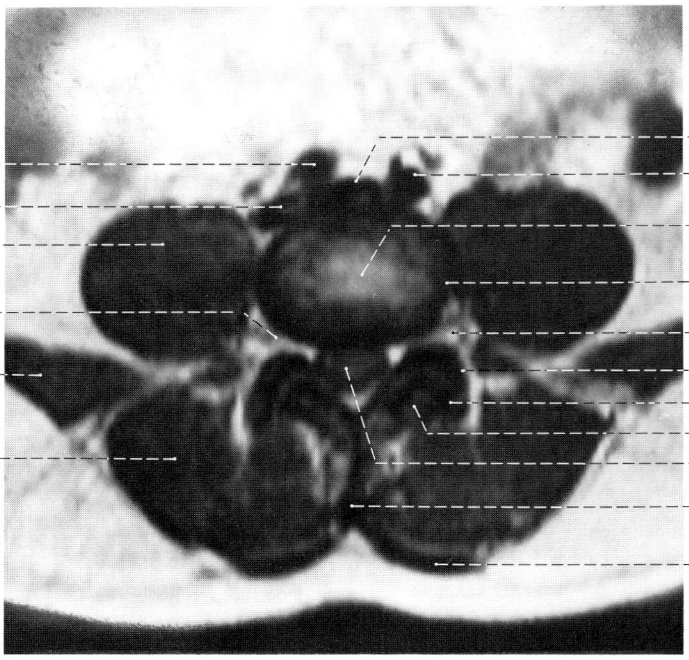

Right

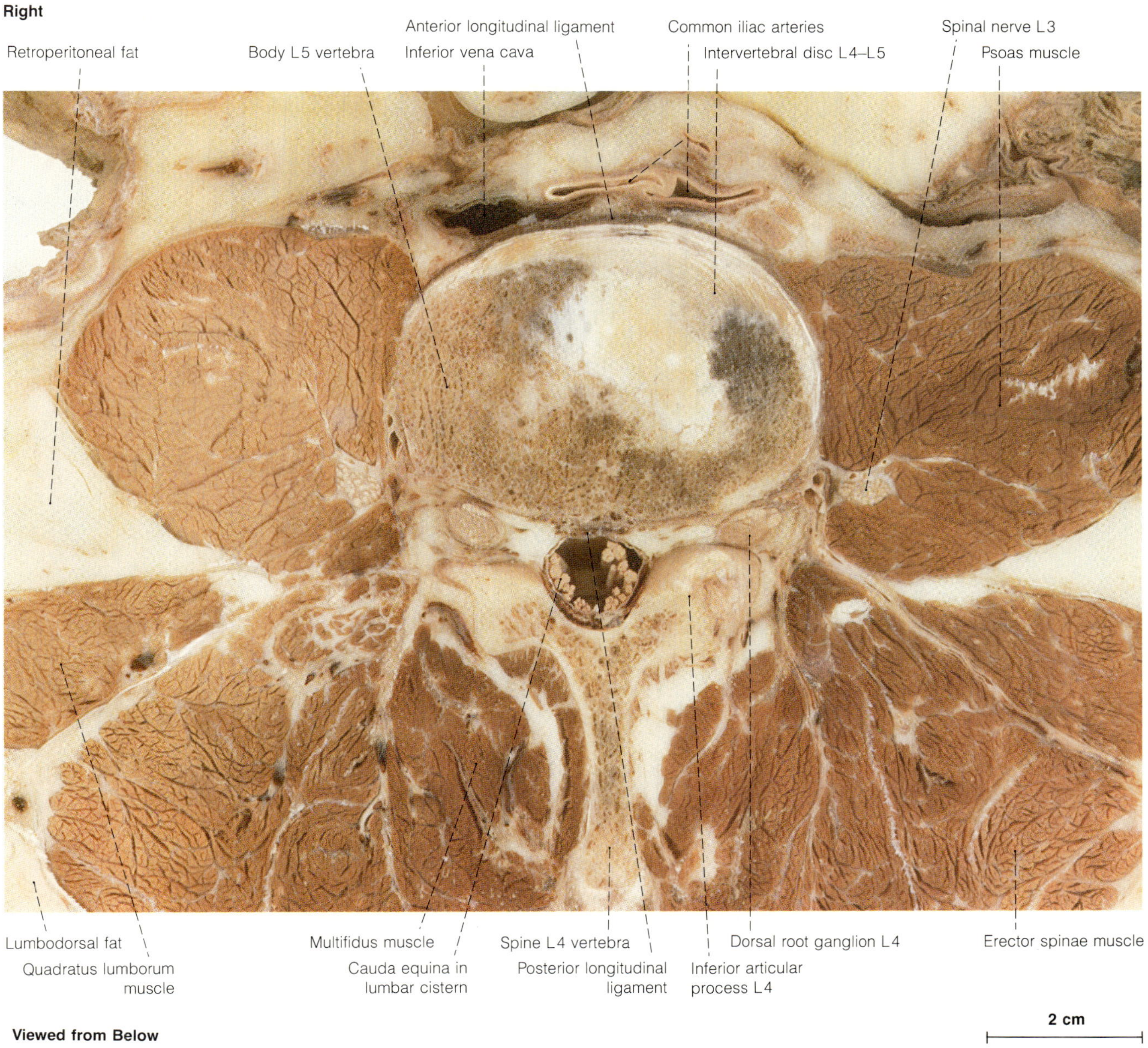

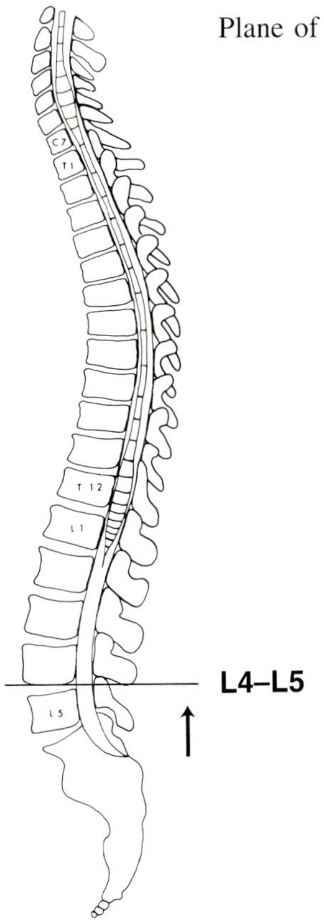

Plane of Section

The lumbosacral areas are particularly important radiologically, and the information available in the axial plane adds greatly to clinical diagnosis. Facets in this region are particularly prone to osteophytic enlargement in response to degenerative changes; because of their oblique orientation, they tend to encroach upon the spinal canal (giving rise to the Taveras-Schlesinger or spinal stenosis syndrome) or upon the lateral recess and the intervertebral foramen (causing nerve root pressure symptoms). Other factors which may contribute to the total canal narrowing include herniated discs, spondylolisthesis, tumors, and arteriovenous anomalies. Disc herniations are clearly seen and their impingement upon Metrizamide®-filled subarachnoid spaces is easily diagnosed with CT. They may also be identified with MRI with the additional possibility of diagnosing early degenerative changes in the nucleus pulposus of the disc itself.

Localization of specific segments of bowel is most difficult because of respiratory motions and the peristaltic movements of the intestines. The fat in the mesenteries may, however, permit identification of blood vessels.

Patient CT Scan

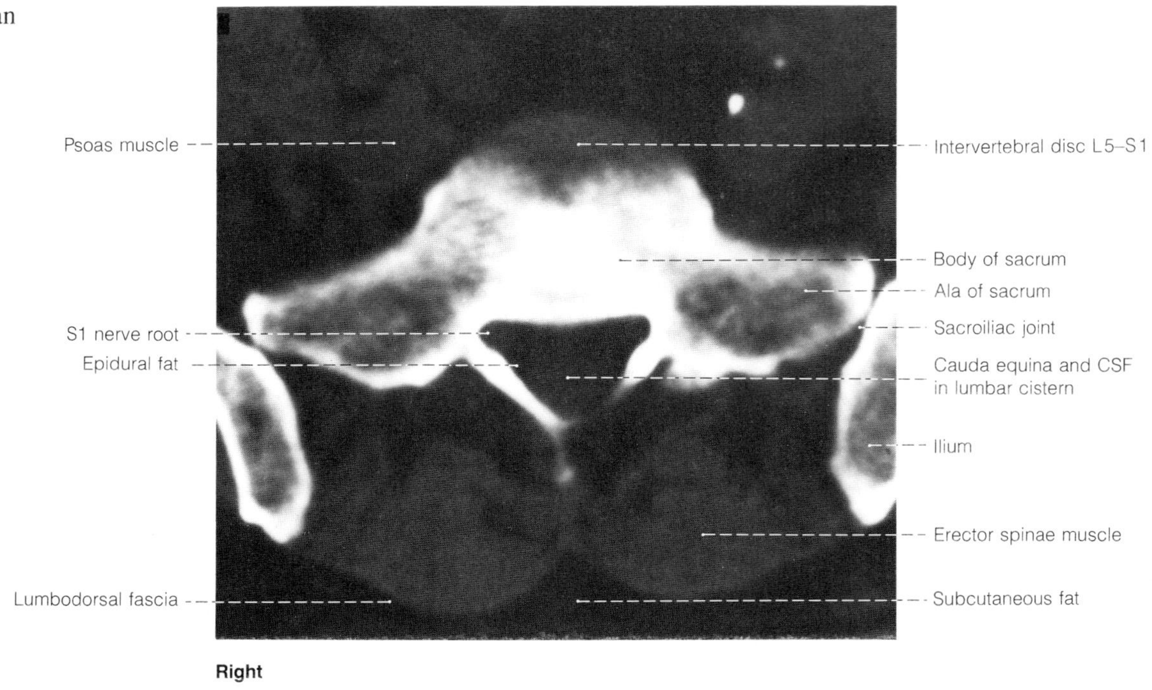

Patient MRI Scan

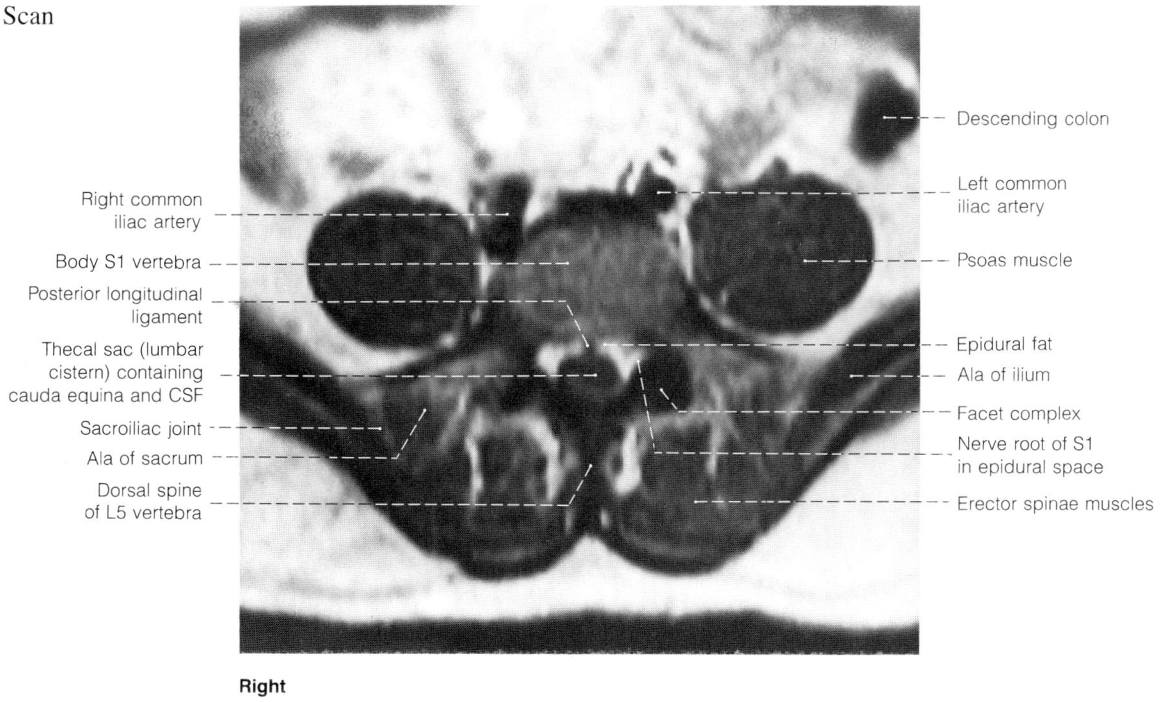

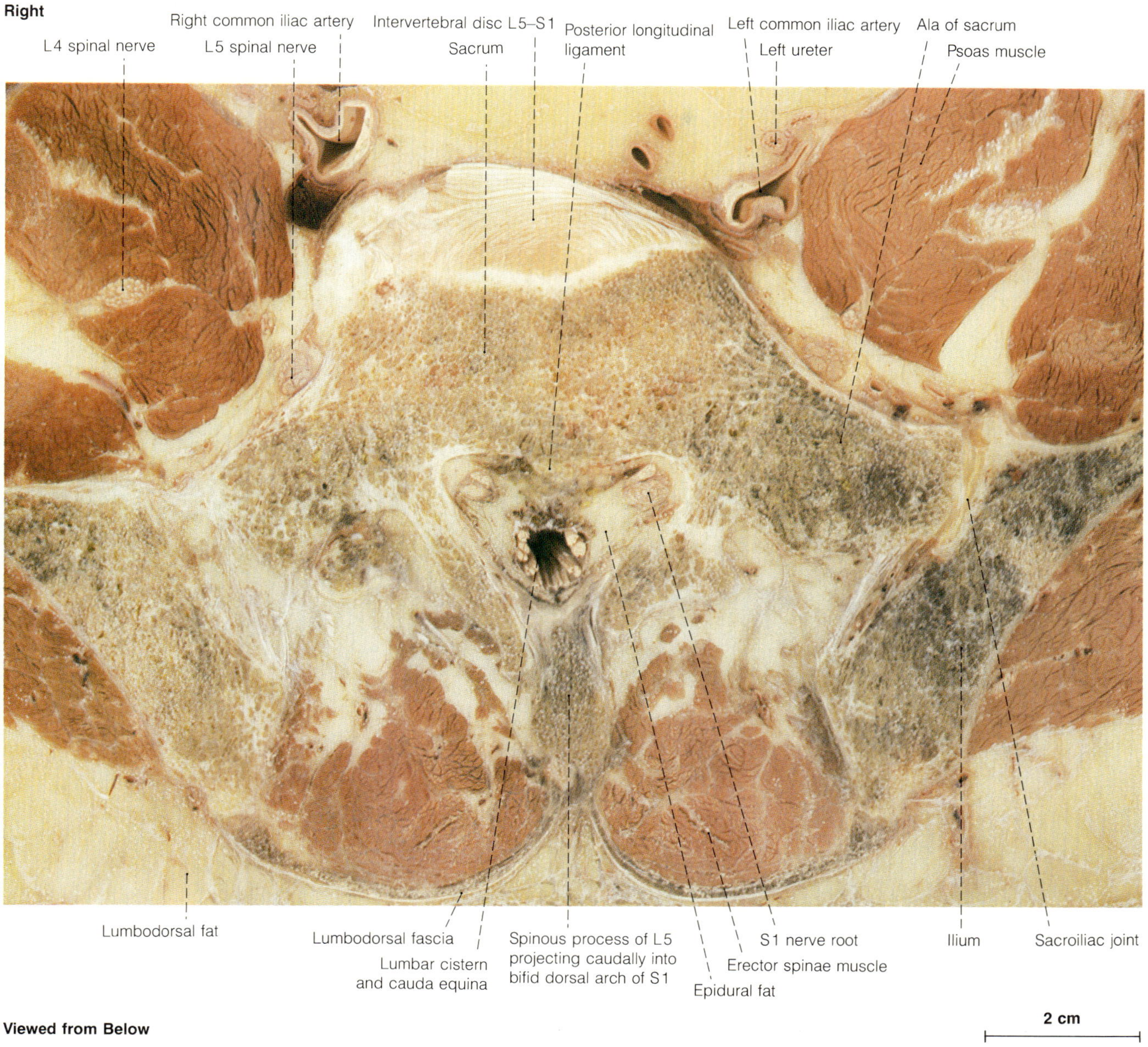

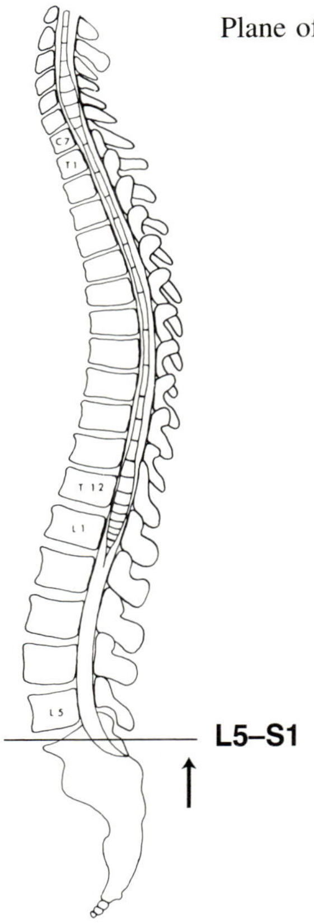

The gross anatomical section at the L5–S1 juncture (in a plane transverse to the body axis) illustrates the lumbar plexus, the lumbar cistern (caudal sac) and the sacroilac joint and ligaments. The projection of the spine of L5 into a bifid sacrum is unusual. Because the usual CT and MRI scans are in a plane parallel to the plane of the intervertebral disc, they demonstrate bony structures differing somewhat from those shown in the gross section. Metrizamide®, if not mixed sufficiently with cerebrospinal fluid, will layer out in the caudal sac making ventral disc herniations difficult to diagnose. Moving blood gives reduced signal with MRI; faster flow has less signal but turbulent blood gives some signal. The high signal produced by fat permits the identification of the large root of S1 in the epidural space.

Addendum

MR images of the spine were all obtained using a 0.5 Telsa MR system and a body coil. The radiofrequency (RF) pulse sequence, Spin Echo (SE), currently used for optimization of image contrast was identical in each case. These were as follows: Echo time (TE) = 30 msec; Repetition time (TR) = 3000 msec; number of averages = 8; slice thickness = 0.75; image magnification = 2. An alternative imaging method, using a surface coil yields images of greater contrast; however, the sensitive volume of the coil is nonuniform.

Selected Bibliography

Anderson, J. E. *Grant's Atlas of Anatomy, 8th ed.* Williams & Wilkins, Baltimore, 1983.

Burrows, E. H., and N. E. Leeds. *Neuroradiology, Vol. 1.* Churchill Livingstone, N. Y., 1981.

Chusid, J. G. *Correlative Neuroanatomy and Functional Neurology.* Lange Medical Publications, Los Altos, California, 1979.

Clemente, C. D. *Anatomy, A Regional Atlas of the Human Body, 2nd ed.* Urban & Schwarzenberg, Baltimore and Munich, 1981.

Crosby E. C., T. Humphrey, and E. W. Lauer. *Correlative Anatomy of the Nervous System.* The Macmillan Co., New York, 1962.

Ferner, H. *Eduard Pernkopf Atlas of Topographical and Applied Human Anatomy, 2nd ed.* Urban & Schwarzenberg, Baltimore and Munich, 1980.

Ferner, H., and J. Staubesand. *Sobotta Atlas of Human Anatomy, 10th English ed.* Translated by W. Hild. Urban & Schwarzenberg, Baltimore and Munich, 1983.

Newton, T. H., and D. G. Potts. *Advanced Imaging Techniques, Modern Neuroradiology, Vol. 2.* Clavadel Press, San Anselmo, Calif., 1983.

Post, J. D., ed. *Radiologic Evaluation of the Spine: Current Advances with Emphasis on CT.* Masson Publishing Co., New York, 1980.

Taveras, J. and E. H. Wood. *Diagnostic Neuroradiology, 2nd ed.* Williams & Wilkins, Baltimore, 1976.

Terry, R. J. and M. Trotter. Section III: Osteology and Section IV: The Articulations. In *Morris' Human Anatomy,* J. P. Schaeffer, ed. Blakiston Co., New York, 1953.

Woodburne, R. T. *Essentials of Human Anatomy.* Oxford University Press, New York, 1978.

Index

Index

D

E

F

G

U

V